This significant new publication provides a summary and overview of the most recent scientific advances in diabetes research, and highlights the role of these developments in advancing clinical practice. Diabetes is one of the major causes of morbidity and mortality in the developed world, and its prevalence elsewhere is on the increase. It affects in excess of 100 million people worldwide. Recent scientific advances have clarified our understanding of the causes and consequences of this devastating disease. These scientific developments are playing an increasingly important role in clinical practice, and could well lead the way to the prevention of complications and even a cure for the disease. An international and authoritative team of authors draws together this knowledge and the most recent developments to provide an up-to-date account which will benefit researchers and clinicians.

# Diabetes: Clinical Science in Practice

# Diabetes: Clinical Science in Practice

Edited by

R. D. G. LESLIE

*St Bartholomew's Hospital and Medical College, London, UK*

and

DAVID C. ROBBINS

*Medlantic Research Institute and George Washington University, USA*

CAMBRIDGE
UNIVERSITY PRESS

Published by the Press Syndicate of the University of Cambridge
The Pitt Building, Trumpington Street, Cambridge CB2 1RP
40 West 20th Street, New York, NY 10011–4211, USA
10 Stamford Road, Oakleigh, Melbourne 3166, Australia



First published 1995

Printed in Great Britain at the University Press, Cambridge

*A catalogue record for this book is available from the British Library*

*Library of Congress cataloguing in publication data*

Diabetes : clinical science in practice / edited by R.D.G. Leslie and
David C. Robbins
p. cm.
Includes index.
ISBN 0–521–45029–2 (hc)
1. Diabetes. I. Leslie, R. D. G. II. Robbins, David C.
[DNLM: 1. Diabetes Mellitus. WK 810 D537504 1995]
RC660.D4446 1995
616.4′62—dc20
DNLM/DLC
for Library of Congress 94–22061 CIP

ISBN 0 521 45029 2 hardback

# Contents

# Preface

Diabetes is one of the commonest chronic illnesses to afflict man. The disease crosses many boundaries, from physicians to geneticists, and represents a major health problem for politicians and health organisations in the next millenium. The World Health Organisation estimated that, in 1990, more than 100 million people had diabetes, that is some 6% of the world population. There are many causes of diabetes, and many complications of the disease ranging from microvascular diseases, such as retinopathy, to macrovascular disease including ischaemic heart disease. The prevalence of diabetes, and the wide-ranging nature of its complications, present a challenge to those students of the disease who wish to assimilate the most recent clinical and scientific advances.

This book provides a forum for distinguished scientists from around the world to elaborate on some of the most recent and exciting observations in diabetes. Particular attention has been paid to the causes and complications of the disease and developments in both their treatment and their prevention. The authors were invited to provide an authoritative analysis of their respective fields of interest and, where possible, to outline the practical implications of recent advances.

We hope that we have provided the reader with an up-to-date and well-balanced vehicle to broaden their view of diabetes. Ultimately, we believe that the successful application of knowledge from any particular discipline of diabetes rests upon a broad understanding of this multifaceted disease.

*David Leslie*
*David Robbins*

# Contributors

S. Amiel,
*Unit for Metabolic Medicine,*
*4th Floor, Hunts House,*
*UMDS,*
*Guy's Hospital Campus,*
*London SE1 9RT, UK*

Jens Friis Bak,
*Department of Endocrinology, University Clinic of Internal Medicine,*
*Aarhus Amtssygehus,*
*Aarhus,*
*and Steno Diabetes Center,*
*Copenhagen,*
*Denmark*

John Bell,
*Institute of Molecular Medicine,*
*John Radcliffe Hospital,*
*Headington,*
*Oxford*
*OX3 9DU, UK*

Peter C. Butler,
*Endocrine Research Unit,*
*5–164 West Joseph,*
*Mayo Clinic,*
*Rochester,*
*MN 55905, USA*

Andrew R. Clark,
*Department of Medicine, University of Birmingham,*
*Queen Elizabeth Hospital,*
*Birmingham,*
*B15 2TH, UK*

Iain C. P. Cranston,
*Unit for Metabolic Medicine,*
*4th Floor, Hunts House,*
*United Medical and Dental Schools*
*Guy's Hospital Campus*
*London SE 19RT, UK*

T. Deckert,
*Steno Memorial Hospital,*
*Niels Steensensvej 2,*
*DK-2820 Gentofte,*
*Denmark*

Kevin Docherty,
*Dept of Medicine,*
*Queen Elizabeth Hospital,*
*Queen Elizabeth Medical Centre,*
*Edgbaston*
*B15 2TH, UK*

Dushan Dvornik,
*Wyeth-Ayerst Research,*
*Radnor,*
*Pennsylvania, and Princeton,*
*New Jersey, USA*

Richard C. Eastman,
*Director, Division of Diabetes, Endocrinology and Metabolic Disorders,*
*National Institutes of Health,*
*9000 Rockville Pike,*
*Bidg. 31, Room 9A-16,*
*Bethesda,*
*MD 20892, USA*

Ele Ferrannini,
*University of Pisa,*
*Via S. Maria 102,*
*Pisa 1–56100,*
*Italy*

E. A. M. Gale,
*Department of Diabetes and Metabolism,*
*3rd Floor, Dominion House,*
*59 Bartholomew Close,*
*West Smithfield,*
*London EC1A 7BE, UK*

Linda S. Geiss,
*Epidemiology and Statistics Branch, Division of Diabetes Translation,*
*National Center for Chronic Disease Prevention and Health Promotion,*
*Centers for Disease Control and Prevention,*
*Atlanta,*
*Georgia, USA*

Leon-Paul Georges,
*The Diabetes Institutes,*
*Eastern Virginia Medical School,*
*Norfolk,*
*Virginia, USA*

Boas Gonen,
*Wyeth-Ayerst,*
*145 King of Prussia Road,*
*Radnor,*
*PA 19087, USA*

Anders Green,
*Institute of Clinical Genetics,*
*J. B. Winslowsvej 17,*
*DK-5000 Odense C,*
*Denmark*

Pernile Mørk Hansen
*Steno Diabetes Center,*
*2, Niels Steensens Vej,*
*DK-2820 Gentofte, Denmark*

William H. Herman,
*Centers for Disease Control,*
*5372 Redfield Drive,*
*Dunwoody,*
*GA 30338, USA*

S. Howell,
*Biomedical Sciences Division,*
*King's College London (University of London),*
*Kensington Campus,*
*Campden Hill Road,*
*London W8, UK*

R. H. Jones,
*Department of Endocrinology,*
*Medway Hospital,*
*Peter Simons Diabetes Centre,*
*Residence 9,*
*Gillingham,*
*Kent ME4 5NY, UK*

David M. Kendall,
*Diabetes Center, Division of Endocrinology and Metabolism, Department of Medicine,*
*University of Minnesota Medical School,*
*Minneapolis,*
*MN 55455, USA*

Patricia A. King,
*Department of Medicine,*
*University of Vermont,*
*Burlington,*
*VT 05405, USA*

Allan Kofoed-Enevoldsen,
*Steno Diabetes Center,*
*2, Niels Steensens Vej,*
*DK-2820 Gentofte, Denmark*

Harold E. Lebovitz,
*Downstate Medical Center,*
*450 Clarkson Ave., Box 1205,*
*Brooklyn,*
*NY 11203, USA*

Steven B. Leichter,
*The Diabetes Institutes,*
*Eastern Virginia Medical School,*
*Norfolk,*
*Virginia, USA*

R. D. G. Leslie,
*Department of Diabetes and Metabolism,*
*Dominion House, 59 Bartholomew Close West,*
*London EC1A 7BE, UK*

Anneke Lucassen,
*Molecular Immunology Group, Nuffield Department of Medicine,*
*Institute of Molecular Medicine,*
*John Radcliffe Hospital,*
*Headington,*
*Oxford OX3 9DU, UK*

Timothy J. Lyons,
*Division of Endocrinology, Diabetes and Metabolism,*
*Medical University of South Carolina,*
*171 Ashley Ave.,*
*Charleston,*
*SC 29425, USA*

David E. Misek,
*Department of Physiology, University of Michigan Medical School,*
*Ann Arbor,*
*Michigan 48109, USA*

Braxton D. Mitchell,
*Health Science Center at San Antonio, The University of Texas,*
*San Antonio,*
*Texas, USA*

C. E. Mogensen,
*Second University Clinic of International Medicine,*
*8000 Aerhus C,*
*Denmark*

Bjarne Myrup,
*Steno Diabetes Center,*
*2, Niels Steensens Vej,*
*DK-2820 Gentofte, Denmark*

John T. O'Brian,
*The Diabetes Institutes, Eastern Virginia Medical School,*
*Norfolk,*
*Virginia, USA*

Kwarne Osei,
*Ohio State University, 485 McCampbell Hall,*
*1581 Dodd Drive,*
*Columbus,*
*OH 43210, USA*

Oluf Pedersen,
*Steno Memorial & Hvidore Hospital,*
*Hagedorn Research Laboratory,*
*2, Niels Steensens Vej,*
*DK 2828 Gentoft, Denmark*

Mark F. Peyrot,
*Loyola College,*
*4501 N. Charles St.,*
*Baltimore,*
*MD 21210, USA*

P. Pozzilli,
*Endocrinologia (I), Istituto II Clinica Medica,*
*University of Rome 'La Sapienza'*
*PO Box 680,*
*00187 Rome,*
*Italy*

Robert E. Ratner,
*George Washington University Medical Center,*
*2150 Pennsylvania Ave., NW,*
*Washington,*
*DC 20037, USA*

R. Paul Robertson,
*Diabetes Center, University of Minnesota,*
*Box 101 UMHC,*
*Minneapolis,*
*MN 55455, USA*

Mary N. Rosholt,
*Department of Medicine, University of Vermont,*
*Burlington,*
*VT 05405, USA*

Richard R. Rubin,
*Department of Pediatrics and Diabetes Center, The Johns Hopkins University School of Medicine,*
*Baltimore, MD 21205, USA*

Alan R. Saltiel,
*Department of Signal Transduction, Parke-Davis Pharmaceutical Research Division,*
*2800 Plymouth Road,*
*Ann Arbor,*
*Michigan 48105, USA*

Timothy Seaton,
*Medical Affairs, Miles Pharmaceuticals, Inc.,*
*4000 Morgan Lane,*
*West Haven,*
*CT 06516, USA*

M. P. Stern,
Division of Clinical Epidemiology,
*Department of Medicine,*
*University of Texas Health Science Center at San Antonio,*
*San Antonio,*
*Texas, USA*

Howard S. Tager,
*Department of Biochemistry and Molecular Biology,*
*920 E. 58th Street,*
*Chicago,*
*IL 60637, USA*

Adrian U. Teuscher,
*Diabetes Center, Division of Endocrinology and Metabolism,*
*Department of Medicine, University of Minnesota Medical School,*
*Minneapolis,*
*MN 55455, USA*

Aaron I. Vinik,
*Diabetes Institute,*
*855 W. Brambleton Avenue,*
*Norfolk,*
*VA 23510, USA*

Alan L. Wagner,
*The Diabetes Institutes, Eastern Virginia Medical School,*
*Norfolk,*
*Virginia, USA*

P. Westermark,
*Department of Pathology, University Hospital,*
*Linköping,*
*Sweden*

# 1 Regulation of Insulin Secretion

S. L. Howell

## INTRODUCTION

Insulin is produced in the body only in the β-cells of the islets of Langerhans. The islets comprise 1–2% of the total volume of the mammalian pancreas and are themselves heterogeneous in composition. The relative proportions of the different endocrine cell types may vary in different anatomical areas of pancreas, but on average there are 70% β-cells, 25% α-cells and 5% δ-cells. The islets may also contain, or be in close proximity to, cells producing pancreatic polypeptide, which may not itself be a hormone. There may be interactions between the three endocrine cell types which contribute to the extent of the response of each to a given stimulus: these are called paracrine relationships. The human pancreas contains ~250 000 individual islets of Langerhans: each containing 3000–4000 β-cells.

## THE CELL BIOLOGY OF THE β-CELL

The ultrastructure of the β-cell is well known from electron microscope studies: it contains many of the features to be expected from a polypeptide secreting cell type. Thus the characteristic feature is the presence of a large number (up to 13 000 per cell) of membrane-limited hormone storage granules which comprise a substantial reservoir of insulin – about 30 pg/cell, sufficient for 24 hours of secretion in the absence of any new synthesis. The dense core of the storage granule contains insulin in a crystalline or paracrystalline form, along with connecting peptide excised during the process of conversion from the biosynthetic precursor proinsulin. These two together comprise about 80–90% of the total granular protein. There are also ~100 additional granule matrix and membrane proteins of varying sizes (1), most of whose functions are unknown. Perhaps the most interesting of these physiologically are:

- *Islet amyloid polypeptide* (IAPP), also called *amylin*: present in β-cells secreted with an abundance of about 5% that of insulin, and localised in β-cells in the granule core (2). The presence of IAPP in β-cells and in particular its deposition outside the cells in amyloid deposits has been much discussed in relation to its possible role in the aetiology of NIDDM (see Chapter 13). High concentrations of IAPP have been reported to inhibit insulin secretion from isolated islets, although the concentrations required to achieve this effect are unlikely to be physiological (3).
- *Betagranin* (abundance 0.1–0.3% of insulin) which has close homology with adrenal chromaffin chromogranin A (4). Its function in β-cells is not known; it may be involved in the segregation of secretory proteins into the granules.

The granules also contain three enzymes responsible for the conversion of pro-insulin to insulin; these have been characterised in considerable detail and comprise two categories: endopeptidases, of which two are known, both active at acid pH but differently dependent on calcium concentrations, and carboxypeptidase H (5). Their differing pH and calcium requirements may serve both to achieve their activation and limit their activities in appropriate compartments of the cell. Carboxypeptidase H removes the basic amino acids which remain in the C terminus of endopeptidase-treated pro-insulin to achieve the insulin structure. A similar enzyme, present mostly as a soluble granule component, is present in many endocrine cell types (6).

Finally, the granules contain a proton-translocating ATPase which serves to lower the pH of the granule interior to 5.0–5.5: this facilitates the limitation of conversion of pro-insulin to insulin by endopeptidases and also allows the crystallisation of insulin within the granule, in the presence of relatively high concentrations of zinc (5). The isoelectric point of insulin, at which crystallisation is most readily achieved, is pH 5.5.

## Pro-insulin biosynthesis

The events involved in the generation of the initial precursor (pre-pro-insulin) which has a half-life of 15 sec within the cell are described in Chapter 1. The initial synthesis occurs in the β-cell endoplasmic reticulum, and is subject to regulation by glucose and possibly by cyclic AMP, but not by the insulin-secreting sulphonylureas. Thus insulin biosynthesis and secretion can be independently regulated. Once in the cisternae of the endoplasmic reticulum, pro-insulin rapidly achieves its three-dimensional configuration with the disulphide bridges correctly formed, and is then transported via microvesicles to the Golgi complex where concentration of the pro-insulin in membrane-limited sacs, and conversion are initiated. These steps are completed by the time the mature granule is formed – within 60 min from the initial biosynthesis of its constituent proteins.

## The secretory mechanism

The major pathway for secretion of insulin from normal β-cells (the regulated pathway) involves transport of granules from the large cytoplasmic pool (sufficient for 24 hours of secretion at normal rates without any new synthesis) to the plasma membrane. Here granule membrane and plasma membrane fuse together with release of the granule contents (in this case predominantly insulin and connecting peptide in equivalent amounts) into the bloodstream.

It is known that the β-cell cytoskeleton, in particular the microtubule network, is involved in this process since its disruption by use of specific drugs serves to inhibit secretion. It seems likely that the microtubules represent a rigid framework along which granules can be transported – they are unlikely themselves to be able to translocate the granules. It has been suggested that the translocation may be activated by actin and myosin, which are known to be present in β-cells (7). Alternative mechanisms known in other cells to be responsible for organelle movement in association with microtubules are members of the kinesin family of microtubule motors. In tumour cells, this regulated pathway may be accompanied by an alternative 'constitutive' secretory pathway which involves direct secretion of insulin via small vesicles which bypass the packaging and storage mechanisms, and therefore bypass the conversion process. This is probably not an important pathway in normal β-cells except conceivably in early IDDM and NIDDM in which high levels of circulating pro-insulin have been detected (see Chapters 10 and 12).

## METABOLIC EVENTS WHICH MAY INFLUENCE INSULIN SECRETION

### Closure of ATP-sensitive potassium channels

These channels, which permit the exit of potassium from the cells down the prevailing concentration gradient were identified in β-cells during patch-clamp experiments (8). The resting membrane potential of the cells is dictated largely by the activity of $K^+$-ATP channels, and between 5 and 25% of channels are activated (i.e. open) in β-cells in the absence of glucose. Addition of glucose causes closing of half the open channels in the presence of 2 mM glucose, while 90% are closed in the presence of 5 mM glucose (9). These concentrations are of course below the range in which insulin secretion is stimulated (5–20 mM). Further experiments have suggested that, rather than simply the absolute concentration of ATP generated from glucose metabolism being important, it may be the ATP/ADP ratio close to the cell membrane which determines the extent of ATP-sensitive potassium ($K^+$-ATP) channel closure (10). This may explain why there is a discrepancy between the concentration of ATP required to close the channels in isolated patches (10 μM) and known intracellular ATP concentrations (3–5 mM)(11).

A number of other agents which are able to alter rates of insulin secretion may act wholly, or in part, through effects on ATP-dependent potassium channels. Amongst these are the insulin-releasing sulphonylureas (12), and diazoxide, an antidiuretic drug (13) which is a reversible inhibitor of insulin secretion, both of which appear to act directly on the potassium channels. Diazoxide does not affect glucose metabolism and does not affect potassium-induced insulin secretion: it seems likely that this effect on potassium channels may be a major mechanism of its action. Galanin (an inhibitor), somatostatin (an inhibitor) or vasopressin (a stimulator of insulin secretion) may act at least in part through effects in opening (inhibitors) or closing (stimuli) potassium channels, although the evidence is not yet conclusive.

In addition to these ATP-sensitive channels, the β-cell contains a number of other potassium channels which are becoming well characterised electrophysiologically. However, they do not seem to be subject to regulation by agents which affect insulin secretion to the same extent as the $K^+$-ATP channels.

### Changes in intracellular calcium concentration

The direct effect of the closure of the ATP-$K^+$ channel by ATP or ATP/ADP is a depolarisation of the β-cell membrane (following reduction of potassium efflux) until the threshold potential for initiation of a change of electrical activity of the membrane, and the entry of calcium into the cells via voltage-sensitive calcium channels, is initiated. This is consistent with much earlier data on the role of calcium which showed that the normal secretory response to glucose requires the presence of calcium outside the cells, and that $^{45}Ca^{2+}$ entry into the cells was increased on stimulation of secretion by a variety of agents. These two facts together led to the proposal that an increase of intracellular free calcium was critically important as a trigger of the insulin secretory mechanism. This hypothesis can now be tested more fully by the use of fluorescent probes such as quin-2 and fura-2 which change the wavelength of their emission with increasing calcium concentrations. Thus it is clear that increasing the glucose concentrations in media in which β-cells are bathed from 5 to 20 mM glucose will at least double the free calcium concentration in the cells (14); the increase in concentration which occurs close to the plasma membrane or in other localised areas of the cell could, of course, be much higher.

The free calcium concentration inside the cell is dependent not only on the balance between influx and efflux as described here but also on the distribution between the various intracellular pools within the organelles which are known to be involved in these regulatory processes. Most important of these quantitatively are probably the mitochondria which act as a site for accumulation of calcium, and can store it at quite high concentrations (15): mitochondrial calcium does not, however, constitute a labile pool of calcium in terms of contributing to regulation of secretion. The endoplasmic reticulum also binds calcium, and this seems more likely to be a regulated pool in that it is known that inositol trisphosphate ($IP_3$) can release calcium from this pool (16) (see p. 6). A number of stimuli of insulin secretion can induce phospholipase-C activation to increase production of both $IP_3$ and diacylglycerol (17). Quantitatively, the major importance of phospholipase-C activation in β-cells seems likely to be in producing diacylglycerol which, in turn, activates protein kinase-C (see below) rather than in mobilisation of calcium by $IP_3$. Many of the actions of calcium in β-cells may be accounted for by activation of calcium–calmodulin dependent protein kinase, which in turn leads to phosphorylation of specific protein substrates (see below).

## Changes of cyclic AMP concentration

Cyclic AMP is one of the classic 'second messengers' and has long been discussed as a possible mediator of the effects of a variety of secretagogues on insulin secretion (18). It is known that addition of exogenous cyclic AMP in a form which can penetrate β-cells will potentiate insulin secretion, and it is likely that agents such as glucagon and other gastrointestinal hormones such as secretin or gastric inhibitory peptide (GIP) may also exert their effects by activating adenylate cyclase and raising intracellular cyclic AMP levels (see below). They will, however, only exert these actions in the presence of a stimulatory (5 mM) glucose concentration. An important question is whether glucose itself exerts its effects on insulin secretion by increasing cyclic AMP concentrations in β-cells. The answer seems to be negative since glucose neither directly affects adenylate cyclase nor cyclic nucleotide specific phosphodiesterase inhibition. Glucose does, in some degree, increase cyclic AMP levels inside β-cells but within a time scale which is not consistent with a regulatory effect on secretion. Conversely, very large increases in cyclic AMP concentration produced, for instance, by the adenylate cyclase activator forskolin have, in the absence of glucose, no effect on secretion. The way in which glucose contributes to raising β-cell cyclic AMP concentrations is unclear; it might involve calcium-calmodulin-mediated alterations of adenylate cyclase or of phosphodiesterase activity (19).

Thus, the role of cyclic AMP seems to be to modulate the secretory responses of the β-cell to glucose; for instance, in the case of the gastrointestinal hormones, these can increase cyclic AMP concentrations and potentiate glucose-induced secretion. This may have some physiological significance since the observation that oral glucose is a more potent stimulus of insulin secretion than intravenous glucose administered at a rate which will produce the same blood glucose concentration, can be explained by the potentiating effect of one or more gastrointestinal hormones. Gastric inhibitory peptide is a likely candidate which results in a higher rate of insulin secretion at any prevailing stimulatory glucose concentration. This relationship between gastrointestinal hormone and the β-cell is called the entero-insular axis (see p. 9).

Cyclic AMP probably exerts its effects in part by activating a specific protein kinase (protein kinase A) following separation of the catalytic and receptor subunits of the kinase (20). The presence of this enzyme and its activation following exposure of β-cells to a variety of agents including cyclic AMP analogues, adenylate cyclase activitors (such as forskolin) or phosphodiesterase inhibitors (such as isobutyl methylxanthine) is readily demonstrable (Fig. 1.1).

## Activation of protein kinase C

The calcium–phospholipid dependent protein kinase (protein kinase C) (PKC) has been identified in islets of Langerhans and its activation, for instance by the phorbol ester phorbol myristate acetate (PMA) can lead (in the presence of glucose) to stimulation of insulin secretion. Similarly, the physiological substrate of PKC, diacylglycerol is generated following exposure of β-cells to a variety of stimuli including carbachol and cholecystokinin. The question therefore arises as to whether PKC activation may play a role in the glucose stimulation of insulin secretion. Three lines of evidence suggest this is not the case:

(a) Inhibitors of PKC do not affect glucose-induced insulin secretion. The specificity of the range of inhibitors used has sometimes led to doubts over the validity of the approach.
(b) Islets in which PKC activity has been reduced by 90% following prolonged exposure to phorbol esters (PKC down regulation) still respond to glucose, but not to phorbol ester, stimulation of insulin secretion (21).
(c) PKC translocation from cytosol to membrane – a necessary concomitant of activation of the enzyme, does not occur following glucose stimulation, although it is readily apparent following PMA stimulation (22).

Thus there is a weight of evidence against the direct involvement of PKC in glucose regulation of insulin secretion. The same techniques have, however, shown that PKC activation may be an important mechanism by which the effects of carbachol and of cholecystokinin are exerted on insulin secretion (23) (Fig. 1.1).

The nature of the endogenous substrates for these three classes of protein kinase, however, remains unclear. Nor does it seem likely that there are substrates in common between calcium calmodulin dependent, cyclic AMP dependent or protein kinase C dependent phosphorylation. Although a substrate of molecular weight 78 kD has been identified in common between cyclic AMP and calcium phospholipid dependent kinases (24), these protein kinase activities did not share substrates in common with $Ca^{2+}$ calmodulin stimulated protein kinase in islets. Thus a common effector substrate for the different pathways of activation cannot be identified at the present time.

## Synthesis of nitric oxide

Nitric oxide has been shown to be a second messenger in a number of systems, following its synthesis from arginine via the enzyme nitric oxide synthase. While there is considerable interest in the possible role of nitric oxide in mediating the potentially lethal effects of cytokines such as interleukin 1 on rodent (although perhaps not human) β-cells, there is little evidence for a role of nitric oxide as a second messenger for glucose or arginine stimulated insulin secretion (25).

## Metabolism of phospholipids

The possible role of phospholipids in the regulation of insulin secretion has been receiving increasing attention in recent years following realisation that their importance may extend far beyond the recognised involvement of phospholipids during the fusion and fission of granule and plasma mechanisms during the exocytosis process (26). Because of lack of sufficient tissue quantities, most studies of phospholipid metabolism in islets have involved radioactive precursors as indicators of their metabolism. This type of approach has shown that inositol metabolism is substantially stimulated during glucose stimulation of insulin secretion and that inositol deprivation of the cells prevents this secretory response. One specific change which occurs is the increased hydrolysis of inositol containing phospholipids in particular phosphoinositol, bisphosphate, probably as a result of activation of the calcium dependent membrane bound enzyme phospholipase C (27); one product of this hydrolysis is inositol trisphosphate ($IP_3$). Whether this activation is a direct effect of glucose, or whether it results from a glucose-induced calcium rise which triggers activation of the calcium-dependent enzyme remains an open question (28). It is possible that glucose exerts its effects via calcium while other stimuli act via a receptor coupled through a membrane-associated GTP-binding protein (G protein) to phospholipase C (29). $IP_3$ can in turn act in many tissues to provoke release of bound calcium from endoplasmic reticulum stores. As discussed above, the importance of this intracellular calcium mobilisation for the activation of insulin secretion remains unclear. It is possible that other products of phosphoinositol hydrolysis may play a significant role in stimulus-secretion coupling in β-cells. In particular as noted above (p. 4), another product of phospholipase C catalysed phospholipid breakdown is diacylglycerol, which when added to islets, can stimulate insulin secretion, and its production is accelerated both by glucose and other stimuli. However, the pathways involved in their generation appear to be different since glucose-induced diacylglycerol synthesis does not lead to activation of PKC, while carbachol induced generation of the same compound does stimulate PKC (see p. 5)(28). This may reflect differences in the pathways and fatty acid composition of the molecules generated in each case.

### Synthesis of arachidonic acid

Arachidonic acid is a major component of islet phospholipids, comprising about 17% of total fatty acid content (28). It can also stimulate insulin secretion when added to islets *in vitro* (30), and its potential action as a membrane fusogen has led to careful evaluation of its role in the secretory process (32,33). In particular, the role of the two pathways of its metabolism (cycloxygenase and lipoxygenase pathways) have been considered in detail. Thus, the major product of the lipoxygenase pathway (12 HETE) has been identified in islets and a range of inhibitors of this pathway has also been employed to assess its role in insulin secretion. Evidence that it is involved in mediating the effects of nutrients on insulin secretion is not yet conclusive (34). *Prostaglandins* (PGs) are products of metabolism of arachadonic acid via the cycloxygenase pathway and in particular $PGI_2$ may be a product of this pathway in islets. However, the available information on the effects of exogenously added prostaglandins – particularly those of the E-series – on insulin secretion is somewhat contradictory and their physiological importance remains uncertain (28). Overall, there is increasing evidence that arachidonic acid itself (rather than its metabolites) may be both an important intermediary and a potential second messenger in insulin secretion (30,31).

*Phospholipase $A_2$* is a calcium dependent enzyme which can catalyse the breakdown of arachidonic acid. It has been identified in islets and there is some evidence of alterations of its activity by inhibitors such as mastaparan which in turn may inhibit insulin secretion, while stimuli such as mellitin may stimulate insulin secretion. However, the role of this enzyme requires further study (28).

## PHYSIOLOGICAL REGULATION OF INSULIN SECRETION

A bewildering array of compounds is known which can alter rates of insulin secretion and, as seen above, many of these are pharmacological agents which are used as tools to examine the importance of different aspects of the various intracellular pathways which have been implicated in its regulation. We review briefly here only those agents which are likely to have physiological relevance.

### Glucose

Glucose is the primary physiological stimulus for insulin secretion and the range of secretory responsiveness of β-cells (see Fig. 1.1) is set optimally for maintenance of blood glucose in the range 5–7 mM. It is clear that glucose must be metabolised by β-cells in order to induce insulin secretion, and the various carbohydrate metabolic pathways which are known are all present in β-cells as in other tissues: in this respect the pattern of glucose metabolism resembles that in liver more than other tissues (35). The probable reason for the exquisite sensitivity of β-cells to glucose lies in the presence of not only a high affinity hexokinase ($K_m$ ~0.1 mM), which is

| Pathway | A | B | C |
|---|---|---|---|
| Stimuli: | Glucagon<br>Gastric inhibitory peptide | Glucose (via metabolism)<br>Arginine | Acetylcholine<br>Cholecystokinin |
| Recognition: | Receptor<br>Gs<br>Adenylate cyclase ↑ | ATP-K$^+$channels (glucose)<br>Depolarisation (arginine)<br>Calcium entry ↑ | Receptor<br>Phospholipase C ↑ |
| Second messenger: | Cyclic AMP ↑ | Intracellular calcium ↑ | Diacylglycerol ↑<br>$Ca^{2+}$ ↑ |
| Effector: | Cyclic AMP dependent Protein kinase ↑ | Ca–calmodulin dependent protein kinase ↑ | Calcium phospholipid dependent protein kinase ↑ |
| | Phosphorylation of proteins | | |
| Outcome: | Activation of secretory mechanism | | |

Fig. 1.1. Summary of the three major signalling pathways which are known to be involved in the regulation of insulin secretion. There are substantial interactions between the pathways.

likely to phosphorylate glucose at all likely physiological concentrations, but also of low affinity glucokinase whose $K_m$ for glucose is set at a level 12 mM which will provide regulation of phosphorylation of glucose in precisely the concentration range at which secretion is stimulated (35). It is interesting that recent genetic studies of the rare MODY (maturity onset diabetes of the young) families have suggested a glucokinase gene defect in those families is a possible cause of the glucose 'blindness' of their β-cells (see p. 11).

Many other aspects of the metabolism of glucose and its regulation in β-cells have been studied in great detail; it is clear that glycolysis provides the major route of metabolism with the pentose phosphate pathway as a minor contributor. Regulation of glycolysis occurs at the phosphofructokinase level by both glucose 1 : 6 bisphosphate and glucose 2 : 6 bisphosphate, as in liver. Compounds feeding into the glycolytic pathway at the triose phosphate level, e.g. glyceraldehyde can also act as potent stimuli of insulin secretion.

Following initial glucose metabolism, predominantly by glycolysis, metabolites feed into the Krebs cycle which is activated to increase ATP production. ATP concentrations in the β-cell are increased as extracellular glucose increases in the range 0–5 mM glucose, but do not increase further as glucose concentrations rise to 20 mM – although the rate of turnover of ATP is presumably increased (36). For instance, ATP will be utilised as a phosphate donor in the phosphorylation of proteins which are activated by protein kinases; in the energy-requiring processes involved both in granule formation and intracellular granule transport prior to exocytosis, in the regulation of calcium efflux from the β-cell and as substrate for adenylate cyclase in the production of cyclic AMP. The role of ATP in regulating potassium entry has been discussed above. Whatever the detailed mechanism which links potassium channel closure to glucose metabolism, the outcome is clear – the cell membranes become depolarized as a result of the net inward current leading to the opening of voltage dependent (L-type) calcium channels and in turn to $Ca^{2+}$ entry into the β-cells (11). This is an important trigger for the insulin secretory mechanism (see Fig. 1.1).

### Amino acids

A number of nutrients other than glucose or the hexoses such as mannose, and trioses such as glyceraldehyde, can stimulate insulin secretion. They share in common a capability to enter and be metabolised by the β-cells (37): the most important are probably amino acids, and in some species fatty acids. The mechanism of action of some of the amino acids is known: leucine and the keto acid 2-ketoisocaproic acid generate ATP by their metabolism which in turn closes ATP sensitive potassium channels, causes depolarisation and calcium entry in a similar way to glucose metabolism. Arginine and other stimulatory basic amino acids may achieve their effects more directly by depolarising the cell on entry, thereby facilitating calcium entry. In experimental situations, the concentrations of amino acids which are used to stimulate insulin secretion are somewhat higher than those which would normally be encountered *in vivo*.

## Regulation of insulin secretion by hormones and neuropeptides

A wide variety of physiologically occurring agents – hormones and neuropeptides – can influence insulin secretion under appropriate conditions, although in some cases it is unclear whether they are likely to be physiologically important in normal man. A range of these are reviewed briefly here, along with notes on their possible mechanisms of action at the β-cell level.

### Catecholamines

β-cell membranes contain adrenergic acceptors, and the catecholamines adrenaline and noradrenaline have long been known to act as potent inhibitors of insulin secretion in response to a whole range of stimuli. This may be important in mediating the physiological responses to stress. It had originally been assumed that catecholamines elicited their effects in β-cells by inhibiting adenylate cyclase and thereby lowering intracellular cyclic AMP concentrations. However, more recent studies have shown that they may act in part at a later stage of the secretory pathway, and can inhibit responses to cyclic AMP or calcium in permeabilized cells in which any effects on adenylate cyclase are effectively bypassed. Interaction with a pertussis toxin sensitive inhibitory G-protein in the β-cell membrane may provide a direct link with a late stage of the secretory mechanism, perhaps at the exocytosis level (38).

### Glucagon

This has long been known to stimulate insulin

secretion, and the close proximity of the pancreatic α- and β-cells suggests that this might effect a form of paracine regulation. The intracellular mechanism is clear: glucagon binds to specific receptors in the β-cell membrane which links via a stimulatory G-protein ($G_s$) to adenylate cyclase. This in turn promotes synthesis of cyclic 3′, 5′ AMP which, as already discussed above, is a regulator of insulin secretion. Similarly, the glucagon-like peptide (GLP-1) released from proglucagon during its cleavage in the small intestine can stimulate insulin secretion *in vitro* (39), through activation of adenylate cyclase. It has a possible role as a hormone of the entero-insular axis (see p. 4).

### Cholecystokinin

This is another potential component of the entero-insular axis and has also been identified in nerve endings in relation to islets. Cholecystokinin and a variety of its fragments stimulate insulin secretion. They also bind to specific β-cell receptors and have been shown to activate protein kinase C following stimulation of plasma membrane bound phospholipase C to produce diacylglycerol (40). It is not known whether cyclic AMP may also be involved in its effects.

### Gastric inhibitory peptide

This is a third candidate for a role in the entero-insular axis and is a potent potentiator of insulin secretion. Like glucagon and cholecystokinin, it is assumed to exert its effects via specific receptors on the β-cell membrane. The mechanism(s) by which it potentiates glucose-induced insulin secretion has been proposed as activation of adenylate cyclase leading to cyclic AMP generation and/or activation of phospholipase C leading to protein kinase C activation (41).

### Somatostatin

This is widely distributed in the body, including the δ-cells of the pancreatic islets. It may act locally within the islets to inhibit both insulin and glucagon secretion (paracrine regulation). The way in which somatostatin acts to inhibit insulin secretion is far from clear. There is evidence that it can lower both intracellular calcium concentrations and decrease cyclic AMP levels. In addition, it may be able to open potassium channels leading to repolarisation of the β-cell membrane, although these do not appear to be the ATP-sensitive channels which are affected by drugs such as the sulphonylureas. Finally, it has been speculated that it may interact with G-proteins involved in the regulation of exocytosis, thus explaining its wide-ranging inhibitory effects on a number of stimuli. Evidence for these possibilities has been reviewed by Berggren (41).

### Pancreastatin

This is a 49 amino acid peptide originally isolated from pig pancreas. It has subsequently been found to be present in β- and δ-cell granules of islets of Langerhans. Insulin release *in vitro* in response to glucose, arginine or sulphonylureas is inhibited by pancreastatin, at least in the rat (42). It may exert these effects within the islets (paracrine effects); there is little information about changes in concentrations of pancreastatin which are circulating in the bloodstream in normal man or in NIDDM, nor about its mechanisms of action at the cellular level, which appear to be multiple (41).

### Opioids

Leu-enkephalin, β-endorphin and other opiates have been identified in the pancreas and have been reported to stimulate (43) or inhibit (44) insulin secretion under various conditions. The importance of opioids in mediating the regulation of insulin secretion by physiological agents remains to be clarified; their possible mechanisms of action are of some interest and a number of opioid receptors has been identified in islet cells.

### Galanin

This is a 29 amino acid peptide which is present in high concentrations in the small intestine. It has also been localised to nerve fibres in both endocrine and exocrine pancreas. Galanin is a potent inhibitor of insulin secretion in rodents and some insulin secreting tumour cell lines, in response to a wide range of stimuli. The physiological relevance of such an inhibition is not clear, since it may not affect insulin secretion in man or pigs. Nor is its mechanism of action fully understood. This action may involve lowering of intracellular calcium concentrations and/or participation of an inhibitory G-protein ($G_1$), in the β-cell plasma membrane, since its effects were abolished by treatment of the cells with pertussis toxin which binds to $G_1$ (45).

### Other neuropeptides

A range of other neuropeptides has also been implicated in the regulation of insulin secretion. For instance, *Neuropeptide Y* is a 36 amino acid peptide originally isolated from brain; it is widely distributed in neurones and may be co-secreted with noradrenaline. It may thus be involved in sympathetic nerve-mediated inhibition of insulin secretion (46); it has also been suggested to play a role in hypothalamic function, specifically regulating food intake in obesity. *Calcitonin gene-related peptide* (CGRP) is present in both nerve fibres and islet endocrine cells. In at least some species it has potent effects in inhibiting glucose-induced insulin secretion (47). *Gastrin releasing peptide* (GRP: bombesin) is also present in nerve endings in pancreatic islets, as well as in the brain and gastric intestinal tract, and is released during stimulation of vagus nerves. Specific antagonists of GRP action have been shown to inhibit part of the response to vagal stimulation of insulin secretion, implying that GRP might play an inhibitory role in parasympathetic control of insulin secretion (48 . Addition of GRP to β-cells has been shown to stimulate insulin secretion, probably by activating phospholipase C, leading to protein kinase C activation. *Vasoactive intestinal peptide* (VIP) is present in pancreatic neurones, some of which reach the pancreatic islets and is the most abundant pancreatic neuropeptide. Vagal stimulation elicits its release. *VIP* (like vagal stimulation) can increase rates of insulin secretion in several species (49) and this peptide may play a role as a neurotransmitter. Similarly, *Substance P* is present in pancreas at low concentrations and in some species is a stimulant of insulin secretion (50).

Summarising the physiological role of the wide range of neuropeptides which has been demonstrated in islet cells or their associated nerves is difficult. We can conclude that, while many of them are of substantial pharmacological interest in investigating the biochemical regulation of insulin secretion, relatively few have a proven physiologically significant role *in vivo*. In this respect, the criteria laid down by Holst (51) to evaluate such a physiological role may provide a useful check list for evaluating the role of the substances in this category: (i) the substance can be demonstrated to be present in islets; (ii) that receptors for it exist in one or more islet cell types; (iii) that the peptide is released from nerves on stimulation; (iv) that release of peptide and response parallel each other; (v) specific interference with peptide action inhibits the response.

## CURRENT TOPICS

Finally, and in order to illustrate the way in which basic knowledge of β-cell physiology can provide essential background information to evaluate important advances in diabetes, brief comments are provided about two topics which will also be found in other chapters of this book. The information here may provide useful background to relate that material to the context of β-cell function.

## Action of the sulphonylureas

Hypoglycaemic sulphonylureas have been used since the 1950s for the treatment of NIDDM, one of their properties being their ability to release insulin from β-cells which had become refractory to those glucose concentrations which are stimulatory in normal β-cells. There was, until recently, little detailed information as to their mechanism of action. At least one of the molecular mechanisms of action of the sulphonylureas is now established: it binds to a specific receptor (52) which is linked closely to, or is itself a part of, the ATP-sensitive potassium channel in the β-cell membrane (53). This binding causes the channel to close, leading, as described above for the actions of glucose, to an influx of calcium and activation of secretion (Fig. 1.2). There is a good correlation between the concentrations of sulphonylureas which are required for half maximal binding to the receptor, for closure of the potassium channel, for $Ca^{2+}$ entry and for the onset of secretion, as reviewed by Nelson *et al.* (53). Thus, it is at last clear how sulphonylureas can bypass one important glucose sensitive regulatory step – closure of the $K^+$ channel following generation of ATP from glucose metabolism – in insulin secretion. Other additional mechanisms of action of sulphonylureas in β-cells cannot, however, be excluded.

## Glucose regulation in NIDDM: glucokinase genes

There has recently been much interest though in the idea that a defect in the glucokinase gene may exist in a proportion of families with a variant of NIDDM called MODY (maturity onset dia-

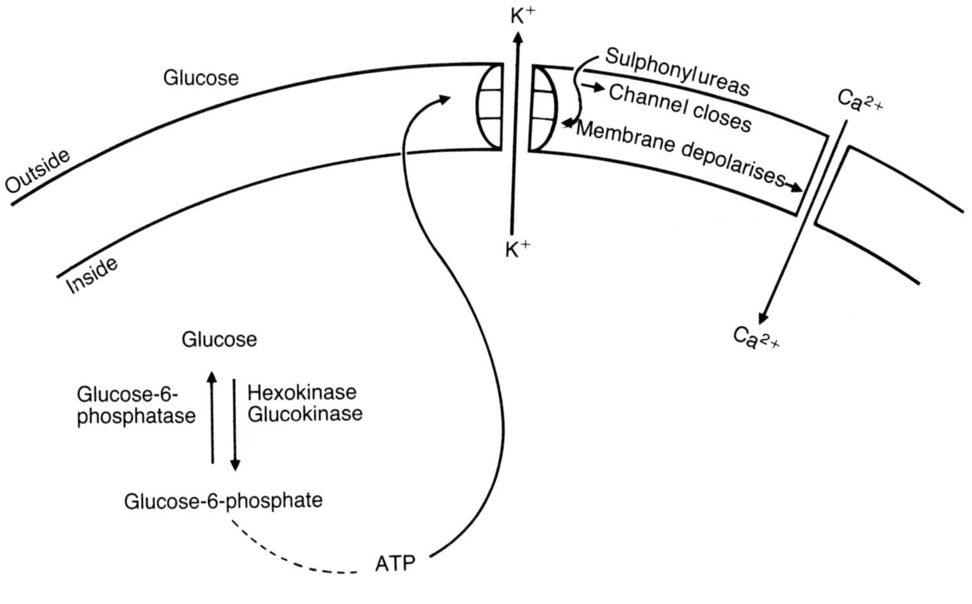


Fig. 1.2. Effects of glucose metabolism leading to ATP generation, and of sulphonylureas binding to specific receptors, leading to closure of potassium channels, depolarisation of β-cell membranes and calcium entry. These steps together may account for some of the actions of glucose and sulphonylureas in stimulating insulin secretion.

betes of the young) (54). There are many similarities (as well as some important differences) in the metabolism of glucose by β-cells and by the liver: the hexose enters both cells via a specific glucose transporter (Glut-2) and is phosphorylated by a pair of enzymes: hexokinase with a $K_m$ of 0.01–0.1 mmol/l (less than 2% of blood glucose concentration) and glucokinase with a $K_m$ of 12 mmol/l. The activity of glucokinase may be critical in eliciting the well-known sigmoidal increase in both glucose metabolism and insulin secretion following increases in extracellular glucose concentration. The dephosphorylation of glucose by glucose-6-phosphatase may also play a regulatory role (3).

Glucokinase is therefore a very attractive candidate for an enzyme which may be defective in NIDDM since at least one of the characteristics of this disease is the inability of the β-cell to respond adequately to increases in blood glucose concentrations. This is despite the presence of normal or even above normal concentrations of insulin in the cells – a glucokinase gene defect would be expected to produce this type of physiological result. However, recent studies on the glucokinase gene in adult-onset NIDDM families have not demonstrated any linkage. It may be that a complex of genes, including perhaps glucose-6-phosphatase and the glucose transporter Glut-2, might together be responsible for some of the genetic component of this, probably rather heterogeneous, disease (34).

Both these examples demonstrate the importance of knowledge derived from 'basic' research for the understanding of clinical problems, and also the great complexity of these problems. There is some way to go before a clear picture of normal and NIDDM β-cell function can be achieved.

## CONCLUSIONS

Our knowledge of the cell biology of the pancreatic β-cell has increased rapidly in the last few years, and we are becoming more confident of our understanding of the way in which glucose and sulphonylureas stimulate insulin secretion. This, in turn, allows the generation of testable hypotheses as to the possible β-cell defects in NIDDM. Beyond this step (and in the future) lie strategies to correct these defects.

## ACKNOWLEDGEMENTS

Financial support from the British Diabetic Association, Medical Research Council and Wellcome Trust is gratefully acknowledged.

## REFERENCES

1 Hutton JC, Penn EJ, Peshavaria M. Isolation and characterisation of insulin secretory granules from a rat islet cell tumour. *Diabetologia* 1982; 23: 365–73.
2 Lukinius A, Wilander E, Westermark GT, Engstrom U, Westermark P. Co-localization of islet amyloid polypeptide and insulin in the B-cell secretory granules of the human pancreatic islets. *Diabetologia* 1989; 32: 240–4.
3 Ohsawa H, Kanatsuka A, Yamaguchi T, Makino H, Yoshida S. Islet amyloid polypeptide inhibits glucose-stimulated insulin secretion from rat pancreatic islets. *Biochem Biophys Res Commun* 1989; 160: 961–967.
4 Hutton JC, Peshavaria M, Johnston CF, Ravazzola M, Orci L. Immunolocalization of betagranin: a chromogranin A related protein of the pancreatic B-cell. *Endocrinology* 1988; 122: 1014–20.
5 Guest PC, Hutton JC. Biosynthesis of insulin secretory granule proteins. In: Flatt PR, ed. *Nutrient regulation of insulin secretion.* Portland Press Ltd, London; 1992; 59–82.
6 Davidson HW, Rhodes CJ, Hutton JC. Intraorganellar Ca and pH control proinsulin cleavage in the pancreatic beta-cell via Arg. Arg and Lys.Arg-specific endopeptidases. *Nature (Lond)* 1988; 333: 93–6.
7 Howell SL, Tyhurst M. The pancreatic B-cell cytoskeleton and insulin secretion. *Diabetes/Metab Rev* 1986; 2: 107–23.
8 Cook DL, Hales CN. Intracellular ATP directly blocks potassium channels in pancreatic B-cells. *Nature (Lond)* 1984; 311: 271–3.
9 Ashcroft FM, Harrison DE, Ashcroft SJH. Glucose induces closure of single potassium channels in isolated rat pancreatic β-cells. *Nature (Lond)* 1984; 312: 446–8.
10 Ashcroft FM, Ashcroft SJH. Properties and functions of ATP-sensitive K-channels. *Cell Sig* 1990; 2: 197–214.
11 Ashcroft FM, Williams B, Smith PA, Fewtrell CMS. Ion channels involved in the regulation of nutrient-stimulated insulin secretion. In: Flatt PR, ed. *Nutrient regulation of insulin secretion.* Portland Press Ltd, London, 1992; 193–212.
12 Sturgess NC, Ashford MLJ, Cook DL, Hales CN. The sulphonylurea receptor may be an ATP-sensitive potassium channel. *Lancet* 1985; ii: 474–5.
13 Trube G, Rorsman P, Ohno-Shosaku T. Opposite effects of tolbutamide and diazoxide on the ATP-dependent

K⁺-channel in mouse pancreatic β-cells. *Pfleugers Arch* 1986; 407: 493–9.
14 Sussman KE, Leitner JW, Draznin B. Cytosolic free-calcium concentrations in normal pancreatic islet cells. *Diabetes* 1987; 36: 571–7.
15 Howell SL, Montague W, Tyhurst M. Calcium distribution in islets of Langerhans: A study of calcium concentrations and of calcium accumulation in β-cell organelles. *J Cell Sci* 1975; 19: 395–409.
16 Prentki M, Wollheim CB. Cytosolic free $Ca^{2+}$ in insulin secretory cells and its regulation by isolated organelles. *Experientia* 1984; 40: 1052–60.
17 Hellman B, Gylfe E, Grapengiesser E, Lund P-E, Marcström A. Cytoplasmic calcium and insulin secretion. In: Flatt PR, ed. *Nutrient regulation of insulin secretion*. Portland Press Ltd, London, 1992; 213–46.
18 Sharp GWG. The adenylate cyclase-cyclic AMP system in islets of Langerhans and its role in the control of insulin release. *Diabetologia* 1979; 16: 287–97.
19 Prentki M, Matschinsky FM. $Ca^{2+}$, cAMP and phospholipid-derived messengers in coupling mechanisms of insulin secretion. *Physiol Rev* 1987; 67: 1185–248.
20 Hughes SJ, Ashcroft SJH. Cyclic AMP, protein phosphorylation and insulin secretion. In: Flatt PR, ed. *Nutrient regulation of insulin secretion*. Portland Press Ltd, London, 1992; 271–289.
21 Hii CST, Jones PM, Persaud SJ, Howell SL. A reassessment of the role of protein kinase C in glucose-stimulated insulin secretion. *Biochem J* 1987; 246: 489–93.
22 Persaud SJ, Jones PM, Sugden D, Howell SL. Translocation of protein kinase C in rat islets of Langerhans: effects of a phorbol ester, carbachol and glucose. *FEBS Lett* 1989; 245: 80–4.
23 Jones PM, Persaud SJ, Howell SL. Protein kinase C and the regulation of insulin secretion from pancreatic B cells. *J Mol Endocrinol* 1992; 6: 121–7.
24 Jones PM, Salmon DMW, Howell SL. Protein phosphorylation in electrically permeabilised islets of Langerhans. Effects of $Ca^{2+}$, cyclic AMP, a phorbol ester and noradrenaline. *Biochem J* 1988; 254: 397–403.
25 Jones PM, Persaud SJ, Bjaaland T, Pearson JD, Howell SL. Nitric oxide is not involved in the initiation of insulin secretion from rat islets of Langerhans. *Diabetologia* 1993; 35: 1020–7.
26 Metz SA. Membrane phospholipid turnover as an intermediary step in insulin secretion. Putative roles of phospholipases in cell signalling. *Am J Med* 1988; 85(5A): 9–21.
27 Biden TJ, Peter-Reisch B, Schlegel W, Wollheim CB. $Ca^{2+}$-mediated generation of inositol 1,4,5-trisphosphate and inositol 1,3,4,5-tetrakisphosphate in pancreatic islets: studies with K⁺, glucose and carbamylcholine. *J Biol Chem* 1987; 262: 3567–71.
28 Morgan NG, Montague W. Phospholipids and insulin secretion. In: Flatt PR, ed. *Nutrient regulation of insulin secretion*. Portland Press Ltd, London: 1992; 125–55.
29 Blachier F, Malaisse WJ. Possible role of a GTP-binding protein in the activation of phospholipase C by carbamylcholine in tumoral insulin-producing cells. *Res Commun Chem Path Pharmacol* 1987; 58: 237–55.
30 Band A, Jones PM, Howell SL. The mechanism of arachidonic acid stimulated insulin secretion. *Biochim Biophys Acta* 1993; in press.
31 Basudev H, Jones PM, Howell SL. Arachidonic acid stimulation of insulin secretion from islets of Langerhans is not mediated by protein phosphorylation. *Mol Cell Endocrinol* 1993; 91: 193–9.
32 Morgan RO, Pek SB. Role of arachidonate lipoxygenase and cyclooxygenase products in insulin and glucagon secretion from rat pancreatic islets. *Metabolism* 1984; 33: 928–35.
33 Turk J, Wolf BA, Lefkowith JB, Stump WT, McDaniel ML. Glucose-induced phospholipid hydrolysis in isolated pancreatic islets: quantitative effects on the phospholipid content of arachidonate and other fatty acids. *Biochim Biophys Acta* 1986; 879: 399–409.
34 Jones PM, Persaud SJ. Arachidonic acid is a second messenger in nutrient induced insulin secretion from pancreatic B cells. *J Endocrinol* 1993; 137: 7–14.
35 Randle PJ. Glucokinase and candidate genes for Type II (non-insulin dependent) diabetes mellitus. *Diabetologia* 1993; 36: 269–75.
36 Ashcroft SJH, Weerasinghe LCC, Randle PJ. Interrelationships of islet metabolism, ATP content and insulin release. *Biochem J* 1973; 132: 223–31.
37 Rasmussen H, Zawalich KC, Ganesan S, Calle R, Zawalich WS. Physiology and pathophysiology of insulin secretion. *Diabetes Care* 1990; 13: 655–66.
38 Persaud SJ, Jones PM, Howell SL. Effect of Bordetella pertussis toxin on catecholamine inhibition of insulin release from intact and electrically permeabilized islets of Langerhans. *Biochem J* 1989; 258: 669–75.
39 Holst JJ, Ørskov C, Nielson OV, Schwartz TW. Truncated glucagon-like peptide I, an insulin releasing hormone from the distal gut. *FEBS Lett* 1987; 211: 169–74.
40 Persaud SJ, Jones PM, Howell SL. Stimulation of insulin secretion by cholecystokinin 8S: the role of protein kinase C. *Pharm Commun* 1994; 3: 39–47.
41 Berggren P-O, Rorsman P, Efendic S *et al.* Mechanisms of action of entero-insular hormones, islet peptides and neural input on the insulin secretory process. In: Flatt PR ed. *Nutrient regulation of insulin secretion*. Portland Press Ltd, London, 1992; 289–318.
42 Efendic S, Tatemoto K, Mutt V, Quan C, Chang D, Östenson C-G. Pancreastatin and islet hormone release. *Proc Natl Acad Sci USA* 1987; 84: 7257–60.
43 Ipp E, Dobbs R, Unger RH. Morphine and beta-endorphin influence the secretion of the endocrine pancreas. *Nature (Lond)* 1978; 276: 190–1.
44 Kanter RA, Ensinck JW, Fujinoto WY. Disparate effects of enkephalin and morphine upon insulin and glucagon secretion by islet cell cultures. *Diabetes* 1980; 29: 84–6.
45 Nilsson T, Arkhammar P, Rorsman P, Berggren P-O. Suppression of insulin release by galanin and somatostatin is mediated by a G-protein: an effect involving repolarization and reduction in cytoplasmic free $Ca^{2+}$ concentration. *J Biol Chem* 1989; 264: 973–80.
46 Sheikh SP, Holst JJ, Skak-Nielsen T *et al.* Release of NPY in pig pancreas: dual parasympathetic and sympathetic regulation. *Am J Physiol* 1988; 255: G46–54.
47 Lewis CE, Clark A, Ashcroft SJH, Cooper GJS, Morris JF. Calcitonin gene-related peptide and somatostatis inhibit insulin release from individual rat B cells. *Mol Cell Endocrinol* 1988; 57: 41–9.
48 Holst JJ, Harling H, Messell T, Coy DH. Identification of the neurotransmitter/neuromodulator functions of the

neuropeptide gastrin-releasing peptide in the porcine antrum, using the antagonist (Leu$^{13}$-ψ-$CH_2$-Leu$^{14}$)-bombesin. *Scand J Gastroenterol* 1990; 25: 89–96.
49 Ahren B, Taborsky GJ, Porte D Jr. Neuropeptidergic versus cholinergic and adrenergic regulation of islet hormone secretion. *Diabetologia* 1986; 29: 827–36.
50 Hermansen K. Effects of substance P and other peptides on the release of somatostatin, insulin and glucagon *in vitro*. *Endocrinology* 1980; 107: 1469–73.
51 Holst JJ. Role of classical and peptidergic neurotransmitters in insulin secretion. In: Flatt PR, ed. *Nutrient regulation of insulin secretion*. Portland Press Ltd, London, 1992; 23–38.
52 Panten U, Burgfeld J, Goerke F *et al*. Control of insulin secretion by sulfonylureas, meglitinide and diazoxide in relation to their binding to the sulfonylurea receptor in pancreatic islets. *Biochem Pharmacol* 1989; 38: 1217–29.
53 Nelson DA, Aguilar-Bryan L, Raef H, Boyd AE III. Molecular mechanisms of sulphonylurea action in the pancreatic B-cell. In: Flatt PR, ed. *Nutrient regulation of insulin secretion*. Portland Press Ltd, London, 1992; 319–39.
54 Froguel Ph, Vaxillaire M, Sun F *et al*. Close linkage of glucokinase locus on chromosome 7p to maturity-onset diabetes of the young (MODY) and mutation screening in late-onset diabetes. *Nature Genetics* 1992; 2: 153–6.

# 2 The Regulation of Insulin Gene Transcription

Kevin Docherty & Andrew R. Clark

## INTRODUCTION

The insulin gene was one of the first hormone genes to be sequenced and characterised in detail (1). Its structure is highly conserved among species consisting of three exons and two introns. Exon 1 is located in the 5′ untranslated region of the gene. Exon 2 contains sequences encoding the signal peptide, the insulin B chain and part of the C-peptide, while exon 3 encodes the remainder of the C-peptide, the insulin A chain and the 3′ untranslated sequences. The insulin gene is present as a single copy in all species with the exception of rat, mouse and *Xenopus*, which have two non-allelic insulin genes. Intron 2 is absent from the rat and mouse insulin I genes. Insulin is a member of a superfamily of structurally related peptides which includes relaxin, insulin-like growth factor I and II and insulin-related peptides from molluscs and insects. Recent reviews have focused on the structure and evolution of the insulin gene (2, 3). This chapter will review current knowledge of the molecular events controlling transcription of the insulin gene. Before addressing these mechanisms, we will briefly describe the regulation of eukaryotic gene expression.

## REGULATION OF GENE TRANSCRIPTION IN EUKARYOTES

Regulation of expression of eukaryotic genes transcribed by RNA polymerase II occurs at the level of initiation. There is little evidence that transcription elongation or termination represent major control points. Regulation of transcription is dependent on the interaction of *cis*-acting DNA sequences close to the specific gene with protein factors (4). These sequences have been classified according to their properties as promoters and enhancers, although this distinction is often blurred.

Promoters are located proximal to the transcription start site, are typically 100 base pairs in length, and represent the site of assembly of the initiation complex, which comprises RNA polymerase II and a number of general transcription factors. Most promoters possess a conserved sequence motif, TATAA (the TATA box), around 20 to 30 nucleotides upstream (−20 to −30) of the transcription start site. This sequence binds the factor TFIID and sets the initiation site. In genes that lack a TATA box, an initiator sequence located at −3 to +5 acts as an alternative TFIID binding site. Enhancers are composed of discrete sequence elements which interact with nuclear regulatory proteins to modulate the activity of the promoter in a positive or negative manner. Gene regulatory proteins can be grouped in structurally related families based on DNA binding or heterodimerisation motifs. These motifs include: helix turn helix, zinc finger, leucine zipper and helix loop helix. Many of these proteins bind to DNA as dimers, and different members of a family bind as homodimers or heterodimers with other members of the same family. It is unclear how multiple enhancer elements interact with the promoter, although models involve protein–protein interactions bringing the DNA-bound regulatory proteins into contact with the transcriptional machinery at the start site. This implies that the DNA is sufficiently flexible to allow bending or looping to occur.

The classical approach to delineating transcriptional control elements involves joining the putative controlling region to a reporter gene (e.g. chloramphenicol acetyltransferase (CAT) or firefly luciferase) and introducing this hybrid construct into cells in culture (5). The cells are then harvested between 24 and 72 hours later and the reporter gene product assayed in the cell extract. The level of reporter gene activity is proportional to the strength of the controlling region inserted upstream of the reporter gene. Fine mapping of regulatory sequences is achieved by deletion or mutation of specific nucleotides within the controlling region of such reporter gene constructs. Protein–DNA interactions can be analysed by DNase footprinting or electrophoretic mobility shift assay (6). In the former, DNA containing the sequence of interest is radiolabelled and incubated with nuclear protein extracts, and the binding of protein monitored by its ability to protect the DNA from DNaseI digestion. The DNase-treated DNA is separated on a polyacrylamide sequencing gel; unbound DNA appears as a ladder of fragments on an autoradiograph, while protein binding generates a space or footprint in the ladder where the DNA is protected from the nuclease. In the electrophoretic mobility shift assay, binding of protein to the radiolabelled DNA fragment affects the mobility of the DNA on a polyacrylamide gel such that retarded bands appear on autoradiographs. There are a number of ways of cloning cDNAs encoding transcription factors. The factor can be purified from nuclear extracts, usually by DNA affinity chromatography using double stranded oligonucleotides containing known protein binding sites, immobilised on an appropriated matrix. The peptide sequence of the purified protein is obtained, and the sequence data used to design oligonucleotide probes to screen cDNA libraries by hybridisation. Alternatively, cDNA expression libraries in bacteriophage λgt 11 can be screened using DNA probes corresponding to the binding site of the factor under study.

## REGULATION OF INSULIN GENE EXPRESSION

The insulin gene provides an excellent model for gene expression in eukaryotes for several reasons. Firstly, sequence information is now available from a large number of different species including primates, rodents, birds, fish and amphibians. This has provided a wealth of comparative data which has been used to search for conserved, and therefore potentially functional, sequences within the non-coding regions adjacent to the gene. As it turns out, most of the regulatory sequences are located close to the gene, making such comparisons particularly informative (7). Secondly, insulin is expressed exclusively in the β-cells of the islets of Langerhans in the adult. Thirdly, expression of the insulin gene is influenced by nutrient and hormonal stimulation of the β-cell. And fourthly, the mechanisms involved in controlling expression of the insulin gene, may also play a role in lineage determination within the developing endocrine pancreas, and in the maintenance of stable islet cell phenotypes in the adult.

In addition to these basic research aspects, studies on insulin gene transcription may be relevant to our understanding of the causes of diabetes. There is evidence that insulin gene mutations and altered insulin gene regulation may contribute to type I (IDDM). Thus, although the major locus for IDDM has been mapped to the HLA complex within chromosome 6, an additional locus on chromosome 11 adjacent to the insulin has been shown to be present in association with HLA-DR4 (8) (see Chapter 9). The sequence of the insulin gene exons is normal in these patients, suggesting that the gene defect may lie within the region regulating expression of the gene. In NIDDM, although most studies have failed to show an association or linkage of the insulin gene with the disease, work on rat models of NIDDM has shown a reduced response to glucose of insulin mRNA accumulation (9). This may be a consequence of a change in the half-life of insulin mRNA or a defect in transcription of the gene.

Before moving on to an account of the mechanisms controlling insulin gene transcription, it is important to point out that these processes are complex. During the past decade, the objectives have been to identify the DNA sequences involved in the control of insulin gene transcription and to purify and characterise the proteins that bind to these sites. Although tremendous progress has been made, we are only just beginning to understand the complexities of the interactions involved. It is therefore impossible at this stage to put forward simplified mechanistic models that will help the uninitiated to understand better these events. What we have attempted to do in this review is pull together the results from a number of laboratories. The field is confounded by the tendency for each research group to develop their own nomenclature system. We have tried where possible to simplify the nomenclature by emphasising shared aspects of sequence elements, e.g. E boxes and TAAT boxes, and by grouping transcription factors into families. The following sections will therefore review the status of current knowledge on the DNA sequences and trans-acting factors involved in regulating transcription of the insulin gene, and attempt to discuss the available data within the context of the tissue-specific, transient, and developmental aspects of insulin gene expression. Most of the published work on insulin gene expression has come from studies on the rat insulin I and II genes, and the human insulin gene. A sequence alignment of the 5′ region of the three genes is shown in Fig. 2.1. Of these, the rat insulin I gene has been studied in greatest detail.

## The rat insulin I gene

Using insulin gene fragments fused to the CAT reporter gene, Walker *et al.*, 1983 showed that sequences between −333 and +51 were sufficient for expression in transfected β cell lines (10). This region contained a proximal promoter and a distal enhancer, both of which could direct tissue-specific gene expression (11), although recent results indicate that the promoter is dispensable for tissue-specific expression in transgenic mice (12). The enhancer was further mapped in detail by a sensitive block mutagenesis study (13). It was found that several mutations had moderate deleterious effects upon transcription, while mutations within three distinct regions decreased the rate of transcription five-fold or more. The first of these was the TATA box (−20 to −30), while the other two coincided with identical eight base pair sequence motifs (GCCATCTG) at −105 and −231. These motifs have been termed the IEB1 (or NIR after a member of the research group) box and the IEB2 (or FAR since it was further from the transcription start site than NIR) box, respectively (Fig. 2.2). A double mutation of the IEB1 and IEB2 motifs effectively abolished transcription.

### The E box

The IEB sequence belongs to a class of regulatory sites, known as E boxes, which have the consensus sequence CANNTG and are implicated in the tissue-specific regulation of genes in muscle,

```
RAT I       CA---GTTCCAGGGACAAAGATACCAGGTCCCC-AACAACTGCAACTTTCTGGGAAATGAGG
RAT II      CAACAGTTCAAGGGACAAAGTTACTAGGTCCCCCAACAACTGCAGCCTCCTGGGGAATGATG
HUMAN       --ACAGC----AGCGCAAAGA-GCCCCGCCCTGCAGC--CTCCAGCTCTCCTGGTC-TAATG
                                    SP1                            CT3

RAT I       TGGAAAA-TGCTCAGCCAAGGAAAAAGAGGGCCTTACCCTCTCTGGGACAAT-GATTG-TGC
RAT II      TGGAAAAATGCTCAGCCAAGGACAAAGAAGGCCTCACCCTCTCTGAGACAAT-GTCCCCTGC
HUMAN       TGGAAAGTGGCCCAGGT---------GAGGGCTTTGCTCTCCTGGAGACATTTGCCCCCAGC
             CORE                                         NRE

                                FAR                  FLAT
RAT I       TGTGAACTGCTTCA--TCAGGCCATCTGGC--CCCTTGTTAATAATCTAATTACCC--TAGG
RAT II      TGTGAACTGGTTCA--TCAGGCCACCCAGGAGCCCCTCTTAAGACTCTAATTACCC--TAAG
HUMAN       TGTGAGCAGGGACAGGTCTGGCCACCGGGC--CCCTGGTTAAGACTCTAATGACCCGCTGGT
                                IEB2/FAR                 CT2

                                                 E3
RAT I       TCTAAGTA-GAGTTGTTGACGTCCAATGAGCGCTTTCTGCAGACTTAGCACTAGGCAAGTG-
RAT II      GCTAAGTA-GAGGTGTTGTTGTCCAATGAGCACTTTCTGCAGACCTAGCACCAGGCAAGTG-
HUMAN       CCTGAGGAAGAGGTGCTGACGACCAAGGAGATCTTCCCACAGACCCAGCACCAGGGAAATGG
                               CRE                                   GG2

RAT I       TTTGGAAATTACAGCTTCAGCCCCTCTCGCCATCTGCCTACCTACCCCTCCTAGAGCCCTTA
RAT II      TTTGGAAACTGCAGCTTCAGCCCCTCTGGCCATCTGCTGATCCACCC----------CCTTA
HUMAN       TCCGGAAATTGCAGCCTCAGCCCC--CAGCCATCTGCCGACCCCCCCACCCCAGG--CCCTA
               GG1                     IEB1/NIR
                                        GAGA
RAT I       ATGGGCCAAACGGCAAAGTCCAGGGGGCAGAGAGGAGGTGCTTTG-GACTATAAAGCTAGTG
RAT II      ATGGGACAAACAGCAAAGTCCAGGGGTCAGGGGGGGGGTGCTTTG-GACTATAAAGCTAGTG
HUMAN       ATGGGCCAGGCGGCAGGGGTTGACAGGTAGGGGAGATGGGCTCTGAGACTATAAAGCCAGCG
            CT1                                                TATA

RAT I       GAGACCCAGTAACTCCC
RAT II      GGGATTCAGTAACCCCC
HUMAN       GGGGCCCAGCAGCCCTC
```

Fig. 2.1. Comparison of sequences in the 5′ regions of the rat and human insulin genes. Characterised sequence elements are boxed. Common names of the identified elements are given above or below the sequence alignment. Further details are provided in the text.

pancreas and lymphoid tissue (14). Several cDNAs have been isolated for protein factors which recognise E boxes. These factors are homologous to one another and to the *myc* family of oncogenes, and are known as helix loop helix (HLH) proteins. They possess a domain capable of forming two amphipathic helices separated by a loop structure, and there is usually an adjacent basic domain. The helix loop helix domain is involved in dimerisation between HLH proteins, while the basic domain mediates DNA binding.

The IEB sequence binds a factor, IEF-1, which was originally shown to be present in β-cells but not in fibroblasts (15). Analysis of a wide range of cell types, however, showed that IEF-1 is present in non-β-cell lines such as α-cells and pituitary cells, though not in non-endocrine cells (16, 17). By screening expression libraries with IEB sequences, cDNA clones for IEB-binding factors have been obtained from mouse, hamster and rat (18–20). All the clones are derived from a single gene, E2A, which generates at least two proteins by alternative splicing (21). The proteins have been named E12/47 for human, A1 and A7 for mouse, Pan 1 and Pan 2 for rat and shPan -1 and shPan-2 for hamster. The participation of HLH proteins in binding to the IEB1 site was demonstrated immunologically using antibodies directed against E2A proteins (17, 22). Using an *in vitro* subunit exchange assay, Park and Walker (1992) obtained data indicating that IEF1 is a heterodimeric HLH complex composed of an E2A gene product and insulin

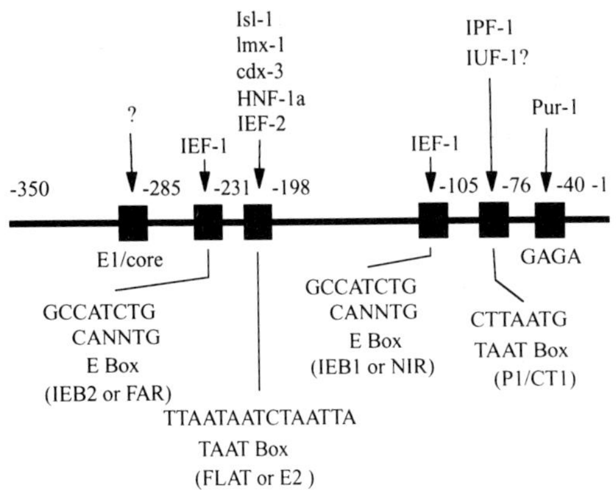


Fig. 2.2. The arrangement of transcriptional regulatory sequences in the rat insulin I gene. The numbers indicate nucleotides upstream of the transcription start site. Information on sequence elements, along with their common names (in parentheses or immediately below the boxed element) is given below the scheme. The names of various DNA binding proteins are given above the scheme.

enhancer specific factor 1 (IESF-1), an HLH protein of $M_r$ 25k (23). Since the E2A proteins are expressed in a wide variety of cells, the restricted expression of the heterodimer IEF-1 may be due to restricted tissue expression of IESF-1. In this case IESF-1 represents an important β-cell transcription factor, and its isolation and characterisation represents an important goal. However, sequences in addition to the IEB sites are also important in controlling transcription of the gene, since combinations of IEB1 and IEB2 fail to confer tissue-specific gene expression in transgenic mice (12).

## The TAAT box

In the rat insulin I gene a highly AT-rich tract around position −198 (the FAR Linked AT rich or FLAT element), contains four copies of the sequence TAAT, three on the upper strand and one on the lower strand (Fig. 2.2) (22). Another TAAT box is located at −77. This promoter-proximal TAAT box binds a factor, IPF-1 (insulin promoter factor 1), which is present in β-cells but not in α-cells (17). The relationship of this factor to a factor, IUF-1 (insulin upstream factor 1), that binds to a corresponding sequence in the human insulin gene will be discussed later. The FLAT region possesses complex regulatory properties. It can be subdivided into two domains which contain the sequence TAATTA (FLAT-E) and TAATAAT (FLAT-F) (24). There is some form of negative interaction between these domains, such that mutation of the FLAT-E motif leads to a substantial increase in the rate of transcription. The simplest explanation of this observation is that factors bound to the FLAT-E region are relatively weak activators of transcription but interfere with the binding of a powerful activator protein at the adjacent FLAT-F region.

In electrophoretic mobility shift assays, using the rat insulin I FLAT region as a probe, several protein–DNA complexes were detected, some of which appeared to be β cell-specific. Using the same region to probe a cDNA library, Edlund and colleagues cloned a DNA binding factor, Isl-1 (25). This factor is related to homeodomain proteins of the nematode *Caenorhabditis elegans* and contains, in addition to its homeodomain, a potential zinc finger domain. The role of Isl-1 in transcriptional regulation of the insulin gene and in islet cell development is not clear. Isl-1 is present in a variety of different cell types (26), and *in vitro* Isl-1 does not appear to bind to the FLAT region (16). It may be an important determinant of a variety of neuroendocrine cells (27). The same group have identified another factor that binds within this region of the rat insulin I gene. Termed IEF-2 (insulin enhancer factor 2), the factor is distinct from Isl-1, and is present in β cells but not in α cells (16).

German *et al.*, 1992 have isolated several cDNAs encoding proteins that bind to the FLAT element (28). Two of these cDNAs, cdx-3 (*caudal*-type homeobox 3) and lmx-1(*LIM*-homeobox 1), represent homeo-box containing mRNAs with restricted patterns of expression. The lmx-1 protein also contains two cysteine/histidine rich regions (LIM domains). Analysis with mutant binding sites demonstrated that both cdx-3 and lmx-1 bind at either the FLAT-E or the FLAT-F site, although both proteins bind best at the FLAT-E site. By Northern blot analysis, the cdx-3 cDNA hybridised with a 2.1 kb mRNA in several endocrine cells but not in the fibroblast cell line BHK21 and CHO. lmx-1 mRNA was absent from non-insulin producing cell lines by Northern analysis; it was present in β cells but its levels were so low that it could only be detected by sensitive RNase protection methods. Another islet cell protein binding to the FLAT-F sequence has been identified as the liver-enriched homeodomain factor HNF-1α (*h*epatocyte *n*uclear *f*actor 1α) (29). In co-transfection experiments, HNF-1α is able to activate transcription of reporter constructs containing the FLAT-F motif.

## The FF mini-enhancer

The E (FAR) box and the TAAT (FLAT) box function synergistically. Neither element can function alone but both are required for enhancer activity, constituting what has been termed the FF (*F*AR/*F*LAT) mini-enhancer (22). This synergism can be seen at the protein level. The E2A protein, E47, which comprises part of the IEF1 heterodimer binding at the FAR box, does not activate the FF mini-enhancer on its own. However, when transfected into fibroblasts expressing lmx-1, E47 causes a dramatic synergistic activation of the mini-enhancer. E47 caused no activation of the mini-enhancer in fibroblasts transfected with cdx-3 or isl-1. Thus a specific interaction of proteins at the FAR (E box) and the FLAT (TAAT box) elements occurs (28). These experiments emphasise the potential importance of lmx-1; it has restricted tissue expression and will interact with E47 to activate transcription of a FF mini-enhancer construct.

## The GAGA box

The GAGA box is a purine-rich stretch of nucleotides at −57 to −40 in the rat insulin I gene. In a systematic mutational analysis, mutation of this sequence resulted in 60% loss of transcription (13), suggesting that the GAGA box may represent an important transcriptional control region. Electrophoretic mobility shift studies, coupled with UV-cross-linking analysis, led to the identification of at least four proteins (50, 80, 100 and 117 kD) that bind sequence specifically to this region. A cDNA encoding a 52 kD, GAGA-box binding protein (Pur-1), has been cloned (30, 31). Pur-1 (*Pu*rine *r*ich 1) is a widely distributed zinc finger protein which exhibits strong transcriptional activatory properties when tested on multimerised GAGA sites as well as on the insulin promoter, in β- and non-β cell lines.

## The E1 to E5 footprints

Mapping of protein binding sites by DNase footprinting identified five binding sites, designated E1 to E5, in the rat insulin I gene 5′ region (Figs. 2.1 and 2.2). These included the promoter-distal E box or FAR element (footprint E4), the promoter- proximal E box or NIR element (footprint E5), the TAAT box or FLAT element (footprint E2), and footprints at: −285 to −332 (E1), and −153 to −174 (E3) (30, 13). E1 is an extensive footprint which remains to be characterised in detail. Although it contains an element similar to the 'enhancer core' (TGTGGAAAG) it is the sequence adjacent to this which is most sensitive to mutation in transcriptional assays (13). Similarly, the results of systematic mutagenesis imply a transcriptional role for footprint E3, which also remains to be characterised.

## The rat insulin II gene

The rat insulin II gene is the ancestral gene. In both rat and mouse, a second insulin gene appears to have arisen by reverse transcription of a rare partially spliced germ line transcript (33). Comparison of the 5′ flanking sequence shows similarity up to 540 base pairs. Although the rat insulin II gene is 80% identical to the insulin I gene within the region −370 to +1 (Fig. 2.1), its regulation clearly differs in a number of respects (Fig. 2.3). Duplication of the

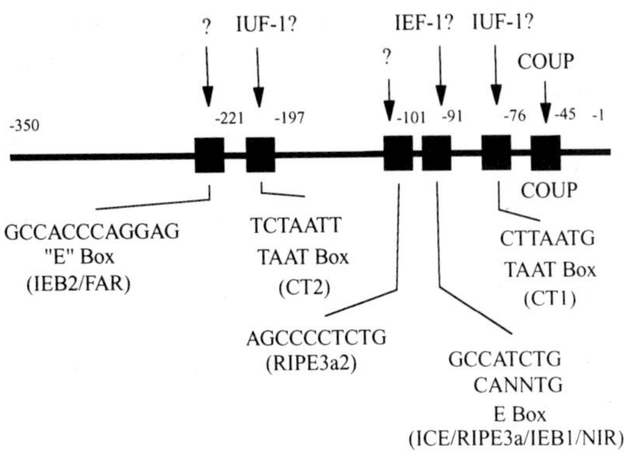


Fig. 2.3. The arrangement of transcriptional regulatory sequences in the rat insulin II gene. The numbers indicate nucleotides upstream of the transcription start site. Information on sequence elements, along with their common names (in parentheses or immediately below the boxed element) is given below the scheme. The names of various DNA binding proteins are given above the scheme.

rat insulin gene has presumably altered the selective pressures operating upon transcriptional regulation. Therefore, the rat insulin genes may not be entirely typical of mammalian insulin genes in this respect. Both genes are expressed equally in normal islets (34–36), though not in foetal yolk sac (37), nor in some insulinoma-derived cells (38).

The rat insulin II gene promoter is strongly active in both insulin-secreting and non-secreting cell lines (39). A β-cell-specific protein binds within the promoter region (40), while a ubiquitous protein related to the chicken ovalbumin upstream promoter (COUP) transcription factor binds to the promoter at position −54 to −45 (41).

Two important transcriptional control elements, which act coordinately, have been mapped within the region −126 to −86 (42–45). This region, which has been referred to as the rat insulin promoter element 3 (RIPE3), contains binding sites for at least three distinct factors. The sequence between −100 and −91 contains an E box identical to the IEB1 sequence in the rat insulin I gene. Known as the insulin control element (ICE), this sequence binds a heterodimeric complex composed of the ubiquitously expressed E2a gene products E12 and/or E47 and a factor with restricted tissue expression (45, 46). It is likely that this factor is IEF-1.

There is no exact equivalent of the rat insulin I gene IEB2 motif, and deletion through the corresponding region has no significant effect upon transcription. One linker scanning mutation which disrupts this region causes a two-fold decrease in transcription, however two other linker scanning mutations within the same area show no significant effect. Thus it remains unclear whether this region is transcriptionally active. Deletion of sequences from −218 to −179 have a marked effect on transcription (41, 43). Interestingly, this region contains a TAAT box, TCTAAT (−210 to −215) similar to that which binds a β-cell specific factor in the human insulin gene, IUF-1 (see below). It remains to be determined whether this TAAT box interacts with adjacent sequences in a manner similar to that observed for the FLAT element in the rat insulin I gene.

Other elements which are sensitive to mutation include: regions of homology to the rat insulin I gene footprints E1 and E3, a region of homology to the rat insulin I gene cAMP response element (see below), and a further uncharacterised site around −185 (Fig. 2.3).

## The human insulin gene

As mentioned previously, the rat insulin genes may not be typical of mammalian insulin genes in terms of transcriptional regulation. Although common regulatory sequences are shared by the rat insulin genes and the human insulin genes, functional differences are observed. If anything a closer similarity exits between the ancestral rat insulin II gene and the human insulin than between the two rat insulin genes. Thus stable transfection of the human insulin gene into the rat islet tumour cell line MSL, which shows differential expression of the two endogenous rat insulin genes under certain conditions, results in preferential co-expression of the rat insulin II gene and the transfected human insulin gene (47). Although sequences downsteam of −258 will confer tissue specific expression of the human insulin gene (18, 48) recent studies on expression of deletion constructs in transfected cells (Clark & Docherty, unpublished observations) and in transgenic mice (49) suggest that regulatory sequences may be located further upstream.

## E boxes and TAAT boxes

The proximal E box or IEB1 site is highly conserved among insulin genes, and is present at −101 to −109 in the human gene (previously designated the GC1 box) (Fig. 2.4). It binds a factor with properties similar to those of IEF-1, i.e. is β-cell enriched and binds to an equivalent sequence in the rat insulin I gene (50). As in the rat insulin II gene, the IEB2 sequence (previously the GC2 box) is not conserved in the human insulin gene. The equivalent sequence (GCCACCGG) at −233 to −239 differs in important respects from the canonical E box consensus sequence, CANNTG. This region, however, is transcriptionally important, since deletion of sequences downstream from −258 reduce transcription markedly (18, 48).

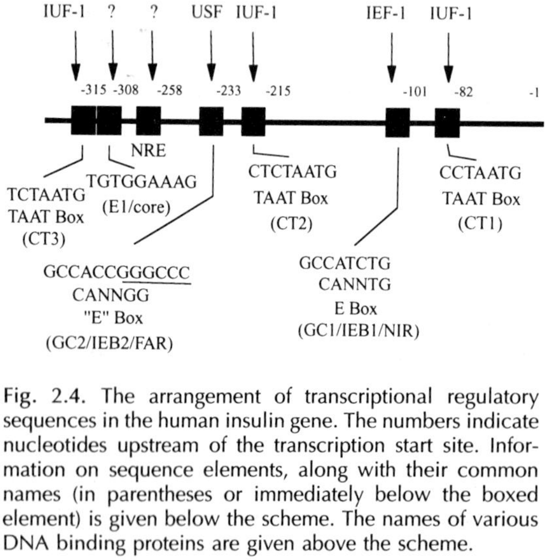


Fig. 2.4. The arrangement of transcriptional regulatory sequences in the human insulin gene. The numbers indicate nucleotides upstream of the transcription start site. Information on sequence elements, along with their common names (in parentheses or immediately below the boxed element) is given below the scheme. The names of various DNA binding proteins are given above the scheme.

Recently, it has been demonstrated that the HLH transcription factor USF (upstream stimulating factor) binds to the IEB2-equivalent sequence in the human insulin gene (50). Another factor binds to the adjacent sequence GGGCCC and to the same sequence in intron 1 between nucleotides +160 and +175 (51) (Fig. 2.4).

There are three important TAAT boxes (CT boxes) in the human insulin gene. These share the consensus sequence [C/T]TAATG, and are located at −82 (CT1), −215 (CT2) and −319 (CT3) (52) (Fig. 2.4). These sites bind a single factor called IUF-1, which is present in β-cell lines, but absent from a wide range of other cell types including pancreatic α-cells (53). IUF-1 is composed of two proteins of $M_r$ 115k and 45k that can be separated by ion exchange chromatography (54). It shares properties with the factor IPF-1 which binds to an equivalent sequence (the P1 site) in the rat insulin I promoter (16). The close association of the TAAT boxes (CT1 and CT2) and the E boxes (IEB1 and IEB2) led to speculation that these sites might constitute a β-cell protoenhancer, similar to the interaction of the A and B domains of the SV40 enhancer (48). Recent preliminary results support this hypothesis. Thus, individually the IEB2 or CT2 motifs exhibit very low transcriptional activity, while higher activity is observed with DNA fragments containing both sequences (Read, Clark & Docherty, unpublished observations). This is reminiscent of the FF mini-enhancer in the rat insulin I gene (24).

## The GG1/GG2 motif

When DNaseI protection assays were performed on the human insulin gene 5′ region, a footprint was observed in the area −153 to −127, which contains two repeats of the six base pair sequence GGAAAT, separated by a short palindromic sequence GGTCC (48). The more promoter-proximal footprint GGAAAT sequence (GG1 box) was protected in all cell lines, whereas the GG2 footprint was only found in β-cell lines. In a linker scanning mutational analysis of the rat insulin 2 gene, the GG1 box was shown to be highly sensitive to mutation (42). These observations suggest that one or both of the GG boxes might play an important role in regulating expression of the human insulin gene.

### The NRE

A negative regulatory element (NRE) exists between −279 and −258 (48). The NRE is active in both β-cells and non-β-cells, and therefore does not appear to play a role in restricting insulin expression to β-cells. It contains at least three protein binding sites. One of these contains the sequence GAGACAT, which is also present in the corresponding position in the rat insulin II gene. Mutagenesis of this sequence in the rat insulin II gene increases the rate of transcription twofold (42), suggesting that this sequence may also act as a negative element in the rat insulin II gene. In the human insulin gene the silencer activity within the NRE is dependent on its position relative to, or interaction with adjacent sequences, and is modulated by an upstream positive element located at −279 to −339 (the CT3/core element). This region contains the CT3 box and the sequence TGTGGAAAG, which is a perfect match to the sequence of the enhancer core, a binding site for the CCAAT-enhancer binding protein (C/EBP) and probably for other factors. There is an interaction between proteins binding at the CT3/core site and the NRE (Clark & Docherty, unpublished observations).

### The insulin linked polymorphic region (ILPR)

The human insulin gene has a polymorphic region at −365, containing variable numbers of tandem repeats of the 14 bp sequence (TCTGGGGAGAGGGG). Population studies have shown that the size of the ILPR can vary. The most common alleles contain 40, 95 or 175 repeat units corresponding to 590, 1320 and 2140 base pairs. These alleles have been referred to as small or class 1, large or class 3, and intermediate sized or class 2. Weak associations of class 3 alleles with type 2 diabetes, and class 1 alleles with type I diabetes in Caucasians have been described. Takeda *et al.* have implicated the ILPR in the negative regulation of the insulin gene in non-β-cells (55). Unfortunately, the description of the constructs used in this study does not make clear whether any sequences flanking the ILPR, which may exert transcriptional effects, were present. Since the same constructs were not tested on β-cells, it is not clear whether the negative effect is restricted to non-β-cells. In an unpublished study from this laboratory, deletion of part of the ILPR resulted in an increase in reporter activity in β-cells, confirming that the ILPR contained negative regulatory activity. Our result raised the possibility that insulin genes adjacent to longer repeat sequences, i.e. class 3 alleles, might be expressed at lower levels than those genes adjacent to short repeat sequences, i.e. class 1 alleles. Interestingly, the ILPR adopts an altered DNA structure (56), which has been characterised as a quadriplex involving interactions between the G residues on the top strand (57). The quadriplex structure is present *in vivo* and in DNA assembled in chromosomes *in vitro* (58, 59). The function of this structure is unknown.

## Negative regulation of insulin gene expression

Negative regulation of the insulin gene in non-β-cell lines was first observed in experiments in which a fibroblast cell line was transfected with a rat insulin I enhancer/CAT construct in the presence or absence of a second plasmid bearing the enhancer alone. The presence of the second plasmid allowed the first construct to become active, presumably by titrating out factors that bound to the enhancer and repressed transcriptional activity (60). Other negative elements in the insulin gene include one located within a long interspersed repetitive sequence (LINES), roughly 3 kb upstream of the rat insulin I gene (61), and the IEB1 box in the rat insulin II gene

(43). The adenovirus five E1a gene products transcriptionally repress several enhancers including those of the insulin genes. A site of action of E1a has been mapped to the IEB1 box of the rat insulin II gene (62), leading to the suggestion that negative regulation of insulin gene expression in non-β-cells may be mechanistically similar to repression by E1a proteins.

An unusual form of negative regulation is associated with multiple copies of the IEB sequence (63). Multiple copies of the IEB sequence, although capable of binding IEF1, showed reduced transcriptional activity over constructs containing two copies. IEB multimers were also able to inhibit *cis*-linked enhancers in β-cells but not in other cell types. The conclusion was that β-cells contain a repressor molecule that functions by regulating access of HLH proteins to multiple E box elements. The insulin gene does not contain multiple E box elements, and so it remains to be determined whether under certain conditions the repressor can recognise monomeric E boxes in the insulin gene, or whether its role is to silence expression of genes containing mutiple E boxes in β-cells.

Negative regulatory elements at −270 and within the ILPR of the human insulin gene have been described above. These elements are functional in both β- and non-β-cell lines and as such their role is unclear. In this respect, it should be pointed out that negative regulation is a common feature of gene expression in eukaryotes (64). In some cases negative regulation may play a role in restricting expression of the insulin gene to the β-cell. Its function may be to prevent low level, ectopic expression of the gene due to the presence of ubiquitous positively acting transcription factors which are able to bind to the insulin enhancer. In other cases where the negative regulatory activity is present in both insulin-secreting and non-secreting cell lines, it may be involved in the modulation of gene expression in response to external signals, or in programmes of cell differentiation that occur during development.

## Hormonal and nutrient control of insulin gene expression

Insulin biosynthesis is regulated by various nutrients and hormones. Glucose, amino acids and glucagon-like peptide 1(7–37) (GLP-1) increase insulin production, while somatostatin decreases it. Several studies have shown that glucose increases insulin mRNA levels (65–69). This response involves increases in both the rate of transcription (70), and the stability of insulin mRNA (71). The exact mechanisms whereby glucose stimulates transcription of the insulin gene are not clearly understood. Glucose metabolism is undoubtedly necessary (72), and anaerobic glycolysis is capable of generating a signal(s) mediating transcriptional control of the insulin gene (73).

It is possible that at least two distinct signalling pathways are involved in the transient control of insulin gene transcription. Thus the effects of cAMP on insulin gene transcription have been mapped to a cAMP response element (CRE) located at −177 to −184 in the rat insulin I gene (74). Deletion or mutagenesis of this sequence abolishes the cAMP stimulatory effect. It is probable that protein kinase A phosphorylation of a CRE-binding protein (CREB) might be involved (75). Thus a 43 kD protein, exhibiting a similar molecular weight to that of CREB (43 kD) has been shown to bind to the insulin gene CRE. The glucose responsive element (GRE) was localised within a fragment of the rat insulin I gene that lacked the CRE (76). The GRE was further mapped to a region −193 to −227 that contained the FLAT element (Fig. 2.2), and was shown to be active in adult rat and human islets (77). A single protein (C1 factor) that bound within this region was identified. The DNA binding activity of C1 is modulated by extracellular glucose with a four- to five-fold increase in binding activity observed when rat islets are incubated for one to three hours in the 20 mM glucose compared with 2 mM glucose. The C1 factor resembles in several respects the factor, IUF-1, that binds to a similar sequence in the human insulin gene enhancer (52, 54). Our own data confirm that there is substantial reduction in the activity of IUF-1 in isolated rat islets incubated for 3 hours in 3 mM compared with 20 mM glucose (W. MacFarlane and K. Docherty, unpublished observations). Further preliminary studies from our laboratory indicate that phosphorylation can modulate the binding of IUF-1 to its DNA recognition sequence in the insulin gene (M. L. Read and K. Docherty, unpublished observations).

The role of $Ca^{2+}$ (72, 77) and phorbol esters in the control of insulin gene transcription is controversial. In HIT T15 β-cells transfected with a rat insulin I gene/CAT construct (−345 to +1), co-incubation with the $Ca^{2+}$ channel blocker verapamil did not significantly decrease the effect of glucose on CAT activity, while raising extracellular $Ca^{2+}$ decreased CAT activity in response to glucose (72). In transfected foetal rat islets, however, verapamil reduced the response of a similar rat insulin I gene fragment (−410 to +1) (77). Phorbol esters affect gene transcription through the binding of a complex, AP1, to the phorbol response element (TRE). AP1 consists of a collection of structurally related transcription factors which belong to the Jun and Fos family. c-Jun can also form heterodimers with members of the CREB family of proteins that bind to CRE's (75). This overlapping specificity of AP1 and CREB may allow the proteins to antagonise or synergise with each other, and may, in part, explain the inhibition of cAMP-stimulated CAT activity in HIT cells co-transfected with a human insulin gene/CAT construct and a plasmid bearing a c-Jun cDNA (78).

## ISLET SPECIFIC GENE EXPRESSION

In addition to insulin, the β-cell expresses a variety of neuroendocrine substances. Of these, islet amyloid polypeptide (IAPP) or amylin, a 37 amino acid peptide structurally related to calcitonin gene related polypeptide, is almost as tightly restricted to the β-cell as insulin. Its expression differs from that of insulin in pluripotent foetal pancreatic endocrine cells and transformed islet cell lines, where it is co-expressed with glucagon and somatostatin (79). Another gene expressed preferentially in α-cells is that encoding glucokinase, a key component of the glucose sensing mechanism (80). The glucokinase gene contains two cell type-specific promoters separated by 15 kilobase pairs. The downstream promoter is active in hepatocytes while the upstream promoter is active in β-cells and in pituitary cells (81). Sufficient data are now available on the regulation of IAPP and glucokinase gene expression for meaningful comparisons to be made with the insulin gene. Such comparisons, when extended to other genes, such as the glucose transporter 2 (GLUT-2), which are expressed in a limited number of cell types including β-cells, or to the genes encoding hormones expressed in other islet cell types, may reveal common sequences and factors involved in cell-specific gene expression in the islets.

What immediately becomes apparent is that there are matches to the CT consensus sequence ([C/T]TAATG) between 80 and 100 bp upstream of the transcription start site, not only in all mammalian insulin genes, but also in the human and rat IAPP genes, the β-cell glucokinase promoter, and the rat somatostatin promoter (Table 2.1). In the rat insulin genes mutations within the CT-1-like region decrease transcription, although not strikingly. In the glucokinase gene this region is mutationally sensitive and binds IUF-1 as demonstrated by competition assays (82). Two further CT boxes (UPE, upstream promoter elements, sites) are found in the glucokinase gene at −130 and −220, but these appear less sensitive to mutation. In the rat somatostatin promoter a complex regulatory region is composed of a CT-1-like TAAT box and an adjacent cAMP response element, which interact co-operatively (83). Mutation within the TAAT sequence abolishes transcriptional activity. Binding of proteins at this TAAT box can be competed using sequences corresponding to the rat insulin I FLAT element. Further evidence suggests an involvement of Isl-1 in acti-

Table 2.1. *E boxes and related sequences in islet-specific promoters*

| | | | | | C | A | N | N | T | G | | | | | E Box consensus |
|---|---|---|---|---|---|---|---|---|---|---|---|---|---|---|---|
| −114 | T | C | G | C | C | A | T | C | T | G | C | C | T | A | Rat insulin I IEB1 or NIR |
| −102 | T | G | G | C | C | A | T | C | T | G | C | T | G | A | Rat insulin II |
| −113 | C | A | G | C | C | A | T | C | T | G | C | T | G | A | Human insulin |
| −240 | A | G | G | C | C | A | T | C | T | G | G | C | C | C | Rat insulin I IEB2 or FAR |
| −230 | A | G | G | C | C | A | C | C | **C** | **A** | G | G | A | G | Rat insulin II |
| −241 | T | G | G | C | C | A | C | C | **G** | G | G | C | C | C | Human insulin |
| −141 | G | A | C | C | C | A | T | C | **C** | G | C | T | T | C | Human IAPP (AN1) |
| −144 | G | C | T | T | C | T | G | C | T | G | C | C | T | G | Human IAPP (AN2) |
| −125 | G | G | C | C | C | A | C | C | T | G | C | T | C | C | Rat IAPP (AN1) |
| −116 | G | C | T | C | C | A | G | C | T | G | C | C | A | A | Rat IAPP (AN2) |
| −135 | T | G | G | C | C | A | T | C | **A** | G | T | C | C | C | Rat β-glucokinase |
| −86 | G | A | C | T | C | A | T | A | T | G | G | C | A | G | Human gastrin |
| −134 | A | C | G | A | C | A | G | C | T | G | G | G | G | G | Rat secretin |
| −87 | T | T | T | A | C | A | G | A | T | G | A | G | A | A | Rat glucagon |

Residues which do map the CANNTG consensus sequence are highlighted.
Reproduced with permission from Ref. 91.

Table 2.2. *TAAT boxes in islet-specific promoters*

| a | | | | | C/T | **T** | **A** | **A** | **T** | G | | | | | IUF1 binding site consensus |
|---|---|---|---|---|---|---|---|---|---|---|---|---|---|---|---|
| −322 | T | G | G | T | C | **T** | **A** | **A** | **T** | G | T | G | G | A | Human insulin (CT3) |
| −219 | G | A | C | T | C | **T** | **A** | **A** | **T** | G | A | C | C | C | Human insulin (CT2) |
| −86 | G | G | C | C | C | **T** | **A** | **A** | **T** | G | G | G | C | C | Human insulin (CT1) |
| −85 | G | C | C | C | T | **T** | **A** | **A** | **T** | G | G | G | C | C | Rat insulin I |
| −85 | C | C | C | C | T | **T** | **A** | **A** | **T** | G | G | G | A | C | Rat insulin II |
| −82 | G | A | C | A | C | **T** | **A** | **A** | **T** | G | A | C | A | C | Rat IAPP |
| −92 | G | A | A | A | T | **T** | **A** | **A** | **T** | G | A | C | A | G | Human IAPP |
| −106 | G | G | C | T | C | **T** | **A** | **A** | **T** | G | A | T | A | G | Rat β-specific glucokinase |
| −100 | G | A | G | G | C | **T** | **A** | **A** | **T** | G | G | T | G | C | Rat somatostatin |

b (Flat-F; Flat-E)

−229 C C C C T T G T **T A A T A A T** C **T A A T T A** C C C T A C G T Rat insulin I
−217 G C C C C T C T T A A G A C T C **T A A T T A** C C C T A C C C Rat insulin II
−161 T G A T G A G T **T T A T** G **T A A T A A T** G A C C C A T C C G Human IAPP

The sequences TAAT and its complement ATTA are highlighted. a: The consensus binding site for the factor IUF1, and matches to this consensus in several islet-specific promoters. b: The complex FLAT element of the rat insulin I 5′ region, and other AT-rich elements containing overlapping TAAT motifs.

Reproduced with permission from Ref. 91.

vating transcription of the somatostatin gene through an interaction at the TAAT. Thus in co-transfection experiments Isl-1 is able to activate a reporter construct bearing multiple copies of the TAAT box sequence. However, because of the abundance of TAAT box-binding factors in islet cell lines, it is not necessarily the case that *in vivo* Isl-1 is the species responsible for activation through the somatostatin CT-1-like TAAT box element.

The human IAPP (hIAPP) gene contains an AT-rich region with multiple TAAT boxes (−172 to −151) adjacent to two transcriptionally active E boxes (AN1 and AN2) at −147 and −140. This region may function as a mini-enhancer similar to the FF mini-enhancer of the rat insulin I gene (24) (Table 2.2). In the hIAPP gene the E boxes are imperfect, i.e. CATCCG (AN1) and CTGCTG (AN2). At the corresponding sequence in the rat IAPP gene, the E boxes fit the perfect consensus sequence, CANNTG, i.e. CACCTG and CAGCTG (84). Competition for binding at the hIAPP E box (AN1) is observed with AN2 and with a FAR-equivalent sequence of the rat insulin II gene, which contains an imperfect E box, but not with sequences containing the rat insulin I E boxes (IEB1/NIR and IEB2/FAR). This leads to the conclusion that a similar factor binds to the E box sequences (AN1 and AN2) in the hIAPP gene and the FAR-equivalent sequence in the rat insulin II gene. The human and rat IAPP genes may therefore resemble the two rat insulin genes in that perfect and imperfect E boxes at equivalent sites may bind different factors.

In the rat glucagon gene, an E box with the sequence CATCTG (on the lower strand) present at position −83, is required for efficient transcription in a glucagon-expressing cell line InR1-G9 and binds a nuclear protein factor present in this and other islet cell lines (85) (Table 2.2). This factor remains to be identified. Finally, it is of interest that two genes expressed transiently in developing islets, gastrin and secretin, contain transcriptionally active E boxes in their promoters (86, 87). It remains to be established whether similar HLH proteins bind to these promoters and to the insulin gene.

## REGULATION OF GENE EXPRESSION DURING ISLET CELL ONTOGENY

The four distinct cell types of the mature islet are believed to be derived from a common pluripotent stem cell. During islet ontogeny the first hormone to be detected is glucagon, followed by insulin, somatostatin, and pancreatic polypeptide (88), although there is evidence that pancreatic polypeptide should be placed at an earlier position in this lineage (89). Islet development is characterised by various stages at which multiple hormone genes are activated followed by selective inactivation of inappropriate genes to yield the final mature islet cell phenotype. Presumably, each stage is marked by a unique complement, or relative concentration of positive- and negative-acting transcription factors.

Myogenesis provides an example of the role of transcription factors in tissue development, and is of particular relevance to a discussion of islet cell development. In myogenesis, several HLH proteins are involved in the differentiation programme (90). These include the cell specifically expressed MyoD gene product and its close relatives myogenin, myf-5 and MRF-4, which can heterodimerise with products of the E2A gene to form complexes that bind to E boxes. The HLH proteins in muscle appear to form a hierarchy in which some are required for the determination of cell fate, while others execute such differentiation decisions, and are unable to bring about myogenesis themselves. Thus transfection of MyoD into the embryonic fibroblast cell line CHO10T1/2 will induce a muscle phenotype. It remains to be determined whether a similar hierarchy of HLH proteins may be involved in the establishment of islet lineages. There is no evidence for such a hierarchy, although the β cell (or endocrine cell) factor IESF-1 may be of particular importance.

Another clue to HLH proteins in islet development comes from studies on HLH proteins in lymphoid tissue. Here, an important lymphoid E box-binding factor (LEF1/BCF1) has been characterised as a homodimer of E2A proteins. This raises the question as to why ubiquitous E2A proteins form cell-specific complexes in lymphoid cells but not in other cell types. A possible explanation comes from the observation that the E2A proteins are highly enriched in lymphoid B cells as compared to pancreatic β cells (91). Thus the preferential accumulation of E2A proteins leads to the formation of homodimeric DNA binding activity, while in muscle and β cells heterodimeric complexes are formed between cell-specific HLH proteins (MyoD and IESF-1) and with E2A proteins which are present at low concentrations in non-lymphoid cells. The relative concentrations of HLH proteins at various stages in development may therefore affect the establishment of islet cell lineages. It will clearly be important to identify and quantify all HLH proteins present in islet cells.

A second paradigm for the regulation of tissue-specific transcription is provided by the homeodomain factors (92). In the dipteran fly *Drosophila*, and in the nematode *Caenorhabditis elegans*, these are required for the establishment of developmental lineages and there is growing evidence for their involvement in mammalian development and tissue-specific regulation. For instance the homeodomain-containing factor Pit-1 is required for the specification of the pituitary phenotype and transcriptional activation of the growth hormone gene (93). Homeodomain proteins commonly bind to motifs that include the TAAT sequence, and, as described above, the proteins binding to the TAAT boxes in the insulin gene all contain homeodomains. The role of Isl-1 in islet cell development is unclear. Assuming that IUF-1 and IPF-1 are homeodomain proteins, then these along with 1mx-1 may be important determinants of islet cell lineage. Their distribution and interaction with HLH proteins at various stages of islet development will represent an expanding area of research over the next few years.

## CONCLUDING REMARKS

Exciting progress has been made in our understanding of the transcriptional control of insulin gene expression. Much of the recent work has highlighted the importance of E boxes and TAAT boxes located within about 300 nucleotides upstream of the transcription start site (94). cDNAs encoding several factors binding at these sites have been cloned and categorised as proteins containing HLH domains or homeodomains. These factors overlap in distribution and differ subtly in their binding specificity and activatory capacity. One potential consequence is that transcription may be fine-tuned by small adjustments in the relative abundance of factors in the nucleus. For instance transcriptional activation through the FLAT region of the rat insulin I gene may be acutely sensitive to the levels of FLAT-E and FLAT-F binding activities. Likewise activation through the IEB/FAR motifs may be very sensitive to the concentration of IEF-1 relative to other E box-binding factors. A second consequence of overlapping patterns of distribution and similar binding specificities of nuclear factors is that truly cell-specific regulators of transcription are difficult to identify. It seems likely that such factors do not exist in the strictest sense. Instead cell-specific programmes of gene expression may be dictated by cell-specific combinations of regulators rather than by regulators which are entirely α cell-specific, D cell-specific or PP cell-specific. Finally, it is clear that *cis*-acting elements other than E boxes and TAAT boxes play important roles in the regulation of islet cell-specific gene expression. These elements include, the GAGA box, CREs, NREs, and core elements among others. They may interact with, and modulate, the activity of the E box and TAAT box elements.

DNA binding proteins can undergo post-translational modification, such as phosphorylation, in response to hormonal or nutrient stimulation of the cell. Such modifications may affect the ability of transcription factors to interact with each other, to bind DNA or to activate transcription. The role of intracellular signalling pathways and their associated kinases and phosphatases in the establishment of patterns of expression or activation of gene regulatory proteins during islet cell ontogeny or in response to changes in circulating nutrients will be another subject of intense research activity during the next few years.

## ACKNOWLEDGEMENTS

A.R.C. was supported by a fellowship from the British Diabetic Association.

## REFERENCES


1 Bell GI, Pictet RL, Rutter WJ, Cordell B, Tischer E, Goodman, HM. Sequence of the human insulin gene. *Nature (Lond)* 1980; 284: 26–32.

2 Steiner DF. The biosynthesis of insulin. In: Cautrecasas P, Jacobs S, eds. *Handbook of experimental pharmacology*, vol. 92, Insulin. Springer Verlag, Berlin, 1990; 67–92.

3 Bell GI, Seino S. The organisation and structure of the insulin gene. In: Okamoto H, ed. *Molecular biology of the islets of Langerhans*. Cambridge University Press, Cambridge, 1990; 9–25.

4 Mitchell PJ, Tjian R. Transcriptional regulation in mammalian cells by sequence-specific DNA binding proteins. *Science* 1989; 245: 371–8.

5 Docherty K., Clark AR. Transcription of exogenous genes in mammalian cells. In: Hames BD, Higgins SJ, eds. *Gene transcription: a practical approach*. IRL Press, Oxford, 1993; 64–123.

6 Boam DSW, Clark AR, Shennan KIJ, Docherty K. The molecular biology of polypeptide hormone expression and biosynthesis. In: Hutton JC, Siddle K, eds. *Peptide hormone secretion: a practical approach*. IRL Press, Oxford, 1990; 271–307.

7 Philippe J. Structure and pancreatic expression of the insulin and glucagon genes. *Endoc Rev* 1991; 12: 252–71.

8 Julier C, Heyer RN, Davies J *et al*. Insulin-IGF2 region on chromosome 11p encodes a gene implicated in HLA-DR4-dependent diabetes susceptibility. *Nature (Lond)* 1991; 354: 155–9.

9 Permutt MA. Genetics of NIDDM. *Diabetes Care* 1990; 13 suppl. 4: 1150–3.

10 Walker MD, Edlund T, Boulet AM, Rutter WJ. Cell-specific expression controlled by the 5′ flanking region of insulin and chymotrypsin genes. *Nature (Lond)* 1983; 306: 557–61.

11 Edlund T, Walker MD, Barr PJ, Rutter WJ. Cell specific expression of the rat insulin gene: evidence for the role of two distinct 5′ flanking sequences. *Science* 1985; 230: 912–16.

12 Dandoy-Dron F, Monthioux E, Jami J, Bucchini D. Regulatory regions of rat insulin I gene necessary for expression in transgenic mice. *Nucl Acids Res* 1991; 18: 4925–30.

13 Karlsson O, Edlund T, Moss LB, Rutter WJ, Walker MD. A mutational analysis of the insulin gene transcription control region: expression in beta cells is dependent on two related sequences within the enhancer. *Proc Natl Acad Sci USA* 1987; 84: 8819–23.

14 Moss LG, Moss JB, Rutter WJ. Systematic binding analysis of the insulin gene transcriptional control region: insulin and immunoglobulin enhancers utilize similar transactivators. *Mol Cell Biol* 1988; 8: 2620–7.

15 Ohlsson H, Karlsson O, Edlund T. A beta cell specific protein binds to two major regulatory sequences of the insulin gene enhancer. *Proc Natl Acad Sci USA* 1988; 85: 4228–31.

16 Ohlsson H, Thor S, Edlund T. Novel insulin promoter- and enhancer-binding proteins that discriminate between pancreatic α and β-cells. *Mol Endocr* 1991; 5: 897–903.

17 Aronheim A, Ohlsson H, Park CW, Edlund T, Walker MD. Distribution and characterisation of helix–loop–helix enhancer-binding proteins from pancreatic β cells and lymphocytes. *Nucl Acids Res* 1991; 19: 3893–9.

18 Walker MD, Park CW, Rosen A, Aronheim A. A cDNA from a mouse pancreatic β cell encoding a putative transcription factor of the insulin gene. *Nucl Acids Res* 1990; 18: 1159–66.

19 Shibasaki Y, Sakura H, Takaku F, Kasuga M. Insulin enhancer binding protein has helix-loop-helix structure. *Biochem Biophys Res Commun* 1990; 170: 314–21.

20 Nelson C, Shen L-P, Meister A, Fodor E, Rutter, WJ. Pan: a transcriptional regulator that binds chymotrypsin, insulin, and AP-4 enhancer motifs. *Genes Dev* 1990; 4: 1035–43.

21 Murre C, McCaw PS, Baltimore D. A new DNA binding and dimerization motif in immunoglobulin enhancer binding, daughterless, MyoD, and myc proteins. *Cell* 1989; 56: 777–83.

22 German MS, Blanar MA, Nelson C, Moss LG, Rutter WJ. Two related helix–loop–helix proteins participate in separate cell-specific complexes that bind the insulin enhancer. *Mol Endocr* 1991; 5: 292–9.

23 Park CW, Walker MD. Subunit structure of cell-specific E box-binding proteins analysed by quantitation of electrophoretic mobility shift. *J Biol Chem* 1992; 267: 15642–9.

24 German MS, Moss LG, Wang J, Rutter WJ. The insulin and amyloid polypeptide genes contain similar cell-specific promoter elements that bind identical β-cell nuclear complexes. *Mol Cell Biol* 1992; 12: 1777–88.

25 Karlsson O, Thor S, Norberg T, Ohlsson H, Edlund T. Insulin gene enhancer binding protein Isl-1 is a member of a novel class of proteins containing both a homeo- and Cys-His domain. *Nature (Lond)* 1990; 344: 879–82.

26 Dong J, Asa SL, Drucker DJ. Islet cell and extrapancreatic expression of the LIM domain gene Isl-1. *Mol Endocr* 1991; 5: 1633–41.

27 Thor S, Ericson J, Edlund T. The homeodomain LIM protein Isl-1 is expressed in subsets of neurons and endocrine cells in the adult. *Neuron* 1991; 7: 881–9.

28 German MS, Wang J, Chadwick RB, Rutter WJ. Synergistic activation of the insulin gene by a LIM-homeodomain protein: building a functional insulin mini-enhancer complex. *Genes Dev* 1992; 6: 2165–16.

29 Emens LA, Landers DW, Moss LG. Hepatocyte nuclear factor 1α is expressed in a hamster insulinoma line and transactivates the rat insulin I gene. *Proc Natl Acad Sci USA* 1992; 89: 7300–4.

30 Kennedy GC, Rutter WJ. Pur-1, a zinc-finger protein that binds to purine-rich sequences, transactivates an insulin promoter in heterologous cells. *Proc Natl Acad Sci USA* 1992; 89: 11498–502.

31 Kennedy GC, Rutter WJ. Characterisation of a cDNA encoding the insulin gene GAGA-binding factor, Pur-1. *Biochem Soc Trans* 1993; 21: 178–80.

32 Ohlsson H, Edlund T. Sequence-specific interactions of nuclear factors with the insulin gene enhancer. *Cell* 1986; 45: 35–44.

33 Soares MB, Schon E, Henderson A *et al*. RNA-mediated gene duplication: the rat preproinsulin I gene is a functional retroposon. *Mol Cell Biol* 1985; 5: 2090–103.

34 Clark JL, Steiner DF. Insulin biosynthesis in the rat: demonstration of two proinsulins. *Proc Natl Acad Sci USA* 1969; 62: 278–85.

35 Giddings SJ, Carnaghi LR. The two nonallelic rat insulin

mRNAs and pre-mRNAs are regulated coordinately *in vivo*. *J Biol Chem* 1988; 263: 3845–9.
36 Koranyi L, Permutt MA, Chirgwin JM, Giddings SJ. Proinsulin I and II gene expression in inbred mouse strains. *Mol Endocr* 1989; 3: 1895–902.
37 Giddings SJ, Carnaghi L. Rat insulin II gene expression by extraplacental membranes. *J Biol Chem* 1989; 264: 9462–9.
38 Fiedorek FT Jr, Carnaghi LR, Giddings SJ. Selective expression of the insulin I gene in rat insulinoma-derived cell lines. *Mol Endocr* 1990; 4: 990–9.
39 Whelan J, Poon D, Weil PA, Stein R. Pancreatic β-cell-specific expression of the rat insulin II gene is controlled by positive and negative cellular transcriptional elements. *Mol Cell Biol* 1989; 9: 3253–9.
40 Sample CE, Steiner DF. Tissue-specific binding of a nuclear factor to the insulin gene promoter. *FEBS Lett* 1987; 222: 332–6.
41 Hwung Y-P, Crowe DT, Wang L-H, Tsai SY, Tsai M-J. The COUP transcription factor binds to a promoter element of the rat II insulin gene. *Mol Cell Biol* 1988; 8: 2070–7.
42 Crowe DT, Tsai M-J. Mutagenesis of the rat insulin II 5′-flanking region defines sequences important for expression in HIT cells. *Mol Cell Biol* 1989; 9: 1784–9.
43 Cordle SR, Whelan J, Henderson E, Masuoka H, Weil PA, Stein R. Insulin gene expression in nonexpressing cells appears to be regulated by multiple distinct negative-acting control elements. *Mol Cell Biol* 1991; 11: 2881–6.
44 Hwung Y-P, Gu Y-Z, Tsai M-J. Cooperativity of sequence elements mediates tissue specificity of the rat insulin II gene. *Mol Cell Biol* 1990; 10: 1784–8.
45 Shieh S-Y, Tsai M-J. Cell-specific and ubiquitous factors are responsible for the enhancer activity of the rat insulin II gene. *J Biol Chem* 1991; 266: 16708–14.
46 Cordle SR, Henderson E, Masuoka H, Weil PA, Stein R. Pancreatic β-cell-type-specific transcription of the insulin gene is mediated by basic helix–loop–helix DNA-binding proteins. *Mol Cell Biol* 1991; 11: 1734–8.
47 Blume N, Petersen JS, Andersen LC *et al.* Immature transformed islet β-cells differentially express C-peptides derived from genes coding for insulin I and II as well as a transfected human insulin gene. *Mol Endocr* 1992; 6: 299–307.
48 Boam DSW, Clark AR, Docherty K. Positive and negative regulation of the human insulin gene by multiple trans-acting factors. *J Biol Chem* 1990; 265: 8285–96.
49 Fromont-Racine M, Bucchini D, Madsen O *et al.* Effect of 5′-flanking sequence deletions on expression of the human insulin gene in transgenic mice. *Mol Endocr* 1990; 4: 669–77.
50 Read ML, Clark AR, Docherty K. The helix loop helix transcription factor USF binds to a regulatory sequence in the human insulin gene enhancer. *Biochem J* 1993; 295: 233–7.
51 Reibel L, Besnard C, Lores P, Jami J, Gacon G. An insulinoma nuclear factor binding to GGGCCC motifs in human insulin gene. *Nucl Acids Res* 1993; 21: 1595–600.
52 Boam DSW, Docherty K. A tissue specific nuclear factor binds to multiple sites in the human insulin gene enhancer. *Biochem J* 1989; 264: 233–9.
53 Clark AR, Petersen HV, Read ML, Scott V, Michelsen B, Docherty, K. Human insulin gene enhancer binding proteins in pancreatic α and β cell lines. *FEBS Lett* 1993; 329: 139–43.
54 Scott V, Clark AR, Hutton JC, Docherty K. Two proteins acts as the IUF1 insulin gene enhancer binding factor. *FEBS Lett* 1991; 290: 27–30.
55 Takeda J, Ishii S, Seino Y, Immamoto F, Imura H. Negative regulation of human insdulin gene expression by the 5′ flanking region in non-pancreatic cells. *FEBS Lett* 1989; 247: 41–45.
56 Hammond-Kosack MCU, Dobrinski B, Lurz R, Docherty K, Kilpatrick MW. The human insulin gene linked polymorphic region exhibits an altered DNA structure. *Nucl Acids Res* 1992; 20: 231–6.
57 Hammond-Kosack MCU, Docherty, K. A consensus repeat sequence from the human insulin gene linked polymorphic region adopts multiple quadriplex structures *in vitro*. *FEBS Lett* 1992; 301: 79–82.
58 Hammond-Kosack MCU, Kilpatrick MW, Docherty K. Analysis of the human insulin gene linked polymorphic region *in vivo*. *J Mol Endocr* 1992; 9: 221–5.
59 Hammond-Kosack MCU, Kilpatrick MW, Docherty K. The human insulin gene linked polymorphic region adopts a quadriplex structure in chromatin assembled *in vitro*. *J Mol Endocr* 1993; 10: 121–6.
60 Nir U, Walker MD, Rutter WJ. Regulation of rat insulin I gene expression: evidence for negative regulation in non-pancreatic cells. *Proc Natl Acad Sci USA* 1986; 83: 3180–4.
61 Laimins L, Holmgren-Konig M, Khoury G. Transcriptional 'silencer' element in rat repetitive sequences associated with the rat insulin I gene locus. *Proc Natl Acad Sci USA* 1986; 83: 3151–5.
62 Stein RW, Whelan J. Insulin gene enhancer activity is inhibited by adenovirus 5 Ela gene products. *Mol Cell Biol* 1989; 9: 4531–4.
63 Leshkovitz D, Aronheim A, Walker MD. Insulin-producing cells contain a cell-specific repressor activity that functions through multiple E-box sequences. *DNA Cell Biol* 1992; 11: 549–58.
64 Clark AR, Docherty K. Negative regulation of transcription in eukaryotes. *Biochem J* 1993; 296: 521–41.
65 Brundstedt J, Chan SJ. Direct effect of glucose on the preproinsulin mRNA level in isolated pancreatic islets. *Biochem Biophys Res Commun* 1982; 106: 1383–9.
66 Giddings SJ, Chirgwin J, Permutt MA. The effects of fasting and feeding on preproinsulin messenger RNA in rats. *J Clin Invest* 1981; 67: 952–60.
67 Nielsen DA, Welsh M, Casadaban MJ, Steiner DF. Control of insulin gene expression in pancreatic β cells and in insulin-producing cell line, RIN-5F. *J Biol Chem* 1985; 260: 13585–9.
68 Hammonds P, Schofield PN, Ashcroft SJH. Glucose regulates preproinsulin messenger RNA levels in a clonal cell line of simian virus 40 transformed B cells. *FEBS Lett* 1987; 213: 149–154.
69 Hammonds P, Schofield PN, Ashcroft SJH, Sutton R, Gray DWR. Regulation and specificity of glucose-stimulated insulin gene expression in human islets of Langerhans. *FEBS Lett* 1987; 223: 131–7.
70 Efrat S, Surana M, Fleischer N. Glucose induces insulin gene transcription in a murine pancreatic β-cell line. *J Biol Chem* 1991; 266: 11141–3.
71 Welsh M, Nielsen DA, MacKreil AJ, Steiner DF. Control of insulin gene expression in pancreatic β cells and in

an insulin producing cell line, RIN-5F. *J Biol Chem* 1985; 260: 13590–4.

72 Goodison S, Kenna S, Ashcroft SJH. Control of insulin gene expression by glucose. *Biochem J* 1992; 285: 563–8.

73 German MS. Glucose sensing in pancreatic islet beta cells: the key role of glucokinase and the glycolytic intermediates. *Proc Natl Acad Sci USA* 1993; 90: 1781–5.

74 Philippe J, Missotten M. Functional characterisation of a cAMP-responsive element of the rat insulin I gene. *J Biol Chem* 1990; 265: 1465–9.

75 Karin M, Smeal T. Control of transcription factors by signal transduction pathways: the beginning of the end. *TIBS* 1992; 17: 418–22.

76 German MS, Moss LG, Rutter WJ. Regulation of insulin gene expression by glucose and calcium in transfected primary islet cultures. *J Biol Chem* 1990; 265, 22063–22066.

77 Melloul D, Ben-Neriah Y, Cerasi E. Glucose modulates the binding of an islet-specific factor to a conserved sequence within the rat I and human insulin promoters. *Proc Natl Acad Sci USA* 1993; 90: 3865–9.

78 Inagaki N, Maekawa T, Sudo T, Ishii S, Seino Y, Imura H. c-Jun represses the human insulin promoter activity that depends on multiple cAMP response elements. *Proc Natl Acad Sci USA* 1992; 89: 1045–9.

79 Madsen OD, Nielsen JH, Michelsen B. Islet amyloid polypeptide and insulin expression are controlled differently in primary and transformed islet cells. *Mol Endocr* 1991; 5: 143–8.

80 Magnusson MA, Jetton TL. Evolutionary conservation of elements in the upstream glucokinase promoter. *Biochem Soc Trans* 1993; 21: 160–3.

81 Magnusson MA, Shelton KD. An alternate promoter in the glucokinase gene is active in the pancreatic β cell. *J Biol Chem* 1989; 264: 15936–42.

82 Shelton KD, Franklin AJ, Khoor A, Beechem J, Magnusson MA. Multiple elements in the upstream glucokinase promoter contribute to transcription in insulinoma cells. *Mol Cell Biol* 1992; 12: 4578–89.

83 Leonard J, Serup P, Gonzalez G, Edlund T, Montminy M. The LIM family transcription factor Isl-1 requires cAMP reponse element binding protein to promote somatostatin expression in pancreatic islet cells. *Proc Natl Acad Sci USA* 1992; 89: 6247–51.

84 van Mansfield ADM, Mosselman S, Höppener JWM *et al.* Islet amyloid polypeptide: structure and upstream sequences of the IAPP gene in rat and man. *Biochim Biophys Acta* 1990; 1087: 235–40.

85 Philippe J, Drucker DJ, Jepeal L, Misulovin Z, Habener JF. Alpha cell-specific expression of the glucagon gene is conferred to the glucagon promoter element by the interactions of DNA-binding proteins. *Mol Cell Biol* 1988; 8: 4877–88.

86 Wang TC, Brand SJ. Islet cell-specific regulatory domain in the gastrin promoter contains adjacent positive and negative DNA elements. *J Biol Chem* 1990; 265: 8908–14.

87 Wheeler MB, Nishitani J, Buchan AMJ, Kopin AS, Chen WY, Chang T-M, Leiter AB. Identification of a transcriptional enhancer important for enteroendocrine and pancreatic islet-cell-specific expression of the secretin gene. *Mol Cell Biol* 1992; 12: 3531–9.

88 Madsen OD, Serup P, Karlsen *et al.* A tumour model for the study of islet cell differentiation. *Biochem Soc Trans* 1993; 21: 142–6.

89 Herrera P-L, Huarte J, Sanvito F, Meda P, Orci L, Vassalli J-D. Embryogenesis of the murine endocrine pancreas: early expression of pancreatic polypeptide gene. *Development* 1991; 113: 1257–65.

90 Olson EN. MyoD family: a paradigm for development? *Genes Dev* 1990; 4: 1454–61.

91 Aronheim A, Shirat R, Rosen A, Walker MD. Cell-specific expression of helix–loop–helix transcription factors encoded by the E2A gene. *Nucl Acids Res* 1993; 21: 1601–6.

92 Affolter M, Schier A, Gehring WJ. Homeodomain proteins and the regulation of gene expression. *Curr Opin Cell Biol* 1990; 2: 485–95.

93 Ingraham HA, Chen R, Mangalan HJ *et al.* A tissue specific factor containing a homeodomain specifies a pituitary phenotype. *Cell* 1988; 55: 519–29.

94 Clark AR, Docherty K. Cell-specific expression in the islets of Langerhans: E boxes and TAAT boxes. *Biochem Soc Trans* 1993; 21: 154–9.

# 3 Molecular Structure of Insulin

Howard S. Tager

## INTRODUCTION AND OVERVIEW

Studies on the molecular properties of insulin have played a major role in our still developing knowledge of insulin function as both a hormone and therapeutic agent. The history of insulin as a defined chemical substance began from the work of Banting, Best and Collip who, in the early 1920s, succeeded in preparing extracts of pancreas that had potent activity in lowering blood glucose levels in diabetic animals (1, 2). This ground-breaking work confirmed earlier suggestions that the pancreas and its internal islets of Langerhans were important in preventing diabetes, and led to the crystallisation of insulin and its eventual identification as a peptide hormone. Methods for the preparation of insulin from animal pancreas were developed by commercial firms, and insulin rapidly became available in sizeable amounts for both the treatment of diabetes and the study of protein biochemistry. Procedures were improved over the years with the result that insulin preparations became more reproducible and more stable. The properties of insulin, especially with respect to its crystallisation in the presence of zinc ions, were studied in great detail with the result that preparations having different pharmacological (as well as physical) characteristics could be produced. These preparations form the base for even contemporary insulin therapy.

Although insulin was recognised early as having the properties of a small protein, the tendency of the hormone to aggregate in ordinary solution led to confusion about its physical state and even about its size. This confusion was lifted by the elegant work of Sanger and his colleagues who published, in the mid-1950s, the complete amino acid sequence of the insulin molecule (3). The sequence of human insulin is shown in Fig. 3.1 in a way that emphasises, but oversimplifies the organisation of the hormone. Insulin consists of two polypeptide chains, an A chain containing 21 amino acid residues and a B chain containing 30 amino acid residues. The two chains are linked by two disulphide bonds, each of which is derived from a cysteine residue on the A chain and from one on the B chain (A7 Cys–B7 Cys and A20 Cys–B19 Cys). An additional disulphide bond occurs in the A chain alone and links A6 Cys to A11 Cys. The methods of insulin isolation and protein sequencing presented above have by now been applied to determining the amino acid sequences of nearly 50 insulins from different animal species. The result is that insulin seems to exhibit a low and common degree of acceptance of amino acid changes, but that relatively few of its 51 amino

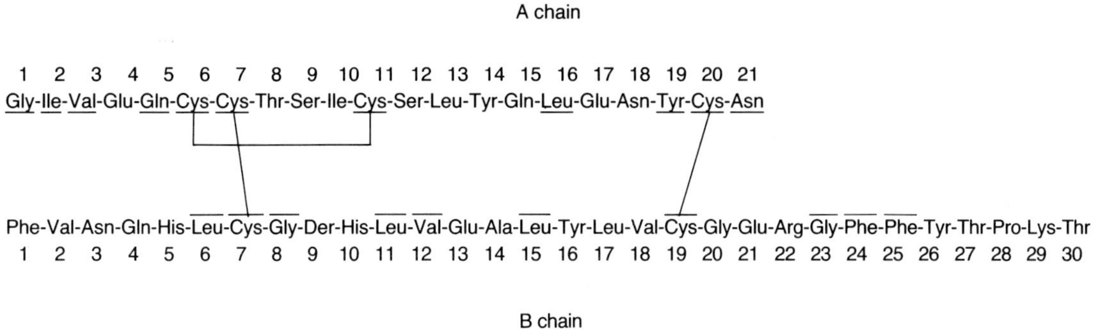


Fig. 3.1. Primary structure and amino acid sequence of human insulin. The amino acid sequences of the insulin A chain (top) and B chain (bottom) are shown. Residues that have remained invariant among various species are indicated by bars above or below the three-letter code for each amino acid. Disulphide bonds linking the A and B chains of the hormone, and occurring within the A chain, are indicated by lines.

acid residues have remained unchanged among all species studied (4, 5). Those that have not changed are in the $NH_2$- and COOH-terminal regions of the A chain, a region in the COOH-terminal domain of the B chain, and regions near the very important disulphide bonds. While some insulins (those from the guinea pig and from various fishes) are quite different from human insulin, others are very similar. For example, pig insulin differs from human insulin only by the replacement of B30 Thr by Ala.

While knowledge of the primary structure of insulin was critical to defining the physical and chemical characteristics of the hormone, it also led to important questions concerning how the hormone is synthesised to produce a 2-chain peptide within pancreatic islets, and what the overall structure and conformation of the hormone really are (given that the interchain disulphide bonds would not easily form in the intracellular environment and would tend to bring the molecule together in a conformation more compact than that implied by the extended diagram of Fig. 3.1). Answers to both questions were provided in the late 1960s and early 1970s when Steiner and his colleagues discovered that insulin is synthesised from a larger precursor (6, 7) and when Dodson, Blundell, Hodgkin and their co-workers presented the first tertiary structure of insulin as determined by X-ray crystallographic methods (5, 8). These areas, in addition to matters related to insulin aggregation and to mutations that have occurred in the human insulin gene, will be discussed later in this chapter. Throughout the 1970s and 1980s, successful efforts were undertaken to improve the production of insulin and to provide ever purer therapeutic preparations of the hormone. Much or most of the insulin used today (actually in stark contrast to the insulin used only a few decades ago) can be considered to be chemically pure.

Methods have been developed that allow insulin to be made in the laboratory or factory by procedures that rely on total chemical synthesis (with the subsequent combination of A and B chains), on enzyme-catalysed semisynthesis (wherein the natural hormone is modified in structure by the action of proteolytic enzymes run in reverse), and on the microbial expression of an insulin gene with the corresponding secretion of peptide product into the growth medium (through the methods applicable to recombinant DNA technology) (9, 10). These methods permit the production of potentially limitless quantities of human insulin for therapeutic use and the preparation of insulin analogues with carefully designed amino acid substitutions. Such analogues are invaluable in asking questions about how insulin combines with receptor, how the physical properties of insulin affect its therapeutic potential, and how alterations in the structure of insulin might lead to the development of better therapeutic agents. Important inroads have been made in these areas, and a few are presented below. The biology, biochemistry and pharmacology of insulin have been intertwined in multiple ways during the 70 years that the molecular and therapeutic characteristics of the hormone have been investigated. In as many ways, all of these areas depend on understanding the structure and properties of the insulin molecule itself, and, these days, on understanding how the structure and properties of insulin can be beneficially changed.

## INSULIN BIOSYNTHESIS

The process through which insulin is synthesised in the β-cell of the pancreatic islet (so that the peptide can be secreted as the correctly folded, active hormone upon appropriate β-cell stimulation) is simultaneously critical to insulin function and complex with respect to the number of steps involved. The process requires nearly simultaneous consideration of the nuclear machinery and molecular biology, protein biosynthesis and cell biology, and peptide structure and enzymology. At this stage, we actually know a great deal about applicable mechanisms. As mentioned above, the discovery of pro-insulin identified that the two peptide chains of insulin are derived from a single-chain precursor protein called pro-insulin (6, 7). The drawing at the top of Fig. 3.2 depicts, in a diagrammatic way, the structure of the insulin precursor. Notably, human pro-insulin is represented by a single polypeptide chain of 86 amino acid residues in which (a) disulphide bonds involving cysteine residues have been correctly formed (see Fig. 3.1), (b) the carboxy terminus of the insulin A chain is linked by the basic amino acid pair Arg–Arg to the amino terminus of a connecting peptide called the C peptide, and (c) the carboxy terminus of the C peptide is linked by the basic amino acid pair Lys–Arg to the amino terminus of the insulin A chain.

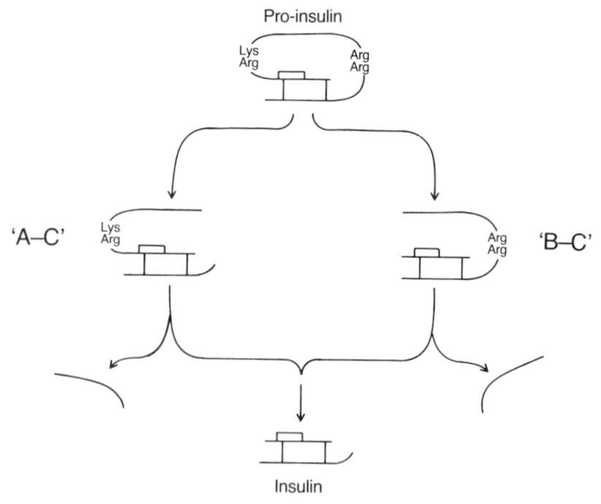


Fig. 3.2. Scheme for the conversion of pro-insulin to insulin through enzyme-catalysed precursor processing. The pairs of basic amino acids that link the insulin B chain to the C peptide (Arg–Arg), and the C peptide to the insulin A chain (Lys–Arg), are shown explicitly. The Figure illustrates how cleavage at either pair to yield one or the other of two pro-insulin processing intermediates, followed by cleavage at the second, ultimately results in the conversion of pro-insulin to insulin plus C peptide. Two enzyme activities (one an endoproteinase activity with specificity for basic amino acid pairs and the other an exoproteinase activity with specificity for COOH-terminal basic amino acids) would be needed to accomplish the conversion.

The molecular structure of pro-insulin contains within it the entire structure of insulin. Accordingly, this organisation of the molecule allows pro-insulin to fold with the correct positioning of disulphide bonds as a favourable unimolecular process, rather than as an unfavourable bimolecular process that would otherwise involve the interaction of separate A and B chains. The processing or conversion of pro-insulin to insulin then requires removal of the C peptide domain of pro-insulin by selective proteolysis to generate the hormone itself. As illustrated in Fig. 3.2, the process of pro-insulin conversion to insulin can be initiated by cleavage between the insulin B chain and the C peptide to yield a so-called 'A–C' intermediate, or by cleavage between the insulin A chain and the C peptide to produce a so-called 'B–C' intermediate (7, 11). A subsequent cleavage of each of these intermediates on the contralateral side of the hormone generates mature insulin and the pro-insulin-derived C peptide. Both of these peptides are stored in secretion granules within the insulin-producing β-cell and are secreted in equimolar amounts upon β-cell stimulation.

In contrast to the great similarity of the insulins from various mammalian species, the C peptides from these species exhibit considerable variability in amino acid sequence and even in length (12). Thus, the importance of the C peptide domain of insulin seems to reside in connecting the two chains of insulin during the unimolecular folding process. Although the excised C peptide apparently has no biological activity of its own, C peptide measurements in blood have proved to be extremely valuable in evaluating β-cell secretory capacity and rates under conditions of exogenous insulin administration or varying endogenous insulin levels (13). The process of pro-insulin conversion to insulin illustrated in Fig. 3.2 normally occurs with about 95% efficiency. Accordingly, small amounts of pro-insulin and the pro-insulin intermediates also appear in blood. These forms have low biological activity (1–5% of that of insulin), however, and do not contribute significantly to the body's ability to regulate glucose metabolism. Interestingly, the elevated immunoreactive insulin levels present in the blood of some Type II diabetics has been attributed in part to higher than expected levels of pro-insulin (14).

The conversion of pro-insulin to insulin in the β-cell secretion granule has long been recognised to require two kinds of enzyme activities: an endoproteinase activity with specificity for paired basic amino acids (to cleave at insulin-C peptide junctions) and an exoproteinase activity with specificity for basic amino acids (to remove COOH-terminal Arg and Lys residues that do not appear in the final products of precursor-processing) (7). Although the identities of these enzymes are still open to some debate, they have been the subject of much recent investigation; in fact, Arg–Arg, Lys–Lys, Lys–Arg and Arg–Lys sequences occur in a great many peptide hormone precursors. A family of proteolytic enzymes having the specificity expected for the endoproteinase has been identified in mammalian systems. All of these enzymes (including those designated as furin, PC1/PC3, PC2 and PACE) exhibit significant homology with the yeast enzyme called Kex2, and all cleave at basic amino acid pairs (15). Whereas Kex2 and furin contain transmembrane domains, the others appear to be soluble, calcium-dependent proteinases of the subtilisin family. Available evidence suggests that PC1/PC3 and PC2 represent the major precursor converting enzymes of endocrine and neuroendocrine secretion granules, and that they function as 'convertases' during the processing of pro-insulin to insulin. Importantly, insulin-like growth factors I and II (hormones that are homologous to pro-insulin with respect to amino acid sequence, disulphide bonds and general character) lack the basic amino acid pairs at sites that would result in the release of a connecting peptide by a PC1/PC3 or PC2 convertase. Accordingly, these peptides are secreted and function as single chain pro-insulin-related peptide hormones.

A more complete view of the stages of insulin biosynthesis is presented in Fig. 3.3. As illustrated at the top of Fig. 3.3, the human insulin gene (one corresponding to about 1500 base pairs in length) can be described as containing (a) a 5′ untranslated region that is split by an intervening sequence, (b) a region corresponding to the sequence of a signal peptide that functions in the translocation of the hormone precursor across the membrane of the endoplasmic reticulum so that the peptide enters the secretory pathway, (c) a region corresponding to the insulin B chain, (d) a region corresponding to the C peptide that is again split by an intervening sequence, (e) a region corresponding to the insulin A chain, and (f) a 3′ untranslated region (12, 15). The 5′ regulatory region of the gene is not shown. Transcription of the insulin gene by the usual nuclear machinery yields a complementary mRNA precursor of the same size that is then modified by capping of the 5′ terminus by 7-methyl-guanosine, by excision of the intervening sequences, and by polyadenylation at the 3′ terminus. The mature mRNA then leaves the nucleus and is translated on membrane-bound ribosomes of the rough endoplasmic reticulum. The initial $NH_2$-terminal segment of the protein (the so-called signal peptide) helps to guide the translocation of the corresponding protein across the membrane into the lumen of the endoplasmic reticulum; this signal sequence is actually removed during the process of translation to yield the pro-insulin molecule (illustrated in Fig. 3.3 by the sequence B–C–A) sequestered from the cytosol. At this stage, pro-insulin folds with the formation of disulphide bonds. As the peptide hormone precursor moves to, and through, the multiple compartments of the Golgi apparatus (as is required of all proteins destined for the regulated secretion pathway), it is mixed with the endo- and exo-proteinases that are necessary for conversion of the precursor to insulin (12). Conversion of pro-insulin to insulin probably begins in the distal portion of the Golgi apparatus and then continues to near completion in secretion granules that are pinched from the Golgi membrane to yield insulin (shown very diagrammatically at the bottom of Fig. 3.3) plus the pro-insulin C peptide.

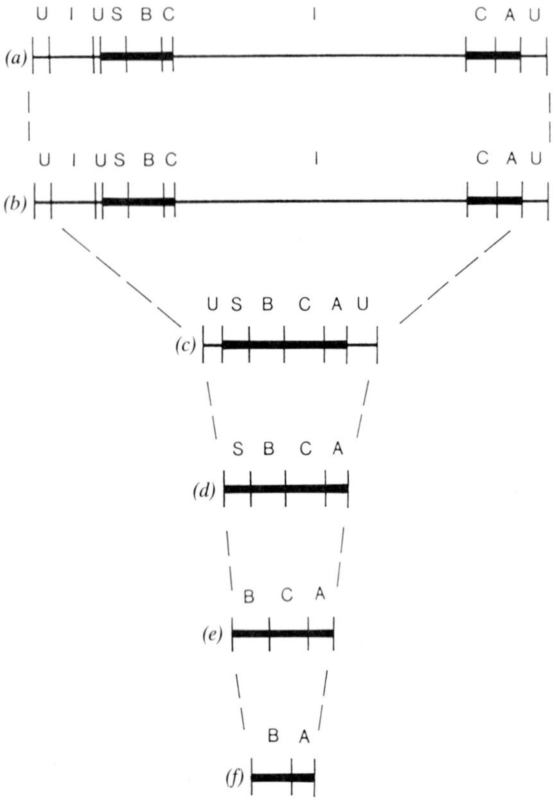


Fig. 3.3. Diagrammatic representation of the structure of the insulin gene and of the steps involved in the production of insulin through gene expression and precursor processing. The structures illustrate, from top to bottom, those of (a) the insulin gene, (b) the initial gene transcript (the mRNA precursor), (c) the mature mRNA (after the excision of intervening sequences and other modifications), (d) prepro-insulin (the co-translationally processed precursor), (e) pro-insulin (the direct hormone precursor) and (f) insulin (after removal of the connecting peptide). The code used to describe the various segments is as follows: U, untranslated region; I, intervening sequence; S, signal peptide; B, insulin B chain; C, pro-insulin connecting peptide; A, insulin A chain.

Importantly, insulin is produced from pro-insulin within the pancreatic β-cell and is secreted as the fully mature and active hormone. The process of pro-insulin biosynthesis, movement through the intracellular secretion apparatus and conversion to insulin takes, on average, about an hour, and requires the input of metabolic energy. Glucose, the major regulator of insulin secretion is also an important regulator of transcription of the insulin gene and of translation of the mature pro-insulin mRNA (12). Taken together, the structures and processes illustrated in Fig. 3.3 identify (a) the complexity of the mechanisms through which insulin comes to be synthesised in pancreatic islets, (b) the importance of nucleic acid and protein structure in these overall mechanisms, (c) the multiple roles of precursor processing and of structural change necessary to arrive at the structure of insulin itself, (d) the interplay of nuclear, cytoplasmic and molecular mechanisms that is required during the biogenesis of the hormone, and (e) the multiplicity of sites both that require close regulation for normal function and that represent loci of potential malfunction during states of inappropriate glucose homeostasis.

## STRUCTURE OF THE INSULIN MONOMER

The simple organisation of insulin shown in Figs. 3.1 and 3.2 actually does not reflect the structure of the hormone as it exists in nature. Fig. 3.4 depicts the structure of the insulin monomer (one molecule of a 2-zinc insulin hexamer) as determined by X-ray crystallographic methods (5, 17). Rather than being linear and extended, insulin really tends to be globular and compact. Important features of the insulin B chain include an $NH_2$-terminal coil region (residues B1–B8), a central α-helical domain (residues B9–B20), a β-turn element (residues B21–B23), and a COOH-terminal β-strand domain (residues B24–B30). Corresponding features of the A chain include an $NH_2$- terminal α-helical domain (residues A1–A8), a central loop (residues A9–A12), and a COOH-terminal α-helical domain (residues A13–A21). In contrast to the representations of Figs. 3.1 and 3.2, Fig 3.4 indicates that the amino terminus of the insulin A chain is close in space to the carboxy terminus of the insulin B chain (the two regions of insulin that are linked by the C peptide in pro-insulin), and that both chains undertake defined secondary structures which identify what can be called a typical insulin fold. Fig. 3.4 also shows that amino acid residues of insulin that do not change among various animal insulins (including the cysteine residues implicated in the formation of disulphide bonds) are dispersed throughout the structure of the hormone. The portion of insulin presented towards the left of Fig. 3.4 (one comprising the $NH_2$- and COOH-terminal domains of the A chain and the COOH-terminal domain of the B chain) has long been placed within what might be called the major receptor binding site of the hormone molecule (8, 18, 19).

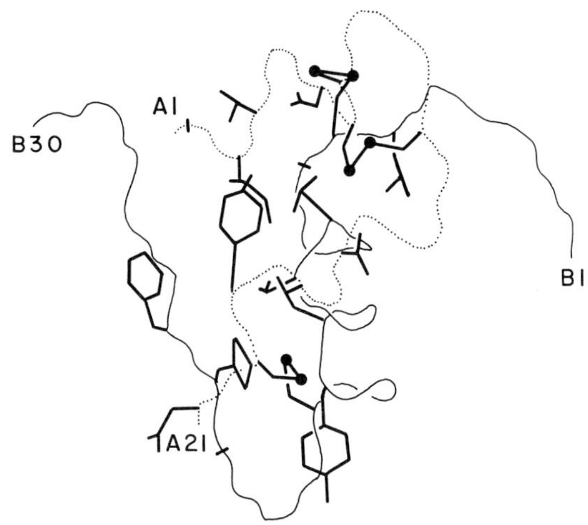


Fig. 3.4. X-ray structure of one molecule of insulin from the 2-zinc insulin hexamer. The A chain is shown by a dotted line and the B chain by a solid line. The $NH_2$- and COOH-termini of the two chains are indicated. Disulphide bonds are indicated by heavier lines and by solid circles. Side chains are shown explicitly only for invariant residues. The view of the molecule is perpendicular to the three-fold crystallographic axis. The diagram is adapted from Ref. 5.

The surface of the insulin monomer is covered by both polar (hydrophilic) and apolar (hydrophobic) side chains, whereas the interior of the molecule (like that of most globular proteins) contains mainly apolar residues. The general fold of the molecule results largely from (a) the central B chain α-helix which is abutted at both ends by cysteine residues in disulphide bond to the A chain, and (b) hydrogen bonds that stabilise the β-turn region of the B chain (illustrated in the lower part of Fig. 3.4). Various studies of insulin conformation, undertaken for example by use of chemical modification and circular dichroic spectroscopy, are consistent with the crystal structure of insulin shown in Fig. 3.4. Most important, the complete structure of insulin has also been determined by nuclear magnetic resonance methods (20). These studies have demonstrated that the conformation of the hormone in solution (i.e. in a state wherein

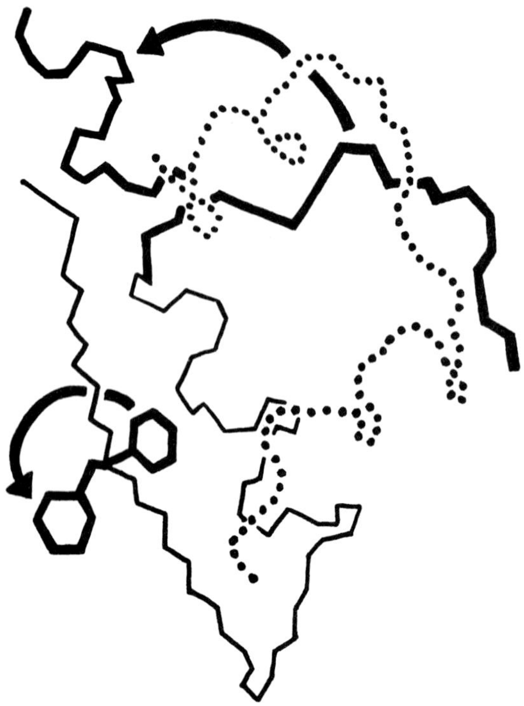

Fig. 3.5. X-ray structure of the insulin monomer designed to illustrate structural changes attending its conversion from the T state to the R state. The A chain is shown by a dotted line and the B chain, by a solid line. The view is similar, but is not identical, to that shown in Fig. 4. The side chain of B25 Phe is shown explicitly. Note that, in the T state, the $NH_2$-terminal domain of the B chain is pointed towards the right in a relatively characterless coil structure, and the side chain of B25 Phe is folded over the top of the molecule. In the R state, the $NH_2$-terminal domain of the B chain assumes an α-helical structure continuous with the central B chain helix and the side chain of B25 Phe points away from the core of the insulin molecule. The diagram is adapted from Refs. 5 and 21.

insulin is capable of binding to receptor) is very close indeed to the conformation of the hormone determined by X-ray crystallography. Although multiple crystal forms of insulins from various species have been examined by X-ray diffraction methods, most (but not all; see below) exhibit very similar structures (21). Accordingly, it seems that the structure of insulin is rather stable, even in solution, and that this structure plays a critical role in determining the receptor binding potency and biological function of the hormone.

Notwithstanding the commonality of insulin structure noted above, in some crystallographic forms of insulin (those that result from hexamer formation in the presence of various anions or phenolic compounds) an important movement in the $NH_2$-terminal portion of the B chain has been observed (21–23). Fig. 3.5 illustrates this movement. In these crystal states of insulin, $NH_2$-terminal residues B1–B8 move from the relatively characterless coil-like structure illustrated in Fig. 3.4 to a tightly packed α-helix that extends into the central α-helical domain of the B chain. Concomitantly, the aromatic side chain of B25 Phe (a side chain of some importance in insulin-receptor interactions) moves away from its usual position on the monomer surface (in molecule 1) to undertake a position extended away from the core of the monomer (in molecule 2). The extent of these movements is large for a molecule as small as insulin. Overall, these structural studies indicate that insulin is simultaneously a relatively stable molecule, but is one with a significant propensity for conformational change. These characteristics of the hormone are important in understanding both insulin self-aggregation and insulin–receptor interactions.

## INSULIN DIMERS AND HEXAMERS

Insulin's ability to self-associate represents a matter of considerable importance both in analysing the structure of the hormone and in evaluating various insulin preparations for their potential therapeutic value. The structures of the insulin monomer presented in Figs. 3.4 and 3.5 in fact represent one molecule of the hormone out of six that occur in various hexameric crystal forms. Most mammalian insulins (including human insulin) exist as monomers only in very dilute solutions (i.e. at concentrations lower than about 1 μM); at higher concentrations, insulin occurs in solution mainly as a mixture of dimers, hexamers and even more highly associated forms. Fig. 3.6 illustrates the process of

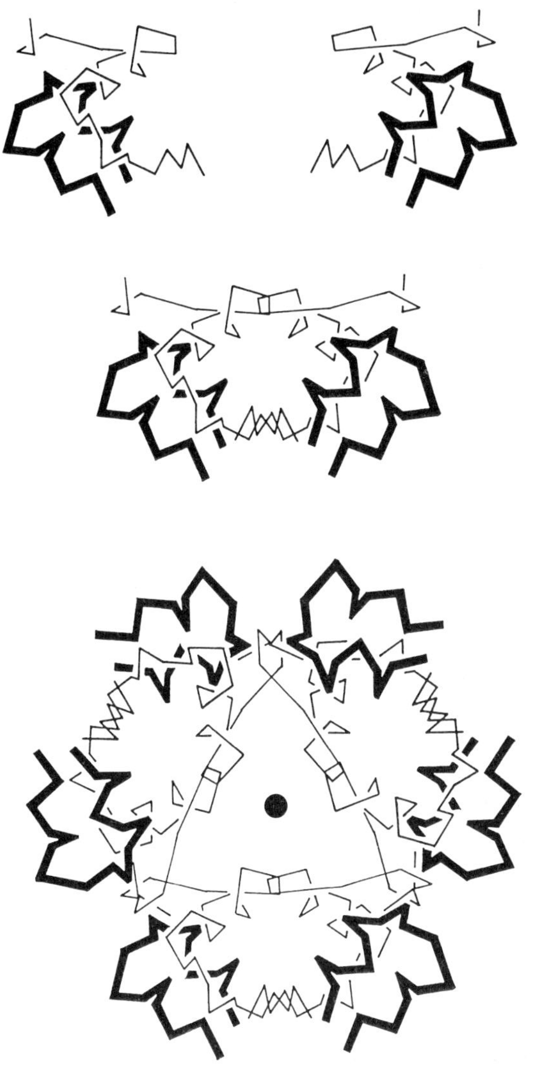

Fig. 3.6. Representation of the process through which insulin monomers form a 2-zinc insulin hexamer. The A chain of insulin is shown by heavy lines and the B chain by light lines. The structures of two insulin monomers in the T state are shown at the top; the molecules have the same structure as illustrated in Fig. 3.4, but have been rotated in space. The structure of an insulin dimer is shown in the middle. The structure of a 2-zinc insulin hexamer (comprising three insulin dimers, each of which comprises two insulin monomers) is shown at the bottom. The solid circle in the bottom drawing represents the two zinc ions viewed on line (one of which appears above the plane of the page and the other of which appears below the plane of the page in this view of the hexamer). The diagram is adapted from Refs. 5 and 21.

insulin association into a 2-zinc insulin hexamer (5, 17, 21). Two monomeric molecules of insulin are shown at the top of Fig. 3.6; the structures of these monomers are actually identical to the structure of insulin shown in Fig. 3.4, but the molecules have been rotated to present a different surface. At appropriate concentrations, the monomer–monomer interfaces of these two molecules come together to form a simple insulin dimer. The two insulin molecules in the dimer are held together by (a) apolar forces that arise, in part, due to the burying of hydrophobic side chains from each molecule, and (b) hydrogen bonds that arise through interactions between the peptide back bones in the regions corresponding to residues B24 to B26 of each monomer within the dimer.

In the presence of zinc ions, three insulin dimers (a total of six molecules) associate to form a 2-zinc insulin hexamer as illustrated at the bottom of Fig. 3.6. The two zinc ions (one above and one below the plane of the paper in the diagram of Fig. 3.6) coordinate with the six B10 histidine residues of the insulin hexamer. Additional hydrophobic side chains become buried when insulin hexamers are formed. Overall, this organisation produces a relatively stable, compact structure with a considerably polar surface. Insulin is known to occur in the secretory granules of the pancreatic islet in a zinc-coordinated microcrystalline state. It is likely that the hexameric structure of the hormone illustrated in Fig. 3.6 actually mirrors the structure of insulin as it exists at its site of synthesis and storage *in vivo*.

The structure of insulin illustrated in Figs. 3.4 and 3.6 (one with an extended B chain $NH_2$-terminal domain) is called the T state. The transition illustrated in Fig. 3.5 leads to the formation of what is called the R state (wherein the $NH_2$-terminal domain of the B chain becomes α-helical) (21, 24). Accordingly, the 2-zinc hexamer shown in Fig. 3.6 is that of a $T_6$ hexamer. Other hexameric states are known, however. The crystallisation of insulin in the presence of chloride ions and excess zinc leads to the formation of a 4-zinc $T_3R_3$ hexamer, with one molecule of the hormone exhibiting the T conformation and the other the R conformation in each of the three dimers of the hexamer (21, 22). This arrangement is well more than a curiosity in that (a) 4-zinc insulin is considerably more stable than 2-zinc insulin (due to the presence of the chloride ion that exists within a deep channel to help coordinate the zinc ions), and (b) crystalline 4-zinc insulin, because of its increased stability, dissolves more slowly than crystalline insulin in the 2-zinc form. Insulin that has been crystallised in the presence of phenol (or similar small compounds) occurs as a 2-zinc $R_6$ hexamer (containing six molecules of phenol that fill six stabilising pockets that would seemingly have been designed for this purpose) (21, 23). The phenol-containing 2-zinc $R_6$ hexamer (like the hexamer formed in the presence of protamine) is again more stable than the 2-zinc $T_6$ insulin hexamer described earlier. As expected, the few insulin forms that exist in crystals as dimers rather than hexamers represent less compact and less stable forms of the hormone.

As noted earlier, the relative stabilities of the various hexameric and crystal forms of insulin described above have therapeutic implications. That is, stable forms of insulin hexamers will be absorbed slowly from sites of administration (the so-called slow-acting insulin preparations), whereas unstable forms of insulin hexamers (or insulin dimers or monomers) will be absorbed rapidly (the so-called fast-acting insulins). Thus, the differing pharmacokinetics of various insulin formulations originally described about 35 years ago (2, 25) have their base in sound physical and structural principles. Much recent attention has been focused on the question of producing and formulating monomeric insulins that might act faster than even so-called Regular Insulin (a preparation that exists mainly in an aggregated, but soluble, state because of insulin's propensity to self-associate). A high potency, monomeric form of insulin would be absorbed quickly and would allow the control of blood glucose to be modulated without hidden (and perhaps somewhat variable) delays. Such preparations would be especially suitable for before-meal insulin injections, for example, or for programmable insulin pumps having the capacity for the simultaneous sensing of blood glucose concentrations and integrated feed-back loops.

Table 3.1. *Amino acid replacements inhibiting insulin self-association*

| Principle | Replacements |
|---|---|
| Charge repulsion | B9 Ser→Asp or B28 Pro→Asp |
| Charge repulsion | B27 Thr→Glu plus A21 Asn→Asp |
| Steric hindrance | B12 Val→Ile |
| Decreased surface hydrophobicity | B26 Tyr→Glu |
| Elimination of metal ion-binding sites | B10 His→Asp |
| Interference with β-sheet formation | B28 Pro→Lys plus B29 Lys→Pro |

Since natural insulin self-associates (essentially under any therapeutically relevant condition) the search for monomeric insulins must necessarily depend on alterations in insulin structure as they can be accomplished by replacing one or more of insulin's 51 amino acid residues by others through the methods of protein engineering. Much activity has recently been focused in related areas (26, 27). Table 3.1 provides a summary of some of the amino acid replacements that have been made in insulin in order to inhibit insulin's propensity to self-associate and to achieve a high potency monomeric insulin. Most important, each of the insulin analogues listed has been prepared by the methods of protein engineering and recombinant DNA technology, and each is based on sound physico-chemical principles that arise from our accumulating knowledge of insulin structure. The principles are based on repulsion by like charges, steric hindrance, decreased surface hydrophobicity, elimination of metal ion-binding sites, or interference with the formation of β-sheets during the combination of two insulin monomers to form dimers. Since we are still at an early stage in the construction and evaluation of high potency monomeric insulins, and since the area is considered elsewhere in this volume, the matter will not be considered further here. Nevertheless, the importance of the interplay between determining, evaluating and changing insulin structure, on the one hand, and of considering and understanding insulin's pharmacodynamics and pharmacokinetics, on the other, cannot be overstated in this respect.

## ABNORMAL HUMAN INSULINS

The complex mechanisms through which insulin is eventually produced as the result of insulin gene transcription (see Figs. 3.2 and 3.3) suggest many places where mutations in the human insulin gene could lead to inappropriate gene expression or the secretion of abnormal products. The first human insulin gene was identified 15 years ago, with the result that a half-dozen different mutations are now known to occur in many different families world-wide (28–30). Important tools for detecting abnormal insulins have included reverse-phase high-performance liquid chromatography coupled with radioimmunoassay to analyse the properties of plasma insulin, restriction fragment mapping of leucocyte DNA by Southern blot analysis to assess the loss or gain in cleavage sites by various restriction enzymes, and, of course, gene cloning and complete sequence determination. Table 3.2 provides a list of natural insulin gene mutations that have been identified in humans. All of these mutations are so-called point mutations resulting in the replacement of a single nucleotide by another, and all result in the concomitant replacement of a favourable amino acid by an unfavourable amino acid within the structure of insulin and/or pro-insulin. The structural and functional implications of these abnormal products of the human insulin gene will be discussed later in this section.

Table 3.2. *Mutant human insulin gene products*

| Name | Codon change | Amino acid change |
|---|---|---|
| Insulin Chicago | TTC→TTG | B25 Phe→Leu |
| Insulin Los Angeles<br>Insulin Montreal | TTC→TCC | B24 Phe→Ser |
| Insulin Wakayama<br>Insulin Osaka<br>Insulin Saitama | GTG→TTG | A3 Val→Leu |
| Pro-insulin Tokyo<br>Pro-insulin Boston<br>Pro-insulin Denver | CGC→CAC | 65 Arg→His |
| Pro-insulin Kyoto | CGC→CTC | 65 Arg→Leu |
| Pro-insulin Providence | CAC→GAC | B10 His→Asp |

All individuals with insulin gene mutations have been found to be heterozygous for normal and abnormal alleles. Since available evidence suggests that both alleles are co-dominantly expressed, it appears that normal insulin (from the normal allele) and mutant insulin (from the mutant allele) are secreted in equimolar amounts from the pancreatic β-cells in affected subjects. The mutant gene and the characteristic of secreting abnormal insulin are inherited in an autosomal fashion (as expected since the insulin gene is located on chromosome 11 in humans) and can often be traced through several generations. Most important, all of the abnormal insulins exhibit severely decreased receptor binding and biological potencies (0.2–5% of the potency of the normal hormone). Since mechanisms for insulin degradation in mammals depend importantly on the initial binding of the hormone to receptors and on subsequent receptor-mediated events, the abnormal insulins are not rapidly cleared from the blood and are seen to rise to relatively high levels (50–200 μunits/ml). Accordingly, affected subjects are found to be hyperinsulinaemic as the result of the slowed degradation of the abnormal forms. In most, but perhaps not all, cases the abnormal insulins do not achieve plasma levels commensurate with their having effect in regulating glucose homeostasis.

While the proband of families associated with

the expression of mutant insulin genes has always presented with hyperglycaemia and mild to moderate glucose intolerance, all family members expressing the mutant gene are not equally affected. For example, in the case of Insulin Los Angeles (see Table 3.2), only one of four family members in a single generation exhibited, at the time of study, symptoms of glucose intolerance (31). Further studies identified that asymptomatic family members compensate for the expression of an abnormal insulin simply by secreting more total insulin (half of which, of course, is the normal hormone). Since the glucose intolerance associated with insulin gene mutations may appear late in life, or perhaps may not appear at all, insulin gene mutations clearly cannot be said to cause diabetes. The association of these mutations with diabetes seems to depend on additional abnormalities that lead to decreased β-cell responses to glucose, or occassionally to varying degrees of peripheral insulin resistance. In most cases, however, glucose-intolerant subjects expressing abnormal insulin genes respond normally to exogenous insulin during an insulin tolerance test and respond well to insulin therapy when it is needed (32). Overall, insulin gene mutations can be considered to be one of several potentially confounding abnormalities that can lead to clinical glucose intolerance in the presence of others. Available evidence suggests that insulin gene mutations are rare within the human population.

While the mutant human insulins have provided clues about the causes of glucose intolerance and about insulin physiology in humans, they have also provided very important information about insulin structure–function relationships. Fig. 3.7 shows a simplified structure of pro-insulin in which the separate sites of amino acid replacements in the naturally occurring mutant insulins have been explicitly identified. In fact, the delineation of these structural changes can be envisioned as a natural screen for critical residues in the pro-insulin and insulin molecules. The substitutions fall into three

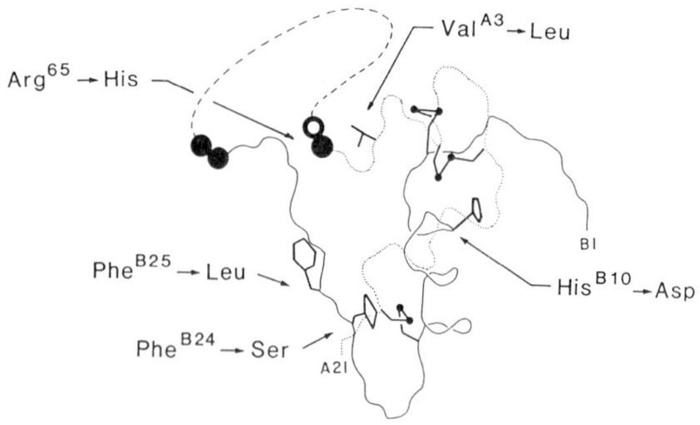


Fig. 3.7. Diagrammatic representation of the structure of human pro-insulin illustrating sites of amino acid substitution due to insulin gene mutations. The insulin A chain is shown by a dotted line, the insulin B chain by a solid line, and the pro-insulin C peptide by a dashed line. Large solid circles represent arginine residues at paired basic amino acid sites for pro-insulin processing to insulin. The large open circle represents the lysine residue at the paired basic site linking the C peptide to the insulin A chain. In each case, the natural residue, along with its position, is shown in conjunction with the relevant amino acid replacement. Note that the five amino acid changes are illustrated on one structure for convenience only; each occurs as a separate molecule in a separate mutant human insulin.

classes: the first identifies the importance of the basic amino acid pair Lys–Arg (one which links the C peptide to the insulin A chain) in the conversion of pro-insulin; the second identifies the importance of three residues of the insulin molecule (A3 Val, B24 Phe and B25 Phe) in directing the affinity of insulin–receptor interactions; the third identifies a special case in suggesting the importance of B10 His (a residue not previously considered to be so critical) in directing both pro-insulin processing and insulin interactions with its receptor. Each of these will be considered below in an abbreviated way.

The substitution of $Arg^{65}$ (a residue at the C peptide/A chain junction) by either His (in Pro-insulin Tokyo/Boston/Denver) or Leu (in Pro-insulin Kyoto) results in a syndrome known somewhat incorrectly as familial hyperpro-insulinaemia (33, 34). In these cases, pro-insulin is synthesised normally within the pancreatic β-cell and is processed correctly at the Arg–Arg pair bridging the insulin B chain and the C peptide (see Fig. 3.2), but is not processed at the site bridging the C peptide and the insulin A chain. Accordingly, individuals with familial hyperpro-insulinaemia are found to secrete an intermediate of pro-insulin conversion in which the C peptide and the insulin A chain remain joined. This material has a molecular weight similar to that of pro-insulin (about 9000) and contains the normal elements of insulin, but cannot be further processed because of the amino acid replacement. The biological activity of the product is diminished to about 5% of that of normal insulin due to the C peptide extention and the blockage of the A1 Gly amino terminus. The residual biological activity of the abnormal pro-insulin conversion intermediate may be sufficient to prevent overt glucose intolerance under most circumstances.

The substitution of A3 Val by Leu (in Insulin Wakayama), B24 Phe by Ser (in Insulin Los Angeles) or B25 Phe by Leu (in Insulin Chicago) leads to fully processed insulins with greatly decreased biological potency (0.2–1% of that of normal insulin) (29, 35). Clinical glucose intolerance is more prevalent in this group, although the penetrance of symptoms is still incomplete in individuals expressing these abnormal insulins. Each of these amino acid substitutions occurs within regions of the insulin molecule thought previously to be relevant to insulin receptor interactions (the $NH_2$-terminal domain of the A chain and the COOH-terminal domain of the B chain) (18, 19), and each occurs at an evolutionarily invariant site. Interestingly, one of these replacements involves a very large change in side chain structure (from the hydrophobic, aromatic side chain of Phe B25 to the hydrophilic side chain of Ser), whereas another involves only a small change in structure (from the hydrophobic, aliphatic side chain of Val to the hydrophobic, aliphatic side chain of Leu). These naturally occurring mutant insulins have formed a base for re-investigating insulin structure–function relationships as presented in the next section.

The substitution of B10 His by Asp (in Pro-insulin Providence) has led to unexpected findings. That is, although the site of substitution is rather distant from pro-insulin processing sites (see Figs. 3.2 and 3.7), the major product resulting from β-cell secretion in this case seems to be the unprocessed mutant pro-insulin. The explanation for this finding probably lies in the importance of His B10 in coordinating zinc ions during the formation of insulin hexamers (see earlier), and in the failure of related molecules to self-associate properly in secretion granules within the β-cell. The overall result seems to lead to the constitutive and unregulated secretion of the unprocessed mutant pro-insulin (36). Interestingly, synthetic insulin with the replacement of B10 His by Asp actually exhibits higher than normal receptor binding potency (37). Nevertheless, limitations in processing of the mutant pro-insulin noted above apparently preclude the formation of sizeable quantities of B10 Asp insulin in individuals expressing the mutant insulin allele.

## INSULIN BINDING SITES

Insulin structure–function relationships have represented an area of intensive investigation for more than two decades. The overriding set of questions relevant to these investigations can be phrased as follows: (a) what elements of insulin structure determine its ability to bind to receptor, (b) which side chains of insulin are critical in contributing free energy to insulin–receptor interactions, and (c) what are the mechanisms through which insulin comes to be receptor bound and through which the signal of receptor-bound ligand is transduced to the interior of insulin target cells? Since insulin is a peptide hormone with relatively stable (but simultaneously adjustable) structure, it represents an excellent model for asking related questions as they apply to peptide hormone–receptor interactions in general. Perhaps because insulin is a relatively tightly packed molecule, few of insulin's 51 amino acid residues can be replaced without some change in the ability of the hormone to bind to receptor. Residues with very little impact on insulin–receptor interactions include those in the very $NH_2$- and COOH-terminal domains of the B chain, a few in the B chain β-turn, and a few in the central loop of the A chain (see Figs. 3.1 and 3.4). Since almost any amino acid replacement in the insulin molecule might be expected to cause some degree of general (and perhaps propagated) change in the structure of the hormone, it is sometimes difficult to know quite how to interpret the effects of a particular amino acid replacement. Is a 2- or 5- or 10-fold decrease in receptor binding potency (a change that, at most, is related to decline in free energy of interaction corresponding to 1.4 kcal/mol – less than that easily attributed to a single hydrogen bond) to be regarded a major or minor, or as important or not? These questions are not easily answered.

Studies based on understanding the molecular basis for the markedly decreased potencies of the naturally occurring mutant human insulins have provided important clues about how insulin binds to receptor (29). Space permits only a summary of related findings. Initial results identified that the replacement of B25 Phe by both Leu and Ser, to give just two examples, yielded analogues with equivalently decreased receptor binding potency (1% of that of insulin). Subsequent findings identified that any residue with a β-aromatic ring served well at position B25 (whether or not the residue represented a natural amino acid), but that a residue with an α- or γ-aromatic ring did not. These results suggested that the loss of the β-aromatic ring of B25 Phe in Insulin Chicago (rather than the character of the substituted amino acid) was instrumental in producing the decreased affinity of the abnormal insulin. They also implied that the natural β-aromatic side chain might directly contact receptor to yield ligand – receptor binding energy. It turns out that this is not the case. Subsequent studies identified that any of several amino acid residues (including Leu and Ser) is acceptable at position B25 as long as the COOH-terminal five residues of the B chain are deleted from the insulin molecule (38). Importantly, deletion of the COOH-terminal five residues of the B chain in insulin itself causes no diminution in the affinity of the resulting analogue for the insulin-receptor (29, 38).

Results related to those presented above led to the conclusion that (a) the side chain of B25 Phe contacts receptor in a way that leads to a concerted conformational adjustment between hormone and receptor, (b) this concerted conformational change eliminates what would otherwise represent a negative interaction between receptor and the COOH-terminal five residues of the hormone, and (c) notwithstanding the importance of B25 Phe in insulin–receptor interactions, the side chain itself does not seem ultimately to contribute to the free energy governing the interaction of the hormone with its receptor. Further studies identified that the negative structural element is localized to the B26 Tyr-B27 Thr peptide bond (see Fig. 3.1). Overall, these studies suggest that the side chain of B25 Phe is indeed critical to insulin–receptor interactions, but that the importance of the residue arises from its ability to induce a change in insulin's structure during the process through which the hormone interacts with receptor (29, 38).

Surprisingly, the role of B24 Phe in insulin–receptor interactions seems to parallel in many ways that of B25 Phe. It turns out that none of various L-amino acids (including Leu, Ser, Ala and Tyr, for example) can replace B24 Phe without major decreases in the receptor binding potencies of the corresponding analogues, but that any of various D-amino acids (including D-Phe, D-Ala and D-Tyr) can replace B24 Phe without loss in receptor binding affinity (39). In fact, analogues with D-amino acids at position B24 exhibit 150–200% of the affinity of natural insulin for binding to receptor. These and related findings suggest that (a) a natural L-directed side chain is not actually necessary for insulin interaction with receptor, (b) the side chain of B24 Phe does not actually contact receptor to induce direct binding energy, and (c) the role of B24

Phe seems to reside in inducing a concerted conformational adjustment in hormone and receptor that results in a favourable D-like (rather than L-like) set of dihedral angles in the insulin peptide backbone in the local region.

The hypothesis presented above was confirmed through the semisynthesis of B24 Gly insulin. This analogue, of course, has no side chain at all at position B24 and can be characterised by its potential ability to undertake with equal facility a set of L- or D-like dihedral angles in the local region. The analogue in fact retains 60–70% of the affinity of insulin for interaction with the insulin receptor. These findings suggest that the critical role of B24 Phe (like that of B25 Phe) lies in its ability to induce a change in the receptor-bound conformation of insulin, rather than in its potential for conferring direct binding energy to insulin–receptor interactions (39). Related studies have indicated that A3 Val may contact receptor to produce a small part of the binding energy characteristic of insulin–receptor interactions, but that it too may function in ways that alter the structure of insulin when the hormone is receptor bound. In this case, the replacement of A3 Val by Gly results in a low potency analogue, notwithstanding that other substitutions that might perturb the structure of the $NH_2$-terminal α-helix of the A chain actually seem to be tolerated rather well (40).

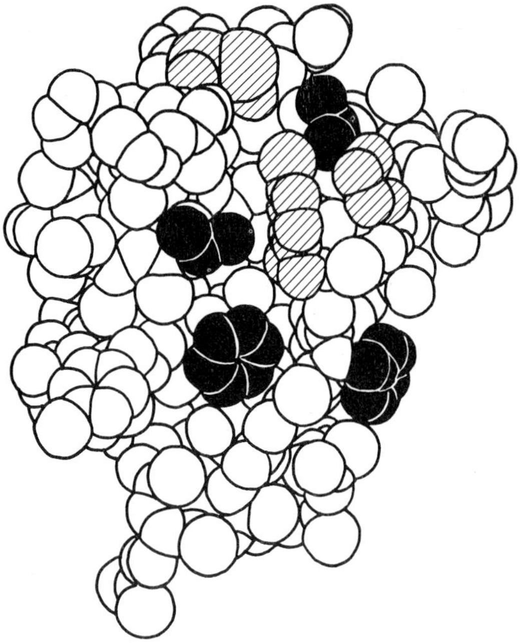

Fig. 3.8. Space-filling model of insulin showing important portions of the dimer-forming interface and the receptor-binding surface of the insulin monomer. The orientation of the monomer is similar to that shown in Fig. 3.4, but the molecule is viewed from the back. Important side chains are shown in black; they include (clockwise from the top) A3 Val, B25 Phe, B24 Phe, and B12 Val. Additional hydrophobic side chains illustrated by hatching include the A7 Cys–B7 Cys disulphide bond and the side chains of B26 Tyr and B28 Pro. The diagram is adapted from Ref. 21.

Fig. 3.8 illustrates a space-filling model of the insulin molecule as it is viewed from the back of the representation provided in Fig. 3.4 (5, 21). This view emphasises both the dimer-forming surface of the insulin monomer and the major portion of what we now envision as the receptor binding surface of the hormone. Importantly, this surface supports the side chains of A3 Val, B24 Phe and B25 Phe (three residues that form the sites of amino acid replacement in the abnormal human insulins) as well as those of a few other residues that have been implicated in insulin–receptor interactions (most notably B12 Val). The surface is hydrophobic in character (21), an observation suggesting that insulin–receptor contacts might mirror in some ways insulin–insulin contacts that are typical of the insulin dimer. The view of insulin illustrated in Fig. 3.8 is static, however; as described above we have reason to believe that adjustments in this structure are necessary for achieving high-affinity insulin–receptor interactions. Interestingly, an analogue that represents insulin cross-linked between residues B29 Lys and A1 Gly by a simple peptide bond (to form a single chain 'minipro-insulin') has been shown to have a crystallographic structure no different from that of insulin as illustrated in Figs. 3.4 and 3.8 (41). Nevertheless, the analogue retains only 0.1% of the receptor binding potency of the natural hormone. This result emphasises that the structure of insulin as we know it cannot represent the receptor-bound structure of the hormone, and that adjustments in this structure are needed to achieve a fully active hormone conformation. The identification of specific contacts between insulin and receptor that are necessary for the formation of high-affinity hormone–receptor complexes must at this stage remain open to speculation.

As noted above, a few insulin analogues have been prepared which exhibit higher potency than insulin for interaction with the insulin receptor *in vitro*. These analogues include B24 D-Phe insulin (200%), B10 Asp insulin (300%), A8 His, B4 His, B10 Glu, B27 His insulin (500%) and B10 Asp, B25 Tyr-amide despentapeptide-(B26-B30) insulin (1000%) (42). Surprisingly, however, many of these analogues exhibit only 100% activity when administered *in vivo* (43). While the full answer is not yet in, it seems that the rapid receptor-mediated clearance of high-affinity analogues precludes them from achieving their full potential as 'super insulins'. Clearly, much work remains to be accomplished in order to understand fully the sites and mechanisms through which insulin comes to be receptor bound and the implications (both *in vitro* and *in vivo*) of structurally altered insulin analogues with unusual and potentially beneficial physical and biological properties.

## CONCLUDING REMARKS

Our knowledge of the molecular structure of insulin has been accumulating for more than 70 years. We have in our hands dozens of X-ray structures of insulins that have been determined through the analysis of insulin crystals, as well as a few nuclear magnetic resonance structures of the hormone that have been determined through the analysis of insulin in solution. Simultaneously, we have information on the perturbation of insulin function that attends the replacement of one or more residues of the hormone as the result of evolution, natural mutation, or the construction of analogues by synthetic, semisynthetic or biosynthetic (recombinant DNA) methods. It is fair to say that more is known about insulin structure and about insulin structure–function relationships than applies to any other peptide hormone. Importantly, insulin analogues with altered characteristics for self-association have been produced, as have analogues with higher than normal receptor binding potency. As is often the case, however, we seem to be in a position of still not knowing quite enough.

The challenges are multiple with respect to understanding not only insulin structure, but also how this structure can change when the hormone binds to receptor, and what the structure of receptor-bound insulin really is. In addition, we must understand more fully how insulin structure influences its (a) physical properties, (b) abilities to self-associate, (c) stability, (d) rate of absorption, (e) rate of transfer from the blood to the local extracellular compartment, (f) receptor binding potency (g) overall biological activity, (h) rate of clearance, (i) immunogenicity, (j) duration of action, (k) pharmacodynamics and pharmacokinetics, (1) undesirable tendencies towards hypoglycaemia, and (m) potentially beneficial interactions directing tissue specificity. While the goal of developing an orally active insulin mimetic with appropriate therapeutic properties seems to be a fair way off, achievement of this goal will clearly depend on understanding even more fully the nuances of insulin structure and its implications in insulin function.

## REFERENCES

1 Banting FG, Best CH. The internal secretion of the pancreas. *J Lab Clin Med* 1922; 7:256–71.
2 Bliss M. *The discovery of insulin*. The University of Chicago Press, Chicago, 1982.
3 Sanger F. Chemistry of insulin. *Science* 1959; 1340–4.
4 Smith LF. Amino acid sequences of insulins. *Diabetes* 1972; 21 (Suppl 2):457–65.
5 Blundell, T, Dodson G, Hodgkin D, Mercola D. Insulin: the structure in the crystal and its reflection in chemistry and biology. *Adv Protein Chem* 1972; 26: 279–402.

6 Steiner DF, Cunningham DD, Spiegelman S, Aten B. Insulin biosynthesis: evidence for a precursor. *Science* 1967; 157:697–700.
7 Steiner DF, Clark JL, Nolan C, Rubenstein AH, Margoliash E, Aten B, Oyer PE. Proinsulin and the biosynthesis of insulin. *Recent Prog Horm Res* 1969; 25:207–82.
8 Dodson GG, Hubbard RE, Reynolds CD. Insulin's structure and its relation to activity. *Biopolymers* 1983; 22: 281–92.
9 Brandenburg D. Insulin chemistry. In: Cuatrecasas P, Jacobs S, eds. *Handbook of experimental pharmacology*, vol. 92. Springer-Verlag, Berlin, 1990; 3–22.
10 Chance RE, Kroeff EP, Hoffman JA, Frank BH. Chemical, physical and biologic properties of biosynthetic human insulin. *Diabetes Care* 1981; 4:147–54.
11 Given BD, Cohen RM, Shoelson SE, Frank BH, Rubenstein AH, Tager HS. Biochemical and clinical implications of proinsulin conversion intermediates. *J Clin Invest* 1985; 76:1398–405.
12 Steiner DF. Insulin today. *Diabetes* 1977; 26:322–40.
13 Polonsky K, Frank B, Pugh W, Addis A, Karrison T, Meier P, Tager H, Rubenstein A. Limitations to the valid use of C-peptide as a marker of the secretion and hepatic extraction of insulin. *Diabetes* 1986; 35:379–86.
14 Temple RC, Carrington CA, Luzio SD, Owens DR, Schneider AE, Sobey WT, Hales CN. Proinsulin levels in NIDDM. *Lancet* 1989; i:293–5.
15 Steiner DF, Smeekens SP, Ohagi S, Chan SJ. The new enzymology of precursor processing endoproteases. *J Biol Chem* 1992; 267: 23435–38.
16 Bell GI, Seino S. The organization and structure of insulin genes. In: Okamoto H, ed. *Molecular biology of islets Langerhans*. Cambridge University Press, Cambridge, 1990; 9–26.
17 Baker EN, Blundell TL, Cutfield JF *et al.* The structure of 2 Zn pig insulin crystals at 1.5 Å resolution. *Phil Trans R Soc Lond* 1988; 319: 369–456.
18 Pullen RA, Lindsay DG, Wood SP *et al.* Receptor-binding region of insulin. *Nature (Lond)* 1976; 259: 369–73.
19 Gammeltoft S. Insulin receptors: binding kinetics and structure–function relationship of insulin. *Physiol Rev* 1984; 61: 1321–78.
20 Hua QX, Shoelson SE, Kochoyan M, Weiss MA. Receptor binding redefined by a structural switch in a mutant human insulin. *Nature* (Lond) 1991; 354: 238–41.
21 Derewenda U, Derewenda ZS, Dodson GG, Hubbard RE. Insulin structure. In: Cuatrecasas P, Jacobs S, eds. *Handbook of experimental pharmacology*, vol. 92. Springer-Verlag, Berlin, 1990; 23–39.
22 Bentley GA, Dodson EJ, Dodson GG, Hodgkin DC, Mercola DA. Structure of 4-zinc insulin. *Nature (Lond)* 1976; 261: 166–8.
23 Derewenda U, Derewenda Z, Dodson EJ, Dodson GG, Reynolds CD, Smith GD, Sparkes C, Swenson D. Phenol stabilizes more helix in a new symmetrical zinc insulin hexamer. *Nature (Lond)* 1989; 338: 594–6.
24 Kaarsholm NC, Ko H-C, Dunn MF. Comparison of solution structural flexibility and zinc binding domains for insulin, proinsulin and miniproinsulin. *Biochemistry* 1989; 28: 4427–43.
25 Schlichtkrull J. Insulin crystals. *Acta Chem Scand* 1956; 10: 1455–69.
26 Brange J, Ribel U, Hansen JF *et al.* Monomeric insulins obtained by protein engineering and their medical implications. *Nature (Lond)* 1988; 333: 679–82.
27 Brange J, Owens DR, Kang S, Volund A. Monomeric insulins and their experimental and clinical implications. *Diabetes Care* 1990; 13: 923–54.
28 Tager HS, Given B, Baldwin D *et al.* A structurally abnormal insulin causing human diabetes. *Nature (Lond)* 1979; 28: 122–5.
29 Tager HS. Abnormal products of the human insulin gene. In: Okamoto H, ed. *Molecular biology of islets of Langerhans*. Cambridge University Press, Cambridge, 1990; 263–86.
30 Steiner DF, Tager HS, Chan S-J, Nanjo K, Sanke T, Rubenstein H. Lessons learned from molecular biology of insulin-gene mutations. *Diabetes* 1990; 13: 600–9.
31 Shoelson SE, Polonsky KS, Zeidler A, Rubenstein AH, Tager HS. Human insulin (Phe → Ser): secretion and metabolic clearance of the abnormal insulin in man and in a dog model. *J Clin Invest* 1984; 73: 1352–58.
32 Haneda M, Polonsky KS, Bergenstal RM *et al.* Familial hyperinsulinemia due to a structurally abnormal insulin: definition of an emerging new clinical syndrome. *N Engl J Med* 1984; 310: 1288–94.
33 Gabbay KH, DeLuca K, Fisher NJ Jr, Mako ME, Rubenstein AH. Familial hyperproinsulinemia: an autosomal dominant defect. *N Engl J Med* 1976; 249: 911–15.
34 Robbins DC, Shoelson SE, Rubenstein AH, Tager HS. Familial hyper-proinsulinemia: two cohorts secreting indistinguishable type II intermediates of proinsulin conversion. *J Clin Invest* 1984; 73: 714–19.
35 Shoelson S, Haneda M, Blix P *et al.* Three mutant insulins in man. *Nature (Lond)* 1983; 302: 540–3.
36 Carroll RJ, Hammer RE, Chan SJ, Swift HH, Rubenstein AH, Steiner DF. A mutant human proinsulin is secreted from islets of Langerhans in increased amounts via an unregulated pathway. *Proc Natl Acad Sci USA* 1988; 85: 8943–7.
37 Schwartz GP, Burke GT, Katsoyanis PG. A superactive insulin: (B10-aspartic acid) insulin (human). *Proc Natl Acad Sci USA* 1987; 84: 6408–11.
38 Nakagawa SH, Tager HS. Role of the phenylalanine B25 side chain in directing insulin interaction with its receptor: steric and conformational effects. *J Biol Chem* 1986; 261: 7332–41.
39 Mirmira RG, Tager HS. Role of the phenylalanine B24 side chain in directing insulin interaction with its receptor: importance of main chain conformation. *J Biol Chem* 1989; 264: 6349–54.
40 Nakagawa SH, Tager HS. Importance of aliphatic side-chain structure at positions 2 and 3 of the insulin A chain in insulin–receptor interactions. *Biochemistry* 1992; 31: 3204–14.
41 Derewenda U, Derewenda Z, Dodson EJ, Dodson GG, Bing X, Markussen J. X-ray analysis of the single chain B29-A1 peptide-linked insulin molecule. *J Mol Biol* 1991; 220: 425–33.
42 Schwartz GP, Burke GT, Katsoyanis PG. A highly potent insulin: des-(B26-B30)-[Asp B10, Tyr B25-$NH_2$] insulin (human). *Proc Natl Acad Sci USA* 1989; 86: 458–61.
43 Ribel U, Hougaard P, Drejer K, Sørensen AR. Equivalent *in vivo* biological activity of insulin analogues and human insulin despite different *in vitro* potencies. *Diabetes* 1990; 39: 1033–9.

# 4 Insulin Receptors

Jens Friis Bak & Oluf Pedersen

## INTRODUCTION

The existence of specific binding sites for insulin was suggested as early as in 1949 in studies of insulin interactions with rat diaphragm (1). This idea was reinforced by the finding that trypsin treatment of cells abolished the action of insulin. Moreover, when insulin was coupled to large polymers its biological actions were retained. In 1970 the introduction of $^{125}$I-labelled insulins allowed for more detailed studies of insulin binding to cells (2, 3). Shortly after the initial insulin binding studies, Cuatrecasas (4) solubilised the insulin receptors by incubating the cellular membranes with Triton X-100 and estimated the molecular mass of the insulin receptor protein to be approximately 300 kD.

The field of insulin receptor research has been expanding. In addition to studies of insulin receptor structure and function, it encompasses examinations of the signal transfer mechanisms including studies of possible endogenous substrates of the insulin receptor kinase, studies of receptor biosynthesis, processing and degradation and examinations of the role of insulin receptors in pathogenesis of disease.

## STRUCTURE

Biochemical studies have shown that the insulin receptor is a transmembrane glycoprotein composed of two 130 kD α-subunits and two 95 kD β-subunits. The two α-subunits which are located exterior to the cell membrane are linked together through S–S bridges. Furthermore, each α-subunit is linked to one β-subunit which has an extracellular portion, a hydrophobic membrane-spanning domain and a cytoplasmic extension that contains a tyrosine kinase. This structure was confirmed when the complete sequence of the insulin receptor cDNA was obtained (5). The receptor for insulin-like growth factor I (IGF-I receptor) is very similar to the insulin receptor showing more than 50% amino acid sequence homology for the total receptor protein and 84% sequence homology in the tyrosine kinase domain (6). In addition, the ligand binding domains of the insulin receptor and the epidermal growth factor (EGF) receptor show homology despite more pronounced differences in overall receptor structure (7, 8). Furthermore, the tyrosine kinase domain of the β-subunit encoded by exons 17–21 shows a considerable homology to oncogenes of the *ras* and *erbB* families (8). The insulin receptor is highly conserved among different species and its overall structure and enzymatic activity are maintained in the fruit fly (9), indicating conservation of its properties for hundreds of millions of years of evolution.

## BIOSYNTHESIS AND PROCESSING

The human insulin receptor gene is located on the short arm of chromosome 19. The gene spans a region of more than 120 kilobase pairs and contains 22 exons (5) (Fig. 4.1). During transcription, one small exon (exon 11) may or may not be included into the mature mRNA (alternative splicing) and, accordingly, two different isoforms (exon 11+) and (exon 11−) of the insulin receptor exist. The initial products of the biosynthesis of the insulin receptor consist of 1382 (exon 11+) (8) or 1370 (exon 11−) (7) amino acids including a 27 amino acid signal peptide (5, 7). These precursors undergo complex glycosylations (10), fatty acylations (11), and disulphide bond formation before cleavage of the proreceptors into α- and β-subunits. Finally, assembly of two α–β heterodimers forms the mature heterotetramer which is inserted into the plasma membrane.

The regulation of insulin receptor biosynthesis is incompletely understood. Insulin may decrease the insulin receptor mRNA level in HepG2 cells (12), whereas glucocorticoids may stimulate insulin receptor synthesis (13).

## INSULIN BINDING

### Ultrastructure of cellular binding locations

According to autoradiographic evidence insulin binding to insulin receptors takes place in relation to microvilli that extend from the cell surface (14). After binding of insulin, the receptor–insulin complex redistributes to non-villous segments where it is internalised through endocytosis (Fig. 4.2). In cytoplasmic endosomes the receptor–insulin complex dissociates under the influence of an acid pH. Insulin is degraded whereas the receptor may recycle back to the cell surface (14). It follows that insulin stimulation of cells may lead to a reduction of the insulin receptor density in the plasma membrane during a process which is known as the acute phase of down-regulation. In addition to the plasma membrane, the nuclear envelope has been reported to possess insulin binding sites (receptors), which may mediate some of the insulin effects on gene regulation (15).

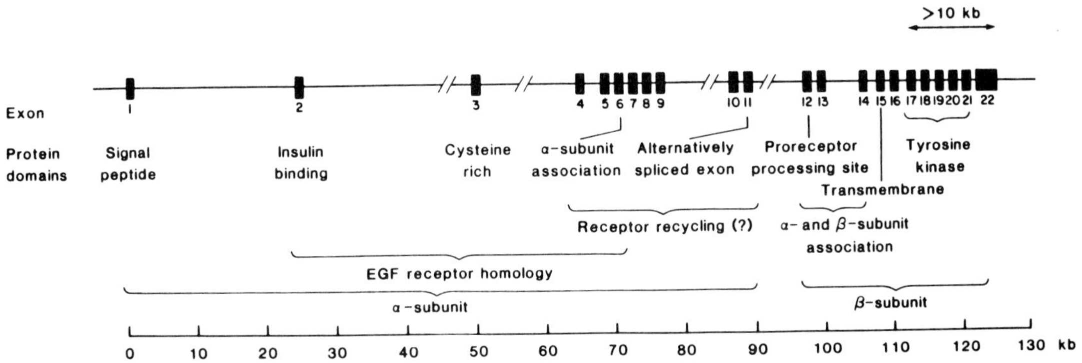


Fig. 4.1. Structural map of the human insulin receptor gene. Locations of exons indicated by vertical bars (adapted and slightly modified from Seino *et al. Diabetes* 1990; 39: 129–33, with permission).

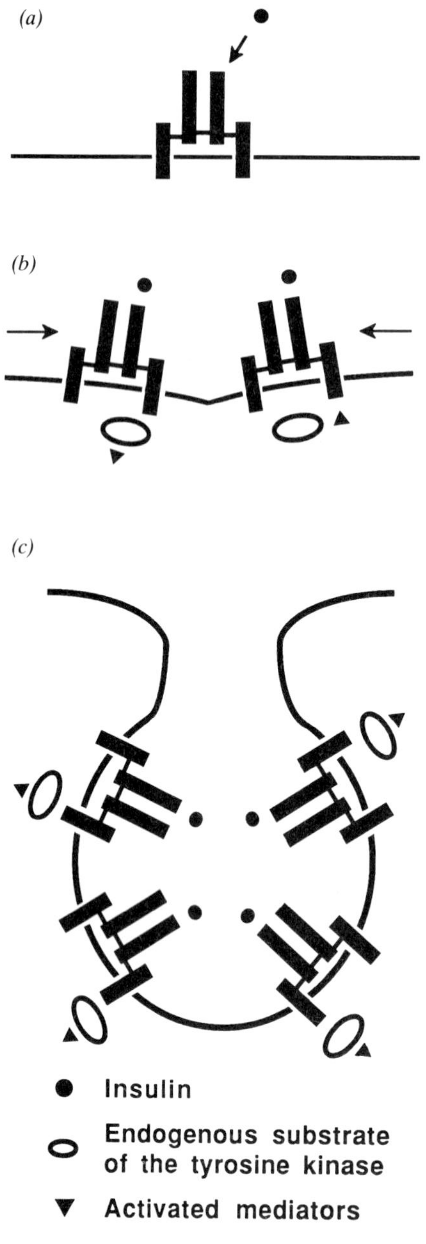


Fig. 4.2. (*a*) Binding of insulin to the membrane receptor. (*b*) Binding induces autophosphorylation with subsequent activation of the intrinsic tyrosine kinase and aggregation of insulin receptors. Endogenous substrates become phosphorylated and mediate propagation of the insulin signal. (*c*) Autophosphorylation and aggregation is followed by internalisation of the receptor–insulin complexes. Finally, insulin is degraded whereas the insulin receptor may recycle back to the cell surface.

## Properties of receptor isoforms

The two splice variants of the insulin receptor are expressed in a tissue-specific manner. Liver cells and perirenal adipose tissue express mainly the exon 11+ isoform form whereas muscle, kidney and placenta express both forms and lymphocytes only the exon 11− form (16–18). The insulin binding affinity is about two-fold higher for the exon 11− isoform as compared to the exon 11+ isoform (19). Furthermore, internalisation after insulin binding proceeds faster for the exon 11− receptor (19). In contrast, insulin-stimulated autophosphorylation and receptor kinase activation of the two receptor isoforms are comparable, and so is their ability to mediate insulin-stimulated glycogen synthesis and thymidine incorporation (19).

## Insulin binding kinetics

The early $^{125}$I-insulin preparations were relatively impure and heterogeneous. The insulin-binding experiments improved considerably when a pure preparation of $^{125}$I-monoiodo-Tyr$^{A14}$-insulin became available. This labelled insulin constitutes an almost ideal insulin tracer ligand with respect to homogeneity, stability, and biological activity (20).

The analysis of insulin binding data is based upon an assumption of insulin interaction with its receptor being a reversible bimolecular reaction where the association reaction and the dissociation reaction lead to a steady state. Therefore, when insulin binding is studied in viable cells, it is mandatory that the internalization of the receptor–insulin complex (see below) is inhibited, e.g. by lowering of the incubation temperature.

### The Scatchard plot

According to the suppositions as outlined above, the binding of a ligand to its receptor

$$R + L \Leftrightarrow RL, \qquad (1)$$

can be considered a bimolecular reaction. $R$ is free receptor (i.e. total receptor − occupied receptor), $L$ is free ligand and $RL$ is receptor bound ligand. When the binding reaction has come to a steady state, the following equation can be derived according to the law of mass action:

$$K_d = [R][L]/[RL] \quad (2)$$

where $K_d$ is the dissociation constant.

The binding of radiolabelled ligand in the presence of various concentrations of unlabelled ligand gives values of bound ($B$) ligand at different total ligand concentrations. In eqn. 2, substitution of $R$ with $(B_{max} - B)$, $L$ with $F$ (free ligand), and $RL$ with $B$ gives after transformation:

$$B/F = -1/K_d(B - B_{max}) \quad (3)$$

where $B_{max}$ is maximal ligand binding, i.e. an estimate of the total receptor number. According to eqn. 3 the plot of $B/F$ versus $B$ (Scatchard plot) is supposed to give a straight line where the intercept of the abscissa ($B/F = O$) gives $B_{max}$ and the slope of the line is $-1/K_d$.

### Negative co-operativity

Several kinetic studies have suggested that the insulin binding event is more complex than expected from a bimolecular reversible first-order reaction. The Scatchard plots of insulin binding data from most cell types are characteristically curvilinear and, in particular, the dissociation of bound (labelled) insulin is accelerated by the addition of excess (unlabelled) insulin. The former observation may have various explanations including assumptions of two-site ligand binding, binding to non-insulin receptors, inaccurate estimates of non-specific binding of the ligand, etc. The latter observation has been interpreted in terms of 'negative co-operativity' although the Hill coefficient of insulin binding data is close to one (21). According to the theory of negative co-operativity as proposed by De Meyts and co-workers (22) the insulin receptor is considered as having different conformations showing different binding affinities: $K_e$ (empty), $K_f$ (fast dissociation, negative co-operativity), and $K_{super}$ (slow dissociation, tight binding). The latter form might be dominating at low ligand concentrations. The change of conformation may explain the slow rate with which 'equilibrium' is obtained at temperatures below 37°C as demonstrated in solubilised muscle-derived insulin receptors (21). The state of 'negative co-operativity' might be caused by site–site interactions at high ligand concentrations.

## Properties of the α-subunit

When exposed to reducing agents (dithiothreitol) insulin receptors dissociate into α–β heterodimers. These may still bind insulin albeit the affinity for insulin binding is lower (23, 24). Moreover, Scatchard analysis of insulin binding to the α–β half receptor disclose no negative cooperative interactions (23, 24). There is a consensus that the $\alpha_2\beta_2$ holoreceptor binds only one insulin molecule with high affinity, but at saturation binds at least a second molecule with low affinity (23–25).

The α-subunit of the insulin receptor contains the domain for insulin recognition and insulin binding. Studies using chimeric receptors composed of IGF-1 receptor portions and insulin receptor portions as well as analysis by site-directed mutagenesis indicate the insulin binding domain to encompass both the N-terminal sequence encoded by exon 2 and a cysteine-rich domain encoded by exon 3 (for review, see ref. 26 and 27). Hydrophobic interactions of residues Phe-B24 and Phe-B25 of insulin with Phe-88 and Phe-89 of the insulin binding domain may be essential (26). In addition, charge interactions are suggested by the pH dependence of insulin binding (21) as well as by studies of modified insulin molecules and mutated insulin receptors (20). In addition, molecular modifications of the receptor α-subunit outside the specific binding region may change the tertiary structure of the α-subunit and thereby interfere with insulin binding kinetics (20). Recently, it has been proposed that insulin is a bivalent ligand bearing two distinct binding surfaces, and that one insulin molecule crosslinks two distinct receptor domains, one on each of the two α subunits (27, 28). It remains to be settled whether synthetic insulin analogues with aberrant affinities for insulin receptor binding may have a role in the treatment of clinical diabetes.

## RECEPTOR AUTOPHOSPHORYLATION AND KINASE ACTIVITY

In 1982, a decade after the first insulin binding studies, it was reported that binding of insulin to the α-subunit was accompanied by autophosphorylation of tyrosine residues of the β-subunit and subsequent activation of a protein tyrosine kinase in the β-subunit (29). Later studies revealed that the β-subunit became autophosphorylated when the α-subunit was digested by trypsin (30). It therefore appears that insulin binding to the α-subunit releases the β-subunit from an inhibitory influence exerted by the α-subunit (30). Studies with anti-receptor antibodies that mimic insulin action have indicated that aggregation of the insulin receptors, which has been known for long periods to be essential for insulin-mediated glucose metabolism (31), is also necessary for receptor kinase activation (32). Further insight into the kinase activation process has come from experiments with insulin interaction with α-β heterodimeric receptors (see above). Such studies have suggested that insulin activation of the protein tyrosine kinase does not occur unless the half-receptors reassociate into the native heterotetrameric complex (33).

### Phosphorylation sites

Thirteen tyrosines are located in the cytoplasmic extension of the β-subunit of the insulin receptor. At least five tyrosine residues of the β-subunit may be autophosphorylated during insulin binding. Three tyrosine residues are in close apposition at residues 1146–1150–1151 (when unit may be autophosphorylated during insulin numbered according to the exon 11− isoform of the receptor). This domain is termed the Tyr 1150 regulatory domain. Full phosphorylation of this domain is important for maximal activation of the receptor tyrosine kinase (34). In mammalian cells, replacement of tyrosine residues 1150 and 1151 of the β-subunit or microinjection of antibodies directed against this domain block insulin stimulation of the receptor kinase and of glucose uptake (35–37) and receptor internalisation (38) but not of mitogenic signalling (36). Furthermore, replacement of tyrosine residue 1146 of the β-subunit blocks insulin-mediated receptor internalisation and DNA synthesis but not insulin stimulation of glycogen synthase activity (39). Phosphorylation of tyrosine residues at the COOH terminus is not required for autoactivation of the tyrosine kinase, but is important for sufficient insulin-mediated metabolic response (40, 41). By contrast, the COOH terminus is an inhibitory regulator of mitogenesis, and removal of the terminal 43 amino acids converts the receptor from a moderately active growth signaller to a very active one (42). The juxtamembrane region of the receptor β-subunit, encoded by exon 16, is required for receptor-mediated internalisation of insulin (43). Substitution of tyrosine 960 within this region does not affect insulin-stimulated receptor autophosphorylation and receptor kinase activation but abolishes insulin-stimulated bioeffects (44). It is apparent therefore, that divergence of signalling pathways for insulin action begins at the receptor level.

During insulin stimulation of isolated solubilised receptors tyrosine residues alone become phosphorylated (45). By contrast, after insulin stimulation of intact cells (i.e. *in situ* insulin stimulation of insulin receptors) analysis of the phosphoamino acids of the α-subunit shows that threonine phosphorylations predominate over tyrosine phosphorylations (46). Serine residues

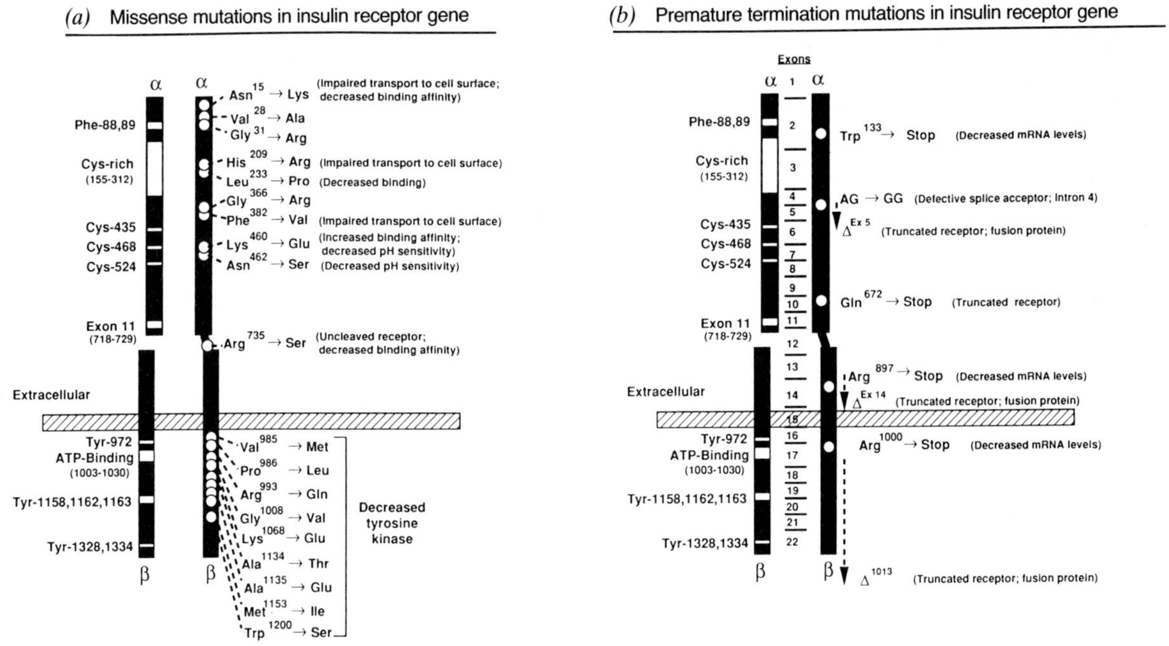


Fig. 4.3. Map of mutations in the insulin receptor gene in severely insulin resistant patients. (*a*) Locations of all the reported missense mutations are indicated in the right half of the drawing of the receptor. (*b*) Locations of all published mutations causing premature chain termination are shown in the right half of the drawing. Locations of the 22 exons are indicated as well. The amino acids are numbered according to the exon 11+ isoform of the receptor (adapted from Taylor SI *et al. J Clin Endocrinol Metab* 1991; 73: 1158–63, with permission).

of the β-subunit may be heavily phosphorylated even in the basal state (45, 46). Incubation of viable cells with catecholamines or phorbol esters attenuates the insulin stimulation of receptor autophosphorylation and receptor kinase activation (47–49). This inhibition seems to be mediated by phosphorylations of serine residues of the β-subunit catalysed by cAMP-dependent kinase and protein kinase C, respectively. It follows that autophosphorylation of the insulin receptor specifically occurs on tyrosine residues whereas serine and threonine residues of the receptor protein may be phosphorylated by other yet unknown protein kinases.

An ATP-binding region which is localised around Lys 1018 is essential to receptor kinase activation (50, 51). Mutations in several other regions of the cytoplasmic extension of the β-subunit may modify, but not abolish, the activity of the tyrosine kinase (Fig. 4.3).

## Endogenous substrates

Identification of endogenous substrates of the insulin receptor kinase has been advanced by the development of high affinity polyclonal and monoclonal antibodies to phosphotyrosines. Such antibodies may identify substrates of tyrosine kinases by immunoblotting and immunoprecipitation. Furthermore, they may be used in affinity chromatography for the purification of substrates of the tyrosine kinase. Numerous peptides become phosphorylated on tyrosine residues during insulin stimulation. This does not indicate that these are substrates for the insulin receptor kinase. The activation of the mitogen activated protein kinases (MAP kinases) illustrates the existence of 'cascades' that may amplify the signal from an activated receptor tyrosine kinase (52).

One peptide with an apparent mass of 185 kD

(pp185) becomes rapidly phosphorylated at tyrosine residues during insulin stimulation of intact cells (53). A component of this peptide has been purified and cloned and is termed IRS-1 (insulin receptor substrate-1). IRS-1 contains six sites which are in Tyr–Met–X–Met motifs (54). These are likely recognition sequences for the insulin receptor kinase (54). Phosphatidylinositol 3-kinase (Ptdlns 3-kinase) is an activator of cell growth which becomes phosphorylated and activated during insulin stimulation. After insulin stimulation PtdIns 3-kinase activity is recovered from immunoprecipitates of anti-insulin receptor antibodies and anti-IRS-1 antibodies (55). Accordingly, IRS-1 may serve as a multisite docking protein for the binding of signal transducing molecules that contain appropriate domains (54, 55).

The concentration of insulin that causes half-maximal stimulation of the insulin receptor kinase (from human muscle) is comparable *in vitro* (21) and *in vivo* (56) at a level of approximately 3 nM, which is far above the physiological range of plasma insulin concentrations. Thus, physiological excursions of plasma insulin may correlate linearly with receptor kinase activation. Furthermore, insulin receptor kinase activity and glucose uptake increase in parallel during insulin stimulation at physiological concentrations in studies of adipocytes and skeletal muscle from rats (57, 58).

Termination of insulin-stimulated receptor kinase activity is likely to require the action of phosphotyrosyl-protein phosphatases (59). However, the identity and regulation of specific phosphatases that act on the insulin receptor are not known.

Although the insulin receptor kinase appears to be a first line signal messenger for insulin binding, some actions of insulin are not related to changes in phosphorylation or kinase activation of the insulin receptor ((60) and references therein). This evidence has come from studies using anti-insulin receptor antibodies which may stimulate glucose uptake, amino acid uptake, and thymidine incorporation without increasing the phosphorylation and kinase activity of the receptor (60). In addition, insulin receptor mutants lacking tyrosine 1150 and 1151 demonstrate no tyrosine kinase activity, whereas such mutants may still be able to mediate thymidine incorporation into DNA in response to insulin stimulation (36).

## INSULIN RECEPTORS AND DIABETES

### Insulin binding studies

Insulin resistance is a characteristic feature of obesity and of insulin-dependent as well as non-insulin-dependent diabetes mellitus. Initial studies of insulin receptors in humans employed monocytes which account for 80–90% of the insulin binding by leucocytes of peripheral blood (61). However, blood cells are not major insulin target cells and therefore, techniques have been developed to study insulin binding in adipocytes after isolation from tissue biopsies using incubation with collagenase (62). This is particularly important as it has been shown that insulin receptor binding in one cell type may not be assumed to reflect insulin binding in other insulin binding tissues (62). Quantification of insulin binding requires an appropriate denominator. Insulin binding (insulin receptor number) may be related to the number of cells, cell surface area, or the content of protein, lipid or nucleic acids. Indirect evidence from studies comparing insulin binding and *in vitro* insulin action in isolated adipocytes has suggested that insulin binding should be expressed per cell surface area (63).

Shortly after the discovery of the insulin receptors their importance for diabetes research was emphasised by findings in monocytes and in isolated adipocytes that insulin receptor binding was decreased in morbidly obese insulin resistant subjects (64). However, in most studies of obese subjects a diabetic state was not associated with any additional (diabetes-specific) impairment of insulin binding to adipocytes (for review see (65)). Accordingly, the reduced insulin action on glucose transport and metabolism seen in isolated adipocytes from diabetic individuals was ascribed to so-called 'post-receptor defects'. In insulin-treated insulin-dependent diabetic patients, insulin binding to adipocytes was reduced with corresponding impairments of insulin-stimulated glucose transport into the isolated cells (66). However, in a study of fat cells obtained from ketotic patients with newly presenting diabetes before initiation of insulin treatment, the insulin binding was normal despite severely impaired insulin-stimulated glucose transport and metabolism (67).

The recognition that the maximal glucose transport into adipocytes is obtained at only 20–25% insulin receptor occupancy ('spare receptors') (68), indicates that a small change in insulin receptor number may only cause a shift in the dose–response curve for insulin action (insulin sensitivity) whereas the maximal responsiveness to insulin is not changed (62). Thus, the moderate reduction in insulin receptor number found in some insulin resistant patients would not explain the severely impaired maximal response to insulin stimulation seen *in vitro* (fat cells) (69) and *in vivo* (70) in these patients. In addition, when day-long experimental hyperinsulinaemia produced insulin resistance in non-obese, healthy volunteers, there was no change in insulin binding to adipocytes and blood cells (71, 72). Furthermore, alleviation of insulin resistance during pharmacological or dietary treatment of NIDDM patients did not lead to consistent changes in the insulin binding to adipocytes (69, 73).

In muscle, which is a major target organ for insulin, insulin binding cannot be easily measured. Insulin binding to human muscle insulin receptors has been assayed using crude membranes or solubilised insulin receptors, but there are obvious limitations to the conclusions that can be drawn from such binding studies (74–76). There is conflicting evidence if the ratio of the two insulin receptor mRNA splice variants in skeletal muscle is altered in non-insulin-dependent diabetes. Thus, Mosthaf and co-workers have reported that only the exon 11–isoform (showing high binding affinity) was present in muscle from normal subjects whereas both isoforms were equally present in NIDDM patients (77). In contrast, Benecke and co-workers found an equal representation of the two isoforms in muscle from diabetic patients and their controls (78).

In liver cells from NIDDM patients there is divergence whether insulin binding to membrane preparations is increased (79) or decreased (80). In the study of Caro and co-workers (80) the binding to intact liver cells was comparable in non-obese and obese patients. However, when differences in cell volume were taken into account the insulin receptor density in the plasma membrane was lower in obese patients with or without diabetes. The insulin action with respect to uptake of α-aminoisobutyric acid was severely impaired in hepatocytes from obese NIDDM patients (80).

In summary, the insulin receptor density in insulin target cells appears not to be a primary pathogenic factor for development of insulin resistance and diabetes. The low insulin binding which may be associated with insulin resistant states might have a secondary origin including metabolic derangement and, perhaps, chronic hyperinsulinaemia and 'down-regulation' of the receptor number. In insulin resistant diabetic patients the reduction in insulin action as demonstrated both *in vivo* and in isolated human adipocytes (glucose transport and metabolism) as well as in skeletal muscle (glycogen synthesis and glycogen synthase activity) is believed to be a result of post-binding abnormalities in insulin action.

## Insulin receptor kinase and diabetes

In diabetes research new light was shed on the insulin receptors when their capability for undergoing autophosphorylation and receptor kinase activation in response to insulin exposure was shown. Numerous studies have been carried out to clarify the importance of insulin receptor kinase activity for insulin resistance. There is some inconsistency among the findings which is largely due to differences in obesity among enclosed patients as well as differences in the tissues that have been examined. One study has examined insulin-stimulated autophosphorylation of insulin receptors isolated from liver, muscle and fat from the same individuals (81). It appears from this study that insulin-stimulated autophosphorylation is most pronounced in receptors from muscle and comparable in receptors from liver and fat (81).

In studies of human muscle-derived receptors, the insulin receptor kinase activity (using an exogenous synthetic substrate as phospho-acceptor) has repeatedly been found to be reduced in lean NIDDM patients as compared to lean control subjects (75, 82, 83). In contrast, no diabetes-specific abnormality of insulin receptor kinase activity has been observed in obese NIDDM patients as compared to obese control subjects (75, 76, 84). In the study of Caro and co-workers (76) autophosphorylation of muscle-derived receptors from obese subjects with, and without, diabetes was comparable to that of lean control subjects. By contrast, studies of lean subjects have demonstrated an impaired autophosphorylation of muscle receptors from patients with NIDDM (82, 83). To elucidate which sites of the β-subunit were insufficiently autophosphorylated in lean NIDDM patients Obermaier-Kusser *et al.* (82) studied the phosphorylation state of tryptic fragments of the β-subunit using high-performance liquid chromatography (HPLC). Despite some heterogeneity in the HPLC-profiles of phosphorylated insulin receptors from diabetic patients there was a strong correlation between receptor kinase activation and tris-phosphorylation of the Tyr 1150 domain of the insulin receptor (82). Amelioration of insulin resistance during treatment of obese NIDDM patients with sulphonylurea or diet caused no change in muscle insulin receptor kinase activity (84, 85).

In normal-weight IDDM patients the insulin receptors from skeletal muscle have shown a normal insulin-stimulated tyrosine kinase activity (86). Likewise, autophosphorylation and receptor kinase activity of insulin receptors from insulin-treated streptozotocin-diabetic rats is normal (87).

Human fat cells are attractive for the study of insulin resistance in humans. In isolated adipocytes several aspects of insulin action can be investigated. Thus, insulin receptor kinase activity has been examined in diabetic patients and their controls. It appears that adipocyte-derived solubilised insulin receptors from obese NIDDM patients have a decreased autophosphorylation and insulin receptor kinase activity towards exogenous substrates as compared to obese control subjects (88, 89), a finding which is at variance with findings in muscle-derived receptors. Moreover, in obese NIDDM patients the kinase activity of adipocyte-derived insulin receptors improves after weight loss (90). Incubation of adipocytes from obese NIDDM subjects with insulin causes rapid phosphorylations of tyrosine residues of a 185 kD cytosolic peptide (91), which is probably identical to the pp 185 found in other cell types. Phosphorylation of this peptide and autophosphorylation of the insulin receptor were reported to be comparably reduced in NIDDM patients (91).

In human liver cell-derived insulin receptors, both receptor autophosphorylation and insulin receptor kinase activity are impaired in obese patients with NIDDM (80).

NIDDM is a hereditary disease and studies of candidate genes responsible for the development of insulin resistance are in progress. However, in the majority of patients with NIDDM the insulin receptor gene is normal both in populations with a high occurrence of this disease such as Pima indians (92) as well as in Caucasians with the common form of NIDDM (93, 94).

## INSULIN RECEPTORS AND EXTREME INSULIN RESISTANCE

Whereas the insulin receptors play only a minor role, if any, in the pathogenesis of insulin-resistant diabetes mellitus there is a subset of diseases in which pathogenesis is closely related to abnormalities of the insulin receptor function. These are the rare syndromes of extreme insulin resistance comprising Leprechaunism, Type A insulin resistance, and the Rabson–Mendenhall syndrome. Leprechaunism is an inborn syndrome characterised by intrauterine growth retardation, acanthosis nigricans, severe insulin resistance and glucose intolerance. Patients usually die within the first year of life. Type A insulin resistance is defined by insulin resistance, acanthosis nigricans and hyperandrogenism in the absence of lipoatrophy. The Rabson–Mendenhall syndrome is characterised by extreme insulin resistance, acanthosis nigricans, abnormalities of teeth and nails and pineal hyperplasia (95). In such syndromes mutations have been recorded at various locations in the insulin receptor gene which may cause serious disturbances in 1) receptor biosynthesis, 2) transport of the receptor to the cell surface, 3) affinity of insulin binding, 4) receptor tyrosine kinase activity and 5) receptor degradation (95) (Fig. 4.3). Clinical diabetes, however, is not a consistent feature of these syndromes. Indeed, patients with Leprechaunism may be hypoglycaemic in the basal state (96), and Type A insulin resistant patients may have normal or elevated fasting glycaemia (96, 97). Type B insulin resistance is another severe insulin resistant state also encompassing acanthosis nigricans and ovarian hyperandrogenism. This syndrome is caused by the presence of blocking anti-insulin receptor antibodies (98, 99) and it may be associated with other autoimmune diseases. Hypoglycaemia may precipitate if the antibodies behave as partial agonists.

## REFERENCES


1 Stadie WC, Haugaard N, Marsh JB, Hills AG. The chemical combination of insulin with muscle (diaphragm) of normal rat. *Am J Med Sci* 1949; 218: 265–74.
2 Freychet P, Roth J, Neville DM Jr. Insulin receptors in the liver: specific binding of [$^{125}$I]insulin to the plasma membrane and its relation to insulin bioactivity. *Proc Natl Acad Sci USA* 1971; 68: 1833–7.
3 Cuatrecasas P, Desbuquois B, Krug F. Insulin-receptor interactions in liver cell membranes. *Biochem Biophys Res Commun* 1971; 44: 333–9.
4 Cuatrecasas P. Properties of the insulin receptor isolated from liver and fat cell membranes. *J Biol Chem* 1972; 247: 1980–91.
5 Seino S, Seino M, Nishi S, Bell GI. Structure of the human insulin receptor gene and characterization of its promotor. *Proc Natl Acad Sci USA* 1989; 86: 114–18.
6 Ullrich A, Gray A, Tam AW *et al.* Insulin-like growth factor I receptor primary structure: comparison with insulin receptor suggests structural determinants that define functional specificity. *EMBO J* 1986; 5: 2503.
7 Ullrich A, Bell JR, Chen EY *et al.* Human insulin receptor and its relationship to the tyrosine kinase family of oncogenes. *Nature* 1985; 313: 756–61.
8 Ebina Y, Ellis L, Jarnagin K *et al.* The human insulin receptor cDNA: the structural basis for hormone-activated transmembrane signalling. *Cell* 1985; 40: 747–58.
9 Rosen OM. Structure and function of insulin receptors. *Diabetes* 1989; 38: 1508–11.
10 Forsayeth J, Maddux B, Goldfine ID. Biosynthesis and processing of the human insulin receptor. *Diabetes* 1986; 35: 837–46.
11 Hedo JA, Collier E, Watkinson A. Myristyl and palmityl acylation of the insulin receptor. *J Biol Chem* 1987; 262: 954–7.
12 Rohilla AMK, Anderson C, Wood WM, Berhanu P. Insulin downregulates the steady-state level of its receptor's messenger ribonucleic acid. *Biochem Biophys Res Commun* 1991; 175: 520–6.
13 McDonald AR, Goldfine ID. Glucocorticoid regulation of insulin receptor gene transcription in IM-9 cultured lymphocytes. *J Clin Invest* 1988; 81: 499–504.
14 Carpentier J-L. The cell biology of the insulin receptor. *Diabetologia* 1989; 32: 627–35.
15 Goldfine ID, Clawson GA, Smuckler EA, Purrello F, Vigneri R. Action of insulin at the nuclear envelope. *Mol Cell Biochem* 1982; 48: 3–14.
16 Moller DE, Yokota A, Caro JF, Flier JS. Tissue-specific expression of two alternatively spliced insulin receptor mRNA's in man. *Mol Endocr* 1989; 3: 1263–9.
17 Seino S, Bell GI. Alternative splicing of human insulin receptor messenger mRNA. *Biochem Biophys Res Commun* 1989; 159: 312–16.
18 Mosthaf L, Grako K, Dull TJ, Coussens L, Ullrich A, McClain DA. Functionally distinct insulin receptors generated by tissue-specific alternative splicing. *EMBO J* 1990; 9: 2409–13.
19 Yamaguchi Y, Flier JS, Yokota A, Benecke H, Backer H, Moller DE. Functional properties of two naturally occurring isoforms of the human insulin receptor in Chinese hamster ovary cells. *Endocrinology* 1991; 129: 2058–66.
20 Gammeltoft S. Insulin receptors: binding kinetics and structure–function relationship of insulin. *Physiol Rev* 1984; 64: 1321–78.
21 Bak JF, Handberg A, Beck-Nielsen H, Pedersen O. Kinetics of insulin binding and kinase activity of the partially purified insulin receptor from human skeletal muscle. *Biochim Biophys Acta* 1990; 1052: 306–12.
22 De Meyts P, Bianco AR, Roth J. Site–site interactions among insulin receptors. Characterization of the negative cooperativity. *J Biol Chem* 1976; 251: 1877–88.
23 Sweet LJ, Morrison BD, Pessin JE. Isolation of func-

tional α-β heterodimers from the purified human placental $\alpha_2\beta_2$ heterotetrameric insulin receptor complex. *J Biol Chem* 1987; 161: 6939–42.

24 Pang DT, Schafer JA. Evidence that insulin receptor from human placenta has a high affinity for only one molecule of insulin. *J Biol Chem* 1984; 259: 8589–96.

25 Markussen J, Halstrom J, Wiberg F, Schäffer L. Immobilized insulin for high affinity chromatography of insulin receptor. *J Biol Chem* 1991; 266: 18814–18.

26 De Meyts P, Gu J-L, Shymko RM, Kaplan BE, Bell GI, Whittaker J. Identification of a ligand-binding region of the human insulin receptor encoded by the second exon of the gene. *Mol Endocr* 1990; 4: 409–16.

27 De Meyts P. The structural basis of insulin and insulin-like growth factor-1 receptor binding and negative cooperativity, and its relevance to mitogenic versus metabolic signalling. *Diabetologia* 1994; 37: in press.

28 Schäffer L. A model for insulin binding to the insulin receptor. *Eur J Biochem* 1994; 221: 1127–32.

29 Kasuga M, Karlsson FA, Kahn CR. Insulin stimulates the phosphorylation of the 95 000-Dalton subunit of its own receptor. *Science* 1982; 215: 185–7.

30 Shoelson SE, White MF, Kahn CR. Tryptic activation of the insulin receptor. Proteolytic truncation of the α-subunit releases the β-subunit from inhibitory control. *J Biol Chem* 1988; 263: 4852–60.

31 Kahn CR, Baird KL, Jarret DB, Flier JS. Direct demonstration that receptor crosslinking or aggregation is important in insulin action. *Proc Natl Acad Sci USA* 1978; 75: 4209–13.

32 Heffetz D, Zick Y. Receptor aggregation is necessary for activation of the soluble insulin receptor kinase. *J Biol Chem* 1986; 261: 889–94.

33 Morrison BD, Swanson ML, Sweet LJ, Pessin JE. Insulin-dependent covalent reassociation of isolated ab heterodimeric insulin receptors into an a2b2 heterotetrameric disulfide-linked. *J Biol Chem* 1988; 263: 7806–13.

34 White MF, Shoelson SE, Keutmann H, Kahn CR. A cascade of tyrosine autophosphorylation in the β-subunit activates the phosphotransferase of the insulin receptor. *J Biol Chem* 1988; 263: 2969–80.

35 Ellis L, Clauser E, Morgan DO, Edery M, Roth RA, Rutter WJ. Replacement of insulin receptor tyrosine kinase residues 1162 and 1163 compromises insulin-stimulated kinase activity and uptake of 2-deoxyglucose. *Cell* 1986; 45: 721–32.

36 Debant A, Clauser E, Ponzio G *et al.* Replacement of insulin receptor tyrosine residues 1162 and 1163 does not alter the mitogenic effect of the hormone. *Proc Natl Acad Sci USA* 1988; 85: 8032–6.

37 Morgan DO, Roth RA. Acute insulin action requires insulin receptor kinase activity: introduction of an inhibitory monoclonal antibody into mammalian cells blocks the rapid effects of insulin. *Proc Natl Acad Sci USA* 1987; 84: 41–45.

38 Carpentier J-L, Paccaud J-P, Gorden P, Rutter WJ, Orci L. Insulin-induced surface redistribution regulates internalization of the insulin receptor and requires its autophosphorylation. *Proc Natl Acad Sci USA* 1992; 89: 162–6.

39 Wilden PA, Backer JM, Kahn CR, Cahill DA, Schroeder GJ, White MF. The insulin receptor with phenylalanine replacing tyrosine-1146 provides evidence for separate signals regulating cellular metabolism and growth. *Proc Natl Acad Sci USA* 1990; 87: 3358–62.

40 McClain DA, Maegawa H, Levy J *et al.* Properties of a human insulin receptor with a COOH-terminal truncation: insulin binding, autophosphorylation, and endocytosis. *J Biol Chem* 1988; 263: 8904–11.

41 Maegawa H, McClain DA, Freidenberg GR *et al.* Properties of a human insulin receptor with a COOH-terminal truncation; truncate receptors have normal kinase activity but are defective in signalling metabolic effects. *J Biol Chem* 1988; 263: 8912–17.

42 Thies RS, Ullrich A, McClain DA. Augmented mitogenesis and impaired metabolic signalling mediated by a truncated insulin receptor. *J Biol Chem* 1989; 264: 12820–5.

43 Backer JM, Kahn CR, Cahill DA, Ullrich A, White MF. Receptor-mediated internalization of insulin requires a 12-amino acid sequence in the juxtamembrane region of the insulin receptor beta-subunit. *J Biol Chem* 1990; 265: 16450–4.

44 White MF, Livingston JN, Backer JM *et al.* Mutation of the insulin receptor at tyrosine 960 inhibits signal transmission but does not affect its tyrosine kinase activity. *Cell* 1988; 54: 641–9.

45 White MF, Takayama S, Kahn CR. Differences in the sites of phosphorylation of the insulin receptor *in vivo* and *in vitro*. *J Biol Chem* 1985; 260: 9470–8.

46 Kasuga M, Zick Y, Blith D, Karlsson FA, Häring HU, Kahn CR. Insulin stimulation of phosphorylation of the β subunit of the insulin receptor. *J Biol Chem* 1982; 257: 9891–4.

47 Häring HU, Kirsch D, Obermaier B, Ermel B, Machicao F. Decreased tyrosine kinase activity of insulin receptor isolated from rat adipocytes rendered insulin-resistant by catecholamine treatment *in vitro*. *Biochem J* 1986; 234: 59–66.

48 Obermaier B, Ermel B, Kirsch D *et al.* Catecholamines and tumour promoting phorbolesters inhibit insulin receptor kinase and induce insulin resistance in isolated human adipocytes. *Diabetologia* 1987; 30:93–9.

49 Takayama S, White MF, Kahn CR. Phorbol ester-induced serine phosphorylation of the insulin receptor decreases its tyrosine kinase activity. *J Biol Chem* 1988; 263:3440–7.

50 Chou CK, Dull TJ, Russell DS *et al.* Human insulin receptors mutated at the ATP-binding site lack protein tyrosine kinase activity and fail to mediate postreceptor affects of insulin. *J Biol Chem* 1987; 262:1842–7.

51 Ebina Y, Araki E, Taira M *et al.* Replacement of lysine residue 1030 in the putative insulin receptor abolishes insulin- and antibody-stimulated glucose uptake and receptor kinase activity. *Proc Natl Acad Sci USA* 1987; 84:704–8.

52 Gomez N, Cohen P. Dissection of the protein kinase cascade by which nerve growth factor activates MAP kinase. *Nature* 1991; 353:170–3.

53 White MF, Maron R, Kahn CR. Insulin rapidly stimulates tyrosine phosphorylation of a $M_r$ = 185,000 protein in intact cells. *Nature* 1985; 318:183–6.

54 Sun XJ, Rothenberg P, Kahn CR *et al.* Structure of the insulin receptor substrate IRS-1 defines a unique signal transduction protein. *Nature* 1991; 352:73–77.

55 Backer JM, Schroeder GG, Kahn CR *et al.* Insulin stimulation of phosphatidyl 3-kinase activity maps to insulin receptor regions required for endogenous substrate phosphorylation. *J Biol Chem* 1992; 267:1367–4.

56 Freidenberg GR, Suter SL, Henry RR, Reichart D, Olefsky JM. *In vivo* stimulation of the insulin receptor kinase in human skeletal muscle. Correlation with insulin-stimulated glucose disposal during euglycemic clamp studies. *J Clin Invest* 1991; 87:2222–9.
57 Bryer-Ash M. Rat insulin-receptor kinase activity correlates with *in vivo* insulin action. *Diabetes* 1989; 38:108–16.
58 Klein HH, Matthaei S, Drenkhan M, Ries W, Scriba PC. The relationship between insulin binding, insulin activation of insulin-receptor tyrosine kinase, and insulin stimulation of glucose uptake in isolated rat adipocytes. *Biochem J* 1991; 274:787–92.
59 King DS, Dalsky GP, Clutter WE *et al.* Effects of lack of exercise on insulin secretion and action in trained subjects. *Am J Physiol* 1988; 254:E537–42.
60 Sung CK. Insulin receptor signalling through non-tyrosine kinase pathways: Evidence from anti-receptor antibodies and insulin receptor mutants. *J Cell Biochem* 1992; 48:26–32.
61 Beck-Nielsen H, Pedersen O, Kragballe K, Sørensen NS. The monocyte as a model for the study of insulin receptors in man. *Diabetologia* 1977; 13:563–9.
62 Pedersen O. Studies of insulin receptor binding and insulin action in humans. *Dan Med Bull* 1984; 31:1–32.
63 Pedersen O, Hjøllund E, Sørensen NS. Insulin receptor binding and insulin action in human fat cells: Effects of obesity and fasting. *Metabolism* 1982; 31:884–95.
64 Olefsky JM. Decreased insulin binding to adipocytes and circulating monocytes from obese subjects. *J Clin Invest* 1976; 57:1165–72.
65 Hjøllund E. Insulin receptor binding and action in human adipocytes. *Dan Med Bull* 1991; 38:252–70.
66 Pedersen O, Hjøllund E. Insulin receptor binding to fat and blood cells and insulin action in fat cells from insulin-dependent diabetics. *Diabetes* 1982; 31:706–15.
67 Hjøllund E, Pedersen O, Richelsen B, Beck-Nielsen H, Sørensen NS. Glucose transport and metabolism in adipocytes from newly diagnosed untreated insulin-dependent diabetics. Severely impaired basal and postinsulin binding activities. *J Clin Invest* 1985; 76:2091–6.
68 Pedersen O, Glieman J. Hexose transport in human adipocytes: factors influencing the response to insulin and kinetics of methylglucose and glucose transport. *Diabetologia* 1981; 20:630–5.
69 Hjøllund E, Pedersen O, Sørensen NS. Adipocyte insulin binding and action in moderately obese NIDDM patients after dietary control of plasma glucose: reversal of post-binding abnormalities. *Diabetes Care* 1987; 10:306–12.
70 Garvey WT, Olefsky JM, Griffin J, Hamman RF, Kolterman OG. The effect of insulin treatment on insulin secretion and insulin action in type II diabetes mellitus. *Diabetes* 1985; 34:222–34.
71 Rizza RA, Mandarino LJ, Genest J, Baker BA, Gerich JE. Production of insulin resistance by hyperinsulinemia in man. *Diabetologia* 1985; 28:70–5.
72 Marangou AG, Weber KM, Boston RC *et al.* Metabolic consequences of prolonged hyperinsulinemia in humans. Evidence for induction of insulin insensitivity. *Diabetes* 1986; 35:1383–9.
73 Kolterman OG, Gray RS, Shapiro G, Scarlett JA, Griffin J, Olefsky JM. The acute and chronic effects of sulfonylurea therapy in type II diabetic subjects. *Diabetes* 1984; 33:346–54.
74 Bonen A, Hood DA, Tan MH, Sopper MM, Begin-Heick N. Insulin binding in human skeletal muscle. *Biochim Biophys Acta* 1984; 801:171–6.
75 Arner P, Pollare T, Lithell H, Livingston JN. Defective insulin receptor tyrosine kinase in human skeletal muscle in obesity and Type 2 (non-insulin-dependent) diabetes mellitus. *Diabetologia* 1987; 30:437–440.
76 Caro JF, Sinha MK, Raju SM *et al.* Insulin receptor kinase in human skeletal muscle from obese subjects with and without noninsulin dependent diabetes. *J Clin Invest* 1987; 79:1330–7.
77 Mosthaf L, Vogt B, Häring HU, Ullrich A. Altered expression of insulin receptor types A and B in the skeletal muscle of non-insulin-dependent diabetes mellitus patients. *Proc Natl Acad Sci USA* 1991; 88:4728–30.
78 Benecke H, Flier JS, Moller DE. Alternatively spliced variants of the insulin receptor protein. Expression in normal and diabetic human tissues. *J Clin Invest* 1992; 89:2066–70.
79 Arner P, Einarsson K, Ewerth S, Livingston J. Studies of the human liver insulin receptor in noninsulin-dependent diabetes mellitus. *J Clin Invest* 1986; 77: 1716–18.
80 Caro JF, Ittoop O, Pories WJ *et al.* Studies on the mechanism of insulin resistance in the liver from humans with noninsulin-dependent diabetes. Insulin action and binding in isolated hepatocytes, insulin receptor structure, and kinase activity. *J Clin Invest* 1986; 78:249–58.
81 Caro JF, Raju SM, Sinha MK, Goldfine ID, Dohm GL. Heterogeneity of human liver, muscle, and adipose tissue insulin receptor. *Biochem Biophys Res Commun* 1988; 151: 123–9.
82 Obermaier-Kusser B, White MF, Pongratz DE *et al.* A defective intramolecular autoactivation cascade may cause the reduced kinase activity of the skeletal muscle insulin receptor from patients with non-insulin-dependent diabetes mellitus. *J Biol Chem* 1989; 264: 9497–504.
83 Maegawa H, Shigeta Y, Egawa K, Kobayashi M. Impaired autophosphorylation of insulin receptors from abdominal skeletal muscles in nonobese subjects with NIDDM. *Diabetes* 1991; 40:815–19.
84 Bak JF, Møller N, Schmitz O, Saaek A, Pedersen O. *In vivo* insulin action and muscle glycogen synthase activity in Type 2 (non-insulin-dependent diabetes): effects of diet treatment. *Diabetologia* 1992; 35:777–84.
85 Bak JF, Schmitz O, Sørensen NS, Pedersen O. Postreceptor effects of sulfonylurea on skeletal muscle glycogen synthase activity in type II diabetic patients. *Diabetes* 1989; 38:1343–50.
86 Bak JF, Jacobsen UK, Jøsrgensen FS, Pedersen O. Insulin receptor function and glycogen synthase activity in skeletal muscle biopsies from patients with insulin-dependent diabetes mellitus: effects of physical training. *J Clin Endocrinol Metab* 1989; 69:158–64.
87 Burant CF, Treutelaar MK, Buse MG. Diabetes-induced functional and structural changes in insulin receptors from rat skeletal muscle. *J Clin Invest* 1986; 77:260–70.
88 Freidenberg GR, Henry RR, Klein HH, Reichart DR, Olefsky JM. Decreased kinase activity of insulin receptors from adipocytes of non-insulin-dependent diabetic subjects. *J Clin Invest* 1987; 79:240–50.
89 Sinha MK, Pories WJ, Flickinger EG, Meelheim D, Caro JF. Insulin-receptor kinase activity of adipose tissue

from morbidly obese humans with and without NIDDM. *Diabetes* 1987; 36:620–5.
90 Freidenberg GR, Reichart DR, Olefsky JM, Henry RR. Reversibility of defective adipocyte insulin receptor kinase activity in non-insulin-dependent diabetes mellitus. Effect of weight loss. *J Clin Invest* 1988; 82:1398–406.
91 Thies RS, Molina JM, Ciaraldi TP, Freidenberg GR, Olefsky JM. Insulin-receptor autophosphorylation and endogenous substrate phosphorylation in human adipocytes from control, obese, and NIDDM subjects. *Diabetes* 1990; 39:250–9.
92 Moller DE, Yokota A, Flier JS. Normal insulin-receptor cDNA sequence in Pima indians with NIDDM. *Diabetes* 1989; 38:1496–1500.
93 Cocozza S, Porcellini A, Riccardi G *et al.* NIDDM associated with mutation in tyrosine kinase domain of insulin receptor gene. *Diabetes* 1992; 41:521–6.
94 Kusari J, Verma US, Buse JB, Henry RR, Olefsky JM. Analysis of the gene sequences of the insulin receptor and the insulin-sensitive glucose transporter (GLUT-4) in patients with common-type non-insulin-dependent diabetes mellitus. *J Clin Invest* 1991; 88:1323–30.
95 Taylor SI, Cama A, Accili D *et al.* Genetic basis of endocrine disease 1. Molecular genetics of insulin resistant diabetes mellitus. *J Clin Endocrinol Metab* 1991; 73: 1158–1163.
96 Kadowaki T, Kadowaki H, Rechler MM *et al.* Five mutant alleles of insulin receptor gene in patients with genetic forms of insulin resistance. *J Clin Invest* 1990; 86: 254–264.
97 Odawara M, Kadowaki T, Yamamoto R *et al.* Human diabetes associated with a mutation in the tyrosine kinase domain of the insulin receptor. *Science* 1989; 245: 66–68.
98 Kahn CR, Flier JS, Bar RS *et al.* The syndromes of insulin resistance and acanthosis nigricans. Insulin receptor disorders in man. *N Engl J Med* 1976; 294: 739–45.
99 Pedersen O, Hjøllund E, Beck-Nielsen H, Kromann H. Diabetes mellitus caused by insulin-receptor blockade and impaired sensitivity to insulin. *N Engl J Med* 1981; 304: 1085–8.

# 5 The Role of Protein Phosphorylation in Insulin Action

David E. Misek & Alan R. Saltiel

## INTRODUCTION

Despite significant advances in molecular and cellular endocrinology over the past few years, our understanding of the molecular events which couple the insulin receptor to the regulation of cellular metabolism lags far behind that of other polypeptide hormones. One likely explanation for this slow progress may lie in the complicated nature of insulin action. Indeed, the cellular effects of insulin are quite diverse, involving modulation of glucose and amino acid transport, activities of key enzymes in intermediary metabolism, rates of protein, DNA and RNA synthesis, transcription of specific genes and cellular growth and differentiation. These different effects are easily distinguished as a function of time course, dose response, the presence or absence of other hormones or the state of differentiation of the cell. This broad diversity of responses makes it improbable that a single mechanism could account for all of the actions of insulin. Instead, it is more likely that insulin action involves a network of interrelated and independent pathways with differing levels of divergence regarding mechanisms of regulation.

As it became clear that the well-recognised mechanisms of signal transduction (i.e. ion channels, cyclic nucleotides) were not primarily responsible for any of the actions of insulin, many investigators focused on the role of protein phosphorylation (1, 2). The insulin receptor itself is a tyrosine kinase that undergoes hormone-dependent autophosphorylation, resulting in increased activity (3, 4). Numerous experiments employing site-directed mutagenesis or anti-receptor antibodies indicate that receptor autophosphorylation is necessary for the full expression of insulin's activities (5–7). However, many of the downstream effects of the hormone appear to require changes in serine and threonine phosphorylation. Complicating matters further, numerous studies have shown that insulin simultaneously produces both the dephosphorylation of some proteins and the phosphorylation of others on serine and threonine residues (2, 8–22). There is general agreement that the dephosphorylation reactions induced by insulin are mediated by the acute stimulation of protein phosphatases (1, 2), and may play a critical role in regulating carbohydrate and lipid metabolism. Many of the metabolic actions of insulin in fat, liver and muscle cells are specifically attenuated by serine/threonine phosphatase inhibitors such as okadaic acid (23–29). The dephosphorylation of catabolic enzymes, such as hormone-sensitive lipase, result in their inactivation, whereas the dephosphorylation of anabolic enzymes, such as glycogen synthetase, result in their activation. The impact of insulin-induced serine phosphorylation on metabolic pathways is less certain, although processes such as glucose transport, protein synthesis and cellular growth may require stimulation of kinase activities (2). These and other observations have led to the emerging concept that two parallel pathways, involving activation of both protein phosphatases and kinases, may mediate many of insulin's actions (Fig. 5.1).

The precise mechanisms involved in translating the tyrosine kinase activity of the insulin receptor into downstream activation of serine/threonine kinases and phosphatases remain uncertain. Two major hypotheses have been proposed for the coupling of the insulin receptor to these enzymes: 1) non-covalent interactions of the receptor with effector proteins that produce diffusible second messengers capable of allosteric modulation of kinases and phosphatases (30), and 2) a phosphorylation cascade, in which the receptor tyrosine kinase phosphorylates intermediate serine/threonine kinases or kinase modulators (31). These two pathways need not be mutually exclusive, and may, in fact, operate synergistically to coordinate the complex pattern of protein phosphorylation that is induced by insulin.

Evaluation of an insulin-induced phosphorylation cascade has centred on the identification of serine/threonine kinases that are regulated by covalent modification in response to insulin. Several such enzymes have been found, providing the groundwork for a well-characterised cas-

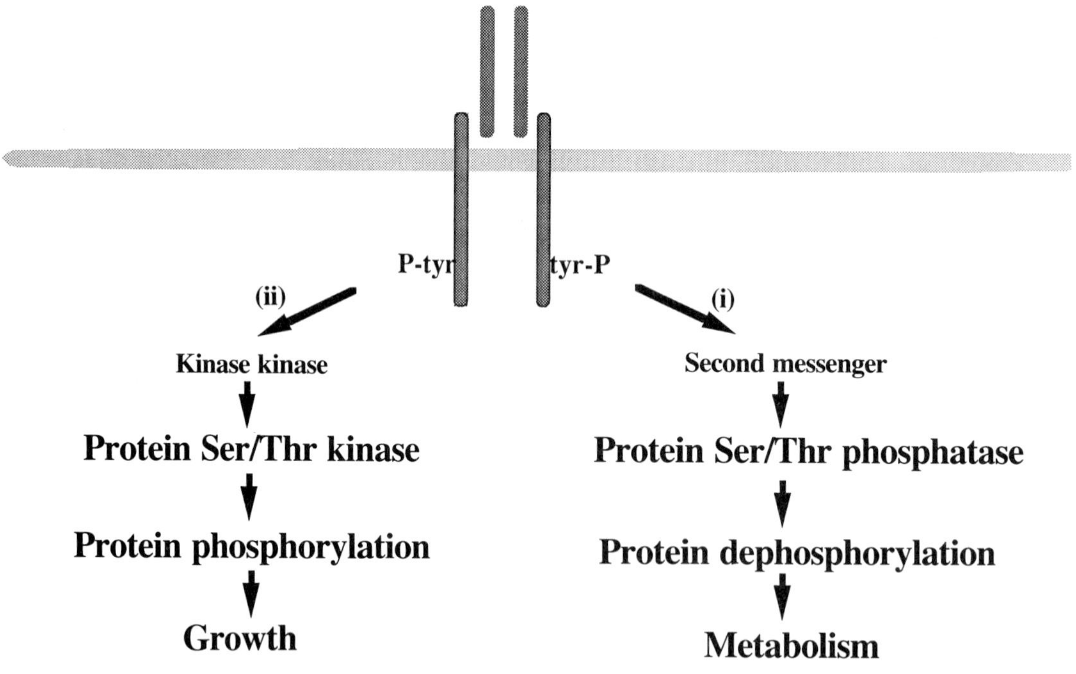


Fig. 5.1. The paradoxical effects of insulin on protein phosphorylation. Insulin simultaneously produces increases in the serine/threonine phosphorylation of some proteins, and decreases in others. This paradoxical effect may result from the activation of both kinases and phosphatases. Depicted here is a hypothetical scheme consisting of two separate biochemical pathways to explain these effects: i) the generation of a soluble second messenger that directly or indirectly activates a serine/threonine phosphatase; and ii) the stimulation of a cascade of protein kinases, resulting in the phosphorylation of cellular proteins.

cade of phosphorylations (4, 32–34). The search for an insulin-dependent 'second messenger' has been underway since the early 1970s. An insulin-sensitive substance was first detected in skeletal muscle that could acutely modulate glycogen synthetase activity *in vitro*, by stimulating the dephosphorylation of the enzyme (30). Similar kinds of extracts or substances of elusive chemical identity were subsequently identified in a variety of cell types and reported capable of regulating the activities of several insulin-sensitive enzymes (35–41). Although these enzyme-modulating activities were detected in several laboratories, there were inconsistencies in their reported properties, and little progress was made in the elucidation of chemical composition or structure.

## INSULIN-DEPENDENT DEPHOSPHORYLATION REACTIONS MAY BE MEDIATED BY NOVEL SECOND MESSENGERS

### Characterisation of glycosyl-phosphatidylinositol

The search for a defined chemical substance that could mediate some of the metabolic actions of insulin resulted initially in the purification of two structurally similar substances that were released from hepatic plasma membranes in response to insulin (42). Their relative hydrophilicity, negative charge, apparent molecular weight of 800–1000 daltons, and sensitivity to periodate and nitrous acid suggested an oligosaccharide phosphate structure. Preliminary compositional analysis revealed inositol as a component, although the known inositol phosphates did not share the chemical properties, chromatographic or electrophoretic behaviour, or insulin sensitivity of this factor, indicating that it might be an unusual derivative containing inositol phosphate.

A potential clue to the structure of this molecule emerged when a glycosylated derivative of inositol was found in certain cell surface proteins. This novel molecular species was shown to result from a covalent bond between certain proteins and phosphatidylinositol (PI), serving as an anchor for attachment to the plasma membrane (43). The protein is coupled via an amide bond to ethanolamine which is then attached through a phosphodiester linkage to an oligosaccharide that exhibits a terminal non-N-acetylated hexosamine glycosidically linked to the inositol ring of PI. The membrane-bound form of the protein can be converted to a water-soluble form that contains a C-terminal glycosyl-inositol phosphate by digestion with a bacterial PI-specific phospholipase C (PLC) (44), with the simultaneous liberation of diacylglycerol.

The first indication that the insulin-dependent enzyme modulators might arise from the hydrolysis of a structurally similar glycolipid emerged from the demonstration that the PI-specific bacterial PLC generated a substance from rat liver plasma membranes that was chemically identical to that produced in response to insulin (42, 45, 46). Moreover, a potential precursor of the PI-PLC-generated glycan was identified in a number of cell types, characterised by enzymatic and chemical means (42, 47–49), as well as sensitivity to hormones (42, 45, 46). This, or similar molecules, have been isotopically labelled with inositol (45, 46), glucosamine (45, 46, 48, 50), phosphate (48, 50, 51), and saturated fatty acids (45, 46, 48, 50), and was chemically labelled with isoethionyl acetimidate (52, 53). In addition to insulin, other hormones and growth factors, including IGF-1, EGF, NGF, ACTH and TSH have been shown to stimulate the turnover of the lipid in a variety of cell types (54–59).

While insulin is known to cause increased labelling of several phospholipids (60–64), it does not acutely stimulate the hydrolysis of the polyphosphoinositides, and it does not induce calcium mobilisation through the generation of inositol trisphosphate (63, 65). These observations suggested that the insulin-sensitive hydrolysis of glycosyl-PI results from the activation of a glycosyl-PI-specific PLC. Such an enzyme was isolated from a plasma membrane fraction of liver, using as an assay the liberation of diacylglycerol from the glycosyl-PI-anchored variant surface glycoprotein (VSG) from *Trypanosoma brucei* (66). The catalytic activity of this enzyme appears to reside in a single polypeptide with an apparent molecular weight of about 52 kD. The enzyme is calcium-independent, and it is specific for glycosyl-PI; no hydrolysis of PI, $PIP_2$, or other phospholipids is observed under a variety of conditions. Although there is still no information available on the primary sequence or sub-cellular localisation of the mammalian glycosyl-PI-specific PLC, the cDNA for an enzyme with similar specificity was cloned and sequenced from *Trypanosoma brucei* (67). Interestingly, both immunohistochemical data and the predicted amino acid sequence indicate a cytoplasmic orientation for this parasitic enzyme.

## Structural features of inositol phosphate glycans

Considerable interest has been focused on the precise structure and biosynthesis of the glycosyl-PI precursor, and on its relationship to the glycosyl-PI protein anchor. Comparison of compositional analyses from several laboratories has indicated certain conserved and variant features. The precursor glycolipid appears to contain a basic core structure of PI-hexosamine. Species identified in T-lymphocyte and $BC_3H1$ cells appear to contain diacylglycerol as the major glycerolipid moiety (45, 46, 68, 69), although in hepatoma cells a 1,2-alkylacylglycerol structure has been suggested (70). More recent studies have indicated the presence of significant but variable amounts of *chiro*inositol, which perhaps accounts for the apparent lack of $[^3H]$*myo*-inositol labelling in some cell types (48, 71). In fact, deficiencies in cellular and circulating *chiro*-inositol levels have recently been proposed to contribute to insulin resistance associated with NIDDM (72–74). Distal to the hexosamine there appears to be considerable heterogeneity in glycan composition, although the structural basis of this heterogeneity is unclear (47).

The insulin-sensitive glycosyl-PI appears to share the core structure of the glycosyl-PI protein anchor. The two types of glycolipid contain similar glycerolipid domains, sensitivity to PI-PLC and nitrous acid, the presence of inositol, non-acetylated glucosamine, and a variable glycan region (43). An antibody raised against a degalactosylated glycan fragment derived from a *T. brucei* VSG membrane anchor selectively inhibited some actions of insulin in intact $BC_3H1$ myocytes (75). Conversely, an antibody raised against an insulin-sensitive glycosyl-PI derived from rat liver recognises hormone-sensitive glycosyl-PI molecules in T-lymphocytes and specifically binds to the Thy-1 glycosyl-PI membrane anchor (47).

Although the topological distribution of the insulin-sensitive glycolipid in the plasma membrane remains uncertain, Alvarez *et al.* (52) have suggested an extracellular location for the lipid, based upon surface labelling experiments. In addition, Romero *et al.* (75) reported that exposure of $BC_3H1$ myocytes to an antibody raised against a glycan fragment from a *Trypanosoma brucei* VSG membrane anchor selectively inhibited some actions of insulin, suggesting that the glycan is released from cells upon insulin addition. In this regard, PI-PLC can exert insulin-like effects on intact cells (76), exogenous addition of purified inositol glycan to intact cells mimics many of the effects of insulin (19, 76–82), and insulin can stimulate the release of certain glycosyl-PI anchored proteins from the cell surface (83, 84). However, the notion that glycosyl-PI hydrolysis and release of the inositol glycan occurs extracellularly remains to be conclusively demonstrated.

## Coupling of the insulin receptor to glycosyl-PI hydrolysis

Despite the purification of a glycosyl-PI-specific PLC, it has thus far been difficult to directly demonstrate the activation of this enzyme by insulin. Two separate studies indicate that the tyrosine kinase activity of the receptor is necessary for glycosyl-PI hydrolysis (85, 86), although we have been unable to detect changes in the phosphorylation state of the enzyme (unpublished observations). It is conceivable that receptor autophosphorylation could catalyse an intramolecular conformational change initiating a non-covalent interaction with some as of yet unidentified regulatory factor, as suggested by studies with insulin-mimetic anti-receptor antibodies that do not stimulate receptor tyrosine kinase activity (87, 88). Although the identity of this coupling factor remains unknown, some evidence indicates a role for heterotrimeric G proteins, as indicated by the blockade of glycosyl-PI hydrolysis (89–91) and insulin-dependent antilipolysis (92, 93) with pertussis toxin.

## The inositol glycan activates a Type 1 serine/threonine phosphatase

Initial studies on the biological activities of the inositol glycan focused on the insulin-sensitive, low $K_m$ cAMP phosphodiesterase in fat cell membranes (94). The activity of this cAMP phosphodiesterase was stimulated acutely by the glycan, as reflected by an increase in the $V_{max}$ of the enzyme, with no appreciable effect on its $K_m$ (49). The purified glycan could also modify *in vitro* other insulin-sensitive enzymes assayed in sub-cellular fractions (42, 49, 95). Although the precise biochemical mechanism(s) involved in the regulation of these enzymes was not determined, some data suggested that phosphorylation of the enzyme or closely related regulatory factors might be involved.

To evaluate the insulin-mimetic properties of the inositol glycans in more detail, these compounds have been added to intact fat, liver or muscle cells. Inositol glycans isolated from insulin-treated cells or membranes mimic the lipogenic (76, 96) and antilipolytic (27, 81) actions of insulin, stimulate pyruvate kinase (78) and pyruvate dehydrogenase (79), inhibit PEPCK transcription (97), hepatic glucose output (27), phosphorylase a (78) and cAMP levels (78), and produce alterations in protein phosphorylation patterns similar to that observed with insulin (77, 98). In order to evaluate the structure/function relationship of these compounds, a structurally similar glycan derived from the VSG glycosyl-PI anchor has been utilised. This glycan mimics the antilipolytic and antigluconeogenic actions of insulin in fat and liver cells (27). Like insulin, this inositol glycan specifically attenuated the phosphorylation of the major isoproterenol-stimulated 70 kD phosphoprotein in adipocytes (98). The differential sensitivity of this dephosphorylation reaction to various inhibitors in intact cells and cellular homogenates indicated that dephosphorylation of the 70 kD protein results from the specific activation of a Type 1 serine/threonine phosphatase in adipocytes. Interestingly, this 70 kD protein was the only phosphoprotein dephosphorylated in response to the glycan (98).

## Inositol glycans as second messengers of insulin action

Despite the progress made in identifying the structure and biogenesis of the inositol glycans, it is still premature to regard these compounds as second messengers for any of the actions of insulin. The apparent insulin dependency, rapidity of action, and extent of the generation of the inositol glycans are consistent with the properties expected for second messengers. However, many questions remain concerning their precise structures as well as the nature of their insulin-mimetic properties. Although the insulin-mimetic actions of the inositol glycan on intact cells suggest that this substance might exert its metabolic effects after entering the cell, its chemical structure suggests that passive transport is unlikely. Interestingly, at millimolar concentrations mannose, glucosamine, and inositol monophosphate block the lipogenic effect of insulin and the inositol glycan in intact adipocytes (76, 96), but are ineffective in attenuating the stimulation of cAMP phosphodiesterase activity in adipocyte membranes (76). This observation suggests the possible existence of an active transport system that specifically recognises the inositol glycan.

Although the inositol glycan appears to be a promising candidate for a second messenger of insulin action, a number of issues remain to be resolved. The ultimate proof of a role for these compounds as second messengers will critically depend, among other things, on the determination of their precise structures. This may be complicated by the chromatographic resolution of multiple species of these molecules, perhaps reflecting the existence of distinct forms with different enzyme-modulating functions. It will also be important to produce these compounds in large quantity and homogeneous form, perhaps by organic synthesis (99). The biosynthetic route, mode of production and degradation, relationship to the insulin receptor, and the precise biochemical actions of these molecules need further exploration. Moreover, the evaluation of the metabolism of glycosyl-PI in pathological states of insulin resistance may lead to the identification of possible critical post-receptor defects in diabetes.

## INSULIN-DEPENDENT PHOSPHORYLATION REACTIONS MAY RESULT FROM A CASCADE OF KINASES

### Tyrosine phosphorylated substrates of the insulin receptor

The tyrosine kinase activity of the insulin receptor has been well characterised, including the mapping of the key autophosphorylation sites (for review, see 3, 4). The search for exogenous tyrosine kinase substrates of the insulin receptor has yielded several phosphoproteins, including major species with $M_r$s of 15, 20, 46, 62, 120 and 185 kD (100–105). cDNAs for two of these proteins have been cloned. The 120 kD protein has been identified as a liver-specific bile glycoprotein, with a single transmembrane domain and an ectoATPase activity (102, 106). Cloning of the cDNA for the 185 kD protein, known as insulin receptor substrate-1 (IRS-1), revealed 14 potential tyrosine phosphorylation sites, many of which reside within a presumed consensus sequence (YMXM) for binding to the *src* homology (SH)2 domain of the 85 kD regulatory subunit of PI-3′kinase (105, 107). Recent data indicate that phosphorylation of IRS-1 initiates its association with p85, resulting in the activation of PI-3′kinase (108–112). This enzyme is similarly activated by virtually all tyrosine kinase receptors (113–120), and may play a role in membrane trafficking (121). Although the precise role of this lipid kinase in insulin action remains unknown, recent experiments indicate that it may be necessary (122), but not sufficient (123, 124), for some of the growth-promoting effects of insulin.

Another substrate of the insulin receptor that has received much attention is the product of the *shc* gene (125–127). The proteins encoded by this gene, with $M_r$s of 46, 52 and 66 kD, are tyrosine phosphorylated in response to insulin in fibroblasts overexpressing the insulin receptor (128). Although the precise functions of these proteins remain unclear, they have been linked to the activation of the $p21^{ras}$ proto-oncogene by growth factors (127, 129). In addition to serving as phosphorylation targets for receptor kinases, these proteins contain SH2 domains, probably mediating interactions with other phosphoproteins. Phosphorylation of Shc induces its association with Grb2/ASH, another SH2 protein thought to be involved in activation of ras (127). Recent experiments indicate that shc phosphorylation and association with Grb2 indeed correlates with *ras* activation in PC-12 cells (124) or quiescent rat embryo fibroblasts (129) expressing growth factor receptors.

### Insulin stimulates serine kinases via a phosphorylation cascade.

A number of different insulin-sensitive serine kinases has been identified, found in both membrane and soluble fractions from insulin-treated cells (reviewed in 32). Among the best characterised are casein kinase II (130–135), glycogen synthase kinase 3 (136), ribosomal S6 kinase I (137) and II (138), the *raf* proto-oncogene (139) and the mitogen activated protein (MAP) kinases or ERKs (140, 141). The cascade of events leading to the activation of this latter class of kinases has been extensively studied. Although the precise role of these enzymes in cellular regulation has yet to be determined, an important role is suggested in the actions of various mitogenic stimuli (142–162). Evaluation of the substrate specificity of MAP kinase *in vitro* revealed that the enzyme can phosphorylate microtubule associated protein-2 (163), myelin basic protein (142, 151, 164, 165), ribosomal S6 kinase II (140, 163, 166–168) and a growing number of transcription factors (169, 170).

MAP kinase requires both tyrosine and threonine phosphorylation for full activation (164, 171–179). These phosphorylations are catalysed by a specific kinase, known as MEK, which is highly specific for MAP kinases (180). MEK is stimulated by exposure of cells to numerous mitogenic and differentiative stimuli (171, 176, 179, 180–183), including insulin (178, 184). A cDNA clone for MEK has been obtained, and it exhibits sequence homology to the byrl and STE7 gene products of *S. pombe* and *S. cerevisiae* (181, 185–187). Although the specific pathways by which growth factors and phorbol esters activate this enzyme remain unknown, recent reports (188, 189) indicate that MEK is itself activated by serine phosphorylation, due to the activity of another upstream kinase. Some experiments have indicated a role for the *raf* protooncogene, a serine kinase activated by both receptor and oncogenic tyrosine kinases, including insulin (189–191) It is important to note, however, that the role of *raf* in the MAP kinase pathway is far from proven, and the possibility remains that an intermediate kinase resides between *raf* and MEK on this pathway.

In addition to the uncertainty regarding the mechanism of MAP kinase activation, the biochemistry of *raf* activation remains an enigma. Increased activity is usually accompanied by enhanced serine and threonine phosphorylation of the enzyme (192–195), although it is still unclear whether this phenomenon reflects autophosphorylation. Considerable evidence now indicates that activation of the *ras* protooncogene is a prerequisite for *raf* activation (196, 197), as well as for activation of MAP kinase and MEK (197–199). Microinjection of neutralising anti-p21$^{ras}$ antibodies (200–202) or expression of dominant negative *ras* mutants (197, 199, 203–206) have revealed an absolute requirement for *ras* activation in the serine/threonine phosphorylations induced by many growth factors (197, 199, 200, 204, 205). Thus, the current dogma for insulin's growth-promoting effects consists of a linear pathway from receptor-shc/Grb2-*ras*-*raf*-X-MEK-MAPK (Fig. 5.2). The likelihood that this simple scheme accurately reflects the myriad of growth factor-induced phosphorylations remains unlikely, however, since it ignores countless numbers of other kinases, such as S6 kinase I, protein kinase C and others, as well as phosphatases, phospholipases and other effector molecules likely to play important modulatory roles.

## SIGNAL TRANSDUCTION IN INSULIN ACTION DIVERGES AT OR NEAR THE INSULIN RECEPTOR

Although the paradoxical ability of insulin to regulate both protein phosphorylation and dephosphorylation may account for its diverse effects on target cells, the precise site at which these signals diverge remains unknown. Differences in insulin's actions have been observed in cells expressing truncated (207–210) or mutant (5, 211–228) receptors, suggesting that discrete signals may emerge from the receptor itself. For example, site-directed mutagenesis of Tyr$^{1158}$ to Phe resulted in deficient receptor endocytosis, but normal stimulation of glycogen synthesis (225). In another study, mutation of two C-terminal tyrosines to phenylalanine resulted in a receptor with a normal glucose uptake and gly-

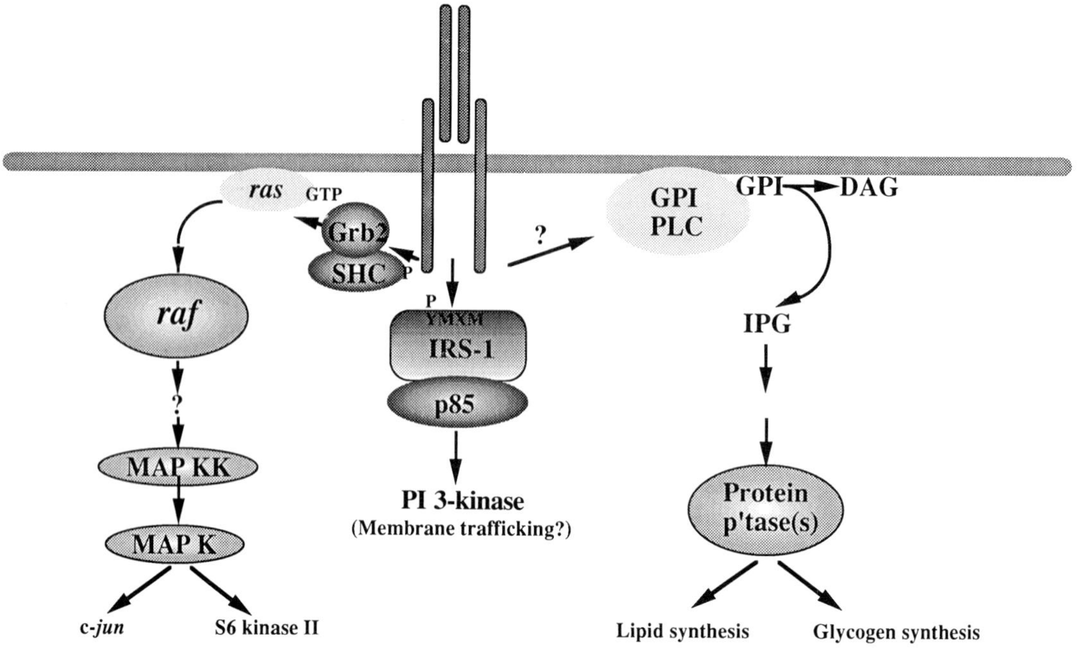


Fig. 5.2. Signal transduction in insulin action. A hypothetical scheme for the bifurcation of signals in insulin action is depicted. The insulin receptor undergoes tyrosine autophosphorylation and subsequent kinase activation upon hormone binding. The receptor phosphorylates intracellular substrates, including IRS1 and Shc proteins, which associate with SH2-containing proteins, such as p85 or Grb2, upon phosphorylation. Formation of the IRS1-p85 complex activates the enzyme PI-3′kinase. Formation of the Shc-Grb2 complex mediates the stimulation of $p21^{ras}$ GTP binding, leading to a cascade of phosphorylations. These phosphorylation events are likely to occur sequentially, involving the *raf* proto-oncogene, MAP kinase kinase, MAP kinase and S6 kinase II. The insulin receptor is separately coupled to the activation of a specific phospholipase C (PLC), that catalyses the hydrolysis of the glycosyl-PI molecules in the plasma membrane. A product of this reaction, inositol phosphate glycan (IPG), may act as an important second messenger, especially regarding activation of serine/threonine phosphatases, and the subsequent regulation of lipid and glucose metabolism.

cogen synthesis response to insulin (220), but enhanced sensitivity regarding mitogenesis (217), ribosomal S6 kinase (218), MAP kinase and MEK (227, 228) activation. A naturally occurring insulin receptor mutant was identified in an insulin resistant patient with a substitution of Ser for $Trp^{1200}$ (211, 213). Overexpression of this mutant receptor, which did not exhibit any insulin-dependent autophosphorylation, resulted in a phenotype that retained responsiveness regarding insulin-stimulated glucose transport and glycogen synthesis resembling that of wild-type transfected cells (213), but with insulin-responsive DNA synthesis (213), $p21^{ras}$) (229) and MAP kinase (158) resembling untransfected cells. Moreover, a PC-12 phaeochromocytoma cell line was described in which insulin was incapable of activating any of the enzymes involved in the MAP kinase pathway, including MAP kinase, MEK, *raf* or $p21^{ras}$ (123). In addition, insulin did not increase the phosphorylation of the shc proteins in these cells (124). In contrast, these cells do express functional insulin receptors that undergo autophosphorylation and produce substantial tyrosine phosphorylation of IRS-1, and activation of PI-3′kinase (120). Moreover, these cells responded metabolically to insulin, regarding glucose, lipid and protein synthesis. Taken together, these observations reinforce the possibility that ser/thr phosphorylation and dephosphorylation pathways play separate functions in insulin action, and furthermore that signalling diverges at, or near, the insulin receptor. However, a more complete understanding of the molecular dynamics of these processes will be required before elucidation of the underlying cellular defects in insulin resistance and related disorders.

## REFERENCES


1 Avruch J, Alexander MC, Palmer JL *et al.* Role of insulin-stimulated protein phosphorylation in insulin action. *Fed Proc* 1982; 41: 2622–33.
2 Denton RM. Early events in insulin actions. *Adv Cycl Nucl Prot Phosphoryl Res* 1984; 26: 293–341.
3 Goldfine ID. The insulin receptor: molecular biology and transmembrane signalling. *Endocr Rev* 1987; 8: 235–55.
4 Rosen, OM. After insulin binds. *Science* 1987; 237: 1452–8.
5 Chou CD, Cull TJ, Russel OS *et al.* Human insulin receptors mutated at the ATP binding site lack protein kinase activity and fail to mediate postreceptor effects of insulin. *J Biol Chem* 1987; 262: 1842–7.
6 Ellis L, Clauser E, Morgan DO, Edery M, Roth RA, Rutter WJ. Replacement of insulin receptor tyrosine residues 1162 and 1163 compromises insulin-stimulated kinase activity and uptake of 2-deoxyglucose. *Cell* 1986; 45: 721–9.
7 Morgan DO, Roth RA. Acute insulin action requires insulin receptor kinase activity: introduction of an inhibitory monoclonal antibody that inhibits the insulin receptor kinase. *Proc Natl Acad Sci USA* 1987; 84:41–5.
8 Larner J. Insulin and glycogen synthase. *Diabetes* 1971; 21:428–38.
9 Villar-Palasi C, Larner J. Insulin mediated effect on the activity of UDPG-glycogen transglucosylase in muscle. *Biochim Biophys Acta* 1960; 39:171–3.
10 Coore HG, Denton RM, Martin BR, Randle PJ. Regulation of adipose tissue pyruvate dehydrogenase by insulin and other hormones. *Biochemistry* 1971; 125: 115–27.
11 Jungas RL. Hormonal regulation of pyruvate dehydrogenase. *Metabolism* 1971; 20:43–53.
12 Stralfors, P, Fredrickson G, Olsson H, Belfrage P. Reversible phosphorylation of hormone-sensitive lipase in the hormonal control of adipose tissue lipolysis. *Horm Cell Regul* 1984; 8:153–62.
13 Claus TH, El-Maghrabi M, Pilkis SJ. Modulation of the phosphorylation state of rat liver pyruvate kinase by allosteric effectors and insulin. *J Biol Chem* 1979; 254: 7855–62.
14 Kennelly PJ, Rodwell VW. Regulation of 3-hydroxy-3-methylglutaryl coenzyme A reductase by reversible phosphorylation-dephosphorylation. *J Lipid Res* 1985; 26:903–14.
15 Jamil H, Madsen NB. Phosphorylation state of acetyl CoA carboxylase. *J Biol Chem* 1987; 262:638–42.
16 Krakower GR, Kim KH. Purification and properties of acetyl CoA carboxylase phosphatase. *J Biol Chem* 1981; 256:2408–13.
17 Thampy KG, Wakil SJ. Activation of acetyl CoA carboxylase. *J Biol Chem* 1985; 260:6318–23.
18 Witters LA. Insulin stimulates the phosphorylation of acetyl CoA carboxylase. *Biochem Biophys Res Commun* 1981; 100:872–8.
19 Witters LA Watts, TD. An autocrine factor from Reuber hepatoma cells that stimulate DNA synthesis and acetyl-CoA carboxylase: characterization of biologic activity and evidence for a glycan structure. *J Biol Chem* 1988; 263:8027–36.
20 Alexander MC, Kowaloff EM, Witters LA, Dennihy DT, Avruch J. Purification of a hepatic 120 000-dalton hormone stimulated $^{32}P$ peptide and its identification as ATP-citrate lyase. *J. Biol Chem* 1979; 256: 8052–6.
21 Brownsey RW, Denton RM. Evidence that insulin activates fat cell acetyl CoA carboxylase by increased phosphorylation at a specific site. *Biochem J* 1982; 202: 77–86.
22 Rosen OM, Rubin CS, Cobb MH, Smith CJ. Insulin stimulates the phosphorylation of ribosomal protein S6 in a cell free system derived from 3T3-L1 adipocytes. *J. Biol Chem* 1981; 256: 3630–3.
23 Aguis L, Peak M. Interactions of okadaic acid with insulin action in hepatocytes: role of protein phosphatases in insulin action. *Biochim Biophys Acta* 1991; 1095: 243–8.
24 Begum N, Sussman K E, Draznin B. Differential effects of diabetes on adipocytes and liver phosphotyrosine and phosphoserine phosphatase activities. *Diabetes* 1991; 40: 1620–9.
25 Corvera S, Japers S, Pasceri M. Acute inhibition of insulin-stimulated glucose transport by the phosphatase inhibitor, okadaic acid. *J Biol Chem* 1991; 266: 9271–5.
26 Hess SL, Suchin, CR, Saltiel AR. The specific protein phosphatase inhibitor okadaic acid differentially modulates insulin action. *J Cell Biochem* 1991; 45: 374–80.
27 Misek DE, Saltiel AR. An inositol phosphate glycan derived from a *Trypanosoma brucei* glycosylphosphatidylinositol mimics some of the metabolic actions of insulin. *J Biol Chem* 1992; 267: 16266–73.
28 Peak M, Aguis L. Insulin alters the sensitivity of glycogen synthesis to inhibition by okadaic acid, a protein phosphatase inhibitor. *Biochem Pharmacol* 1992; 43: 2307–11.
29 Rutter GA, Borthwick AC, Denton, RM. Effects of protein phosphatase inhibitors on the regulation of insulin-sensitive enzymes within rat epididymal fat pads and cells. *Biochem J* 1991; 276: 649–54.
30 Larner J, Galasko G, Cheng K *et al.* Generation by insulin of a chemical mediator that controls protein phosphorylation and dephosphorylation. *Science* 1979; 206: 1408–10.
31 Kasuga M, Karlsson FA, Kahn CR. Insulin stimulates the phosphorylation of the 95 000 dalton subunit of its own receptor. *Science* 1982; 215: 185–7.
32 Czech MP, Klarlund JK, Yagaloff KA, Bradford AP, Lewis, RE. Insulin receptor signaling. *J Biol Chem* 1988; 263: 11017–20.

33 Pillion DJ, Kim SJ, Kim H, Meezan E. Insulin signal transduction: the role of protein phosphorylation. *Am J Med Sci* 1992; 303: 40–52.
34 Saltiel AR. Second messengers of insulin action. *Diabetes Care* 1990; 13: 244–56.
35 Kiechle FL, Jarett L, Kotagal N, Popp DA. Isolation from rat adipocytes of a chemical mediator for insulin activation of pyruvate dehydrogenase. *Diabetes* 1980; 29: 852–5.
36 Saltiel AR, Jacobs S, Siegel M, Cuatrecasas P. Insulin stimulates the release from liver plasma membranes of a chemical modulator of pyruvate dehydrogenase. *Biochem Biophys Res Commun* 1981; 102: 1041–7.
37 Seals JR, Czech MP. Evidence that insulin activates an intrinsic plasma membrane protease in generating a secondary chemical mediator. *J Biol Chem* 1980; 255: 6529–31.
38 Parker JC, Kiechle FL, Jarett L. Partial purification from hepatoma cells of an intracellular substance which mediates the effects of insulin on pyruvate dehydrogenase and low $K_m$ cAMP phosphodiesterase. *Arch Biochem Biophys* 1982; 215: 339–44.
39 Saltiel AR, Siegel MI, Jacobs S, Cuatrecasas P. Putative mediators of insulin action: regulation of pyruvate dehydrogenase and adenylate cyclase activities. *Proc Natl Acad Sci USA* 1982; 79: 3513–17.
40 Saltiel AR, Doble A, Jacobs S, Cuatrecasas P. Putative mediators of insulin regulate hepatic acetyl CoA carboxylase activity. *Biochem Biophys Res Commun* 1983; 110: 789–95.
41 Suzuki S, Toyoto T, Suzuki H, Goto Y. A putative second messenger of insulin action regulates hepatic microsomal glucose-6-phosphatase. *Biochem Biophys Res Commun* 1984; 118: 40–6.
42 Saltiel AR, Cuatrecasas P. Insulin stimulates the generation from hepatic plasma membranes of modulators derived from an inositol glycolipid. *Proc Natl Acad Sci USA* 1986; 83: 5793–7.
43 Low MG, Saltiel AR. Structural and functional roles of glycosyl-phosphatidylinositol in membranes. *Science* 1988; 239: 268–75.
44 Low MG, Finean JB. Release of alkaline phosphatase from membranes by a phosphatidylinositol-specific phospholipase C. *Biochem J* 1977; 167: 281–4.
45 Saltiel, AR, Fox J A, Sherline P, Cuatrecasas P. Insulin stimulated hydrolysis of a novel glycolipid generates modulators of cAMP phosphodiesterase. *Science* 1986; 233: 967–72.
46 Saltiel AR, Sherline P, Fox JA. Insulin-stimulated diacylglycerol production results from the hydrolysis of a novel phosphatidylinositol glycan. *J Biol Chem* 1987; 262: 1116–21.
47 Gaulton GN. Differential regulation of glycosylated phosphatidylinositol subtypes by insulin. *Diabetes* 1991; 40: 1297–304.
48 Mato JM, Kelly KL, Abler A, Jarett L. Identification of a novel insulin-sensitive glycophospholipid from H35 hepatoma cells. *J Biol Chem* 1987*a*; 262: 2131–7.
49 Saltiel AR. Insulin generates an enzyme modulator from hepatic plasma membranes: regulation of cAMP phosphodiesterase, pyruvate dehydrogenase and adenylate cyclase. *Endocrinology* 1987; 120: 967–72.
50 Igareshi Y, Chambaz EM. A novel inositol glycophospholipid (IGPC) and the serum dependence on its metabolism in bovine adrenocortical cells. *Biochem Biophys Res Commu* 1987; 145: 249–56.
51 Merida I, Corrales FJ, Clemente R, Ruiz-Albusar JM, Villalba M, Mato JM. Different phosphorylated forms of an insulin-sensitive glycosylphosphatidylinositol from rat hepatocytes. *FEBS Lett.* 236: 251–5.
52 Alvarez JF, Varela I, Ruiz-Albusac JM, Mato JM. Localisation of the insulin-sensitive phosphatidylinositol glycan at the outer surface of the cell membrane. *Biochem Biophys Res Commun* 1988; 152: 1455–62.
53 Varela I, Alvarez JF, Clemente R, Ruiz-Albusac JM, Mato JM. Asymmetric distribution of the phosphatidylinositol-linked phospho-oligosaccharide that mimics insulin action in the plasma membrane. *Eur J Biochem* 1990; 188: 213–18.
54 Chan BL, Chao MV, Saltiel AR. Nerve growth factor stimulates the hydrolysis of glycosyl-phosphatidylinositol in PC-12 cells: a mechanism of protein kinase C regulation. *Proc Natl Acad Sci USA* 1989; 86: 1756–60.
55 Kojima I, Kitaoka M, Ogata E. Insulin-like growth factor-1 stimulates diacylglycerol production via multiple pathways in Balb/c 3T3 cells. *J Biol Chem* 1990; 265: 16846–50.
56 Merida I, Pratt JC, Gaulton GN. Regulation of interleukin 2-dependent growth responses by glycosylphosphatidylinositol molecules. *Proc Natl Acad Sci USA* 1990; 87: 9421–5.
57 Eardley DD, Koshland ME Glycosylphosphatidylinositol: a candidate system for interleukin-2 signal transduction. *Science* 1991; 251: 78–81.
58 Martiny L, Antonicelli F, Thuilliez B, Lambert B, Jacquemin C, Haye B. Control by thyrotropin of the production by thyroid cells of an inositol phosphate-glycan. *Cell Signalling* 1990; 2: 21–7.
59 Represa J, Avila MA, Miner C *et al.* Glycosylphosphatidylinositol/inositol phosphoglycan: a signaling system for the low-affinity nerve growth factor receptor. *Proc Natl Acad Sci USA* 1991; 88: 8016–19.
60 Detorrontegui G, Berthet J. The action of insulin on the incorporation of [$^{32}$P] phosphate in the phospholipids of rat adipose tissue. *Biochim Biophys Acta* 116: 477–81.
61 Farese RV, Cooper DR, Konda TS, Nair G, Standart ML, Pollet RJ. Insulin provokes coordinated increases in the synthesis of phosphatidylinositol, phosphatidylinositolphosphates and the phosphatidylinositol-glycan in $BC_3H1$ myocytes. *Biochem J* 1988*a* 256:185–8.
62 Manchester KL. Stimulation by insulin of incorporation of [$^{32}$P] phosphate and [$^{14}$C] acetate into lipid and protein of isolated rat diaphragm. *Biochim Biophys Acta* 1963; 70: 208–10.
63 Penington SR, Martin BR. Insulin-stimulated phosphoinositide metabolism in isolated fat cells. *J Biol Chem* 1985; 260: 11309–405.
64 Stein JM Hale CN. The effect of insulin on $^{32}$P incorporation into rat-fat cell phospholipids. *Biochim Biophys Acta* 1974; 337: 41–9.
65 Farese RV, Davis JT, Barnes DE *et al.* The de novo phospholipid effect of insulin is associated with increases in diacylglycerol, but not inositol phosphates or cytosolic Ca. *Biochem J* 1985*b*; 231: 269–78.
66 Fox JA, Soliz NM, Saltiel AR. Purification of a phosphatidylinositol-glycan specific phospholipase C from

liver plasma membranes: a possible target of insulin action. *Proc Natl Acad Sci USA* 1987; 84: 2663–7.
67 Hereld D, Hart, GW, Englund PT. cDNA encoding the glycosyl-phosphatidylinositol-specific phospholipase C of *Trypanosoma brucei*. *Proc Natl Acad Sci USA* 1988 85: 8914–18.
68 Gaulton GN, Kelly KL, Pawlowski J, Mato JM, Jarett L. Regulation and function of an insulin-sensitive glycosyl-phosphatidylinositol during T lymphocyte activation. *Cell* 1988; 538: 963–70.
69 Farese RV, Cooper DR, Konda TS *et al*. Mechanisms whereby insulin increases diacylglycerol in $BC_3H1$ myocytes. *Biochem J* 1988*b*; 256: 175–84.
70 Mato JM, Kelly KL, Abler A *et al*. Partial structure of an insulin-sensitive glycophospholipid. *Biochem Biophys Res Commun* 1987*b*; 146: 764–72.
71 Larner J, Huang LC, Schwartz CFW *et al*. Rat liver insulin mediator which stimulates pyruvate dehydrogenase phosphatase contains galactosamine and d-*chiro*-inositol. *Biochem Biophys Res Commun* 1988; 151: 1416–26.
72 Ortmeyer HK, Bodkin NL, Lilley K, Larner J, Hansen BC. Chiroinositol deficiency and insulin resistance. I. Urinary excretion rate of chiroinositol is directly associated with insulin resistance in spontaneously diabetic rhesus monkeys. *Endocrinology* 1993*a*; 132: 640–5.
73 Ortmeyer HK, Huang LC, Zhang L, Hansen BC, Larner J. Chiroinositol deficiency and insulin resistance. II. Acute effects of d-chiroinositol administration in streptozotocin-diabetic rats, normal rats given a glucose load, and spontaneously insulin-resistant rhesus monkeys. *Endocrinology* 1993*b*; 132: 646–1.
74 Huang LC, Fonteles MC, Houston DB, Zhang C, Larner J. Chiroinositol deficiency and insulin resistance. III. Acute glycogenic and hypoglycemic effects of two inositol phosphoglycan insulin mediators in normal and streptozotocin-diabetic rats *in vivo*. *Endocrinology*, 1993; 132: 652–7.
75 Romero G, Gamez G, Huang LC, Lilley K, Luttrell L. Anti-inositol glycan antibodies selectively block some of the actions of insulin in intact $BC_3H1$ cells. *Proc Natl Acad Sci USA* 1990; 87: 1476–80.
76 Saltiel AR, Sorbara-Cazan LR. Inositol glycan mimics the action of insulin on glucose utilization in rat adipocytes. *Biochem Biophys Res Commun* 1987; 149: 1084–92.
77 Alemany S, Mato JM, Stralfors P. Phosphodephospho control by insulin is mimicked by a phospho-oligosaccharide in adipocytes. *Nature (Lond)* 1987; 330: 77–9.
78 Alvarez JF, Cabello MA, Feliu JE, Mato JM. A phospho-oligosaccharide mimics insulin action on glycogen phosphorylase and pyruvate kinase activities in isolated rat hepatocytes. *Biochem Biophys Res Commun* 1987; 147: 765–71.
79 Gottschalk WK, Jarret L. The insulinomimetic effect of the polar head group of an insulin-sensitive glycophospholipid on pyruvate dehydrogenase in both subcellular and whole cell assays *Arch Biochem Biophys* 1988; 261: 175–185.
80 Kelly KL, Merida I, Wong EHA, DiCenzo D, Mato JM. A phospho-oligasaccharide mimics the effect of insulin to inhibit isoproterenol-dependent phosphorylation of phospholipid methyltransferase in isolated adipocytes. *J Biol Chem* 1987*a*; 262:15285–90.
81 Kelly KL, Mato JM, Merida I, Jarett L. Glucose transport and antilipolysis are differentially regulated by the polar head group of an insulin sensitive glycophospholipid. *Proc Natl Acad Sci USA* 1987*b*; 84: 6404–7.
82 Witters LA, Watts TD, Gould GW, Lienhard GE, Gibbs EM. Regulation of protein phosphorylation by insulin and an insulin-mimetic oligosaccharide in 3T3-L1 adipocytes and FaO hepatoma cells. *Biochem Biophys Res Commun* 1987; 153: 992–8.
83 Chan BL, Lisanti MP, Rodriguez-Boulan E, Saltiel AR. Insulin-stimulated release of lipoprotein lipase by metabolism of its phosphatidylinositol anchor. *Science* 1988; 241: 1670–72.
84 Lisanti, MP, Darnell JC, Chan BL, Rodriguez-Boulan E, Saltiel AR. The distribution of glycosyl-phosphoinositol anchored proteins is differentially regulated by serum and insulin. *Biochem Biophys Res Commun* 1989; 164: 824–32.
85 Suzuki S, Taneda Y, Hirai S, Yamamoto-Honda R, Toyota T. Mutated insulin receptor $val^{996}$ reduces insulin-dependent generation of inositol glycan and diacylglycerol. *Diabetes* 1992; 41: 1373–9.
86 Villalba M, Alvarez JF, Russel DS, Mato JM, Rosen OM. Hydrolysis of glycosyl-phosphatidylinositol in response to insulin is reduced in cells bearing kinase-deficient insulin receptors. *Growth Factors* 1990; 2:91–7.
87 Forsayeth JR, Caro JF, Sinha MK, Maddux BA, Goldfine ID. Monoclonal antibodies to the human insulin receptor that activate glucose transport but not insulin receptor kinase activity. *Proc Natl Acad Sci USA* 1987; 84:3448–53.
88 Hawley DM, Maddux BA, Patel RG *et al*. Insulin receptor monoclonal antibodies that mimic insulin action without activating tyrosine kinase. *J Biol Chem* 1989; 264:2438–44.
89 Luttrell L, Kilgour E, Larner J, Romero G. A pertussis toxin-sensitive G-protein mediates some aspects of insulin action in BC3H1 murine myocytes. *J Biol Chem* 1990; 265:16873–9.
90 Vila MC, Milligan G, Standaert ML, Farese RV. Insulin activates glycerol-3-phosphate acyltransferase (de novo phosphatidic acid synthesis) through a phospholipid-derived mediator. Apparent involvement of Gi alpha and activation of a phospholipase C. *Biochemistry* 1990; 29:8735–40.
91 Kilgour E, Larner J, Romero G. The generation of inositolglycan mediators from rat liver plasma membranes: the role of guanine nucleotide binding proteins. *Biochem Biophys Res Commun* 1992; 186:1151–7.
92 Lonnqvist F, Wennlund A, Arner P. Antilipolytic effects of insulin and adenylate cyclase inhibitors on isolated human fat cells. *Int J Obes* 1989; 13:137–6.
93 Saulnier-Blache JS, Dauzats M, Daviaud D *et al*. Late expression of alpha 2-adrenergic-mediated antilipolysis during differentiation of hamster preadipocytes. *J Lipid Res* 1991; 32:1489–9.
94 Saltiel AR, Steigerwalt RW. Purification of a putative insulin-sensitive cAMP phosphodiesterase or its catalytic domain from rat adipocytes. *Diabetes* 1986; 35: 698–704.
95 Kelly KL, Mato JM, Jarett L. The polar head group of a

novel insulin-sensitive glycophospholipid mimics insulin action on phospholipid methyltransferase. *FEBS Lett* 1986; 209:238–42.

96 Machicao F, Mushack J, Seffer E, Ermel B, Haring HU. Mannose, glucosamine and inositol monophosphate inhibit the effects of insulin on lipogenesis. Further evidence for a role for inositol phosphate-oligosaccharides in insulin action. *Biochem J* 1990; 266:909–16.

97 Alvarez L, Avila MA, Mato JM, Castano JG, Varela-Nieto I. Insulin-like effects of inositol phosphate-glycan on messenger RNA expression in rat hepatocytes. *Mol Endocrinol* 1991; 5:1062–8

98 Misek DE, Saltiel AR. An inositol phosphate glycan derived from a *Trypanosoma brucei* glycosyl-phosphatidylinositol activates a type-1 protein serine/threonine phosphate in rat epididymal adipocytes. *Endocrinology* (in press).

99 Plourde R, d'Alarcao M, Saltiel AR. Synthesis and characterization of insulin-mimetic disaccharide. *J Organic chem* 1992; 57: 2606–10.

100 Haring HU, White MF, Machicao F, Ermel B, Schleider E, Obermaier B. Insulin rapidly stimulates phosphorylation of a 46-kDa membrane protein on tyrosine residues as well as phosphorylation of several soluble proteins in intact fat cells. *Proc Natl Acad Sci USA* 1987; 84: 113–17.

101 Hresko RC, Hoffman RD, Flores-Riveros JR, Lane, MD. Insulin receptor tyrosine kinase-catalyzed phosphorylation of 422 (aP2) protein. Substrate activation by long-chain fatty acid. *J Biol Chem* 1990; 265: 21075–85.

102 Margolis RN, Tanner K, Seminara D, Taylor SI. Insulin receptors in developing rat liver. Receptor autophosphorylation and phosphorrylation of the endogenous substrate pp120/HA4 (ecto-ATPase) in fetal and neonatal liver. *biol Neonate* 1990; 58: 227–35.

103 Okamoto M, Karasik A, White MF, Kahn CR. Coordinate phosphorylation of insulin-receptor kinase and its 175,000-$M_r$ endogenous substrate in rat hepatocytes. *Diabetes* 1991; 40: 66-72.

104 Rothenburg PL, Lane WS, Karasik A, Backer J, White M, Kahn CR. Purification ans partial sequence analysis of pp185, the major cellular substrate of the insulin receptor tyrosine kinase. *J Biol, Chem* 1991; 266: 8302–11.

105 Sun XJ, Rothenberg P, Kahn CR *et al.* Structure of the insulin receptor substrate IRS-1 defines a unique signal transduction protein. *Nature Lond* 1991; 352: 73–7.

106 Najjar SM, Accili D, Philippe N, Jernberg J, Margolis R, Taylor SI. pp120/ecto-ATPase, an endogenous substrate of the insulin receptor kinase, is expressed as two variably spliced isoforms. *J Biol Chem* 1993; 268: 1201–6.

107 Myers MG Jr, Backer JM, Sun XJ *et al.* IRS-1 activates phosphatidylinositol 3′-kinase by associating with src homology 2 domains of p85. *Proc Natl Acad Sci USA* 1992; 89: 10350–4.

108 Backer JM, Myers MG Jr, Shoelson SE *et al.* Phosphatidylinositol 3′-kinase is activated by association with IRS-1 during insulin stimulation. *EMBO J* 1992; 11: 3469–79.

109 Giorgetti S, Ballotti R, Kowalski-Chauvel A, Cormont M, Van Obberghan E. Insulin stimulates phosphatidylinositol-3′-kinase activity in rat adipocytes. *Eur J Biochem* 1992; 207: 599–606.

110 Hadari YR, Tzahar E, Nadiv O *et al.* Insulin and insulinomimetic agents induce activation of phosphatidylinositol 3′-kinase upon its association with pp185 (IRS-1) in intact rat livers. *J Biol Chem* 1992; 267: 17483–6.

111 Hayashi H, Kamohara S, Nishioka Y *et al.* Insulin treatment stimulates the tyrosine phosphorylation of the 85-kDa subunit of phosphatidylinositol 3′-kinase *in vivo. J Biol Chem* 1992; 267: 22575–80.

112 Yonezawa K, Ueda H, Hara K *et al.* Insulin-dependent formation of a complex containing an 85-kDa subunit of phosphatidylinositol 3-kinase and tyrosine-phosphorylated insulin receptor substrate 1. *J Biol Chem* 1992; 267: 25958–66.

113 Bjorge JD, Chan T, Antczak M, Kung H, Fugita DJ. Activated type 1 phosphatidylinositol kinase is associated with the epidermal growth factor (EGF) receptor following EGF stimulation. *Proc Natl Acad Sci USA* 1990; 87: 3816–20.

114 Cantley LC, Auger KR, Carpenter C *et al.* Oncogenes and signal transduction. *Cell* 1991; 64: 281–302.

115 Endemann G, Yonezawa K, Roth RA. Phosphatidylinositol kinase or an associated protein is a substrate for the insulin receptor tyrosine kinase. *J Biol Chem* 1990; 265: 396–400.

116 Escobedo JA, Kaplan DR, Kavanaugh WM, Turck CW, Williams LT. A phosphatidylinositol-3′ kinase binds to platelet-derived growth factor receptors through a specific receptor sequence containing phosphotyrosine. *Mol Cell Biol* 1991; 11: 1125–32.

117 Hu P, Margolis B, Skolnick EY, Lammers R, Ullrich A, Schlessinger J. Interaction of phosphatidylinositol 3-kinase-associated p85 with EGF and PDGF receptors. *Mol Cell Biol* 1992; 12: 981–90.

118 Kaplan DR, Whitman M, Schaffhausen B *et al.* Common elements in growth factor stimulation and oncogenic transformation: 85 kD phosphoprotein and phosphatidylinositol kinase activity. *Cell* 1987; 50: 1021–9.

119 Ruderman N, Kapeller R, White MF, Cantley LC. Activation of phosphatidylinositol 3-kinase by insulin. *Proc Natl Acad Sci USA* 1990; 87: 1411–15.

120 Ohmichi M, Decker SJ, Saltiel AR. Activation of phosphatidylinositol-3 kinase by nerve growth factor involves indirect coupling ot the *trk* protooncogene with *src* homology 2 domains. *Neuron* 1992*a*; 9: 769–77.

121 Panayotou G, Waterfield MD. Phosphatidylinositol 3-kinase: a key enzyme in diverse signaling processes. *Trends Cell Biol* 1992; 2: 358–60.

122 Rose DW, Saltiel AR, Decker SJ. Majumdar M, Olefsky JM. IRS-1 is required for insulin-mediated mitogenic signal transduction. *Proc Natl Acad Sci USA* 1994; 91: 797–801.

123 Ohmichi M, Pang L, Ribon V, Saltiel AR. Divergence of signaling pathways for insulin in PC-12 pheochromocytoma cells. *Endocrinology* 1993; 133: 46–56.

124 Ohmichi M, Matuoka K, Takenawa T, Saltiel AR. Growth factors differentially stimulate the phosphorylation of shc proteins and their association with Grb2 in PC-12 pheochromocytoma cells. *J Biol Chem* 1994; 269: 1143–8.

125 Pelicci G, Lanfrancone L, Grigani F *et al.* A novel transforming protein (SHC) with an SH2 domain is implicated in mitogenic signal transduction. *Cell* 1992; 70: 93–104.

126 McGlade J, Cheng A, Pelicci PG, Pawson T. Shc proteins are phosphorylated and regulated by the v-Src and v-Fps protein-tyrosine kinases. *Proc Natl Acad Sci USA* 1992; 89: 8869–73.
127 Rozakis-Adcock M, McGlade J, Mbamalu *et al.* Association of the Shc and Grb2/Sem5 SH2-containing proteins is implicated in activation of the Ras pathway by tyrosine kinases. *Nature (Lond)* 1992; 360:689–92.
128 Pronk GJ, McGlade J, Pelicci G, Pawson T, Bos JL. Insulin-induced phosphorylation of the 46- and 52-kDa Shc proteins. *J Biol Chem* 1993; 268: 5748–5753.
129 Lowenstein EJ, Daly RJ, Batzer A *et al.* The SH2 and SH3 domain-containing protein GRB2 links receptor tyrosine kinases to ras signaling. *Cell* 1992; 70: 431–42.
130 Alemany S, Puerta J, Guadano A, Mato JM. Modulation of casein kinase II activity by the polar head group of an insulin-sensitive glycosyl-phosphatidylinositol. *J Biol Chem* 1990; 265: 4849–2.
131 Diggle TA, Schmitz-Peiffer C, Borthwick AC, Welsh GI, Denton RM. Evidence that insulin activates casein kinase 2 in rat epididymal adipocytes and that this may result in the increased phosphorylation of an acid-soluble 22 kDa protein. *Biochem J* 1991; 279: 545–1.
132 Klarlund JK, Czech MP. Insulin-like growth factor I and insulin rapidly increase casein kinase II activity in Balb/c 3T3 fibroblasts. *J Biol Chem* 1988; 263: 15872–5.
133 Maeda R, Raz I, Zurlo F, Sommercorn J. Activation of skeletal muscle casein kinase II by insulin is not diminished in subjects with insulin resistance. *J Clin Invest* 1991; 87: 1017–22.
134 Sommercorn J, Mulligan JA, Lozeman FJ, Krebs EG. Activation of casein kinase II in response to insulin and to epidermal growth factor. *Proc Natl Acad Sci USA* 1987; 84: 8834–8.
135 Villa-Moruzzi E, Crabb JW. Stimulation of FA and casein kinase II by insulin in 3T3-L1 cells. *Biochem Biophys Res Commun* 1991; 177: 1019–24.
136 Dent P, Lavoinne A, Nakielny S, Caudwell FB, Watt P, Cohen P. The molecular mechanism by which insulin stimulates glycogen synthesis in mammalian skeletal muscle. *Nature (Lond)* 1990; 348: 302–8.
137 Price DJ, Gunsalus JR, Avruch J. Insulin activates a 70-kDa S6 kinase through serine/threonine-specific phosphorylation of the enzyme polypeptide. *Proc Natl Acad Sci USA* 1990; 87: 7944–8.
138 Erikson E, Maller JL. *In vivo* phosphorylation and activation of ribosomal protein S6 kinases during *Xenopus* oocyte maturation. *J Biol Chem* 1989; 264: 13711–17.
139 Blackshear PJ, Haupt DM, App H, Rapp UR. Insulin activates the Raf-1 protein kinase. *J Biol Chem* 1990; 265: 12131–4.
140 Ray LB, Sturgil TW. Rapid stimulation by insulin of a serine/threonine kinase in 3T3-L1 adipocytes that phosphorylates microtubule-associated protein-2 *in vitro*. *Proc Natl Acad Sci USA* 1987; 84: 1502–6.
141 Ray LB, Sturgill TW. Characterization of insulin-stimulated microtubule-associated protein kinase. *J Biol Chem* 1988; 263: 12721–7.
142 Ahn NG, Weiel JE, Chan CP, Krebs EG. Identification of multiple epidermal growth factor-stimulated protein serine/threonine kinases from swiss 3T3 cells. *J Biol Chem* 1990; 265: 11487–94.
143 Bading H, Greenberg ME. Stimulation of protein tyrosine phosphorylation by NMDA receptor activation. *Science* 1991; 253: 912–14.
144 Bird TA, Sleath PR, deRoos PC, Dower SK, Virca GD. Interleukin-1 represents a new modality for the activation of extracellular signal-related kinases/microtubule-associated protein-2 kinases. *J Biol Chem* 1991; 266: 22661–70.
145 Boulton TG, Nye SH, Robbins DJ *et al.* ERKs: a family of protein-serine/threonine kinases that are activated and tyrosine phosphorylated in response to insulin and NGF. *Cell* 1991; 65: 663–75.
146 Cahill AL, Perlman RL. Activation of a microtubule-associated protein-2 kinase by insulin-like growth factor-I in bovine chromaffin cells. *J Neurochem* 1991; 57: 1832–9.
147 Campbell GS, Pang L, Miyasaka T, Saltiel AR, Carter-Su C. Stimulation by growth hormone of MAP kinase activity in 3T3-F442A fibroblasts. *J Biol Chem* 1992; 267: 6074–80.
148 Ely CM, Oddie KM, Litz JS *et al.* A 42-kD tyrosine kinase substrate linked to chromaffin cell secretion exhibits an associated MAP kinase activity and is highly related to a 42-kD mitogen-stimulated protein in fibroblasts. *J Cell Biol* 1990; 110:731–42.
149 Gomez N, Tonks NK, Morrison C, Harmer T, Cohen P. Evidence for communication between nerve growth factor and protein tyrosine phosphorylation. *FEBS Lett* 1990; 271:119–22.
150 Gotoh Y, Nishida E, Sakai H. Okadaic acid activates microtubule-associated protein kinase in quiescent fibroblastic cells. *Eur J Biochem* 1990*a*; 193:671–4.
151 Gotoh Y, Nishida E, Yamashita T, Hoshi M, Kawakami M, Sakai H. Microtubule-associated-protein (MAP) kinase activated by nerve growth factor and epidermal growth factor in PC12 cells. Identity with the mitogen activated MAP kinase of fibroblastic cells. *Eur J Biochem* 1990*b*; 193:661–9.
152 Haystead TAJ, Weiel JE, Litchfield DW, Tsukitani Y, Fischer EH, Krebs EG. Okadaic acid mimics the action of insulin in stimulating protein kinase activity in isolated adipocytes. *J Biol Chem* 1990; 265:16571–80.
153 Hoshi M, Nishida E, Sakai H. Activation of a $Ca^{2+}$-inhibitable protein kinase that phosphorylates microtubule-associated protein 2 *in vitro* by growth factors, phorbol esters, and serum in quiescent cultured human fibroblasts *J Biol Chem* 1980; 263:5396–401.
154 L'Allemain G, Sturgill TW, Weber MJ. Defective regulation of mitogen-activated protein kinase activity in a 3T3 cell variant mitogenically nonresponsive to tetradecanoyl phorbol acetate. *Mol Cell Biol* 1991; 11:1002–8.
155 Miyasaka T, Chao MV, Sherline P, Saltiel AR. Nerve growth factor stimulates a protein kinase in PC-12 cells that phosphorylates microtubule-associated protein-2. *J Biol Chem* 1990; 265:4730–5.
156 Nel A, Hanekom C, Rheeder A *et al.* Stimulation of MAP-2 kinase activity in T lymphocytes by anti-CD3 or anti-Ti monoclonal antibody is partially dependent on protein kinase C. *J Immunol* 1990; 144:2683–9.
157 Ohmichi M, Pang L, Decker SJ, Saltiel AR. Nerve growth factor stimulates the activities of the raf-1 and the mitogen-activated protein kinases via the trk protooncogene. *J Biol Chem* 1992*b* 267:14604–10.
158 Pang L, Lazar DF, Moller DE, Flier JS, Saltiel AR. The stimulation of pp42 map kinase by insulin does not

correlate with its metabolic actions in cells overexpressing mutant insulin receptors. *Biochem Biophys Res Commun* 1993; 196: 301–10.
159 Pavlovic-Surjancev B, Cahill AL, Perlman RL. Nicotinic agonists, phorbol esters, and growth factors activate two extracellular signal-related kinases, ERK1 and ERK2, in bovine chromaffin cells. *J Neurochem* 1992; 59: 2134–40.
160 Pelech SL, Tombes RM, Meijer L, Krebs EG. Activation of myelin basic protein kinases during echinoderm oocyte maturation and egg fertilization. *Dev Biol* 1988; 130: 28–36.
161 Sanghera J, Paddon H, Bader S, Pelech S. Purification and characterization of a maturation-activated myelin basic protein kinase from sea star oocytes. *J Biol Chem* 1990; 265: 52–7.
162 Tsao H, Aletta JM, Greene LA. Nerve growth factor and fibroblast growth factor selectively activate a protein kinase that phosphorylates high molecular weight microtubule-associated proteins. *J Biol Chem* 1990; 265: 15471–80.
163 Sturgill TW, Ray LB, Erikson E, Maller JL. Insulin-stimulated MAP-2 kinase phosphorylates and activates ribosomal protein S6 kinase II. *Nature* (*Lond*) 1988; 334: 715–18.
164 Anderson NG, Maller JL, Tonks NK Sturgill TW. Requirement for integration of signals from two distinct phosphorylation pathways for activation of MAP kinase. *Nature (Lond)* 1990; 343: 651–3.
165 Hoshi M, Nishida E, Sakai H. Characterization of a mitogen-activated, $Ca^{2+}$-sensitive microtubule-associated protein-2 kinase. *Eur J Biochem* 1989; 184: 477–6.
166 Ahn NG, Krebs EG. Evidence for an epidermal growth factor-stimulated protein kinase cascade in swiss 3T3 cells. *J Biol Chem* 1990; 265: 11495–501.
167 Chung J, Pelech SL, Blenis J. Mitogen-activated swiss mouse 3T3 RSK kinases I and II are related to $pp44^{mpk}$ from sea star oocytes and participate in the regulation of $pp90^{rsk}$ activity. *Proc Natl Acad Sci USA* 1991; 88: 4981–5.
168 Gregory JS Boulton TG, Sang BC, Cobb MH. An insulin-stimulated ribosomal protein S6 kinase from rat liver. *J. Biol Chem* 1989; 264: 18397–41.
169 Pulverer BJ, Kyriakis JM, Avruch J, Nikolakaki E, Woodgett JR. Phosphorylation of c-jun mediated by MAP kinases. *Nature (Lond)* 1991; 353: 670–4.
170 Alvarez E, Northwood IC, Gonzales FA *et al.* Pro–leu–ser/thr–pro is a consensus primary sequence for substrate protein phosphorylation. *J Biol Chem* 1991; 266: 15277–85.
171 Crews CM, Erikson RL. Purification of a murine protein-tyrosine/threonine kinase that phosphorylates and activates the ERK-1 gene product: relationship to the fission yeast byrl gene product. *Proc Natl Acad Sci USA* 1992; 89:8205–9.
172 Crews CM, Alessandrini A, Erikson RL. ERKS: their fifteen minutes has arrived. *Cell Growth Different* 1992*a*; 3:135–42.
173 Thomas G. MAP kinase by any other name smells just as sweet. *Cell* 1992; 68:3–6.
174 Pelech SL, Sanghera JS, Daya-Makin M. Protein kinase cascades in meiotic and mitotic cell cycle control. *Biochem Cell Biol* 1990; 68:1297–30.
175 Cobb MH, Boulton TG, Robbins DJ. Extracellular signal-related kinases: ERKS in progress. *Cell Regul* 1991; 2:965–78.
176 Adams PD, Parker PJ. Activation of mitogen-activated protein (MAP) kinase by a MAP kinase-kinase. *J Biol Chem* 1992; 267:13135–7.
177 Haystead TA, Dent P, Wu J, Haystead CM, Sturgill TW. Ordered phosphorylation of $p42^{mapk}$ by map kinase kinase. *FEBS Lett* 1992; 306:17–22.
178 Nakielny S, Cohen P, Wu J, Sturgill T. MAP kinase activator from insulin-stimulated skeletal muscle is a threonine/tyrosine kinase. *EMBO J* 1992; 11:2123–9.
179 Rossomando A, Wu J, Weber MJ, Sturgill TW. The phorbol ester-dependent activator of the mitogen-activated protein kinase $p42^{mapk}$ is a kinase with specificity for the threonine and tyrosine regulatory sites. *Proc Natl Acad Sci USA* 1992; 89:5221–5.
180 Seger R, Ahn NG, Posada J *et al.* Purification and characterization of mitogen-activated protein kinase activator(s) from epidermal growth factor-stimulated A431 cells. *J Biol Chem* 1992*a*; 267:14373–81.
181 Seger R, Seger D, Lozeman FJ *et al.* Human T-cell mitogen-activated protein kinase kinases are related to yeast signal transduction kinases. *J Biol Chem* 1992*b*; 267:25628–31.
182 Alessandrini A, Crews CM, Erikson RL. Phorbol ester stimulates a protein-tyrosine/threonine kinase that phosphorylates and activates the ERK-1 gene product. *Proc Natl Acad Sci USA* 1992; 89: 8200–8204.
183 L'Allemain G, Her J-H, Wu J, Sturgill TW, Weber MJ. Growth factor-induced activation of a kinase activity which causes regulatory phosphorylation of p42/microtubule-associated protein kinase. *Mol Cell Biol* 1992; 12: 2222–29.
184 Tobe K, Kadowaki T, Hara *et al.* Sequential activation of MAP kinase activator, MAP kinases and S6 peptide kinase in intact rat liver following insulin injection. *J Biol Chem* 1992; 267: 21089–97.
185 Crews CM, Allessandrini A, Erikson RL. The primary structure of MEK, a protein kinase that phosphorylates the ERK gene product. *Science* 1992b; 258: 478–80.
186 Ashworth A, Nakielny S, Cohen P Marshall C. The amino acid sequence of a mammalian MAP kinase kinase. *Oncogene* 1992; 7: 2555–6.
187 Wu J, Harrison JK, Vincent LA *et al.* Molecular structure of a protein–tyrosine/threonine kinase activating p42 mitogen-activated protein (MAP) kinase: MAP kinase kinase. *Proc Natl Acad Sci USA* 1993; 90: 173–7.
188 Kyriakis J, Brautigan DL, Ingebritsen TS, Avruch J. pp54 microtubule-associated protein-2 kinase requires both tyrosine and serine/threonine phosphorylation for activity. *J Biol Chem* 1991; 266: 10043–6.
189 Kyriakis J, App H, Zhang X-F *et al.* Raf-1 activates MAP kinase-kinase. *Nature* (*Land*) 1992; 358: 417–21.
190 Dent P, Haser W, Haystead TA, Vincent LA, Roberts TM, Sturgill TW. Activation of mitogen-activated protein kinase kinase by v-Raf in NIH 3T3 cells and *in vitro. Science* 1992; 257: 1404–7.
191 Lee RM, Cobb MH, Blackshear PJ. Evidence that extracellular signal-related kinases are the insulin-activated Raf-1 kinase kinases. *J Biol Chem* 1992; 267: 1088–92.
192 Izumi T, Tamemoto H, Nagao M, Kadowaki T, Takaku F, Kasuga M. Insulin and platelet-derived growth factor stimulate phosphorylation of the c-raf product at

serine and threonine residues in intact cells. *J Biol Chem* 1991; 266: 7933–9.
193 Kovacina KS, Yonezawa K, Brautigan DL *et al.* Insulin activates the kinase activity of the Raf-1 proto-oncogene by increasing its serine phosphorylation. *J Biol Chem* 1990; 265: 12115–18.
194 Lee RM, Rapp UR, Blackshear PJ. Evidence for one or more Raf-1 kinase kinase(s) activated by insulin and polypeptide growth factors. *J Biol Chem* 1991; 266: 103551–7.
195 Sozeri O, Vollmer K, Liyanage M *et al.* Activation of the c-Raf protein kinase by protein kinase C phosphorylation. *Oncogene* 1992; 7: 2259–62.
196 Troppmair J, Bruder JT, App H *et al.* Ras controls coupling of growth factor receptors and protein kinase C in the membrane to Raf-1 and B-Raf protein serine kinases in the cytosol. *Oncogene* 1992; 7: 1867–73.
197 Wood KW, Sarnecki C, Roberts TM, Blenis J. Ras mediates nerve growth factor receptor modulation of three signal-transducing protein kinases: MAP kinase, Raf-1, and RSK. *Cell* 1992; 68: 1041–50.
198 Hattori S, Fukuda M, Yamashita T, Nakamura S, Gotoh Y, Nishida E. Activation of mitogen-activated protein kinase and its activator by ras intact cells and in a cell-free system. *J Biol Chem* 1992; 267: 20346–51.
199 Thomas SM, DeMarco M, D'Arcangelo G, Halegoua S Brugge JS. Ras is essential for nerve growth factor- and phorbol ester-induced tryosine phosphorylation of MAP kinases. *Cell* 1992; 68: 1031–40.
200 Hagag N, Halegona S, Viola M. Inhibition of growth factor-induced differentiation of PC12 cells by microinjection of antibody to ras p21. *Nature (Lond)* 1986; 319: 680–2.
201 Mulcahy LS, Smith MR, Stacey DW. Requirement for ras proto-oncogene function during serum-stimulated growth of NIH 3T3 cells. *Nature (Lond)* 1985; 313: 241–8.
202 Williams NG, Roberts TM, Li P. Both $p21^{ras}$ and pp60v-src are required, but neither alone is sufficient, to activate the Raf-1 kinase. *Proc Natl Acad Sci USA* 1992; 89: 2922–26.
203 Robbins DJ, Cheng M, Zhen E, Venderbilt CA, Feig LA, Cobb MH. Evidence for a Ras-dependent extracellular signal-related protein kinase (ERK) cascade. *Proc Natl Acad Sci USA* 1992; 89: 6924–68.
204 Szeberenyi J, Cai H, Cooper GM. Effect of a dominant inhibitory Ha-ras mutation on neuronal differentiation of PC12 cells. *Mol Cell Biol* 1990; 10: 5324–32.
205 de Vries-Smits AM, Burgering BM, Leevers SJ, Marshall CJ, Bos JL. Involvement of p21ras in activation of extracellular signal-regulated kinase 2. *Nature (Lond)* 1992; 357: 602–4.
206 Medema RH, de Vries-Smits AM, Van der Zon GC, Maassen JA, Bos JL. Ras activation by insulin and epidermal growth factor through enhanced exchange of guanine nucleotides on $p21^{ras}$. *Mol Cell Biol* 1993; 13: 155–62.
207 McClain DA. Insulin action in cells expressing truncated or kinase-defective insulin receptors. Dissection of multiple hormone-signaling pathways. *Diabetes Care* 1990; 13: 302–16.
208 McClain DA, Maegawa H, Lee J, Dull TJ, Ullrich A, Olefsky JM. A mutant insulin receptor with defective tyrosine kinase displays no biologic activity and does not undergo endocytosis. *J Biol Chem* 1987; 262: 14663–71.
209 Thies RS, Ullrich A, McClain DA. Augmented mitogenesis and impaired metabolic signaling mediated by a truncated insulin receptor. *J Biol Chem* 1989; 264: 12820–5.
210 Maegawa H, McClain DA, Freidenberg G *et al.* Properties of a human insulin receptor with a COOH-terminal truncation. *J Biol Chem* 1988; 263: 8912–17.
211 Moller DE, Yokota A, Ginsberg-Fellner F, Flier JS. Functional properties of a naturally occuring trp1200–ser1200 mutation of the insulin receptor *Mol Endocrinol* 1990*a*; 4: 1183–91.
212 Moller DE, Yokota A, White MF, Pazianos AG, Flier JS. A naturally occuring mutation of insulin receptor alanine 1134 impairs tyrosine kinase function and is associated with dominantly inherited insulin resistance. *J Biol Chem* 1990*b*; 265: 14979–85.
213 Moller DE, Benecke H, Flier JS. Biologic activities of naturally occurring human insulin receptor mutations. *J Biol Chem* 1991; 266: 10995–1001.
214 Kadowaki T, Kadowaki H, Accili D, Yazaki Y, Taylor SI. Substitution of lysine for asparagine at position 15 in the α-subunit of the human insulin receptor. *J Biol Chem* 1990; 265: 19143–50.
215 Kadowaki T, Kadowaki H, Accili D, Yazaki Y, Taylor SI. Substitution of arginine for histidine at position 209 in the α-subunit of the human insulin receptor. *J Biol Chem* 1991; 266: 21224–31.
216 Rafaeloff R, Maddux BA, Brunetti A *et al.* Transmembrane signalling by insulin via an insulin receptor mutated at tyrosines 1158, 1162, and 1163. *Biochem Biophys Res Commun* 1991; 179: 912–18.
217 Takata Y, Webster NJ and Olefsky JM. Mutation of the two carboxyl-terminal tyrosines results in an insulin receptor with normal metabolic signaling but enhanced mitogenic signaling properties. *J Biol Chem* 1991; 266: 9135–9.
218 Takata Y, Webster NJ, Olefsky JM. Intracellular signaling by a mutant human insulin receptor lacking the carboxyl-terminal tyrosine autophosphorylation sites. *J Biol Chem* 1992; 267: 9065–70.
219 Accili D, Mosthaf L, Ullrich A, Taylor SI. A mutation in the extracellular domain of the insulin receptor impairs the ability of insulin to stimulate receptor autophosphorylation. *J Biol Chem* 1991; 266: 434–9.
220 Reynet C, Caron M, Magre J *et al.* Mutation of tyrosine residues 1162 and 1163 of the insulin receptor affects hormone and receptor internalization *Mol Endocrinol* 1990; 4: 304–11.
221 Odawara M, Kadowaki T, Yamamoto R *et al.* Human diabetes associated with a mutation in the tyrosine kinase domain of the insulin receptor. *Science* 1989; 245: 66–8.
222 White MF, Livingston JN, Backer JM *et al.* Mutation of the insulin receptor at tyrosine 960 inhibits signal transmission but does not affect its tyrosine kinase activity. *Cell* 1988; 54: 641–9.
223 Hari J, Roth RA. Defective internalization of insulin and its receptor in cells expressing mutated insulin receptors lacking kinase activity. *J Biol Chem* 1987; 262: 15341–4.
224 Cama A, Quon MJ, de la Luz-Sierra M, Taylor SI. Substitution of isoleucine for methionine at position 1153

in the beta-subunit of the human insulin receptor. A mutation that impairs receptor tyrosine kinase activity, receptor endocytosis, and insulin action. *J Biol Chem* 1992; 267: 8383–9.
225 Wilden PA, Siddle K, Haring E, Backer JM, White MF, Kahn CR. The role of insulin receptor kinase domain autophosphorylation in receptor-mediated activities. Analysis with insulin and anti-receptor antibodies. *J Biol Chem* 1992; 267: 13719–27.
226 Wilden PA, Kahn CR, Siddle K, White MF. Insulin receptor kinase domain autophosphorylation regulates receptor enzymatic function. *J Biol Chem* 1992; 267: 16660–8.
227 Ando A, Momomura K, Tobe K *et al.* Enhanced insulin-induced mitogenesis and mitogen-activated protein kinase activities in mutant insulin receptors with substitution of two COOH-terminal tyrosine autophosphorylation sites by phenylalanine. *J Biol Chem* 1992; 267: 12788–96.
228 Dickens M, Chin JE, Roth RA, Ellis L, Denton RM, Tavare JM. Characterization of insulin-stimulated protein serine/threonine kinases in CHO cells expressing human insulin receptors with point and deletion mutations. *Biochem J* 1992; 287: 201–9.
229 Osterop APRM, Medema RH, Bos JL *et al.* Relation between the insulin receptor number in cells, autophosphorylation and insulin-stimulated ras-GTP formation. *J Biol Chem* 1992; 267: 14647–53.

# 6 Glucose Transport Mechanisms

Mary N. Rosholt & Patricia A. King

## INTRODUCTION

D-Glucose is the major carbohydrate fuel used by mammalian cells. Some tissues, such as red blood cells and brain, depend almost entirely on glucose for their metabolic fuel. Others such as muscle and adipose use multiple fuels, with the use of glucose dependent on the presence of hormones such as insulin. The liver, on the other hand, can synthesise glucose (gluconeogenesis) as well as store glucose as glycogen. Whole-body glucose homeostasis is maintained jointly by these tissues through interactions with hormones and other systemic factors.

The transport of glucose across cell membranes is essential to its metabolism in the cell. There are two major types of glucose transporters: the Na-dependent transporters and the facilitative or Na-independent transporters. These membrane proteins provide transmembrane pathways for the hydrophilic glucose that would otherwise have poor permeability across the lipid bilayer. The Na-dependent glucose transporter is present in epithelia and is involved in the transepithelial movement of glucose in tissues such as the intestine and kidney. This transporter cotransports Na and glucose and concentrates glucose inside the cell. The facilitative transporters promote the movement of glucose down its concentration gradient, and include the insulin responsive transporters in muscle and adipose tissue. In the present chapter, both types of transporters are reviewed with respect to their cellular physiology, mechanism of operation, structure, and regulation.

## Na-DEPENDENT GLUCOSE TRANSPORT

### Cell physiology

Na-dependent glucose transport has been described in a number of epithelial tissues including the small intestine and kidney proximal tubule (1–3). These tissues are characterised by a Na-dependent transepithelial movement of glucose from the luminal solution to the blood, resulting in absorption in the intestine and reabsorption by the kidney. The Na-dependent transporter is located at the luminal membrane and couples the transport of glucose and sodium into the cell (Fig. 6.1). In this process, Na movement down its electrochemical gradient promotes the transport of glucose against its concentration gradient, resulting in glucose accumulation in the cell. The mechanism is defined as secondary active transport since net transport is dependent on the Na-gradient which is maintained by the

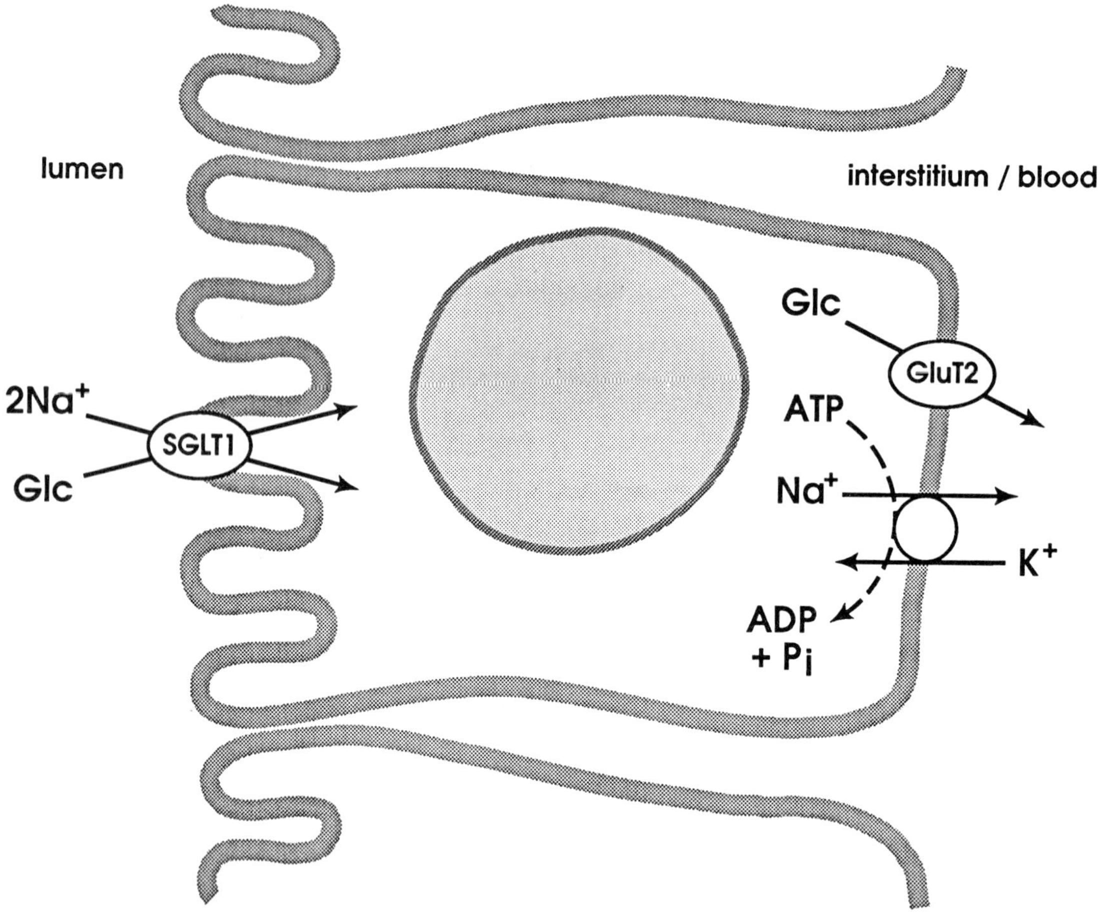


Fig. 6.1. Transepithelial transport of glucose. SGLT1 is the Na and glucose cotransporter located in the luminal membrane. GluT2 is a Na-independent transporter isoform located in the basolateral membrane. The Na–K ATPase is present in the basolateral membrane.

membrane Na–K ATPase. To complete the transepithelial flux, glucose inside the cell moves down its concentration gradient across the basolateral membrane, via a facilitative (Na-independent) glucose transporter. It is clear that the segregation of Na-dependent and Na-independent transporters to the luminal and basolateral membranes, respectively, is critical for efficient transepithelial transport. The polarity of epithelial cells and the targeting of proteins to the luminal vs. basolateral membrane is an area of current investigation (4).

Multiple Na-dependent glucose transporters have been identified in intestine and kidney, based on kinetic characteristics. For the intestine, functional studies have suggested the presence of two types of Na-dependent glucose transporters but only a single transporter, named SGLT1, has been cloned (5, 6). This transporter is present in both human and rabbit intestine, with 94% similarity in amino acid structure (7). Functional studies of SGLT1 expressed in Xenopus oocytes indicate that the transporter has a high affinity for glucose and transports two Na per one glucose (8). In humans, SGLT1 appears to account for the majority of intestinal glucose uptake. A specific missense mutation in SGLT1 is associated with glucose/galactose malabsorption, a human autosomal recessive disease in which there is a selective failure to absorb dietary glucose and galactose from the intestine (9). In the rodent kidney, there is functional and molecular evidence for two distinct Na-dependent glucose transporters (10–12). One is located in the early proximal convoluted tubule, and is responsible for the reabsorption of the bulk of the glucose filtered at the glomerulus. This transporter has a relatively high capacity but low affinity for glucose, and is characterised by a 1 : 1 stoichiometry for Na and glucose transport. The second transporter is located in the late proximal tubule and is responsible for the reabsorption of the final portion of glucose. This transporter is characterised by a lower capacity but higher affinity, and a 2 : 1 Na : glucose stoichiometry. The latter probably corresponds to SGLT 1 (12). Additional cloning studies indicate that a family of SGLT1-related proteins may exist (13).

## Mechanism

The Na-dependent glucose transporter is a cotransport system. Both Na and glucose are transported, and presence of one solute stimulates the transport of the other. Hopfer (2) has reviewed models for the kinetic mechanism of Na–glucose cotransport. These systems are complex and many assumptions are made in attempting to simplify them for analysis. In addition, variability in the reported stoichiometries of Na : glucose transported makes it difficult to present a single scheme. In general, the working models consider that the transporter can exist with the binding sites facing outward (extracellular) or inward (cytoplasmic), and with substrates bound or not bound. Transport then occurs by a sequence in which Na and glucose bind to the empty outward-facing transporter, followed by a conformational change that renders the binding site with bound substrates inward facing, followed by the dissociation of substrates from the transporter. Most kinetic data indicate an ordered, not random, sequence of Na and glucose binding in which the order of binding at one side of the membrane and dissociation at the other side are the same (14).

## Structure

Low abundance, hydrophobic membrane proteins like the Na–glucose cotransporter have been difficult to purify and therefore impossible to clone using traditional methods involving antibodies or oligonucleotide probes for screening cDNA libraries. As an alternative, Hediger and Wright (5,6), employed expression cloning in which poly-$(A)^+$-RNA from rabbit intestine was injected into *Xenopus laevis* oocytes, resulting in expression of Na-dependent glucose transport. After size selection of poly-$(A)^+$-RNA, the mRNA coding for the cotransporter was found to be in a 2.3 kb fraction. The complementary DNA was synthesised and further screened. A cDNA clone corresponding to the transporter, SGLT1, contained an open reading frame of 602 amino acids. Similar proteins have been identified in human intestine (7) and rabbit kidney (15), which share greater than 90% identity of amino acid sequences. Surprisingly, initial cDNA screening studies of human kidney have not identified a protein with equally high amino acid identity in this tissue (16). The primary structure of SGLT1 predicts a 73 kD protein with 11–12 membrane spanning signals. Radiation-inactivation studies (17,18) indicate that the cotransporter *in situ* in the brush border membrane functions as a 290 kD homotetramer comprised of four independent 73 kD subunits.

## Regulation of Na-dependent glucose transport

The Na-dependent glucose transporter(s) is generally thought to be insulin insensitive, although there are some reports of regulation of the intestinal brush border transporter by insulin, diet, and experimental diabetes. In animal models, both high carbohydrate diet and streptozotocin-induced diabetes result in increased intestinal glucose uptake associated with an increase in the number of Na-dependent glucose transporters in the luminal membrane (19, 20). Hyperinsulinaemia in rats has also been associated with increased intestinal glucose uptake, but the membrane site of regulation is not known (21).

Inherited disorders of Na-dependent glucose transport are known for both the kidney and intestine. Renal glycosuria is inherited as an autosomal trait, with both dominant and recessive patterns of inheritance in different families (22, 23). In this disorder glucose is excreted in the urine even though blood glucose concentrations are normal. The abnormality in tubular transport is specific for glucose and is not associated with impaired glucose transport in the intestine. In most cases, this disorder is benign.

Glucose–galactose malabsorption is an autosomal recessive trait characterised by a failure to absorb glucose and galactose from the intestinal lumen (23). The abnormality presents within the first weeks of life and is characterised by severe diarrhoea and dehydration. The problem is corrected by substituting fructose for glucose and galactose in the diet. Turk *et al.* (9) have found that the SGLT1 gene of these patients is characterised by a single missense mutation that results in a complete loss of Na-dependent glucose transport when tested *in vitro*.

## Na-INDEPENDENT (FACILITATIVE) GLUCOSE TRANSPORTER

### Cell physiology

The Na-independent or facilitative glucose transporter promotes the downhill movement of glucose across plasma membranes. These transporters are widely distributed in tissues, and recent studies from a number of laboratories have demonstrated that the proteins represent a family of glucose transporter proteins that are structurally related but have different kinetic and biochemical characteristics. Seven isoforms have been identified. The isoforms of the glucose transporter demonstrate tissue specificity and have been named by two conventions, one based on the order in which they were cloned and sequenced and the other on the tissue(s) in which they predominate (Table 6.1).

The GluT-1 and GluT-3 transporters are thought to have a fairly ubiquitous distribution, suggesting that these transporters play an important role in constitutive glucose transport. GluT-1 is detected to some degree in all tissues and is expressed in highest numbers in foetal tissues, brain, placental, and human red blood cells (24–26). In addition, it is the predominant transporter expressed by cells in culture. GluT-3 is expressed in greatest concentrations in brain, kidney, and placenta (27). Both transporters are characterised by a relatively high affinity for glucose, a property that is important in assuring an adequate supply of glucose to the brain and to the developing foetus *in utero*. It has been suggested that these transporters may serve separate functions in the brain, GluT-1 for glucose transport across the blood–brain barrier and GluT-3 for glucose uptake into neuronal cells (28).

GluT-2 is found in the liver, the pancreatic β-cell, and epithelial tissues such as the kidney and intestine (29). Unlike GluT-1 and GluT-3, GluT-2 is characterized by a relatively low affinity (30) which is important to the function of these tissues. The high $K_m$ value ensures that glucose transport will be fairly linear with glucose concentrations in the physiological range, making these cells more responsive to changes in plasma and cellular glucose. In kidney and intestinal cells these transporters are concentrated on the basolateral membrane and facilitate the movement of glucose from the cell, where it has been concentrated, into the extracellular space and blood (Fig. 6.1). In the liver, glucose may enter or exit the cell depending on the net balance of gluconeogenesis or glycogen synthesis/breakdown, and therefore the concentrations of glucose inside and outside the cell. In

Table 6.1. *Characteristics of glucose transporters*

| Numerical designation | Other names | Tissue distribution | Function | Kinetic properties | Insulin stimulation |
|---|---|---|---|---|---|
| SGLT1 | Na-dependent transporter | Intestine, kidney, other epithelia | Intestinal abs., renal reabsorption | Concentrative glucose transport with Na cotransport | – |
| GluT-1 | Erythrocyte, brain, HepG2 | Ubiquitous; highest in human RBC, brain, placenta | Basal glucose transport | High affinity | + |
| GluT-2 | Liver | Liver: β-cell: intestine, kidney | Uptake and release Glucose sensor Basolateral transport | Low affinity | – |
| GluT-3 | Foetal muscle | Brain, kidney, placenta | Basal glucose transport | High affinity | ? |
| GluT-4 | Insulin-regulatable (IRGT), fat/muscle | Skeletal muscle, adipocytes, heart | Hormone-responsive glucose transport | High affinity | +++ |
| GluT-5 | Fructose transporter | Intestine, spermatozoa | Fructose transport | Specific for fructose | – |
| GluT-6 | Pseudogene | | | | |
| GluT-7 | $T_3$ of the G-6-Pase system | Liver | Transport across endoplasmic reticulae | | – |

addition, after meals the liver and other tissues of the splanchnic bed are exposed to higher glucose concentrations via the portal system. For the pancreatic β-cell, a low affinity (high $K_m$) for glucose transport allows glucose entry into the cell to act as a sensor for changes in extracellular glucose concentration.

GluT-4 is found in the insulin-sensitive tissues, fat, skeletal muscle, and heart (31–35). This transporter isoform is specifically involved in the ability of insulin to stimulate glucose uptake, and also appears to be involved in the stimulation of glucose transport by exercise. The first studies of GluT-5 demonstrated a great abundance of this protein in the intestine where it was localised to the luminal membrane (36). It is now known that GluT-5 is specific for the transport of fructose (37), supporting the previous findings of Sigrist-Nelson and Hopfer (38) that fructose and glucose/galactose move across the intestinal brush border membrane by separate pathways. In addition, GluT-5 has been found to be in very high concentrations in human spermatozoa, and is likely responsible for the uptake of fructose by these cells (37).

GluT-6, cloned from human jejunum and foetal skeletal muscle libraries, has been identified as a pseudogene (36). The nucleotide sequence has approximately 80% identity with the GluT-3 transporter and the mRNA shows variable expression in all tissues. However, due to the presence of multiple nonsense codons and frameshifts, the sequence cannot encode a functional glucose transporter.

The GluT-7 isoform was cloned from a rat liver cDNA library (39). The amino acid sequence shows 68% identity with the GluT-2 isoform, with six extra amino acids at the C-terminus that include a consensus motif for retension of transmembrane proteins in the endoplasmic reticulum. Expression studies indicate that GluT-7 encodes a functional glucose transporter located in the endoplasmic reticulum that may be part of the glucose-6-phosphatase system.

## Mechanism

The mechanism of facilitative glucose transport has been studied most extensively for the GluT-1 transporter in human red blood cells (40, 41). In the working model of the transport mechanism, the transporter can exist in one of two alternating conformations, outward facing or inward facing (Fig. 6.2). In the outward facing conformation, $T_o$, the binding site for glucose is exposed to the extracellular medium. Following the binding of glucose ($T_oG$), the protein undergoes a conformational change converting to the inward facing conformation with glucose bound ($T_iG$). This transition involves small changes in the protein conformation, not gross flip flops or rotations of the transporter–substrate complex in the membrane. Glucose then dissociates from the transporter, forming $T_i$. The inward facing transporter ($T_i$) can then reconvert to form $T_o$ ((a) in Fig. 6.2) or can bind another glucose ($T_iG$), reconvert, and dissociate ((b) in Fig. 6.2). In the former case, a net transport of glucose will occur while in the latter, glucose will be exchanged across the membrane with no net transport. The rate of the total cycle of transport at saturating substrate concentration determines the carrier turnover number or intrinsic activity of the transporter.

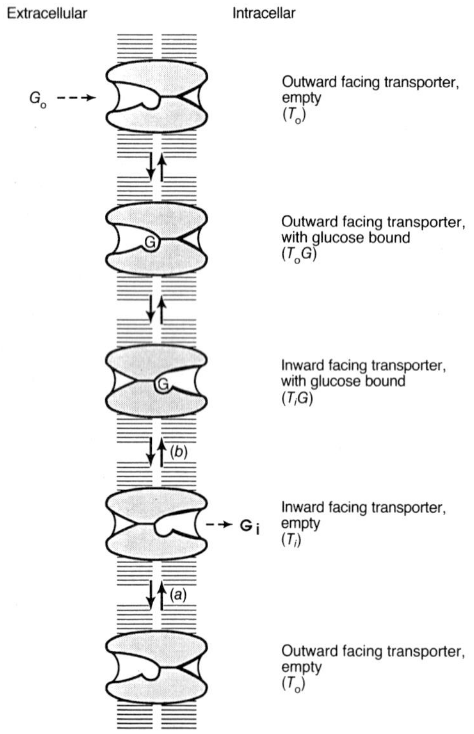


Fig. 6.2. Schematic representation of the mechanism of glucose transport by the facilitative (Na-independent) glucose transporter. The mechanism and (a) and (b) are described in the text.

Physiologically, the transporter will move glucose down its concentration gradient, but depending on the concentration of glucose inside and outside the cell, this process may involve net transport or net transport plus exchange of glucose. Thus in skeletal muscle, where intracellular free glucose is very low due to its rapid phosphorylation to glucose-6-phosphate, the gradient for glucose influx is high and net transport predominates. In the liver, on the other hand, intracellular glucose and extracellular glucose approach the same concentrations, and exchange activity as well as net transport will occur.

Several characteristics of the glucose transporter resulting from this mechanism are important for our understanding of transport measurements. First, the maximal velocity of influx ($V_{max}$) as well as the measured affinity of the transporter for substrate ($K_m$) are different when transport is measured under imposed conditions of net transport (no glucose on the opposite side of the membrane) versus equilibrium exchange transport (glucose present at equal concentrations on both sides). A very early observation of this transporter was that the presence of glucose inside the cell (equilibrium exchange) accelerates the uptake of glucose from the outside (42), likely reflecting a faster reconversion for the loaded carrier ($T_iG \rightarrow T_oG$) versus the unloaded carrier ($T_i \rightarrow T_o$). The $K_m$ is affected because, under equilibrium exchange conditions, one must consider substrate binding at both sides of the membrane. In addition, the architecture of the outward facing site is different from that of the inward facing site, with the result that the glucose affinities for $T_o$ versus $T_i$ can be different (43). In the future, the use of molecular techniques to modify protein structure, together with functional measurements, will lead to a much greater understanding of the biophysical characteristics of these proteins.

### Structure

GluT-1 was originally purified from human red blood cells. Antibodies directed against this protein were then used in the cloning of the transporter from human HepG2 hepatoma and rat brain cDNA libraries (24, 25). These cloned cDNAs predicted GluT-1 to have a sequence of 492 amino acids that is highly conserved between the two species. Based on a hydropathy plot of the predicted amino acid sequence, together with results of chemical and proteolytic digestion experiments performed on the native membrane-bound protein, Mueckler *et al.* (24) proposed a model for the membrane orientation of the transporter. In this model, the protein has 12 membrane spanning segments with the $NH_2$- and COOH-termini on the intracellular side of the membrane. Radiation inactivation studies of red blood cells suggest that GluT-1 *in situ* exists as a homotetramer (44).

Using the human and rat GluT-1 cDNAs as probes, cDNA libraries from a variety of tissues have been screened, leading to the identification of the family of glucose transporters described above. All are separate gene products and are, in large part, located on different chromosomes (45). In general, these proteins have a similar size and orientation in the plasma membrane. The most divergent regions are the $NH_2$- and COOH-termini, and a large extracellular loop between the first and second membrane spanning regions. These regions are likely to contribute differences in kinetic properties among the transporters ($K_m$ and turnover number) as well as targeting of the proteins to different cellular locations. Several excellent reviews of the molecular structure of the isoforms have been published (28, 45, 46).

## REGULATION OF Na-INDEPENDENT (FACILITATED) GLUCOSE TRANSPORT

### Introduction

Tissues that use glucose as a primary energy source consume the majority of circulating glucose during the basal, post-absorptive state. Of these tissues, the brain and other nervous tissue account for 70% of non-insulin mediated glucose disposal in humans (47). Transport into these cell types may be saturated at basal plasma glucose concentrations, and the absolute amounts of glucose uptake and usage do not change greatly during hyperglycaemia or hyperinsulinaemia.

The most significant acute regulator of glucose uptake is insulin. As blood glucose and insulin concentrations increase after meals, the insulin-responsive tissues, which include the heart, adipose tissue, and skeletal muscle, increase their rates of glucose transport to dispose of the majority of glucose that exceeds basal uptake. The processes that link insulin binding to cellular events are just beginning to be understood (see the chapters on Insulin Receptors and Second Messengers). Analogous to the effects of insulin, exercise acutely increases glucose uptake in the heart and skeletal muscle, providing fuel for contractile activity.

The regulation of glucose transporters has been most thoroughly studied in insulin-sensitive tissues and in a number of tissue culture models which show both acute and chronic regulation of transport. It is now accepted that acute control involves an increase in the number of glucose transporters in the plasma membrane. Many cell types also show short-term regulation of the intrinsic activity of plasma membrane transporters. Chronic regulation is mainly through altered transporter expression, which may involve pre- or post-translational modifications.

## Acute regulation: insulin action

### Translocation

Glucose transporters are located in both the plasma membranes and in intracellular membranes of insulin-responsive tissues, and these subcellular fractions may be redistributed for readily reversible, acute regulation of glucose uptake. Insulin stimulation causes transporters to be relocated from the intracellular compartments to the plasma membrane by a process called translocation, or recruitment (Fig. 6.3). This process was initially described by Cushman *et al.* (48), and Kono *et al.* (49) from studies of the effects of insulin on adipocytes. This process has subsequently been demonstrated in skeletal (50, 51) and cardiac muscle (52). Translocation is thought to be related to the mechanism of exocytosis, and involves docking of post-Golgi vesicles containing transporters with the plasma membrane, fusion of these membranes, and eversion to expose the transporters to the interstitial space. GluT-4, also known as the insulin regulatable glucose transporter or IRGT, accounts for most of the changes associated with translocation. This transport protein is found only in insulin-responsive tissues, and is pre-

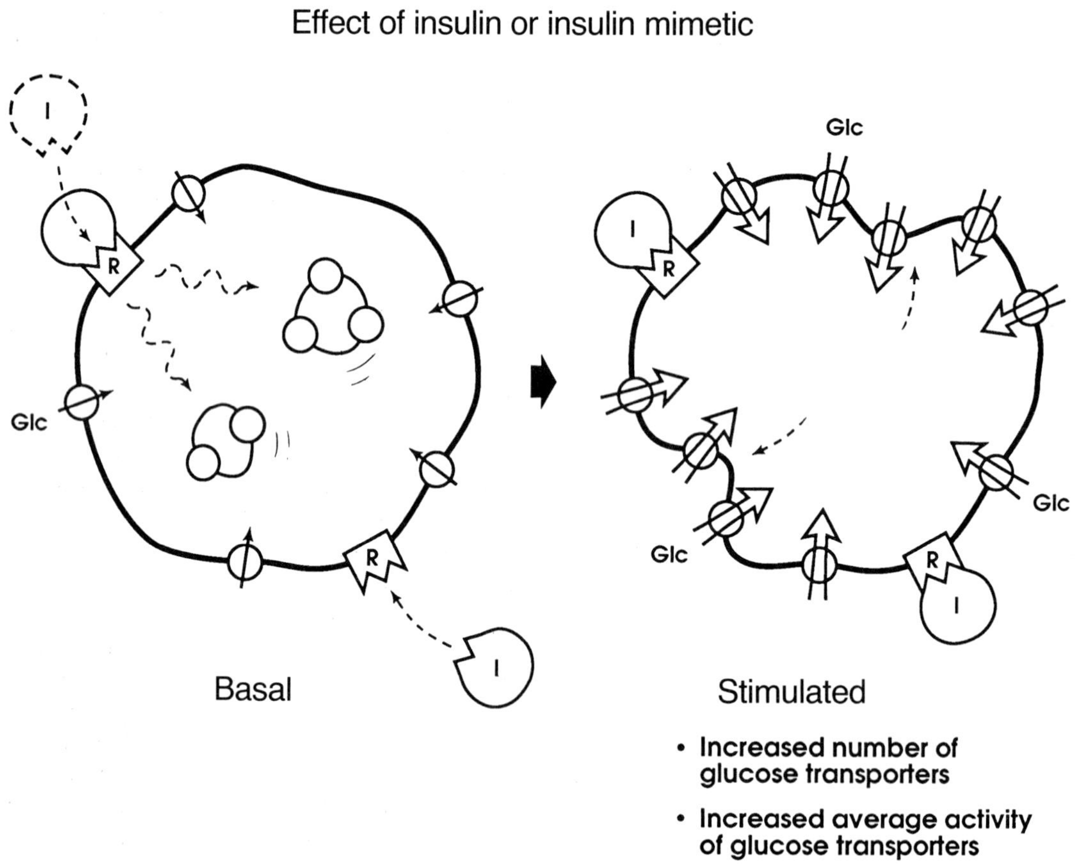


Fig. 6.3. Mechanism of insulin or insulin mimetic factors to stimulate glucose transport in insulin-sensitive tissues (adipose and muscle).

dominantly located in intracellular membranes in the absence of insulin. A relocation of Glut-4 to the plasma membrane is a post-binding event of insulin stimulation. In contrast, the ubiquitous GluT-1 protein is located primarily in the plasma membrane of most tissues, and is thought to be affiliated with basal glucose transport. However, some translocation of GluT-1 has been shown in adipose cells. After GluT-1 and GluT-4 proteins are synthesized and processed in the Golgi apparatus, there may be specific targeting of GluT-1 to the plasma membranes of most cell types, and of GluT-4 to intracellular membranes. Two major models of the control of cellular distribution have been proposed (for review see Birnbaum (53)).

The transporter redistribution that follows acute insulin stimulation reverses within 30 minutes (54). As the stimulus dissipates, a decrease in glucose transport corresponds directly to the loss of transporters from the plasma membrane (55). This selective removal of GluT-4 from the plasma membrane may be conferred by structural elements of the terminal ends of the protein (56). Although glucose transport via the GluT family of membrane proteins does not require energy, the translocation process is ATP dependent, as is reverse translocation (49).

## Intrinsic activity

There is increasing evidence that changes in glucose transporter intrinsic activity are involved in the acute regulation of transport, in addition to the processes that increase transporter numbers in the plasma membrane. Rapid increases in glucose uptake rates have been observed after insulin stimulation of fibroblasts without increases in plasma membrane transporter protein (57). In insulin responsive tissues, the translocation response is insufficient to explain the increase in transport after stimulation by cholera toxin or cadmium (58), or after insulin stimulation in some physiological conditions (59). The increases in plasma membrane transporters after *in vivo* insulin stimulation explain only half of the increase of *in vitro* glucose transport into plasma membrane vesicles isolated from normal rat muscle (60–62). There is a time lag between the increase in transporter number and the stimulation of glucose transport into rat adipocytes (55), indicating that a separate activation step may occur after translocation. Therefore, both GluT-1 and GluT-4 proteins may be regulated partially through changes in turnover number.

The mechanism by which intrinsic activity increases is not known, but several hypotheses have been proposed. An apparent activation could occur through disinhibition of the transporter function, possibly by detachment of a putative regulating metabolite, protein or peptide (for review see Czech *et al.* (63)). It is also possible that newly translocated tranporters have higher intrinsic activity than those customarily located in the plasma membrane, and therefore raise the average rate of calculated transport per identifiable transporter.

## Counter-regulation

The actions of other hormones may either enhance or antagonize the effects of insulin. Antagonism, or counter-regulation, by epinephrine and other β adrenergic agonists are the best known of these. Isoproterenol reduces insulin-stimulated glucose uptake in adipocytes, but not transporter redistribution. This could result from changes in transporter intrinsic activity (64) or from non-functional, 'cryptic' translocation of GluT-4 proteins, i.e. intracellular vesicles that attach to the plasma membrane without concomitant exposure of the transporters to the cell surface (65). In contrast, counter-regulation by steroid hormones and their agonists appears to acutely inhibit translocation, and may actually stimulate reverse translocation (66). Chronic exposure to dexamethasone also diminishes GluT-4 transporter expression (67). These hormones may influence the responsiveness of the transporters themselves, or may act through the mediating pathways of insulin (for review see Birnbaum (53)).

## Acute regulation: exercise

In animal studies, acute exercise also stimulates glucose transporter translocation and intrinsic activity in the heart and skeletal muscle. The presence of insulin is not necessary for the exercise effect, and either acute *in vivo* exercise or *in vitro* contractions produce similar changes in glucose transport (68). Insulin and exercise may cause recruitment from a common pool of intracellular transporters (69), or there may be discrete, additive pools for these stimuli (70). Hypoxia also increases the GluT-4 content of the muscle plasma membrane through translocation, although the process is slower to develop and slower to reverse after hypoxia than after exercise (71, 72). The translocation stimulated by hypoxia apparently is additive with insulin stimulation, but not exercise (71), which would suggest that exercise and hypoxia activate the same pool of transporters. Unlike insulin, the increase in plasma membrane GluT-4 after a bout of exercise may persist for at least 24 hours (73, 74). Therefore, studies of chronic exercise allow a 'rest' period of 36–48 hours, in which subjects are relatively sedentary, to avoid the effects due to acute exercise. A shorter period is required to return to the basal rate of glucose uptake and resting transporter distribution if the animals are fed carbohydrate during or after an acute exercise bout (75). This supports a theory that acute exercise-stimulated glucose uptake supplies energy for contraction, and the effects persist longer than those of insulin to replenish the intramuscular glycogen stores that have been depleted by exercise (75).

## Chronic regulation

The tissue concentrations of glucose transporter isoforms are regulated through pre- and post-translational mechanisms in response to chronic changes in glucose availability or hormone concentrations. In some cells, this regulation results in chronic changes in the number of transporters present in the plasma membrane and, therefore, the on-going rate of glucose transport. In insulin-responsive tissues, an increase in GluT-4 transporter expression enhances the capacity of that tissue to respond to acute stimuli, i.e. an increase in the reserves of translocatable proteins amplifies the potential response to insulin or exercise.

Pretranslational changes in expression occur through the inhibition or stimulation of gene transcription, or by changes in the relative stability of the messenger RNA. Comparative levels of the mRNAs specific to single transporter isoforms can be quantitated using Northern blots, i.e. total tissue RNA is isolated, subjected to electrophoresis, and hybridised to $^{32}P$ labelled cDNA. These studies have been more extensively reviewed elsewhere (28, 53).

Changes in mRNA concentrations may predict the protein content of the tissue, as is the case with decreased GluT-4 in long-term streptozotocin diabetes in skeletal muscle and in fat tissue (76, 77). In cell culture systems, the addition of a number of different growth factors, including tumour promoters, rapidly induces the expression of both glucose transporter mRNA and protein (78). However, in a study including a variety of conditions with modified insulin responsiveness, no general relationship was found between the mRNA concentration and the protein content of GluT-4 in skeletal muscle (77).

Post-translational effects may occur through differences in the rates of transporter degradation, or in other steps of processing subsequent to protein synthesis. These effects are more difficult to investigate *in vivo*, but may explain changes in protein content without concomitant differences in mRNA content. The mechanisms are more easily studied in *in vitro* conditions, where inhibitors of transcription or translation can be added. For example, the increases in glucose transporter numbers that occur after glucose starvation in cultured fibroblasts do not require protein synthesis, and therefore may be due to a decrease in the degradation rate of GluT-1 proteins (79).

## Tissue specialisation

### Insulin-sensitive tissues

The literature about cellular glucose transport has emerged and changed rapidly. *In vitro* studies using adipocytes isolated with collagenase digestion have been widely used to examine the relationship of function (glucose uptake rate), glucose transporter protein concentrations, and regulation by insulin. Initially, the findings of these studies were extrapolated to other insulin sensitive tissues that are more difficult to study, because some work showed similar responses of muscle and adipose tissue to various *in vitro* conditions. Muscle and adipose tissue are now known to differ in their responses to chronic changes in insulin and glucose levels, sometimes reacting in opposite directions. Furthermore, information about rat or cultured adipocytes should not be applied directly to the human condition. Rat adipocytes are known to use glucose for *de novo* lipogenesis, which does not occur to any extent in humans. The glucose uptake by human adipocytes may serve mainly as a source for glycerol-3-phosphate for fatty acid esterification.

### Skeletal muscle

GluT-4 is the predominant transporter isoform in adult skeletal muscle, and is mainly associated with intracellular membranes in resting, non-insulin stimulated conditions. GluT-1, and very small amounts of GluT-3, have also been identified in this tissue. Most of the GluT-1 proteins that are present in muscle tissue may be associated with the perineural sheath or red blood cells rather than with the myocytes themselves (80, 81).

In the post-absorptive state, resting muscle is responsible for about 20% of the total glucose disposal in normal humans. During experimental hyperglycaemia and moderate insulinaemia, as might occur after meals, muscle tissue accounts for 85% of glucose disposal (47). Since membrane transport is rate-limiting for glucose utilisation in insulin-sensitive tissues in physiological conditions (82, 83), the fluctuations of glucose uptake in muscle are mediated through GluT-4 proteins. Therefore, the magnitude of the translocation/activation response in muscle is a major determinant of peripheral insulin responsiveness or resistance. Impairment in the GluT-4 response is currently believed to be the cause of post-prandial hyperglycaemia in glucose intolerance and in diabetes (47).

The concentrations of transporter isoforms in muscle may vary with the muscle type, customary exercise, and the age of the subject (84). The rate of glucose uptake following insulin stimulation is directly proportional to the total number of GluT-4 transporters contained in the tissues of normal adult rats and humans (32), i.e. greater intracellular GluT-4 pools expand the capacity of the tissue to acutely increase the number of transporters in the plasma membrane through translocation. The heart has a higher insulin-stimulated glucose uptake rate and higher numbers of transporters than skeletal muscle. Likewise, muscles made up of predominantly red, oxidative fibres contain higher levels of glucose transporters than white, glycolytic muscles. Glucose transporter expression may increase in all fibre types after training, but the relative effect is more pronounced in glycolytic fibres (85, 86). Therefore, the capacity for glucose transport may reflect the fibre type and the customary activity of that muscle, with the highest concentrations of transporters in heart and diaphragm, followed by postural muscles. An enforced sedentary lifestyle in rats decreases the expression of GluT-4 proteins (87); similarly, extended bedrest decreases muscle glucose uptake in human skeletal muscle (88). In addition to increasing the GluT-4 content in some muscle types (60, 85), chronic exercise training is thought to improve insulin responsiveness in rats (86). The effectiveness of exercise in insulin resistant humans as a treatment independent of diet or drug therapy is less clear (89).

The concentrations of transporter isoforms may be modulated throughout life. Foetal tissues have high basal glucose requirements, and contain mostly GluT-1 transporters. During the neonatal period, GluT-1 protein concentrations decline while the GluT-4 proteins increase ((90), reviewed in (91)). During weaning in rats, GluT-4 protein content is increased to adult levels through rapid increases in mRNA (92). As rats age, there is a progressive decline in GluT-4 expression and insulin responsiveness in skeletal muscles in rats (93) but older animals remain capable of increasing transporter concentrations in response to training (94).

A variety of changes in glucose transporter regulation has been identified in insulin resistant animals. In older rats, insulin resistance is associated with a decreased translocation of transporters to the plasma membrane of the skeletal muscles (95). In streptozotocin diabetic rats, insulin-stimulated transporter translocation is decreased and the intracellular GluT-4 protein pools and associated mRNA are reduced (96). However, insulin resistance is apparent before the decrease of protein occurs (97), implying that the impairment in the translocation precedes the reduction in transporter protein. The transporters in plasma membranes isolated from insulin-resistant obese Zucker rats respond to insulin stimulation with activation only, but no significant translocation (98). However, obese Zuckers respond normally to acute exercise, with both activation and translocation of skeletal muscle transporters (50), so the responses to exercise and insulin stimuli appear to be independent.

The regulation of glucose transport in skeletal muscles is extremely complex. Both acute and chronic control are affected by glucose concentration, insulin, exercise, and hypoxia, which are interrelated factors. Therefore, experimental conditions have been devised to help clarify the individual effects. For example, experiments with the hyperglycaemic clamp technique have shown that acute elevation of blood glucose increases the rates of both insulin dependent and independent glucose uptake in muscle (47). This has led to speculation that the hyperglycaemia of diabetes may partially override the requirement for insulin. However, for cultured muscle cells, exposure to high glucose in the medium acutely decreases the rate of basal glucose uptake (79), and subsequently suppresses GluT-1 expression without changing GluT-4 concentration or mRNA (99). A down-regulation of glucose uptake with chronic hyperglycaemia is also seen with *in vivo* experiments in rats and humans ((100), for review see (99, 101)). This may have a protective effect in preventing glucose toxicity, or the accumulation of free glucose, within the cell (for reviewed see (101).

## Adipose tissue

Approximately 90% of the total glucose transporters in rat adipocytes are GluT-4 proteins, which are located in intracellular compartments in the basal state. The remaining transporters are GluT-1, which are equally distributed between plasma membranes and intracellular membranes in the basal condition. Currently, translocation is thought to be the major process that regulates transport activity in adipocytes. After insulin stimulation, the plasma membrane content of glucose transporters may increase by 20–30-fold (102). Transporter activation may also be involved (for review see (28)). A cell line of transformed fibroblast, 3T3-L1, differentiates into adipocytes in culture, and has been extensively used to study glucose transporters. GluT-1 is the sole transporter in preadipocytes, but during differentiation the total cellular content of GluT-1 declines and GluT-4 increases (103). The rates of basal and insulin-stimulated glucose transport change in proportion to the respective levels of GluT-1 and GluT-4. This change in isoform concentration predicts the maturation process in adipocytes of newborn rats, which initially have predominantly GluT-1 proteins, and low sensitivity to insulin (90, 104). GluT-4 protein expression is rapidly induced in rat adipose tissue with weaning from milk, which is a high fat food, to high carbohydrate foods (92). Older rats typically show a decline of adipocyte total GluT-4 content and translocation in response to insulin (105). However, the insulin resistance in the adipose tissue of ageing rats can be delayed by chronic food restriction and exercise to prevent the fat cell hypertrophy characteristic of old, sedentary animals (106). Therefore, it is possible that obesity and cell size may govern adipocyte insulin responsiveness more than ageing *per se*.

Obese humans (107) and animals (108) show adipose tissue insulin resistance, with decreases in GluT-4 transporter translocation (107) and expression (109). However, the adipose tissue from growing Zucker obese rats has a period of insulin hyper-responsiveness associated with increased adipocyte content of GluT-4 protein and mRNA (108). As these rats become obese, transporters decrease, and the rats become insulin resistant. Although the average fat cell size in lean Zuckers also increased with age, adipocyte size was about 25% of age-matched obese rats, and the GluT-4 protein and mRNA content did not change significantly in ageing lean rats (108). It has been postulated that a chronic elevation of plasma insulin increases the capacity of adipose tissue to store glucose (102, 107, 110). When insulin levels are raised by injection or minipump implants, GluT-4 expression and glucose uptake increase in adipose tissue (110, 111). During the hyperphagic phase of hypothalamic obesity, GluT-4 expression and glucose uptake are also increased in adipose tissue (112). However, as fat cells become enlarged, they become insulin resistant with an associated decrease in glucose transporter protein content and translocation (107, 109).

Both glucose and insulin concentrations are likely to have roles in the chronic regulation of glucose transport in adipose tissue (31). Hypoinsulinaemia through starvation and streptozotocin diabetes decreases GluT-4 mRNA and protein levels, which are restored by refeeding starved rats, and by insulin treatment of diabetic rats (113). In contrast, treatment of diabetic rats with phlorizin to reduce blood glucose by inhibiting renal glucose transport and thus re-absorption, has no effect on adipocyte GluT-4 expression, although insulin responsiveness and glucose transport are enhanced (114).

## Control of glucose transporters in insulin-sensitive tissues under various conditions

### Diabetes

Streptozotocin treatment, which selectively kills pancreatic β-cells, has been widely used as a model of chronic hypoinsulinaemia and insulin-dependent diabetes (IDDM). In severely diabetic animals there is impairment of transporter translocation and a diminished expression of GluT-4 in the muscle (77, 96); peripheral insulin resistance may precede the changes in the GluT-4 protein content (97). A decrease in insulin-stimulated transport without changes in muscle GluT-4 content has been reported after milder streptozotocin treatment (97). Therefore, insulin appears to have a role in maintaining transporter expression that is distinct from its function in acute glucose uptake. Insulin therapy in diabetic rats normalises both the transporter content and glucose uptake in muscle and in adipose tissue (97).

The role of glucose transporters in human diabetes is not clear. In fat biopsies from non-insulin dependent diabetic (NIDDM) patients, GluT-4 transporter proteins are reduced by approximately 85% compared to non-diabetic controls; by contrast, in weight-matched non-diabetic obese subjects, there was a 40% reduction compared to non-diabetic, non-obese controls subjects. These changes are associated with a decrease in mRNA content of the adipocytes (109, 115). Less than 20% of insulin-mediated glucose uptake is by adipose tissue even in obese subjects, so the significance of these changes is not known. Skeletal muscle accounts for most of insulin-mediated glucose disposal, and the GluT-4 content in muscle biopsies is not generally different than control in NIDDM patients (116, 117), although a significant reduction in transporter protein was reported in one study (118). Likewise, glucose transporter protein expression in muscle has been reported to be unchanged in insulin-dependent diabetics (76, 119). However, skeletal muscle insulin resistance has been shown repeatedly in human obesity, IDDM, and NIDDM. In the absence of consistent evidence for altered expression of GluT-4, several metabolic regulators of transporter function have been proposed (76), such as chronic hyperfatty-acidaemia, hyperglycaemia, hyperinsulinaemia, or blood flow changes (for reviews see Kahn, (117) and Garvey, (120)).

Insulin resistance has been reported to improve with weight loss and calorie restriction, which are frequently recommended for the treatment of carbohydrate intolerance in obesity and NIDDM (121). Since the involvement of skeletal muscle glucose transporters in human insulin resistance is not completely clear, the changes involved in improvement are only beginning to be defined. In a study of morbidly obese people before and after gastric bypass surgery to cause weight losses of more than 40 kg, Friedman *et al.* reported a marked improvement in insulin responsiveness, with a three-fold increase in insulin stimulation of whole-body glucose disposal (122). This was associated with increased *in vitro* insulin-stimulated 2-deoxyglucose uptake by muscle biopsies. However, there was no change in the cellular content of the muscle GluT-4 protein compared to normal subjects. Therefore, the altered glucose metabolism associated with even extreme changes in body weight seem to be mediated through post-translational regulation rather than through the expression of glucose transporter protein.

Oral hypoglycaemic agents have effects on peripheral insulin responsiveness that appear to be independent of the well-known enhancement of insulin secretion. Sulphonylureas enhance the insulin-induced recruitment of GluT-4 to the plasma membrane of skeletal muscle (123) and may also increase GluT-1 expression in other tissues (103). These effects are further discussed in the section on NIDDM treatment.

## Dietary changes

Alterations in diet patterns may produce dramatic changes in the glucose transporter expression and function in muscle and adipose tissue. In acute and prolonged starvation (more than 2 days) in rats, the concentrations of the GluT-4 mRNA and protein decrease in adipose cells (31, 124). The GluT-4 protein concentration in white and red muscle has been reported to be relatively unaffected by 48 hours of fasting (124, 125), but the mRNA and protein content of red skeletal muscle increases after prolonged fasting (31, 77). However, both fat and muscle show *in vivo* resistance to insulin stimulation of glucose transport. Therefore, metabolic factors may be involved in the regulation of glucose transport in skeletal muscle during starvation (31, 124). With refeeding after prolonged starvation, GluT-4 expression decreases to normal levels in skeletal muscle, but there is a period of overshoot in adipocytes, i.e. transport and transporter proteins are at higher than normal levels after refeeding (31, 59).

High fat diets produce insulin resistance in the adipose tissue and skeletal muscle of rats (126, 127). In muscle, the relative amounts of GluT-4 transporter proteins (51, 128) and GluT-4 mRNA (129) are unchanged by a diet with 60% of the calories from fat. Transporters are translocated after an insulin or acute exercise stimulus, but show no apparent activation of intrinsic activity (51, 128). In adipose tissue, the total number of glucose transporters is depleted as a result of a decrease in the intracellular pool (130). Rats that were fed diets with 80% of calories from fat have been reported to have decreased GluT-4 expression in both adipose tissue (131) and skeletal muscle (132), but these rats were hypoinsulinaemic, did not grow well, and may not be representative of attainable, balanced diets.

During the suckling period, a time of high fat feeding, insulin resistance is observed in rats (104). In the suckling-to-weanling transition, GluT-4 transporter expression is rapidly induced. The GluT-4 mRNA content of skeletal muscle increases three-fold within 12 hours of carbohydrate feeding, and doubles in adipose tissue within 6 hours (92). The GluT-4 protein content is approximately three-fold higher in carbohydrate-weaned rat muscle compared to either suckling rats or rats weaned on a high fat diet, and is directly related to the levels of insulin responsiveness observed in these animals (133).

### Control in liver and β cells

The major glucose transporter in hepatocytes is GluT-2, which has a high $V_{max}$ and $K_m$, i.e. high capacity for transport but low affinity for glucose at euglycaemia. This allows the liver to effectively remove large amounts of glucose from the portal blood following a high carbohydrate meal to help prevent post-prandial hyperglycaemia (91). Transport is not rate-limiting for glucose metabolism in the liver and most of the other splanchnic tissues, unlike muscle and fat. When gluconeogenesis and glycogenolysis are stimulated by hormonal or metabolite changes in the post-absorptive period, the transporters facilitate a net efflux of glucose to the extracellular space to maintain euglycaemia. Perivenous hepatocytes contain both GluT-2 and GluT-1 transporters, which allows the efflux of glucose from hepatocytes over a wide range of intracellular glucose concentrations (134). During starvation, the concentrations of high-affinity GluT-1 proteins are increased in these cells. Refeeding reverses these changes (134, 135). The expression of GluT-1 is also increased in diabetic rats, and decreased by subsequent insulin treatment (135, 136). Hepatic concentrations of the predominant GluT-2 protein are relatively unaffected by fasting and diabetes in rats, although GluT-2 mRNA levels change with fasting and refeeding (135). The role of altered glucose transporter expression in the increases of hepatic glucose output associated with diabetes and starvation is not known.

Pancreatic β-cells also contain high numbers of GluT-2 transporters. The $K_m$ of this transporter protein is higher than the glucose concentrations found in the splanchnic blood under most conditions, and, as a result, transport is likely to be linear with the plasma glucose concentration (137). Therefore, the cytoplasmic glucose concentration in the β-cell may serve as an accurate sensor for a wide range of blood glucose levels, which is coupled to the requirement for insulin. Intracellular β-cell glucose metabolism has been correlated to insulin secretion (for review see (91), described in the Insulin Secretion chapter). The expression of β-cell glucose transporter proteins has been reported to correlate well with the chronic insulin secretory function in a variety of conditions (91). Also, a link between the expression and function of GluT-2 transporters and the appearance of NIDDM has been postulated ((120), see chapters on Insulin Secretion and NIDDM).

## ACKNOWLEDGEMENTS

We thank L. Del Hagen for assistance in preparing the manuscript. The authors are supported by the National Institute of Arthritis and Musculoskeletal and Skin Diseases (AR41149 to PAK) and the National Institute of Diabetes, Digestive and Kidney Diseases (DK08648 to MNR).

## REFERENCES

1 Ullrich KJ. Sugar, amino acid, and Na cotransport in the proximal tubule. *Ann Rev Physiol* 1979; 41:181–5.

2 Hopfer, U. Membrane transport mechanisms for hexoses and amino acids in the small intestine. In: *Physiology of the gastrointestinal tract*, Johnson LR, ed. Raven Press, New York; 1987: 1499–526.

3 Haase W, Koepsell H. Electron microscopic immunohistochemical localization of Na-cotransporters along the rat nephron. *Eur J Cell Biol* 1989; 48:360–74.

4 Rodrigues-Boulan E, Nelson WJ. Morphogenesis of the polarized epithelial cell phenotype. *Science* 1989; 245: 718–25.
5 Hediger M, Ikeda T, Coady M, Gunderson C, Wright E. Expression of site-selected mRNA encoding the intestinal Na/glucose cotransporter in *Xenopus laevis* oocytes. *Proc Natl Acad Sci USA* 1987; 84:2634–7.
6 Hediger M, Coady M, Ikeda T, Wright E. Expression cloning and cDNA sequencing of the Na/glucose cotransporter. *Nature (Lond)* 1987; 330:379–81.
7 Hediger MA, Turk E, Wright EM. Homology of the human intestinal $Na^+$/glucose and *Escherichia coli* $Na^+$/ proline cotransporters. *Proc Natl Acad Sci USA* 1989; 86: 5748–52.
8 Ikeda TS, Hwang ES, Coady MJ, Hirayama BA, Hediger MA, Wright EM. Characterization of a $Na^+$/glucose cotransporter cloned from rabbit small intestine. *J Membrane Biol* 1989; 110:87–95.
9 Turk E, Zabel B, Mundlos S, Dyer J, Wright EM. Glucose/galactose malabsorption caused by a defect in the $Na^+$/glucose cotransporter. *Nature (Lond)* 1991; 356: 354–6.
10 Barfuss D, Schafer J. Differences in active and passive glucose transport along the proximal tubule. *Am J Physiol* 1981; 241:F322–32.
11 Turner RJ, Moran A. Further studies of proximal tubular brush border membrane D-glucose transport heterogeneity. *J Membrane Biol* 1982; 70:37–45.
12 Pajor AM, Hirayama BA, Wright EM. Molecular evidence for two renal $Na^+$/glucose cotransporters. *Biochim Biophys Acta* 1992; 1106:216–20.
13 Pajor AM, Wright EM. Cloning and functional expression of a mammalian Na+/nucleoside cotransporter. *J Biol Chem* 1992; 267:3557–60.
14 Hopfer U, Groseclose R. The mechanism of $Na^+$-dependent D-glucose transport. *J Biol Chem* 1980; 255:4453–62.
15 Coady MJ, Pajor AM, Wright EM. Sequence homologies among intestinal and renal Na+/glucose cotransporters. *Am J Physiol* 1990; 259:C605–10.
16 Wells RG, Pajor AM, Kanai Y, Turk E, Wright EM, Hediger MA. Cloning of a human kidney cDNA with similarity to the sodium-glucose cotransporter. *Am J Physiol* 1992; 263:F459–65.
17 Stevens BR, Fernandez A, Hirayama B, Wright EM, Kempner ES. Intestinal brush border membrane $Na^+$/ glucose cotransporter functions *in situ* as a homotetramer. *Proc Natl Acad Sci USA* 1990; 87:1456–60.
18 Takahashi M, Malathi P, Preiser H, Jung CY. Radiation inactivation studies on the rabbit kidney sodium-dependent glucose transporter. *J Biol Chem* 1985; 260: 10551–6.
19 Ferraris RP, Diamond JM. Use of phlorizin binding to demonstrate induction of intestinal glucose transporters. *J Membrane Biol* 1986; 94:77–82.
20 Fedorak RN, Gershon MD, Field M. Induction of intestinal glucose carriers in streptozotocin-treated chronically diabetic rats. *Gastroenterology* 1989; 96:37–44.
21 Westergaard H. Insulin modulates rat intestinal glucose transport: effect of hypoinsulinemia and hyperinsulinemia. *Am J Physiol* 1989; 256:G911–18.
22 Elsas LJ, Rosenberg LE. Familial renal glycosuria: a genetic reappraisal of hexose transport by kidney and intestine. *J Clin Invest* 1969; 48:1845–54.
23 Desjeux J-F. Congenital selective Na, D-glucose transport defects leading to renal glycosuria and congenital selective intestinal malabsorption of glucose and galactose. In: *The metabolic basis of inherited disease*, McGraw-Hill, New York; 1989: 2463–78.
24 Mueckler M, Caruso C, Baldwin SA *et al.* Sequence and structure of a human glucose transporter. *Science* 1985; 229:941–5.
25 Birnbaum M, Haspel H, Rosen O. Cloning and characterization of a cDNA encoding the rat brain glucose-transporter protein. *Proc Natl Acad Sci USA* 1986; 83: 5784–8.
26 Bell GI, Kayano T, Buse JB *et al.* Molecular biology of mammalian glucose transporters. *Diabetes Care* 1990; 13,3:198–208.
27 Kayano T, Fukumoto H, Eddy R *et al.* Evidence for a family of human glucose transporter-like proteins. Sequence and gene localization of a protein expressed in fetal skeletal muscle and other tissues. *J Biol Chem* 1988; 263:15245–8.
28 Pessin JE, Bell GI. Mammalian facilitative glucose transporter family: structure and molecular regulation. *Annu Rev Physiol* 1992; 54:911–30.
29 Thorens B, Cheng Z-Q, Brown D, Lodish HF. Liver glucose transporter: a basolateral protein in hepatocytes, intestine and kidney cells. *Am J Physiol* 1990; 259: C279–85.
30 Gould GW, Thomas HM, Jess TJ, Bell GI. Expression of human glucose transporters in Xenopus oocytes: kinetic characterization and substrate specificities of the erythrocyte, liver and brain isoforms. *Biochemistry* 1991; 30:5139–45.
31 Charron MJ, Kahn BB. Divergent molecular mechanisms for insulin-resistant glucose transport in muscle and adipose cells *in vivo*. *J Biol Chem* 1990; 265:7994–8000.
32 James DE, Strube M, Mueckler M. Molecular cloning and characterization of an insulin-regulatable glucose transporter. *Nature (Lond)* 1989; 338:83–7.
33 Fukumoto H, Kayano T, Buse JB, Edwards Y, Pilch PF *et al.* Cloning and characterization of the major insulin-responsive glucose transporter expressed in human skeletal muscle and other insulin-responsive tissues. *J Biol Chem* 1989; 264:7776–9.
34 Birnbaum MJ. Identification of a novel gene encoding an insulin-responsive glucose transporter protein. *Cell* 1989; 57:305–15.
35 Kaestner KH, Christy RJ, McLenithan JC, Braiterman LT, Cornelius P *et al.* Sequence, tissue distribution, and differential expression of mRNA for a putative insulin-responsive glucose transporter in mouse 3T3-L1 adipocytes. *Proc Natl Acad Sci USA* 1989; 86:3150–4.
36 Kayano T, Burant CF, Fukumoto H *et al.* Human facilitative glucose transporters. Isolation, functional characterization, and gene localization of cDNAs encoding an isoform (GluT-5) expressed in small intestine, kidney, muscle, and adipose tissue and an unusual glucose transporter pseudogene-like sequence (GluT-6). *J Biol Chem* 1990; 265:13276–82.
37 Burant CF, Takeda J, Brot-Laroche E, Bell GI, Davidson NO. Fructose transporter in human spermatozoa and small intestine is GluT-5. *J Biol Chem* 1992; 267: 14523–6.

38 Sigrist-Nelson K, Hopfer U. A distinct fructose transport system in isolated brush-border membrane. *Biochim Biophys Acta* 1974; 367:247–54.
39 Waddell ID, Scott H, Burchell A. Identification and characterization of a hepatic microsomal glucose transport protein. *Biochem J* 1991; 275:363–7.
40 Welmsley A. The dynamics of the glucose transporter. *Trends Biochem Sci* 1988; 13(6):226–31.
41 Baldwin S, Lienhard G. Glucose transport across plasma membranes: facilitated diffusion systems. *Trends Biochem Sci* 1981; 6:208–11.
42 Stein W. *Transport and diffusion across cell membranes*. Academic Press, Orlando, FL, 1986.
43 Gorga FR, Lienhard G. Equilibria and kinetics of ligand binding to the human erythrocyte glucose transporter. Evidence for an alternating conformation model for transport. *Biochemistry* 1981; 20: 5108–13.
44 Cuppoletti J, Jung CY, Green FA. Glucose transport carrier of human erythrocytes. Radiation target size measurement based on flux inactivation. *J Biol Chem* 1981; 256: 1305–6.
45 Elsas LJ, Longo N. Glucose transporters. *Annu Rev Med* 1992; 43: 377–93.
46 Silverman M. Structure and function of hexose transporters. *Annu Rev Biochem* 1991; 60: 757–94.
47 Baron AD, Brechtel G, Wallace P, Edelman SV. Rates and tissue sites of non-insulin- and insulin-mediated glucose uptake in humans. *Am J Physiol* 1988; 255: E769–74.
48 Cushman SW, Wardzala LJ. Potential mechanism of insulin action on glucose transport in the isolated rat adipose cell: apparent translocation of intracellular transport systems to the plasma membrane. *J Biol Chem* 1980; 255: 4758–62.
49 Kono T, Suzuki K, Dansey LE, Robinson RW, Blevins TL. Energy-dependent and protein synthesis-independent recycling of the insulin-sensitive glucose transport mechanism in fat cells. *J Biol Chem* 1981; 256: 6400–7.
50 King PA, Betts JJ, Horton ED, Horton ES. Acute exercise, unlike insulin, promotes glucose transporter translocation in the obese (fa/fa) Zucker rat muscle. *Am J Physiol* 1993; 265: R447–52.
51 Rosholt MN, King PA, Horton ES. High fat diet reduces glucose transporter response to insulin and acute exercise. *Am J Physiol* 1994; 266: R95–101.
52 Wheeler TJ. Translocation of glucose transporters in response to anoxia in heart. *J Biol Chem* 1988; 263: 19447–54.
53 Birnbaum MJ. The insulin-sensitive glucose transporter. *Intl Rev Cytol* 1992; 137A: 239–97.
54 Karnieli E, Chernow B, Hissin PJ, Simpson IA, Foley JE. Insulin stimulates glucose transport in isolated human adipose cells through a translocation of intracellular glucose transporters to the plasma membrane: a preliminary report. *Hormone Metab Res* 1986; 18: 867–8.
55 Clark AE, Holman GD, Kozka IJ. Determination of the rates of appearance and loss of glucose transporters at the cell surface of rat adipose cells. *Biochem J* 1991; 278: 235–41.
56 Piper RC, Tai C, Slot JW *et al.* The efficient intracellular sequestration of the insulin-regulatable glucose transporter (GluT-4) is conferred by the $NH_2$ terminus. *J Cell Biol* 1992; 117:729–43.
57 Harrison SA, Buxton JM, Clancy BM, Czech MP. Evidence that erythroid-type glucose transporter intrinsic activity is modulated by cadmium treatment of mouse 3T3-L1 cells. *J Biol Chem* 1991; 266:19438–49.
58 Clancy BM, Czech MP. Hexose transport stimulation and membrane redistribution of glucose transporter isoforms in response to cholera toxin, dibutyryl cyclic AMP, and insulin in 3T3-L1 adipocytes. *J Biol Chem* 1990; 265:12434–43.
59 Kahn B, Simpson I, Cushman S. Divergent mechanisms for the insulin resistant and hyperresponsive glucose transport in adipose cells from fasted and refed rats. *J Clin Invest* 988; 82:691–9.
60 Goodyear LJ, Hirshman MF, Valyou PM, Horton ES. Glucose transporter number, function, and subcellular distribution in rat skeletal muscle after exercise training. *Diabetes* 1992; 41:1091–9.
61 King PA, Hirshman MF, Horton ED, Horton ES. Glucose transport in skeletal muscle membrane vesicles from control and exercised rats. *Am J Physiol* 1989; 257:C1128–34.
62 Sternlicht E, Barnard RJ, Grimditch GK. Mechanism of insulin action on glucose transport in rat skeletal muscle. *Am J Physiol* 1988; 254:E633–8.
63 Czech MP, Clancy BM, Pessino A, Woon C-W, Harrison SA. Complex regulation of simple sugar transport in insulin-responsive cells. *Trends Biochem Sci* 1992; 17:197–201.
64 James DE, Hiken J, Lawrence JC Jr. Isoproterenol stimulates phosphorylation of the insulin-regulatable glucose transporter in rat adipocytes. *Proc Natl Acad Sci USA* 1989; 86:8368–72.
65 Vannucci SJ, Nishimura H, Satoh S, Cushman SW, Holman GD, Simpson IA. Cell surface accessibility of GluT-4 glucose transporters in insulin-stimulated rat cells. *Biochem J* 1992; 288:325–30.
66 Carter-Su C, Okamoto K. Effect of glucocorticoids on hexose transport in rat adipocytes. *J Biol Chem* 1985; 260:11091–8.
67 Garvey WT, Huecksteadt TP, Monzon R, Marshall S. Dexamethasone regulates the glucose transport system in primary cultured adipocytes: different mechanisms of insulin resistance after acute and chronic exposure. *Endocrinology* 1989; 124:2063–73.
68 Richter EA, Ploug T, Glabo H. Increased muscle glucose uptake after exercise: no need for insulin during exercise. *Diabetes* 1985; 34:1041–8.
69 Goodyear LJ, King PA, Hirshman MF, Thompson CM, Horton ED, Horton ES. Contractile activity increases plasma membrane glucose transporters in absence of insulin. *Am J Physiol* 1990; 258: E667–72.
70 Douen AG, Ramlal T, Rastogi S *et al.* Exercise induces recruitment of the 'insulin-responsive glucose transporter'. Evidence for distinct intracellular insulin- and exercise-recruitable transporter pools in skeletal muscle. *J Biol Chem* 1990; 265: 13427–30.
71 Cartee GD, Douen AG, Ramlal T, Klip A, Holloszy JO. Stimulation of glucose transport in skeletal muscle by hypoxia. *J Appl Physiol* 1991; 70: 1593–600.
72 Instrom JP, Rennie MJ, Schersten T, Bylund-Fellenius A-C. Membrane transport in relation to net uptake of glucose in the perfused rat hindlimb: stimulatory effect of insulin, hypoxia and contractile activity. *Biochem* J 1986; 233: 131–7.

73 Cartee GD, Young DA, Sleeper MD, Zierath J, Wallberg-Henriksson H, Holloszy JO. Prolonged increase in insulin-stimulated glucose transport in muscle after exercise. *Am J Physiol* 1989; 256: E494–9.
74 Holloszy JO, Ivy JL. Persistent increase in glucose uptake by rat skeletal muscle following exercise. *Am J Physiol* 1981; 241: C200–3.
75 Reed MJ, Brozinick JT Jr, Lee MC, Ivy JL. Muscle glycogen storage postexercise: effect of mode of carbohydrate administration. *J Appl Physiol* 1989; 66: 720–6.
76 Kahn BB, Rosen AS, Bak JF *et al.* Expression of GluT-1 and GluT-4 glucose transporters in skeletal muscle of humans with insulin-dependent diabetes mellitus: regulatory effects of metabolic factors. *J Clin Endocrinol Metab* 1992; 74: 1101–9.
77 Bourey RE, Koranyi L, James DE, Mueckler M, Permutt MA. Effects of altered glucose homeostasis on glucose transporter expression in skeletal muscle of the rat. *J Clin Invest* 1990; 86: 542–7.
78 Hiraki Y, Rosen OM, Birnbaum MJ. Growth factors rapidly induce expression of the glucose transporter gene. *J Biol Chem* 1988; 263: 13655–2.
79 Haspel HC, Wilk EW, Birnbaum MJ, Cushman SW, Rosen OM. Glucose deprivation and hexose transporter polypeptides of murine fibroblasts. *J Biol Chem* 1986; 261: 6778–89.
80 Hardy RW, Ladenson JH, Henriksen EJ, Holloszy JO, McDonald JM. Palmitate stimulates glucose transport in rat adipocytes by a mechanism involving translocation of the insulin sensitive glucose transporter (GluT-4). *Biochem Biophys Res Commun* 1991; 177: 343–9.
81 Froeher SC, Davies A, Baldwin SA, Lienhard GE. The blood–nerve barrier is rich in glucose transporter. *J Neurocytol* 1988; 17: 173–8.
82 Furler SM, Jenkins AB, Storlien LH, Kraegen EW, Barnett D. *In vivo* location of the rate-limiting step of hexose uptake in muscle and brain tissue of rats. *Am J Physiol* 1991; 261:E337–47.
83 Rossetti L, Giaccari A. Relative contribution of glycogen synthesis and glycolysis to insulin-mediated glucose uptake. A dose-response euglycemic clamp study in normal and diabetic rats. *J Clin Invest* 1990; 85: 1785–92.
84 Marette A, Richardson JM, Ramlal T *et al.* Abundance, localization, and insulin-induced translocation of glucose transporters in red and white muscle. *Am J Physiol Cell Physiol* 1992; 263:C443–52.
85 Rodnick KJ, Holloszy JO, Mondon CE, James DE. Effects of exercise training on insulin-regulatable glucose-transporter protein levels in rat skeletal muscle. *Diabetes* 1990; 39:1425–9.
86 Rodnick KJ, Henriksen EJ, James DE, Holloszy JO. Exercise training, glucose transporters, and glucose transport in rat skeletal muscles. *Am J Physiol* 1992; 262:C9–14.
87 Fushiki T, Kano T, Inoue K, Sugimoto E. Decrease in muscle glucose transporter number in chronic physical inactivity in rats. *Am J Physiol* 1991; 260:E403–10.
88 Mikines KJ, Richter EA, Dela F, Galbo H. Seven days of bed rest decrease insulin action on glucose uptake in leg and whole body. *J Appl Physiol* 1991; 70:1245–54.
89 Segal KR, Edano A, Abalos A *et al.* Effect of exercise training on insulin sensitivity and glucose metabolism in lean, obese, and diabetic men. *Am J Physiol* 1991; 71(6):E2402–11.
90 Studelska DR, Campbell C, Pang S, Rodnick KJ, James DE. Developmental expression of insulin-regulatable glucose transporter GluT-4. *Am J Physiol* 1992; 263: E102–6.
91 Devaskar SU, Mueckler MM. The mammalian glucose transporters. *Pediatr Res* 1992; 31:1–13.
92 Leturque A, Postic C, Ferre P, Girard J. Nutritional regulation of glucose transporter in muscle and adipose tissue of weaned rats. *Am J Physiol* 1991; 260: E588–93.
93 Lin J-L, Asano T, Shibasaki Y *et al.* Altered expression of glucose transporter isoforms with aging in rats-Selective decrease in GluT-4 in the fat tissue and skeletal muscle. *Diabetologia* 1991; 34:477–82.
94 Kern M, Dolan PL, Mazzeo RS, Wells JA, Dohm GL. Effect of aging and exercise on GluT-4 glucose transporters in muscle. *Am J Physiol* 1992; 263:E362–7.
95 Barnard RJ, Lawani LO, Martin DA, Youngren JF, Singh R, Scheck SH. Effects of maturation and aging on the skeletal muscle glucose transport system. *Am J Physiol* 1992; 262: E619–26.
96 Klip A, Ramlal T, Bilan PJ, Cartee GD, Gulve EA, Holloszy JO. Recruitment of GluT-4 glucose transporters by insulin in diabetic rat skeletal muscle. *Biochem Biophys Res Commun* 1990; 172: 728–36.
97 Kahn BB, Rossetti L, Lodish HF, Charron MJ. Decreased *in vivo* glucose uptake but normal expression of GluT-1 and GluT-4 in skeletal muscle of diabetic rats. *J Clin Invest* 1991; 87: 2197–206.
98 King PA, Horton ED, Horton ES. Insulin resistance in obese Zucker rat (fa/fa) skeletal muscle is associated with a failure of glucose transporter translocation. *J Clin Invest* 1992; 90: 1568–75
99 Klip A, Marette A. Acute and chronic signals controlling glucose transport in skeletal muscle. *J Cell Biochem* 1992; 48: 51–60.
100 Dimitrakoudis D, Ramlal T, Rastogi S, Vranic M, Klip A. Glycaemia regulates the glucose transporter number in the plasma membrane of rat skeletal muscle. *Biochem J* 1992; 284: 341–8.
101 Rossetti L, Giaccari A, DeFronzo RA. Glucose toxicity. *Diabetes Care* 1990; 13: 610–30.
102 Kahn BB, Cushman SW. Cell biology of insulin's stimulatory action on glucose transport and its perturbation in altered metabolic states. *Ann NY Acad Sci* 1986; 488: 356–69.
103 Tordman KM, Leingang KA, James DE, Mueckler MM. Differential regulation of two distinct glucose transporter species expressed in 3T3-L1 adipocytes: effect of chronic insulin and tolbutamide treatment. *Proc Natl Acad Sci USA* 1989; 86: 7761–5.
104 Issad T, Coupe C, Ferre P, Girard J. Insulin resistance during suckling period in rats. *Am J Physiol* 1987; 253: E142–48.
105 Ezaki O, Fukuda N, Itakura H. Role of two types of glucose transporters in enlarged adipocytes from aged obese rats. *Diabetes* 1990; 39: 1543–9.
106 Craig BW, Garthwaite SM, Holloszy JO. Adipocyte insulin resistance: effects of aging, obesity, exercise, and food restriction. *J Appl Physiol* 1987; 62(1): 95–100.
107 Salans LB, Bray GA, Cushman SW *et al.* Glucose metabolism and the response to insulin by human adipose tissue in spontaneous and experimental obesity. Effects

of dietary composition and adipose cell size. *J Clin Invest* 1974; 53: 848–56.
108 Pedersen O, Kahn CR, Kahn BB. Divergent regulation of the GluT-1 and GluT-4 glucose transporters in isolated adipocytes from Zucker rats. *J Clin Invest* 1992; 89:1964–1973
109 Garvey WT, Maianu L, Hueckstеadt TP, Birnbaum MJ, Molina Joseph M, Ciaraldi TP. Pretranslational suppression of a glucose transporter protein causes insulin resistance in adipocytes from patients with non-insulin-dependent diabetes mellitus and obesity. *J Clin Invest* 1991; 87:1072–81.
110 Cusin I, Terrettaz J, Rohner-Jeanrenaud F, Zarjevski N, Assimacopoulos-Jeannet F, Jeanrenaud B. Hyperinsulinemia increases the amount of GluT-4 mRNA in white adipose tissue and decreases that of muscles: a clue for increased fat depot and insulin resistance. *Endocrinology* 1990; 127:3246–8.
111 Kahn BB, Horton ES, Cushman SW. Mechanism for enhanced glucose transport response to insulin in adipose cells from chronically hyperinsulinemic rats. *J Clin Invest* 1987; 79:853–8.
112 Thurlby PL, Ellis RDM. Differences between the effects of noradrenaline and the beta-adrenoceptor agonist BRL 28410 in brown adipose tissue and hind limb of the anaesthetized rat. *Can J Physiol Pharmacol* 1986; 64: 1111–14.
113 Kahn BB, Charron MJ, Lodish HF, Cushman SW, Flier JS. Differential regulation of two glucose transporters in adipose cells from diabetic and insulin-treated diabetic rats. *J Clin Invest* 1989; 84:404–11.
114 Kahn BB, Shulman GI, DeFronzo RA, Cushman SW, Rossetti L. Normalization of blood glucose in diabetic rats with phlorizin treatment reverses insulin-resistant glucose transport in adipose cells without restoring glucose transporter gene expression. *J Clin Invest* 1991; 87:561–70.
115 Garvey WT, Maianu L, Hancock JA, Golichowski AM, Baron A. Gene expression of GluT-4 in skeletal muscle from insulin-resistant patients with obesity, IGT, GDM, and NIDDM. *Diabetes* 1992; 41:465–75.
116 Pedersen O, Bak JF, Andersen PH *et al.* Evidence against altered expression of GluT-1 or GluT-4 in skeletal muscle of patients with obesity or NIDDM. *Diabetes* 1990; 39:865–70.
117 Kahn BB. Facilitative glucose transporters: regulatory mechanisms and dysregulation in diabetes. *J Clin Invest* 1992; 89:1367–74.
118 Dohm GL, Elton CW, Friedman JE *et al.* Decreased expression of glucose transporter in muscle from insulin-resistant patients. *Am J Physiol* 1991; 260:E459–63.
119 Yki-Jarvinen H, Vuorinen-Markkola H, Koranyi L *et al.* Defect in insulin action on expression of the muscle/adipose tissue glucose transporter gene in skeletal muscle of type-1 diabetic patients. *J Clin Endocrinol Metab* 1992; 75:795–9.
120 Garvey WT. Glucose transport and NIDDM. *Diabetes Care* 1992; 15: 396–413.
121 American Diabetes Association. Position statement: nutritional recommendations and principles for individuals with diabetes mellitus. *Diabetes Care* 1990; 13 (suppl.1): 18–25.
122 Friedman JE, Dohm GL, Leggett-Frasier N *et al.* Restoration of insulin responsiveness in skeletal muscle in morbidly obese patients after weight loss. *J Clin Invest* 1992; 89: 710–5.
123 Jacobs DB, Jung CY. Sulfonylurea potentiates insulin-induced recruitment of glucose transport carrier in rat adipocytes. *J Biol Chem* 1985; 260: 2593–6.
124 Camps M, Castello A, Munoz P *et al.* Effect of diabetes and fasting on GluT-4 (muscle/fat) glucose transporter expression in insulin-sensitive tissues. *Biochem J* 1992; 282: 765–72.
125 Smith DM, Bloom SR, Sugden MC, Holness MJ. Glucose transporter expression and glucose utilization in skeletal muscle and brown adipose tissue during starvation and re-feeding. *Biochem J* 1992; 282: 231–5.
126 Kraegen EW, Clark PW, Jenkins AB, Daley EA, Chisholm DJ, Storlien LH. Development of muscle insulin resistance after liver resistance in high-fat-fed rats. *Diabetes* 1991; 40: 1397–403.
127 Storlien LH, James DE, Burleigh KM, Chrisholm DJ, Kraegen EW. Fat feeding causes widespread *in vivo* insulin resistance, decreased energy expenditure, and obesity in rats. *Am J Physiol* 1986; 251, 14: E576–83.
128 Rosholt MN, King PA, Horton ES. High fat diet reduces glucose transporter response to insulin in wheelcage-trained rats. *Diabetes* 1992; 41 (suppl.1): 108a.
129 Wake SA, Sowden JA, Storlien LH *et al.* Effects of exercise training and dietary manipulation on insulin-regulatable glucose-transporter mRNA in rat muscle. *Diabetes* 1991; 40: 275–9.
130 Hissin PJ, Karnieli E, Simpson IA, Salans LB, Cushman SW. A possible mechanism of insulin resistance in the rat adipose cell with high fat/low-carbohydrate feeding: depletion of intracellular glucose transport systems. *Diabetes* 1982; 31: 589–92.
131 Pederson O, Kahn CR, Flier JS, Kahn BB. High fat feeding causes insulin resistance and a marked decrease in the expression of glucose transporters (GluT-4) in fat cells of rats. *Endocrinology* 1991; 129: 771–7.
132 Kahn BB, Pederson O. Supression of GluT-4 expression in skeletal muscle of rats that are obese from high fat feeding but not from high carbohydrate feeding of genetic obesity. *Endocrinology* 1993; 132: 13–22.
133 Issad T, Coupe C, Pastor-Anglada M, Ferre P, Girard J. Development of insulin-sensitivity at weaning in the rat; role of the nutritional transition. *Biochem J* 1988; 251:685–90.
134 Tal M, Schneider DL, Thorens B, Lodish HF. Restricted expression of erythroid/brain glucose transporter isoform to perivenous hepatocytes in rats. *J Clin Invest* 1990; 86:986–92.
135 Thorens B, Flier JS, Lodish HF, Kahn BB. Differential regulation of two glucose transporters in rat liver by fasting and refeeding and by diabetes and insulin treatment. *Diabetes* 1990; 39:712–19.
136 Tal M, Kahn BB, Lodish HF. Expression of the low Km GluT-1 glucose transporter is turned on in perivenous hepatocytes in rats with diabetes mellitus. *Endocrinology* 1991; 129:1933–41.
137 Mueckler M. Family of glucose-transporter genes: implication for glucose homeostasis and diabetes. *Diabetes* 1990; 39:6–11.

# 7 Glucose Homeostasis

Peter C. Butler

## INTRODUCTION

In health, the plasma glucose concentration is maintained within the range of 3–8 mmol despite major perturbation in the rate that glucose enters (meals) and leaves (exercise) the plasma pool. Homeostasis of plasma glucose concentration is clearly important since hypo- and hyperglycaemia both have well-recognised adverse consequences. This homeostasis is achieved by regulation of both the rate of hepatic glucose release and tissue glucose uptake. In this chapter, I will first briefly review the metabolic pathways involved in glucose uptake and release; secondly, review some of the methods that have been employed to measure regulation of glucose homeostasis in humans; and thirdly, review the *in vivo* regulatory factors important in glucose homeostasis in the post-absorptive/fasted versus the post-prandial state.

## METABOLIC PATHWAYS OF GLUCOSE METABOLISM

### Glucose uptake (Fig. 7.1)

Glucose taken up by a cell and phosphorylated has several potential fates. In tissue with the enzyme glucose-6-phosphatase (e.g. liver, kidney, GI mucosa) it may be de-phosphorylated and promptly re-released into the circulation; one of the so-called glucose (or futile) cycles. Alternatively, glucose-6-phosphate may be converted to the storage form of glucose in mammals, glycogen (**glycogen synthesis**) or undergo partial oxidation (**glycolysis**) to pyruvate. From the latter it may be further oxidized in the mitochondria to carbon dioxide and water (**glucose oxidation**).

There are several important regulatory steps in these metabolic pathways of glucose disposal that contribute to glucose homeostasis (Fig. 7.1, Table 7.1). The transport of water soluble glucose from the extracellular to intracellular aqueous environments requires transport of glucose through the hydrophobic lipid cell membrane. This is achieved by a family of glucose transporter proteins which are characterised by numerous membrane spanning sequences (1). These glucose transporter proteins differ in their tissue distribution as well as their sensitivity to insulin. Thus, the insulin sensitive glucose transporter-4 (GLUT-4) is the predominant transport protein present in skeletal muscle while glucose transporter protein-2 (GLUT-2) is the predominant transport protein in liver (2). Since glucose uptake across these transporter proteins is, in part, dependent upon mass action, the higher

Table 7.1. *Hormonal control of glucose homeostasis*

| Effect | Insulin | Glucagon | Epinephrine | Growth hormone | Cortisol |
|---|---|---|---|---|---|
| Glucose uptake | ↑ | ↓ | ↓ | ↓ | ↓ |
| Glucose production | | | | | |
| Glycogenolysis | ↓ | ↑ | ↑ | ↑ | ↑ |
| Gluconeogenesis | ↓ | ↑ | ↑ | ↑ | ↑ |

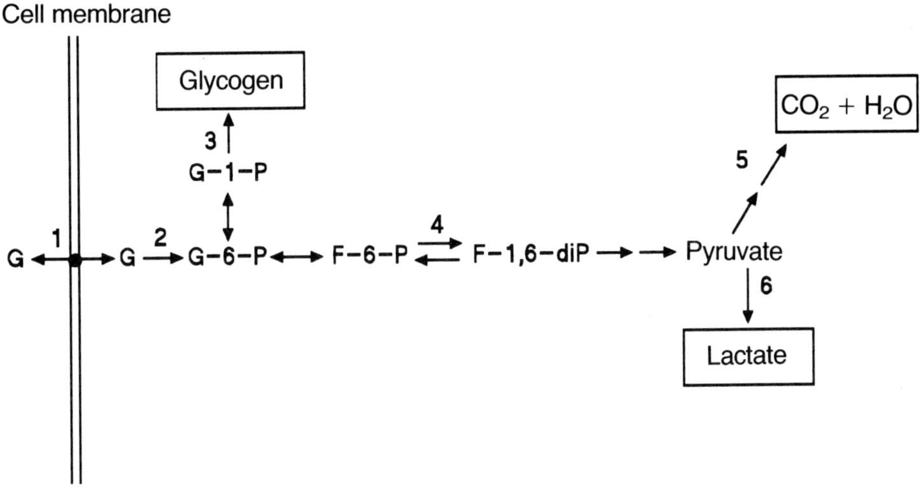


Fig. 7.1. Key regulatory steps of cell glucose uptake and metabolism. Glucose uptake requires transport of glucose across the hydrophobic cell membrane by glucose transporter proteins (1). In insulin sensitive tissue, flux of glucose via this transporter is stimulated by insulin. Glucose may then be phosphorylated (2 = glucokinase) and stored as glycogen (3 = glycogen synthetase) or undergo glycolysis (4 = phosphofructokinase). Following glycolysis, pyruvate may be oxidised (5 = pyruvate dehydrogenase and enzyme of the tricarboxylic cycle) or converted to lactate (6 = lactate dehydrogenase).

the glucose concentration the more rapid the flux is into cells (3). It should be noted, however, that prolonged hyperglycaemia results in decreased GLUT-4 transporter number (4) and glucose transport (5) in skeletal muscle. In addition, insulin stimulates glucose flux through GLUT-4 transporter protein in part by mobilising the protein to the cell membrane and, in part, by other as yet unrecognised mechanisms (6).

After glucose has gained access to a cell, it is rapidly phosphorylated by glucokinase (hexokinase in the liver and pancreatic β cells) to glucose-6-phosphate. The fate of glucose-6-phosphate is also subject to regulation. Thus, glycogen synthesis is favoured under conditions of high glucose uptake and high cell energy status (e.g. high NADPH/NADP, NADH/NAD, ATP/ADP) and in the presence of sufficient insulin to activate glycogen synthetase. The concentration of insulin required to activate glycogen synthetase appears to differ in different tissues (7). In contrast, the rate of glycolysis is increased under conditions of low energy stores (e.g. exercising skeletal muscle). The rate of glucose oxidation under conditions of increased glycolysis depends upon provision of oxygen (enhanced by adequate blood supply and myoglobin in Type II muscle fibres). The key regulatory steps in the pathways of glucose disposal are summarised in Fig. 7.1 and will be referred to in the discussion of glucose regulation during the post-absorptive versus post-prandial state below.

## Glucose release

In the post-absorptive state, glucose can only enter the circulation from the release of stored glycogen (**glycogenolysis**) or newly synthesised glucose (**gluconeogenesis**). Both of these pathways converge on glucose-6-phosphate (Fig. 7.2), with the exception of the small quantity of free glucose liberated by the enzyme (amylo-1,6-glycosidase) that degrades the branch points in glycogen. Since glucose-6-phosphate cannot be transported through the glucose transporters, only tissues with the enzyme glucose-6-phosphatase (which catalyses the dephosphorylation of glucose-6-phosphate) are capable of releasing glucose into the extracellular space.

The key regulatory steps of glucogenic and glycogenolytic pathways are shown in Fig. 7.2. It has been estimated that, in the post-absorptive state, gluconeogenesis accounts for approximately 25% of hepatic glucose release. Organ catheterisation studies suggests that the relative contribution of the three carbon precursors towards gluconeogenesis in the post-absorptive state are lactate ~60%, glycerol ~13%, amino acids ~15%, and pyruvate ~1% (8–10). Lactate is derived from glycolysis, particularly in the skin, red blood cells, intestinal mucosa, exercising Type II muscle fibres, adipose tissue, and perivenous hepatocytes (11, 12). Alanine and glutamine are the most important precursor amino acids for gluconeogenesis and together provide ~50% of the amino acids released by skeletal muscle (13, 14). While alanine is the predominant amino acid taken up by the liver (15), glutamine is the principal amino acid taken up by the kidney and gut (16).

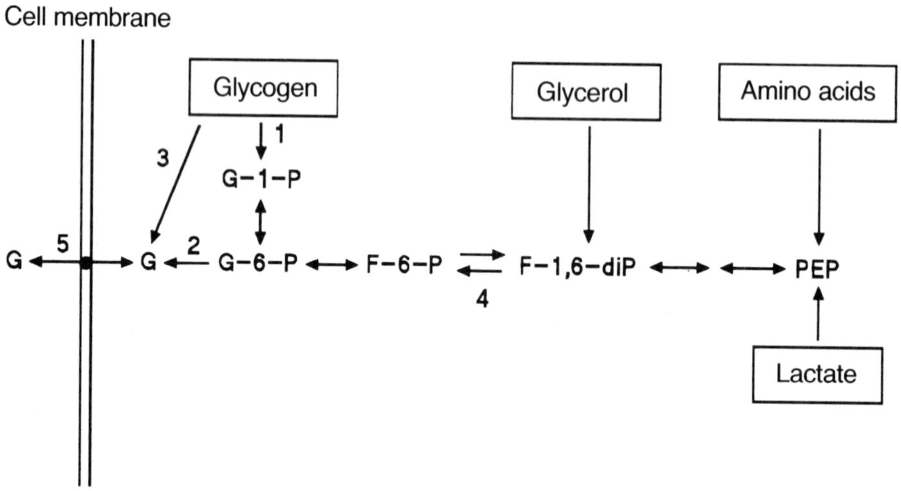


Fig. 7.2. Pathways of cell glucose release. The gluconeogenic precursors lactate, glycerol, and amino acids may undergo gluconeogenesis to generate glucose-6-phosphate. Glycogen may be degraded to G-6-P (1 = glycogen phosphorylase). G-6-P must be dephosphorylated (2 = glucose-6-phosphatase) before export by glucose transporter protein (5) across the cell membrane. A small portion of glycogen (the 1–6 branch points degraded by amylo-1, 6-glycosidase = 3) may be converted directly to glucose.

## METHODS EMPLOYED TO MEASURE GLUCOSE HOMEOSTASIS IN HUMANS

The role of insulin and other key regulatory hormones in the regulation of glucose metabolism in humans has been extensively investigated by various combinations of the hyperinsulinaemic, euglycaemic clamp, isotope dilution technique, cross-organ perfusion studies (e.g. hepatic vein catheterisation, forearm catheterisation), indirect calorimetry, and tissue biopsies to measure enzyme activities. Despite this impressive array of techniques, several important questions concerning the regulation of glucose metabolism in health and disease remains unclear.

Confusion arose when it became clear that the isotope dilution technique, employed to measure hepatic glucose release and total glucose uptake, was seriously flawed (17). These flaws were particularly problematic under conditions of high glucose turnover when errors due to non-steady state (18) and contaminants present in commercially available glucose (19) become particularly troublesome. Unfortunately, these errors cast into doubt many conclusions drawn from studies comparing the hepatic versus extrahepatic response to insulin in health versus disease (19). In general, the errors resulted in an underestimate of the absolute rate of hepatic glucose release and an overestimate in the rate of activation of insulin on suppression of hepatic glucose release (20). Numerous studies that employed the isotope dilution technique also employed other techniques to derive additional information from these studies. Thus, the combination of the isotope dilution technique and indirect calorimetry has been extensively employed to estimate the rate of glycogen synthesis (non-oxidative glucose disposal) versus oxidative glucose disposal. Glucose oxidation has also been measured by tracing the generation of labelled carbon dioxide from labelled glucose (20). To the extent that methods employed to measure glucose turnover have been erroneous, these derived methods will also have been subject to error.

Probably the most frequently used method of measuring the response of hepatic glucose release versus glucose uptake to insulin has been the hyperinsulinaemic, euglycaemic clamp technique (21). This method, which employs a constant insulin infusion to achieve steady-state hyperinsulinaemia, does not mimic conditions present *in vivo*. Unfortunately, the prolonged hyperinsulinaemia employed in hyperinsulinaemic clamp studies most likely obscures differences in the rate of activation of insulin action between groups. Thus, provision of insulin in a profile that mimics post-prandial insulin concentrations may result in different conclusions from those seen during a constant hyperinsulinaemia (22).

Fortunately, the errors that have confounded the isotope dilution technique can now largely be avoided. Furthermore, the availability of pumps which can be programmed to provide insulin as a variable profile that mimics post-prandial insulin concentrations allows for more physiological studies of the homeostasis glucose metabolism (23).

## POST-ABSORPTIVE/FASTED STATE

In the post-absorptive state (6 hours after feeding) blood glucose concentrations are maintained at ~4–5 mmol. Glucose uptake is ~6 μmol/kg/min of which half is due to obligate uptake by neural tissue as well as the other non-insulin-dependent tissues (24). At rest, skeletal muscle glucose uptake is approximately 30% but this increases by as much as 20-fold during intense exercise (10). Perturbations in the rate of glucose uptake in the post-absorptive state result in changes in insulin, glucagon, and growth hormone concentrations which in turn restore glucose homeostasis. Insulin is the key glucoregulatory hormone: even small changes in insulin concentration in the fasting state lead to relatively large changes in the rate of hepatic glucose release and suppression of glucose (25).

Thus, a decrease in insulin concentration results in increased rates of glycogenolysis and gluconeogenesis so that the total rate of hepatic glucose release increases (Fig. 7.2). Insulin suppresses glycogenolyses by inhibiting the activities of the enzyme hepatic phosphorylase (26). Insulin also inhibits gluconeogenesis by decreasing the circulating concentrations of gluconeogenic precursors (27) and by inhibiting the gluconeogenic pathway. Thus, when the plasma insulin concentration falls, the resulting increased rates of gluconeogenesis and glycogenolysis result in increased availability of glucose-6-phosphate. In the presence of the low insulin and increased glucagon concentrations present under conditions of fasting, the glucose-6-phosphate thereby generated is preferentially dephosphorylated and made available for release to the systemic circulation (Fig. 7.2).

Glucagon, which stimulates glycogenolysis (28) and gluconeogenesis (29) while inhibiting glycolysis (30), acts in concert with insulin to increase rates of hepatic glucose release under conditions of increased glucose uptake in the fasting state. Glucagon stimulates glycogenolysis via a cyclic AMP-dependent mechanism which results in a reciprocal increase in phosphorylase and a decrease in glycogen synthetase activity (28, 31). Since insulin has the opposite effect on the activity of these enzymes by a cyclic AMP-independent mechanism, the prevailing ratio of glucagon and insulin concentrations in the hepatic sinusoid blood determine the rate of hepatic glucose release. The effect of increased concentrations of glucagon on stimulating glycogenolysis is transient (32) in contrast to the effect on stimulating gluconeogenesis which is sustained (33). Thus, a rapid increase in the rate of glucose uptake during fasting (with a consequent decrease in glucose concentration) causes a rise in glucagon concentration which stimulates a transient increase in the rate of glycogenolysis to restore the plasma glucose concentration. However, if the increased rate of glucose uptake was sustained, increased rates of gluconeogenesis would be called into play to provide the prolonged increased rate of hepatic glucose released required to maintain the plasma glucose concentration.

Growth hormone is also an important modulator of carbohydrate metabolism. Following meal ingestion, the growth hormone concentration is decreased but, as the glucose concentrations falls during the second hour after meal ingestion, there is a secretory surge of growth hormone (34). Since growth hormone stimulates both gluconeogenesis and glycogenolysis (35), the increase in growth hormone concentration that coincides with transition to the post-absorptive state contributes to the restoration of the rate of hepatic glucose release to the post-absorptive levels. In addition, growth hormone inhibits glucose uptake by insulin sensitive tissues and increases the rate of lipolysis which most likely also decreases glucose requirements through substrate competition (35).

Epinephrine, norepinephrine, and corticosteroids all increase the rate of hepatic glucose release (29, 30). However, under resting conditions in the post-absorptive state, catecholamines do not appear to have an important role in sustaining hepatic glucose release. However, during exercise, they play an important role in mobilising sufficient glucose to maintain glycaemic control (36, 37). The rise in plasma cortisol following the overnight secretory burst of ACTH stimulates both gluconeogenesis and glycogenolysis (38) and therefore appears to decrease insulin sensitivity in the morning. The importance of corticosteroids in maintaining hepatic glucose release is apparent in patients with cortisol deficiency who are prone to fasting hypoglycaemia (39). Similarly, patients with cortisol excess are prone to fasting hyperglycaemia (40).

In addition to the effects of circulating hormones in maintaining plasma glucose regulation, it is becoming clear that there is also an important role of neural regulation upon carbohydrate metabolism. For example, the brain appears to have areas specifically sensitive to the circulating glucose concentration (41). Release of the neurotransmitter calcitonin and gene-related peptide in skeletal muscle under conditions of stress appears to markedly decrease glucose uptake (42). While this is a difficult field to study, it is likely there will be increasing information available in the future on the impact of the nervous system on glucose release and uptake.

## POSTPRANDIAL STATE

Following meal ingestion, glucose is absorbed for approximately six hours (43). Thus, the post-prandial state far exceeds the period of increased glucose concentrations that follows meal ingestion, reflecting the impressive mechanisms in place to restore glycaemia despite continuing increased rates of glucose appearance from the gut. It should also be noted that, since the post-prandial state lasts for six hours, most humans are in the post-prandial state for at least 75% of the 24-hour cycle. Therefore, although most studies of carbohydrate metabolism and regulation have focused on the post-absorptive state, the post-prandial state is actually more important in terms of day-to-day carbohydrate regulation.

Following meal ingestion, the increase in glucose concentration, together with other factors that are still poorly understood (the so-called incretin effect), results in a very rapid increase in circulating insulin concentration (44). Recent studies have shown that the majority of insulin secreted following meal ingestion is due to insulin secretory burst activity (i.e. pulsatile insulin secretion) (45). Following meal ingestion, there is a transient fall in both the glucagon and growth hormone concentration. From the above discussion, it will be clear that these changes result in decreased rates of glycogenolysis and gluconeogenesis and therefore the rate of hepatic glucose release decreases. Since the rate of hepatic glucose uptake appears to depend upon glucose concentration in the setting of adequate insulin (46), portal vein hyperglycaemia stimulates glucose uptake which, in turn, is channelled in large part to glycogen. In healthy subjects, following ingestion of a mixed meal containing 50 grams of glucose, initial splanchnic glucose uptake (glucose cleared primarily by the liver that does not reach the systemic circulation) accounts for approximately 10 grams of glucose. Hepatic glucose uptake continues during subsequent circulation of the glucose through the liver via the hepatic artery (47). The increase in insulin concentration and decrease in glucagon concentration serve to change conditions within the liver from glycogen breakdown to glycogen synthesis.

However, it would appear that this is not complete with at least a small proportion of glucose cycling through hepatic glycogen and being re-released.

The increased insulin concentration together with glucose concentration following meal ingestion both serve to increase glucose uptake in extrahepatic tissues, primarily skeletal muscle (47). In the non-exercising state, most of this glucose is primarily diverted to skeletal muscle glycogen stores. The increased insulin concentration, consequent upon meal ingestion, also results in inhibition of lipolysis and a switch of fuel oxidation in insulin-sensitive tissues from fat to carbohydrate (48). Thus, following meal ingestion, rates of carbohydrate oxidation increase and fat oxidation decline. Following meal ingestion, glucose uptake also increases markedly within adipose tissue where it is converted primarily to lactate which in turn is made available for subsequent gluconeogenesis within the liver (49). After meal ingestion, skeletal muscle also releases a small proportion of the glucose cleared from the circulation as lactate which in turn is also made available for gluconeogenesis (the so-called Cori cycle) (50).

## MECHANISM OF HYPERGLYCAEMIA IN DIABETES MELLITUS

Following the development of the insulin assay, patients with diabetes mellitus were subdivided into those with no insulin secretion (Type 1 diabetes mellitus) versus those with insulin secretion present (Type 2 diabetes mellitus). The mechanism of hyperglycaemia in untreated Type 1 diabetes mellitus has generally been described to the failure of insulin secretion as a consequence of autoimmune induced β-cell destruction (51). The difficulty of establishing glycaemic control in patients with Type 1 diabetes mellitus is further ascribed to the difficulty of reproducing normal insulin secretion profiles with sub-cutaneous insulin therapy.

Thus, insulin is secreted in a pulsatile manner with very rapid increases of insulin concentrations following meal ingestion (52). Since even regular sub-cutaneous insulin does not achieve a peak until two to four hours following injection therapy, it is not possible to reproduce this profile of insulin secretion using subcutaneous insulin therapy. As emphasised previously, most humans are in the fed state for 75% or more of the day; and since it is post-prandial insulin secretion that is impossible to reproduce, it is not surprising that postprandial glycaemic control is suboptimal. Furthermore, patients with insulin-dependent diabetes mellitus also have insulin resistance that appears to be related to hyperglycaemia *per se* (53). The latter further complicates restoration of glycaemic control. It has been debated whether provision of insulin through the systemic versus portal route is also a contributory factor to impaired glycaemic control in patients with Type 1 diabetes mellitus. However, a number of studies suggests that glycaemic control can be normalised with peripheral insulin delivery. Thus, patients with pancreatic transplants into the systemic circulation are able to achieve comparable carbohydrate metabolism to patients on similar anti-rejection medication (54). In addition, dogs which have had the pancreatoduodenal vein diverted to the inferior vena cava have carbohydrate tolerance that is distinguishable from dogs in which the pancreatoduodenal vein drains into the portal vein (55).

The mechanism of hyperglycaemia in patients with Type 2 diabetes mellitus has been considerably more controversial. This has in part been due to confusion that has arisen concerning the abnormalities of insulin secretion present in Type 2 diabetes mellitus. In fact, as long ago as the 1960s, Perley and Kipnis (56) pointed out that insulin secretion was grossly impaired in patients with Type 2 diabetes mellitus if the glucose concentration was matched to normal controls. More recently, it has become clear that the increased circulating concentrations of proinsulin and other split products of insulin have also probably resulted in an overestimate of insulin secretion present in patients with Type 2 diabetes mellitus (57). The mechanism of impaired insulin secretion in Type 2 diabetes mellitus is unclear. However, there is a loss of a significant proportion of β-cells in this disease which is associated with the appearance of islet amyloid polypeptide (IAPP) induced islet amyloidosis (58). It is likely that the loss of β-cell mass, at least in part, contributes to impaired insulin secretion in Type 2 diabetes mellitus, but it is unlikely to be the sole cause of this deficiency. With the progression of Type 2 diabetes mellitus from its earlier stages (glucose intolerance) to fully established diabetes mellitus, there is a decline in both the rate as well as the extent of insulin secreted in response to meal ingestion which is also associated with failure of glucagon suppression (Fig. 7.3). Together, impaired insulin secretion and inadequate glucagon suppression following meal ingestion result in failure to appropriately suppress hepatic glucose release, which is the principal cause of postprandial hyperglycaemia in Type 2 diabetes mellitus (59). While it has been suggested that futile cycling of glucose through hepatic glycogen contributes to this postprandial hyperglycaemia, this is probably only quantitatively small (47). Insulin resistance in extrahepatic insulin sensitive tissues in Type 2 diabetes mellitus (i.e., primarily skeletal muscle) is largely overcome following meal ingestion by the increased effect of hyperglycaemia on glucose disposal (59). Thus, it appears that, if insulin secretion could be

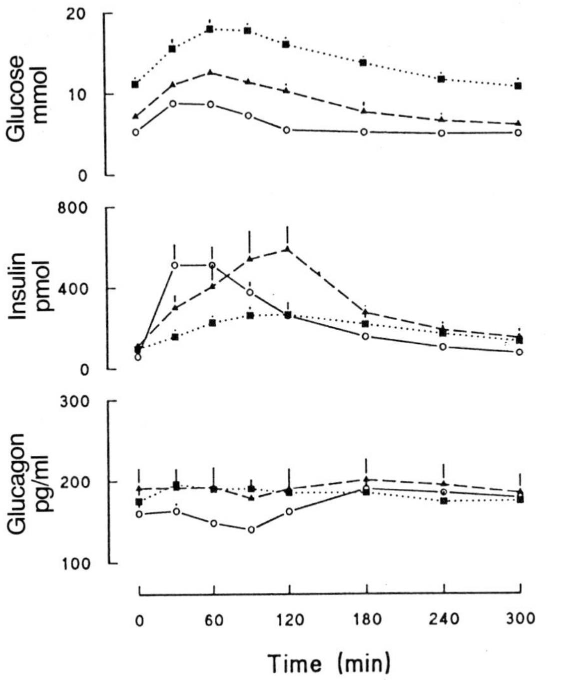


Fig. 7.3. Glucose, insulin and glucagon concentrations before and after meal ingestion in non-diabetic (○), glucose-intolerant (▲), and Type 2 diabetes mellitus (■) subjects. Note the progressive decrease in rate and magnitude of insulin response to meal ingestion, and the associated failure of suppression of glucagon (from Butler PC, Rizza RA. *Diabetes* 1991; 40: 73–81 with permission).

restored in patients with Type 2 diabetes mellitus, glycaemic control would also be restored.

In conclusion, numerous factors contribute to glucose homeostasis in health. While there appears to be redundancy in these overlapping systems, insulin has a unique and essential role. Thus, provision of adequate quantities of insulin in an appropriate profile is essential to restore glycaemic control in patients with either complete (i.e. Type 1 diabetes mellitus) or partial (i.e. Type 2 diabetes mellitus) β cell failure.

## ACKNOWLEDGEMENT

Dr Butler is supported by PHS grants DK-44341, RR-00585, and Mayo Foundation.

## REFERENCES


1 Kayano T, Fukumoto H, Eddy RL *et al.* Evidence for a family of human glucose transporter-like proteins. *J Biol Chem* 1988; 263: 15245–8.

2 Thorens B, Sarker HK, Kaback HR, Lodish HF. Cloning and functional expression in bacteria of a novel glucose transporter present in liver, intestine, kidney, and β-pancreatic islet cells. *Cells* 1988; 55: 281–90.

3 Verdonk CA, Rizza RA, Gerich JE. Effects of plasma glucose concentration on glucose utilization and glucose clearance in normal man. *Diabetes* 1981; 30: 535–7.

4 Ramlal T, Rastogi S, Vranic M, Klip A. Decrease in glucose transporter number in skeletal muscle of mildly diabetic (Streptozotocin-treated) rats. *Endocrinology* 1989; 125: 890–7.

5 Vuorinen-Markkola H, Koivisto VA, Yki-Jarvinen H. Mechanisms of hyperglycemia-induced insulin resistance in whole body and skeletal muscle of Type I diabetic patients. *Diabetes* 1992; 41: 571–80.

6 Friedman JE, Dudek RW, Whitehead DS *et al.* Immunolocalization of glucose transporter GLUT4 within human skeletal muscle. *Diabetes* 1991; 40: 150–4.

7 Nuttall F, Gannon M, Larner J. Oral glucose effect on glycogen synthase and phosphorylase in heart, muscle and liver. *Physiol Chem Phys* 1972; 4: 497–515.

8 Dietze G, Wichlmayr M, Hepp K *et al.* On gluconeogenesis of human liver: accelerated hepatic glucose formation by increased precursor supply. *Diabetologia* 1976; 12:555–61.

9 Nilsson L, Hultman E. Liver glycogen in man: the effect of total starvation on a carbohydrate-poor diet followed by carbohydrate refeeding. *Scand J Clin Lab Invest* 1973; 32:325–30.

10 Wahren J, Felig P, Ahlborg G *et al.* Glucose metabolism during leg exercise in man. *J Clin Invest* 1971; 50:2715–25.

11 Kreisberg RA. Glucose-lactate interrelationships in man. *N Engl J Med* 1972; 287:132–7.

12 Jungerman K. Metabolic zonation of liver parenchyma: significance for the regulation of glycogen metabolism, gluconeogenesis, and glycolysis. *Diabetes Metab Rev* 1987; 3:269–93.

13 Odessey R, Khaerallah EA, Goldberg AL. Origin and possible significance of alanine production by muscle. *J Biol Chem* 1974; 23:7623–29.

14 Ruderman NB, Berger M. The formation of glutamine and alanine in skeletal muscle. *J Biol Chem* 1974; 249: 5500–6.

15 Felig P. The glucose-alanine cycle. *Metabolism* 1973; 22: 179–207.

16 Matsulaka H, Arkawa T, Yamamato H *et al.* Gluconeogenesis and amino acid metabolism. III. Uptake of glutamine and output of alanine and ammonia by nonhepatic splanchnic organs of fasted rats and their metabolic significance. *J Biochem* 1973; 74: 1019–29.

17 Bergman R, Finegood D, Ader M. Assessment of insulin sensitivity *in vivo*. *Endocr Rev* 1985; 6: 45–86.

18 Cobelli C, Mari A, Ferrannini E. Non-steady state: error analysis of Steele's model and developments for glucose kinetics. *Am J Physiol* 1987; 252: 679–89.

19 Schwenk WF, Butler PC, Haymond MW, Rizza RA. Underestimation of glucose turnover corrected with

high-performance liquid chromatography purification of [6-$^3$H]glucose. *Am J* Physiol 1990; 258: E228–33.
20 Butler PC, Caumo A, Zerman A, O'Brien PC, Cobelli C, Rizza RA. Methods for assessment of the rate of onset and offset of insulin action during nonsteady state in humans. *Am J Physiol* 1993; 264 (*Endocrinol Metab* 27): E548–60.
21 DeFronzo RA, Tobin JD, Andres R. The glucose clamp technique. A method for the quantification of beta cell sensitivity to glucose and of tissue sensitivity to insulin. *Am J Physiol* 1979; 237: E214–23.
22 Doeden B, Rizza R. Use of a variable insulin infusion to assess insulin action in obesity: defects in both the kinetics and amplitude of response. *J Clin Endocrinol Metab* 1987; 64: 902–908.
23 Katz H, Butler P, Homan M *et al.* Hepatic and extrahepatic insulin action in humans: measurement in the absence of non-steady-state error. *Am J Physiol* 1993; 264: E561–6.
24 Owen O, Morgan A, Kemp H *et al.* Brain metabolism during fasting. *J Clin Invest* 1967; 46: 1589–95.
25 Rizza RA, Mandarino LJ, Gerich JE. Dose-response characteristics for the effects of insulin on production and utilization of glucose in man. *Am J Physiol* 1981; 240: E630–E9.
26 Hems DA, Whitton PD. Control of hepatic glycogenolysis. *Physiol Rev* 1980; 60: 1–50.
27 Manchester KL. The control by insulin of amino acid accumulation in muscle. *Biochem J* 1970; 117: 457–65.
28 Hers HG. The control of glycogen metabolism in the liver. *Ann Rev Biochem* 1976; 45: 167–89.
29 Exton JH. Gluconeogenesis. *Metabolism* 1972; 21: 945–89.
30 Rognstad R, Katz J. Control of glycolysis and lipogenesis in the liver by glucagon at the phosphofructokinase-fructose 1,6-diphosphatase site. *Arch Biochem Biophys* 1980; 203: 642–6.
31 Larner J, Lawrence J, Walkenbach R *et al.* Insulin control of glycogen synthesis. *Adv Cycl Nucl Res* 1978; 9: 425–39.
32 Bomboy J, Lewis S, Lacy W *et al.* Transient stimulatory effect of sustained hyperglucagonemia on splanchnic glucose production in normal and diabetic man. *Diabetes* 1977; 26: 177–84.
33 Cherrington AD, Williams PE, Shulman GI *et al.* Differential time course of glucagon's effect on glycogenolysis and gluconeogenesis in the conscious dog. *Diabetes* 1981; 30: 180–7.
34 Conover CA, Butler PC, Wang M, Rizza RA, Lee PDK. Lack of growth hormone effect on insulin-associated suppression of insulin-like growth factor binding protein-1 in humans. *Diabetes* 1990; 39: 1251–6.
35 Butler PC, Kryshak EJ, Rizza RA. Mechanism of growth hormone-induced postprandial carbohydrate intolerance in humans. *Am J Physiol* 1991; 260: E513–20.
36 Galbo HJ, Holst J, Christensen NJ. Glucagon and plasma catecholamine response to graded and prolonged exercise in man. *J Appl Physiol* 1975; 38: 70–6.
37 Silverberg AB, Shah SD, Haymond MW, Cryer PE. Norepinephrine: hormone and neurotransmitter in man. *Am J Physiol* 1978; 234: E252–6.
38 Dinneen S, Alzaid A, Miles J, Rizza RA. The metabolic effects of the nocturnal rise in cortisol on carbohydrate metabolism in normal humans. *J Clin Invest* 1993; In Press.
39 Malerbi D, Liberman B, Giurno-Filho A, Giannellaneto D, Wajchenberg BL. Glucocorticoids and glucose metabolism: hepatic glucose production in untreated Addisonian patients and on two different levels of glucocorticoid administration. *Clin Endocrinol* 1988; 28: 415–22.
40 McMahon M, Gerich J, Rizza R. Effects of glucocorticoids on carbohydrate metabolism. *Diabetes Metab Rev* 1988; 4: 17–30.
41 Kjæer M, Engfred K, Fernandes A, Secher NH, Glabo H. Regulation of hepatic glucose production during exercise in humans: role of sympathoadrenergic activity. *Am J Physiol* 1993; 265: E275–E83.
42 Leighton B, Cooper GJS. Pancreatic amylin and calcitonin gene-related peptide cause resistance to insulin in skeletal muscle *in vitro*. *Nature* 1988; 335: 632–5.
43 McMahon M, Marsh H, Rizza R. Comparison of the pattern of postprandial carbohydrate metabolism following ingestion of a liquid glucose drink or a solid mixed meal. *J Clin Endocrinol Metab* 1989; 68: 647–653.
44 Ensinck JW, D'Alessio DA. The enteroinsular axis revisited. A novel role for an incretin. *N Engl J Med* 1992; 326: 1352–53.
45 Butler PC, Vore SJ, Acock D. Glucose ingestion causes increased frequency and amplitude of insulin pulsatility. *Diabetologia* 1992; 35: 140 (Abstr.).
46 Bergman R, Bucolo R. Interaction of insulin and glucose in the control of hepatic glucose balance. *Am J Physiol* 1974; 227: 1314–22.
47 Butler PC, Rizza RA. Contribution to postprandial hyperglycemia and effect on initial splanchnic glucose clearance of hepatic glucose cycling in glucose-intolerant or NIDDM patients. *Diabetes* 1991; 40: 73–81.
48 Elia M, Folmer P, Schlatmann A, Goren A, Austin S. Carbohydrate, fat and protein metabolism in muscle and in the whole body after mixed meal ingestion. *Metabolism* 1988; 37: 542–51.
49 Coppack SW, Fisher RM, Gibbons GF *et al.* Postprandial substrate deposition in human forearm and adipose tissue *in vivo*. *Clin Sci* 1990; 79: 339–48.
50 Jackson RA, Roshania R, Hawa M, Sim P, DiSilvio L. Impact of glucose ingestion in hepatic and peripheral glucose metabolism in man: an analysis based on simultaneous use of forearm and double isotope techniques. *J Clin Endocrinol Metab* 1986; 63: 541–9.
51 Bottazzo GF, Dean BM, Gorsuch AN, Cudworth AG. Complement fixing islet cell antibodies in Type 1 diabetes. Possible monitors of active β-cell damage. *Lancet* 1980; i: 668–72.
52 Balks HJ, Schmidt A, Prank K, Hemmer F, von zur Mühlen A, Brabant G. Temporal pattern of pancreatic insulin and C-peptide secretion and of plasma glucose levels after nutritional stimulation. *J Clin Endocrinol Metab* 1992; 75: 1198–203.
53 Yki-Järvinen H, Koivisto VA. Natural course of insulin resistance in Type I diabetes. *N Engl J Med* 1986; 315: 224–30.
54 Katz H, Homan M, Velosa J, Robertson P, Rizza R. Effects of pancreas transplantation on postprandial glucose metabolism. *N Engl J Med* 1991; 325: 1278–83.
55 Kryshak EJ, Butler PC, Marsh C *et al.* Pattern of postprandial carbohydrate metabolism and effects of portal and peripheral insulin delivery. *Diabetes* 1990; 39: 142–18.
56 Perley M, Kipnis DM. Plasma insulin responses to glucose and tolbutamide of normal weight and obese dia-

betic and nondiabetic subjects. *Diabetes* 1966; 15: 867–74.
57 Schmidli RS, Hagan C, Scott RS, Livesey J, Forbes LV. Plasma proinsulin in recently diagnosed type 2 diabetes mellitus. *Diabetes Res Clin Pract* 1993; 20: 133–18.
58 O'Brien TD, Butler PC, Westermark P, Johnson KH. Islet amyloid polypeptide: a review of its biology and potential roles in the pathogenesis of diabetes mellitus. *Vet Pathol* 1993; 30: 317–32.
59 Firth R, Bell P, Marsh H, Hansen I, Rizza R. Postprandial hyperglycemia in patients with noninsulin dependent diabetes mellitus: role of hepatic and extrahepatic tissue. *J Clin Invest* 1986; 77: 1525–32.

# 8 Epidemiology of Insulin-Dependent Diabetes Mellitus (IDDM)

Anders Green

## INTRODUCTION

Diabetes mellitus represents a group of syndromes, all characterised by abnormal glucose tolerance due to impaired insulin secretion and function. Of the major forms of diabetes, insulin-dependent diabetes mellitus (IDDM) afflicts only a relatively small proportion of all diabetic patients. Nevertheless, since IDDM predominantly develops in children and young adults and is associated with increased risk of disabling macrovascular and microvascular complications as well as of premature death, the disease represents a severe burden to patients and society. With the possible exemption of some native populations, IDDM is prevalent in all populations but with marked variations in its geographical distribution.

It has been well established from family and twin studies that IDDM develops on the basis of genetic susceptibility (1). Although probably multifactorial of nature, the genetic susceptibility has its major contribution from the HLA-complex on the short arm of chromosome 6 (see elsewhere in the present volume). There are several lines of evidence indicating the involvement of environmental factors in the aetiology of IDDM. The concordance rate of IDDM among monozygotic twins is about 30–50% (2, 3, unpublished data from the Danish Diabetes Twin Study), and only one in six HLA identical siblings will develop diabetes by the age of 25. The documentated rise in the IDDM incidence as reported from several European populations (4) cannot possibly be explained by increased reproduction among diabetic patients (1) but must be the result of increased occurrence of diabetogenic non-genetic determinants and/or increased individual susceptibility to such factors.

Although the exact nature of the environmental determinants and the way they interact with the genetic factors remain to be clarified, it is generally believed that the process leading to overt IDDM by destruction of the insulin-producing beta-cells of the pancreas is mediated by immune mechanisms (see elsewhere in this volume).

The complex aetiology and pathogenesis of IDDM, combined with the individual and public health impact of the disease, makes IDDM an excellent 'model' disease for epidemiological and aetiological research. The epidemiological approach to research in IDDM is important for several reasons. First, the description of the geographical distribution and determinants of IDDM provides the foundation of generation of hypothesis of aetiology aiming at identifying ways of possible prevention. Secondly, epidemiological knowledge of IDDM is needed to provide the basis for optimal planning and dimensioning of health care in diabetes.

The last decades have seen an almost explosive development in the epidemiological research of IDDM. This trend reflects the recognised need of improved and more detailed knowledge (5), the establishment of standard protocols and guidelines for research in the epidemiology of IDDM (6, 7), and the creation of large international research networks like the WHO DIAMOND Multinational Project on Childhood Diabetes (7) and the EURODIAB ACE programme (8).

This chapter reviews the epidemiology of IDDM. Focus is put on incidence rather than prevalence, since the former more closely reflects events related to disease inception, whereas the latter is determined by both incidence and course of the disease. Furthermore, the review will concentrate on childhood onset IDDM because most epidemiological studies on IDDM have been carried out in paediatric populations. The epidemiology of late complications to IDDM will be presented elsewhere in this volume.

## GEOGRAPHICAL DISTRIBUTION OF IDDM

In spite of the rapidly increasing amount of research in the epidemiology of IDDM, the geographical distribution of IDDM is known for only 5% of the global population (9). Most of the studies have been performed in the Northern hemisphere, particularly in Europe and North America (10).

### Europe

Europe is the part of the world for which the epidemiology of IDDM has been studied most extensively. Until recently, there was a general belief of a 'north–south' gradient in the IDDM incidence (9, 11), with North Europe showing the highest rates reported worldwide. New information, notably arising from the EURODIAB ACE study (8), has changed the picture. Table 8.1 summarises incidence rates, expressed as sex-specific standardised rates for the age group 0–14 years in Europe. In addition to data from recent surveys (8, 10) information has been obtained from the Baltic region (12), Norway (13), Sweden (14), Iceland (15), United Kingdom (16, 17), Luxembourg (18), Austria (19), Italy (20), Spain (21) and Russia (22).

Certainly, the high incidence level in the Nordic countries, particularly in Finland, is evident as compared with the rest of Europe. Overall, Europe is characterised by an almost ten-fold difference in incidence, ranging from almost 40 new cases (Finland) to about 4–5 new cases (Poland, Romania) per 100 000 children annually. Rather than being characterised by a simple north-to-south incidence gradient, the geographical pattern reflects a remarkable variation with sharp contrasts between neighbouring regions. Thus, Sardinia represents a 'hot spot' with an incidence approaching that in Finland and which is several folds higher than the surrounding Mediterranean regions. The Baltic region represents another area of contrasts. Estonia, with its ethnic and cultural similarities with Finland, has an incidence level almost three times less than in Finland. Iceland, founded many centuries ago by migration from Western Norway, has incidence rates much smaller than the rates in Norway, and even smaller than the rates in the UK from where there might have been genetic admixture to the Icelandic population. Although epidemiological information from Germany is limited, there seems to be evidence of an almost three-fold difference in incidence between Denmark and Germany.

From the EURODIAB ACE Study, new information has been obtained from South Europe, indicating incidence levels comparable with Central Europe or possibly somewhat higher (as seen in Sicily and Spain, compared with France, Austria, Hungary and mainland Italy).

It remains to be established whether the huge

Table 8.1. *Recently reported standardised* incidence rates of IDDM (per 100 000 per year) in Europe. Age group 0–14 years*

| Country (region) | Period | Boys | Girls | Reference |
|---|---|---|---|---|
| *Nordic countries* | | | | |
| Finland: | | | | |
| Whole nation | 1971–75 | 26.1 | 23.6 | 10 |
| Whole nation | 1976–80 | 30.0 | 27.4 | 10 |
| Whole nation | 1981–85 | 34.7 | 29.3 | 10 |
| Whole nation | 1983–88 | 36.9 | 31.6 | 12 |
| Two counties | 1989–90 | 47.0 | 38.8 | 8 |
| Norway: | | | | |
| Whole nation | 1973–77 | 19.5 | 17.3 | 13 |
| Whole nation | 1978–82 | 23.3 | 20.7 | 13 |
| Eight counties | 1989–90 | 22.3 | 19.3 | 8 |
| Sweden: | | | | |
| Whole nation | 1977–83 | 24.2 | 22.0 | 14 |
| Denmark: | | | | |
| Three counties | 1970–76 | 14.5 | 13.5 | 10 |
| Two counties | 1989–90 | 21.5 | 21.4 | 8 |
| Iceland: | | | | |
| Whole nation | 1970–79 | 9.3 | 6.6 | 15 |
| Whole nation | 1980–89 | 10.5 | 11.1 | 15 |
| *Baltic region* | | | | |
| Estonia: | | | | |
| Whole nation | 1983–88 | 10.7 | 10.0 | 12 |
| Latvia: | | | | |
| Whole nation | 1983–88 | 6.4 | 6.7 | 12 |
| Lithuania: | | | | |
| Whole nation | 1983–88 | 6.5 | 7.0 | 12 |
| *British Isles* | | | | |
| England: | | | | |
| Leicestershire | 1965–81 | 8.6 | 8.6 | 10 |
| Oxford | 1985–86 | 17.3 | 13.9 | 16 |
| Oxford | 1989–90 | 17.8 | 14.9 | 8 |
| Scotland: | | | | |
| Whole region | 1977–83 | 20.1 | 19.6 | 17 |
| Tayside | 1980–83 | 21.5 | 18.2 | 10 |
| Northern Ireland: | | | | |
| Whole region | 1989–90 | 17.8 | 15.4 | 8 |
| *Central Europe* | | | | |
| The Netherlands: | | | | |
| Whole nation | 1978–80 | 9.9 | 9.5 | 10 |
| Five counties | 1989–90 | 11.2 | 10.8 | 8 |
| Belgium: | | | | |
| Antwerp region | 1989–90 | 9.2 | 10.4 | 8 |
| France: | | | | |
| Four provinces | 1989–90 | 7.8 | 7.8 | 8 |
| Luxembourg: | | | | |
| Whole nation | 1977–86 | 12.4 | 8.7 | 18 |
| Whole nation | 1989–90 | 12.1 | 12.6 | 8 |
| Germany: | | | | |
| Former GDR | 1982–84 | 7.0 | 7.0 | 10 |
| Austria: | | | | |
| Whole nation | 1979–84 | 7.9 | 7.3 | 19 |

Table 8.1. (*cont.*)

| Country (region) | Period | Boys | Girls | Reference |
|---|---|---|---|---|
| Hungary: | | | | |
| Eighteen counties | 1989–90 | 7.7 | 7.5 | 8 |
| Slovenia: | | | | |
| Whole nation | 1989–90 | 5.2 | 7.7 | 8 |
| *East Europe* | | | | |
| Russia: | | | | |
| Novosibirsk district | 1983–89 | 4.6 | 4.9 | 22 |
| Poland: | | | | |
| Wielkopolska region | 1971–75 | 3.3 | 3.7 | 10 |
| | 1976–80 | 4.9 | 4.1 | 10 |
| | 1981–85 | 6.0 | 6.6 | 10 |
| Nine western provinces | 1989–90 | 5.3 | 5.8 | 8 |
| Three cities | 1989–90 | 5.7 | 6.0 | 8 |
| Romania: | | | | |
| Bucharest region | 1989–90 | 4.6 | 5.7 | 8 |
| *South Europe* | | | | |
| Italy: | | | | |
| Turin | 1984–86 | 7.8 | 9.1 | 20 |
| Lombardia | 1989–90 | 7.6 | 5.9 | 8 |
| Lazio | 1989–90 | 7.2 | 5.8 | 8 |
| Eastern Sicily | 1989–90 | 11.2 | 9.0 | 8 |
| Sardinia | 1989–90 | 33.5 | 26.9 | 8 |
| Portugal: | | | | |
| Three districts | 1989–90 | 10.1 | 4.9 | 8 |
| Greece: | | | | |
| Athens region | 1989–90 | 10.9 | 7.7 | 8 |
| Thessaloniki region | 1989–90 | 5.3 | 3.8 | 8 |
| Spain: | | | | |
| Madrid | 1985–88 | 11.8 | 10.9 | 21 |
| Catalonia | 1989–90 | 10.5 | 10.6 | 8 |

* The standard population assumes sex and age classes (0–4; 5–9; 10–14 yr) of equal sizes.

variation in the IDDM within Europe can be ascribed to variation in genetic susceptibility factors, to differential distribution of environmental disease determinants, or a combination of these. However, the considerable variation between genetically similar populations (Finland versus Estonia and Hungary; Norway versus Iceland), and even within countries of assumedly homogeneous composition (Norway (13); Sweden (14)) strongly suggests that environmental factors contribute substantially to the geographical variation. On the other hand, the Russian population residing in Estonia seems to exhibit a disease risk considerably lower than the native Estonians (23) but higher than Russians residing in Siberia (24). It remains to be established whether the difference is caused by genes or environment. Unfortunately, no migrant studies have been performed in Europe to elucidate the extent to which the individual risk will be changed by shifting environment.

## IDDM incidence outside Europe

The epidemiology of IDDM outside Europe has been reviewed recently (9, 25). With the contribution of new data from Australia (26), available information on the incidence of childhood-onset IDDM is summarized in Table 8.2. The general picture is that, in North America, the incidence level compares well with that found in the UK and Central Europe. In Australia, the same

Table 8.2. *Recently reported standardised* incidence rates of IDDM (per 100 000 per year) outside Europe. Age group 0–14 years*

| Country (region) | Period | Boys | Girls | Reference |
|---|---|---|---|---|
| *North America* | | | | |
| United States: | | | | |
| Allegheny Co., PA | 1978–83 | 12.1 | 14.8 | 9 |
| Colorado | 1978–83 | 13.8 | 16.4 | 9 |
| Jefferson Co., AL | 1979–83 | 8.8 | 14.4 | 9 |
| North Dakota | 1979–83 | 16.0 | 19.5 | 9 |
| Rochester, MN | 1970–79 | 19.7 | 22.1 | 9 |
| San Diego, CA | 1978–80 | 9.6 | 9.1 | 9 |
| Canada: | | | | |
| Montreal | | 9.0 | 9.4 | 9 |
| Prince Edward Island | | 25.6 | 25.1 | 9 |
| *Asia and Oceania* | | | | |
| Australia: | | | | |
| Western Australia | 1985–89 | 13.2 (Sexes combined) | | 26 |
| New Zealand: | | | | |
| Auckland | 1982–85 | 8.2 | 7.2 | 9 |
| Canterbury | 1982–85 | 10.2 | 12.9 | 9 |
| Japan: | | | | |
| Hokkaido | 1985–87 | 2.3 (Sexes combined) | | 25 |
| Korea: | | | | |
| Seoul | 1985–86 | 0.5 | 0.6 | 25 |
| *Middle East* | | | | |
| Israel: | | | | |
| Whole nation | 1989–90 | 4.4 | 6.7 | 8 |

* Adjusted to the world population as described in Ref. 9.

seems to be the case, although estimates based on prevalence data from Tasmania suggest a somewhat smaller level (27).

All Asian populations studied so far exhibit extremely low incidence levels. Also, for the non-white populations in US, rates are smaller than for whites (reviewed in (25)).

For many native populations, like the Inuit in the Circumpolar region, diabetes in childhood is extremely rare (28, 29).

Many areas and populations in Asia, Africa and the Americas remain to be described in terms of their IDDM epidemiology. Combined with information from migrant studies, such descriptive epidemiological research would be extremely important for the generation of hypotheses of the IDDM aetiology.

## TEMPORAL TRENDS

Until a decade ago it was generally believed that IDDM was stable in terms of incidence and individual risk. With the subsequent reporting of long-term studies of populations, a much more differentiated pattern has emerged. The temporal trend in IDDM incidence has two components: trends in the calendar time of diagnosis, and seasonality of clinical onset of IDDM.

### Calendar time

The first well-established evidence of increasing incidence of IDDM came from Sweden (30), Denmark (31) and The Netherlands (11). Further support and characterisation of the calendar time trend have been obtained from Sweden (32), Finland (33), Denmark (34), The Netherlands (35), Hungary (36) and, most recently, Sardinia (37). In Poland, an apparent epidemic of IDDM in the mid-1980s has been reported (38) but, otherwise, the trend has in general been described as a steadily increasing incidence during the last several decades (34), corresponding in some instances to an estimated doubling in incidence per generation (4). The increasing incidence has predominantly been reported from Europe and some Caucasian populations in North America, whereas the large Pittsburgh study did not find evidence of major secular trends (39).

Although attempts have been made to correlate the changing incidence to environmental factors, like changing breast-feeding habits (40), no obvious explanations have been identified. In elegant epidemiological–mathematical models neither the Swedish (32) nor the Finnish (33) studies could find support for a cohort effect to explain the increasing incidence, which would otherwise have been predicted by the breast-feeding hypothesis. Since there is no possible way of attributing the increasing incidence to improved survival and reproductiveness among patients with IDDM (1), the secular trend must be caused by changes in the occurrence of so far unknown environmental determinants and/or by changes in individual susceptibility to IDDM. The subject represents one of the major challenges for future research in IDDM epidemiology.

### Seasonality of IDDM onset

In the northern hemisphere it has consistently been found that relatively more cases of childhood IDDM are diagnosed during the autumn and winter season as compared with the spring and summer seasons (e.g. 13, 14, 16, 18, 19, 38, 41). The same feature has been identified in Chile from the southern hemisphere (42).

Some studies have reported evidence that this seasonal trend is seen particularly at age levels around puberty and less evidently during the first years of life (11, 17, 19, 41, 43–45). On the other hand, detailed analysis of the EURODIAB ACE data base (8) has indicated that the effect of seasonality applies equally to all sex and age classes, without evidence of heterogeneity across the populations studied.

Since the destruction of the beta cells of the pancreas may be induced several years prior to clinical onset of the disease, the characteristic seasonality of IDDM onset may reflect seasonal variations in individual susceptibility to certain environmental, precipitating factors. Another possibility may be increased demand of endogenous insulin during winter months, thereby precipitating clinical disease in subjects with partially destroyed beta cells. This is to some extent supported by the finding that glucose tolerance deteriorates slightly, as indicated by seasonal variations in glycosylated haemoglobin levels, in winter months in normal subjects (46).

Alternatively, the variation may be explained by heterogeneity of natural history, i.e. that some cases represent epidemic cases with rapid development particularly in winter months, whereas the remaining cases represent a more prolonged natural history (47). Within this context, some studies (48, 49) have found that cases with onset in the youngest age class (0–4 years) and with less marked seasonal variation experienced increased cumulative rates of complete beta cell destruction at follow-up after 2–3 years as compared with cases having onset at higher ages.

## ENVIRONMENTAL DETERMINANTS

The identification of environmental determinants of IDDM is of particular importance, since they are potentially modifiable for the purpose of disease prevention. Although the search for environmental determinants of IDDM has been intensified, the results have not so far led to a unified hypothesis of the non-genetic contribution to IDDM. The research has focused on exposure to infectious diseases and immunisations, nutritional factors, socio-economic status and stressful life events. The evidence for viral determination has been reviewed recently (50) and will be discussed elsewhere in this volume. The present review will comment on the remaining issues.

## Nutrients

Several studies have focused on the possible role of dietary factors in the aetiology of IDDM. It has been suggested, in a study from Iceland, that exposure to nitrosamines in women at the time of conception may increase the risk of IDDM in the offspring, particularly males (51). Some support to this concept has come from Sweden (52), but the finding needs confirmation and does not explain the high IDDM incidence level in populations where exposure to nitrosamines is less common than in Iceland.

The association between IDDM and breast-feeding habits has been extensively studied since Borch-Johnsen *et al.* (40) found evidence that reduced length of breast-feeding during infancy seems to be associated with increased risk of developing IDDM. Subsequently, some studies have confirmed this possibility (53, 54), whereas another Danish study (55) has been unable to do so. In general, the associations described have been weak and, if causal, can only explain the development of diabetes in a limited number of cases. Furthermore, changes in breast-feeding habits over time as well as the possible operation of recall biases in such case-control studies are potential confounders that are difficult to control.

Nevertheless, the breast-feeding hypothesis has experienced its come-back, following the identification of a much higher occurrence of antibodies to cow's milk protein in newly onset diabetic children as compared with control subjects (56). Accordingly, the increased IDDM risk among children with lack of, or with reduced duration of, breast-feeding might be explained by early introduction to a protein that acts as a trigger for the immunological destruction of the beta-cells. At present, this hypothesis represents a possible major concept of the aetiology and pathogenesis of IDDM since it incorporates elements from epidemiology, immunology and molecular genetics into one unified model. It is, however, likely that this mechanism is only one of several possible mechanisms to explain the causation of IDDM.

## Socio-economic status

Conflicting results have been reported regarding the influence of socio-economic status on the risk of developing IDDM. After attempts to stratify their study populations according to income level and other indicators of socio-economic status, Christau *et al.* (57) in the Copenhagen area, Denmark, found higher incidence of IDDM in regions with relatively low average income level, whereas Siemiatycki *et al.* (58) found an opposite trend. In both studies, however, the incidence differences between social classes were rather modest only, and neither of the studies applied a case-control technique to evaluate the extent to which the individual cases from the various sub-areas in fact were representative of those particular status levels. In a Swedish case-control study, Blom *et al.* (54) found a positive, but rather weak association between IDDM and low educational and income level.

The results from studies of associations between indicators of socio-econmic status and IDDM are difficult to interpret. First, comparisons between studies are hampered by differences in definitions, study design and methods of data analysis. Secondly, as proposed by Blom *et al.* (54), such associations are probably explained by unknown events and factors in life-style that influence the risk of developing IDDM as well as the socio-economic status.

## Stressful life events

A few studies have addressed the possible aetiological role of psychological factors and stressful life events in the period preceding clinical onset of disease. Although with rather weak associations, several reports have provided consistent evidence of such possible influence (59–61). It is most likely that stressful life events and psychological dysfunction may, through elevated stress hormone levels, increase the demand for endogenous insulin production and thereby accelerate clinical precipitation of IDDM in individuals with ongoing beta-cell destruction.

## DETERMINANTS OF INDIVIDUAL SUSCEPTIBILITY

The most important determinant of individual susceptibility to IDDM is the genome of a given subject. The genetic contribution to the aetiology of IDDM is reviewed elsewhere in this volume and will not be addressed in details in this chapter. Similarly, the influence on individual disease risk by presence of immune markers of beta-cell destruction will be described elsewhere. From an epidemiological viewpoint, the remaining major determinants of individual susceptibility relate to gender and age.

### Gender

Until recently, it has been a consistent finding that boys exhibit a slightly increased risk of IDDM as compared to girls (e.g. 11, 13, 14, 16). It appears that these studies originate from populations of high or intermediate risk. The new information on the detailed epidemiology of IDDM in populations at low risk suggests, as evident from Table 8.1, that in these populations the two genders have similar risks. Apparently, the influence of gender on the IDDM risk interacts with other determinants. These are most likely to be non-genetic in nature since advanced genetic analysis has failed to demonstrate any gender difference in the genetic susceptibility to IDDM (62, 63).

### Age

Detailed analyses of large study materials have repeatedly found that, within the first 15 years of the age span, IDDM incidence shows certain peaks at pre-school age and around puberty. This trend is similar for the two sexes, but the peak around puberty appears to occur slighty earlier among girls (e.g. 19). As with the influence by gender, the age dependency may reflect that humans are particularly susceptible at certain age levels and/or that exposure to environmental aetiological factors is associated with age.

The incidence of IDDM beyond childhood has only been studied to a limited extent, probably reflecting ascertainment difficulties in adulthood. In their population-based Swedish study Östman *et al.* (64) found that the incidence of IDDM in the age interval 15–34 years remains rather constant at a relatively low level. A remarkable and so-far unexplained finding from studies in high risk areas is that males in adulthood seem to carry a considerably higher disease risk than females; this has been found in Sweden (64) and, most recently, in Sardinia (65). Presently, studies on the IDDM incidence among adults in low risk populations are highly needed.

## THE EPIDEMIOLOGY OF IDDM: FUTURE CHALLENGES

The most noble task of epidemiology is to provide clues to a better understanding of disease causation, thereby leading to possible ways of prevention. Despite intensive epidemiological and aetiological research in IDDM, we are still far away for a clear understanding of the detailed elements and mechanism causing this severe disease. The future challenges for epidemiology are, first of all, represented by the need to obtain a better and more detailed picture of the disease variation according to populations, ethnic groups and time. Secondly, continued epidemiological efforts may hopefully identify environmental disease determinants that are subject to potential modification. The ultimate goal is to be able to characterise an individual's disease risk according to genetic and immunological status and environmental exposure, in order to be able to identify groups of individuals at high disease risk and in whom measures of intervention might be appropriate.

Given the obvious complex causation of IDDM, these goals can only be achieved by collaborative efforts with the involvement of epidemiologists, immunologists, clinicians, population geneticists and molecular geneticists.

## REFERENCES


1 Green A. The role of genetic factors in the development of insulin-dependent diabetes mellitus. In: Bækkeskov S, Hansen B, eds. *Current topics in microbiology and immunology, vol. 164: Human diabetes: genetic, environmental and autoimmune etiology.* Springer-Verlag; 1990: 3–16.
2 Leslie RDG, Lo SSS, Hawa M, Tun RYM. Lessons on the etiology of insulin-dependent diabetes from twin studies. In: Levy-Marchal C, Czernichow P, eds. *Epidemiology and etiology of insulin-dependent diabetes in the young.* Karger, Basel; 1992: 91–106.
3 Kaprio J, Tuomilehto J, Koskenvuo M, *et al.* Concordance for Type 1 (insulin-dependent) and Type 2 (non-insulin-dependent) diabetes mellitus in a population-based cohort of twins in Finland. *Diabetologia* 1992; 35: 1060–7.
4 Bingley PJ, Gale EAM. Rising incidence of IDDM in Europe. *Diabetes Care* 1989; 12: 289–95.
5 LaPorte RE, Tajima N, Åkerblom HK *et al.* Geographic differences in the risk of insulin-dependent diabetes mellitus: the importance of registries. *Diabetes Care* 1985; 8 Suppl 1: 101–7.
6 Green A, King HOM, LaPorte RE. Workshop on diabetes registers: the role of IDDM registers in diabetes research and care. In: Serrano Rios M, Lefébvre JP, eds. *Diabetes, 1985.* Elsevier; Amsterdam, 1985: 443–8.
7 WHO DIAMOND Project Group. WHO Multinational Project for Childhood Diabetes. *Diabetes Care* 1990; 13: 1062–8.
8 Green A, Gale EAM, Patterson CC for the EURODIAB ACE Study Group. Incidence of childhood-onset insulin-dependent diabetes mellitus: the EURODIAB ACE study. *Lancet* 1992; 339: 905–9.
9 Diabetes Epidemiology Research International Group. Geographic patterns of childhood insulin-dependent diabetes mellitus. *Diabetes* 1988; 37: 1113–19.
10 Rewers M, LaPorte RE, King H, Tuomilehto J. Trends in the prevalence and incidence of diabetes: Insulin-dependent diabetes mellitus in childhood. *World Health Statistics Quart* 1988; 41: 179–89.
11 Vaandrager GJ, Bruining GJ, Veenhof FJ, Drayer NM. Incidence of childhood diabetes in The Netherlands: a decrease from north to south over North-Western Europe? *Diabetologia* 1984; 27: 203–6.
12 Tuomilehto J, Podar T, Brigis G *et al.* Comparison of the incidence of insulin-dependent diabetes mellitus in childhood among five Baltic populations 1983–1988. *Int J Epidemiol* 1992; 21: 518–27.
13 Joner G, Søvik O. Increasing incidence of diabetes mellitus in Norwegian children 0–14 years of age 1973–1982. *Diabetologia* 1989; 32: 79–83.
14 Dahlquist G, Blom L, Holmgren G *et al.* The epidemiology of diabetes in Swedish children 0–14 years – a six-year prospective study. *Diabetologia* 1985; 28: 802–8.
15 Helgason T, Danielsen R, Thorsson AV. Incidence and prevalence of Type 1 (insulin-dependent) diabetes mellitus in Icelandic children 1970–1989. *Diabetologia* 1992; 35: 880–3.
16 Bingley PJ, Gale EAM. Incidence of insulin dependent diabetes in England: a study in the Oxford region, 1985–6. *Br Med J* 1989; 298: 558–60.
17 Patterson CC, Smith PG, Webb J, Heasman MA, Mann JI. Geographical variation in the incidence of diabetes mellitus in Scottish children during the period 1977–1983. *Diabetic Med* 1988; 5: 160–5.
18 de Beaufort CE, Michel G, Glaesener G. The incidence of type 1 (insulin-dependent) diabetes mellitus in subjects aged 0–19 years in Luxembourg: a retrospective study from 1977 to 1986. *Diabetologia* 1988; 31: 758–61.
19 Schober E, Frisch H. Incidence of childhood diabetes mellitus in Austria 1979–1984. *Acta Pæd Scand* 1988; 77: 299–302.
20 Bruno G, Merletti F, Pisu E, Pastore G, Marengo C, Pagano G. Incidence of IDDM during 1984–1986 in population aged <30 yr; residents of Turin, Italy. *Diabetes Care* 1990; 13: 1051–6.
21 Rios M, Moy CS, Serrano RM *et al.* Incidence of Type 1 (insulin-dependent) diabetes mellitus in subjects 0–14 years of age in the Comunidad of Madrid, Spain. *Diabetologia* 1990; 33: 422–4.
22 Shubnikov E, Podar T, Tuomilehto J, Nikitin Y. Low incidence of childhood IDDM in District of Novosibirsk (Russia). *Diabetes Care* 1992; 15: 915–7.
23 Podar T, Tuomilehto-Wolf E, Tuomilehto J, LaPorte RE, Adojaan B. Insulin-dependent diabetes mellitus in native Estonians and immigrants to Estonia. *Am J Epidemiol* 1992; 135: 1231–6.
24 Podar T, LaPorte RE, Tuomilehto J, Shubnikov E. Risk of childhood Type 1 diabetes for Russians in Estonia and Siberia. *Int J Epidemiol* 1993; 22: 262–7.
25 Tajima N, LaPorte RE on behalf of WHO DIAMOND project group. Incidence of IDDM outside Europe. In: Levy-Marchal C, Czernichow P, eds. *Epidemiology and etiology of insulin-dependent diabetes in the young.* Karger, Basel; 1992: 31–41.
26 Kelly HA, Byrne GC. Incidence of IDDM in Western Australia in children aged 0–14 yr from 1985 to 1989. *Diabetes Care* 1992; 15: 515–17.
27 King H, Dixon J, Senator G, Schooneveldt M, Zimmet P. Type 1 (insulin-dependent) diabetes in Tasmania: prevalence and apparent regional differences. *Diabetologia* 1988; 31: 93–7.
28 Young TK, Schraer CD, Shubnikoff EV, Szathmary EJE, Nikitin YP. Prevalence of diagnosed diabetes in circumpolar indigenous populations. *Int J Epidemiol* 1992; 21: 730–6.
29 Kromann N, Green A. Epidemiological studies in the Upernavik District, Greenland. Incidence of some chronic diseases 1950–1974. *Acta Med Scand* 1980; 208: 401–6.
30 Hägglöf B, Holmgren G, Wall S. Incidence of insulin-dependent diabetes mellitus among children in a North-Swedish population 1938–1977. *Hum Hered* 1982; 32: 408–17.
31 Green A, Andersen PK. Epidemiological studies of diabetes mellitus in Denmark: 3. Clinical characteristics

and incidence of diabetes among males aged 0 to 19 years. *Diabetologia* 1983; 25: 226–30.
32 Nyström L, Dahlquist G, Rewers M, Wall S. The Swedish Childhood Diabetes Study. An analysis of the temporal variation in diabetes incidence 1978–1987. *Int J Epidemiol* 1990; 19: 141–6.
33 Tuomilehto J, Rewers M, Reunanen A *et al.* Increasing trend in Type 1 (insulin-dependent) diabetes mellitus in childhood in Finland. Analysis of age, calendar time and birth cohort effects during 1965 to 1984. *Diabetologia* 1991; 34: 282–7.
34 Green A, Andersen PK, Svendsen AJ, Mortensen K. Increasing incidence of early onset Type 1 (insulin-dependent) diabetes mellitus: a study of Danish male birth cohorts. *Diabetologia* 1992; 35: 178–82.
35 Drykoningen CEM, Mulder ALM, Vaandrager GJ, LaPorte RE, Bruining GJ. The incidence of male childhood Type 1 (insulin-dependent) diabetes mellitus is rising rapidly in The Netherlands. *Diabetologia* 1992; 35: 139–42.
36 Soltész G, Madácsy L, Békefi D, Dankó l, the Hungarian Childhood Diabetes Epidemiology Group. Rising incidence of Type 1 diabetes in Hungarian children (1978–1987). *Diabetic Med* 1990; 7: 111–14.
37 Songini M, Loche M, Muntoni Sa *et al.* Increasing prevalence of juvenile onset Type 1 (insulin-dependent) diabetes mellitus in Sardinia: the military service approach. *Diabetologia* 1993; 36: 547–52.
38 Rewers M, LaPorte RE, Walczak M, Dmochowski K, Bogaczynska E. Apparent epidemic of insulin-dependent diabetes mellitus in Midwestern Poland. *Diabetologia* 1987: 36: 106–13.
39 LaPorte RE, Fishbein HA, Drash AL *et al.* The Pittsburgh insulin-dependent diabetes mellitus (IDDM) registry. The incidence of insulin-dependent diabetes mellitus in Allegheny County, Pennsylvania (1965–1976). *Diabetes* 1981; 30: 279–84.
40 Borch-Johnsen K, Mandrup-Poulsen T, Zachau-Christiansen B *et al.* Relation between breast-feeding and incidence rates of insulin-dependent diabetes. A hypothesis. *Lancet* 1984; 4: 1083–6.
41 Fishbein HA, LaPorte RE, Orchard TJ, Drash AL, Kuller LH, Wagener DK. The Pittsburgh insulin-dependent diabetes mellitus registry: seasonal incidence. *Diabetologia* 1982; 23: 83–5.
42 Durruty P, Ruiz F, Garcia de los Rios M. Age at diagnosis and seasonal variation in the onset of insulin-dependent diabetes in Chile (southern hemisphere). *Diabetologia* 1979; 17: 357–60.
43 Gray RS, Duncan LJP, Clarke BF. Seasonal onset of insulin dependent diabetes in relation to sex and age at onset. *Diabetologia* 1979; 17: 29–32.
44 Gleason RE, Kahn CB, Funk IB, Craighead JE. Seasonal incidence of insulin-dependent diabetes (IDDM) in Massachusetts, 1964–1973. *Int J Epidemiol* 1982; 11: 39–45.
45 Allen C, Palta M, D'Alessio DJ. Incidence and differences in urban-rural seasonal variation of type 1 (insulin-dependent) diabetes in Wisconsin. *Diabetologia* 1986; 29: 629–33.
46 MacDonald MJ, Liston L, Carlson I. Seasonality in glycosylated hemoglobin in normal subjects. Does seasonal incidence in insulin-dependent diabetes suggest specific etiology? *Diabetes* 1987; 36: 265–8.
47 Ludvigsson J, Afoke AO. Seasonality of type 1 (insulin-dependent) diabetes mellitus: values of C-peptide, insulin antibodies and haemoglobin $A_{1c}$ show evidence of a more rapid loss of insulin secretion in epidemic patients. *Diabetologia* 1989; 32: 84–91.
48 Dahlquist G, Blom L, Persson B, Wallensteen M, Wall S. The epidemiology of lost β-cell function in short term diabetic children. *Acta Paed Scand* 1988; 77: 852–9.
49 Schiffrin A, Suissa S, Poussier P, Guttmann R, Weitzner G. Prospective study of predictors of β-cell survival in Type 1 diabetes. *Diabetes* 1988; 37: 920–5.
50 Yoon J-W, Pak CY, Lee M, MacArthur RG. Is viral infection an initiating factor for insulin-dependent diabetes mellitus? In: Levy-Marchal C, Czernicow P, eds. *Epidemiology and etiology of insulin-dependent diabetes in the young.* Basel: Karger, 1992; 218–31.
51 Helgason T, Jonasson MR. Evidence for a food additive as a cause of ketosis-prone diabetes. *Lancet* 1981; ii: 716–20.
52 Dahlquist G, Blom L, Lönnberg G. The Swedish Childhood Diabetes Study – a multivariate analysis of risk determinants for diabetes in different age groups. *Diabetologia* 1991; 34: 757–62.
53 Mayer EJ, Hamman RF, Gay EC, Lezotte DC, Savitz DA, Klingensmith J. Reduced risk of IDDM among breastfed children. The Colorado IDDM Registry. *Diabetes* 1988; 37: 1625–32.
54 Blom L, Dahlquist G, Nyström L, Sandström A, Wall S. The Swedish childhood diabetes study – social and perinatal determinants for diabetes in childhood. *Diabetologia* 1989;32:7–13.
55 Kyvik KO, Green A, Svendsen A, Mortensen K. Breast feeding and the development of type 1 diabetes mellitus. *Diabetic Med* 1992;9:233–5.
56 Karjalainen J, Martin JM, Knip M *et al.* A bovine albumin peptide as a possible trigger of insulin-dependent diabetes mellitus. *N Engl J Med* 1992;327:302–7.
57 Christau B, Kromann H, Andersen OO *et al.* Incidence, seasonal and geographic patterns of juvenile-onset insulin-dependent diabetes mellitus in Denmark. *Diabetologia* 1977;13:281–4.
58 Siemiatycki J, Colle E, Campbell S, Dewar R, Aubert D, Belmonte MM. Incidence of IDDM in Montreal by ethnic group and by social class and comparisons with ethnic groups living elsewhere. *Diabetes* 1988;37:1096–102.
59 Robinson N, Fuller JH. Role of life events and difficulties in the onset of diabetes mellitus. *J Psychosomatic Res* 1985;29:583–91.
60 Siemiatycki J, Colle E, Campbell S, Dewar RAD, Belmonte MM. Case-control study of IDDM. *Diabetes Care* 1989;12:209–16.
61 Hägglöf B, Blom L, Dahlquist G, Lönnberg G, Sahlin B. The Swedish childhood diabetes study: indications of severe psychological stress as a risk factor for Type 1 (insulin-dependent) diabetes mellitus in childhood. *Diabetologia* 1991;34:579–83.
62 Green A, Svejgaard A, Platz P *et al.* The genetic susceptibility to insulin-dependent diabetes mellitus (IDDM): Combined segregation and linkage analysis. *Genet Epidemiol* 1985;2:1–15.

63 Pascoe L, Sherman S, Wu D, Becker M, Falk C. Combined segregation and linkage analysis for IDDM and HLA-DR under several ascertainment assumptions. *Genet Epidemiol* 1989;6:131–6.
64 Östman J, Arnqvist H, Blohmé G *et al.* Epidemiology of diabetes mellitus in Sweden. Results of the first year of a prospective study in the population age group 15–34 years. *Acta Med Scand* 1986;220:437–45.
65 Muntoni S, Songini M, Sardinian Collaborative Group for Epidemiology of IDDM. High incidence rate of IDDM in Sardinia. *Diabetes Care* 1992;15:1317–22.

# 9 Genetics of Insulin-dependent Diabetes

Anneke Lucassen & John Bell

## INTRODUCTION

Insulin dependent diabetes mellitus (IDDM) or Type I diabetes is a chronic autoimmune disease resulting from the selective destruction of pancreatic beta cells. As with many autoimmune diseases, both genetic and environmental factors seem to play a role in susceptibility. Inheritance of IDDM is complex with no clear Mendelian pattern. However, the disease does run in families and siblings of a diabetic individual are at increased risk of developing diabetes over the general population (6% (1) versus 0.4% (2)). The risk to siblings is increased to 12% (1) if they are HLA identical, and to 36% for monozygotic twins (3). These figures indicate that there is a definite genetic component to susceptibility with the HLA (human leucocyte antigen) locus providing some, but not all of the genetic component. However, since the concordance rate for genetically identical twins is much less than 100%, other non-genetic factors must also be involved. These other factors may be either environmental, or alternatively may relate to the stochastic processes of gene rearrangements which occur during lymphocyte ontogeny and which produce differences in immunoglobulin and T cell repertoires even in individuals with identical genetic backgrounds. Twin studies in humans and evidence from mouse and rat models of IDDM suggest that there are several different genes, which may interact or function independently, encoding susceptibility. This chapter focuses on the genetic loci that have been identified to date in Type I diabetes.

## IDDM IS A POLYGENIC DISEASE

Evidence from both animal models and humans, suggests that several different genetic loci are involved in the susceptibility to IDDM. In humans, large multiply affected extended pedigrees are rare and there is a high frequency of non-familial disease. HLA is an important component of genetic susceptibility: 60% of the diabetic siblings of a patient are HLA identical (4) and the risk of developing IDDM is greater for HLA identical than non HLA identical siblings (see above). However, theoretical studies show that the HLA region genes can not explain the total genetic susceptibility to IDDM. For example, Risch showed that the increased risk of IDDM in siblings of diabetics compared with the general population risk was not fully accounted for by sharing of HLA haplotypes (2). Risch's calculations suggested that of the 15-fold increased relative risk to siblings of an IDDM patient (6%/0.4%) only approximately 25% is accounted for by HLA. The remaining familial factors are likely to consist of both genetic loci outside the HLA and non-genetic factors. Furthermore, as already mentioned, the concordance rate for monozygotic twins is higher than for HLA identical siblings implying that other genes outside the MHC (major histocompatibility complex) must also provide susceptibility to IDDM (5). Evidence for the involvement of several genes in IDDM susceptibility also comes from animal models. Two animal models of diabetes exist; the non-obese diabetic (NOD) mouse (6) and the biobreeding (BB) rat (7). The NOD mouse was derived from selective inbreeding of mice being bred for the study of cataracts, who spontaneously developed hyperglycaemia. Backcross experiments have shown that the MHC locus is important in susceptibility, but more than five genes outside the MHC are thought also to contribute (8–12). Similar studies in the BB rat show that the MHC and presence of a lymphopenic trait are not sufficient to account for all of the genetic susceptibility to diabetes (13).

## APPROACHES TO IDENTIFYING A GENETIC LOCUS

The two main approaches to identifying a genetic locus in humans are either by association studies or linkage studies. Association studies look at the association of a particular marker with the disease in a population of patients and controls. Differences in marker frequencies can be expressed as a relative risk or odds ratio and its statistical significance evaluated. For a marker to be associated with the disease, it must lie relatively close to the disease gene. In a population over the generations there are many opportunities for genetic recombination between a marker and an adjacent disease locus and eventually a state of equilibrium will be reached where there is no association between marker and disease gene. If this state of equilibrium is not reached, the loci are said to be in linkage disequilibrium (LD) with each other. LD can arise through several mechanisms. For example: (a) the markers lie very close to each other and/or (b) there may be few DNA sequences between the markers that allow recombination. (c) If a new mutation occurs, it will be in LD with the alleles on the haplotype on which it occurs, or (d) there may be evolutionary selection pressures on particular markers to remain together on the same haplotype. An example of this occurs in the HLA region (see below) where several genes occur together on the same haplotypes more frequently than expected based on their individual allele frequencies. A population association may, however, reflect population stratification or lack of ethnic homogeneity rather than close proximity to the disease locus and, for this reason, independent confirmation of linkage in families is generally considered to be necessary to prove a genetic association. Linkage studies follow the segregation of a marker with the disease in families. As there are relatively few meioses within a family, the marker can lie at quite large chromosomal distances from the disease gene and because markers are examined within families, environmental influences are neutralised. Traditionally linkage studies are performed on large multi-generation pedigrees with many affected individuals and LOD scores are calculated to measure the degree of linkage. However, large pedigrees are rare in IDDM and therefore small nuclear pedigrees with two affected siblings are usually studied using the affected sib-pair (ASP) method. This method involves identifying four distinguishable haplotypes in parents (a,b,c,d see Fig. 9.1) and the inheritance of each haplotype identical by descent can be traced in affected offspring pairs. Random expectations would be that offspring share 2,1 or 0 haplotypes respectively 25%, 50%, 25% of the time. Significant deviation from these expectations supports linkage. ASP analyses have been shown to produce results equivalent to multi-generation pedigrees and have the advantage that no genetic model of inheritance is required (14–16). The power to detect linkage depends on the number of multiplex families studied, the degree of polymor-

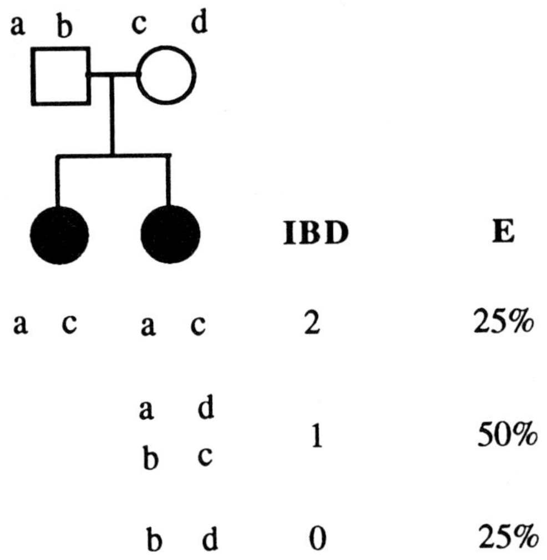


Fig. 9.1 The affected sib pair method. Families are selected where parents are heterozygous for alleles a–d such that the parental origin of alleles in affected offspring can be determined. The amount of shared alleles (or alleles identical by descent IBD) is compared with the Mendelian expected proportions (E). a–d can represent different alleles or different haplotypes (series of markers situated close to each other on a chromosome).

phism of the marker and the contribution that the locus makes to susceptibility (16–18).

## IDDM IS AN AUTOIMMUNE DISORDER

Evidence that IDDM is an autoimmune process comes from both animal models and humans. In humans, examination of the diabetic pancreas reveals immune cell infiltrates in the islets of Langerhans (19–21) and pancreatic graft survival is dependent on immunosuppressive drugs (22). There are distortions of lymphocyte subsets (23, 24) and lymphocytes from diabetic patients have been shown to be cytotoxic to insulinoma cells *in vitro* (25). Autoantibodies against specific islet cell antigens have been detected: for example, insulin autoantibody (IAA) (26), islet cell autoantibody (ICA) (26, 27), autoantibodies directed against glutamic acid decarboxylase (GAD) (28) and autoantibodies directed against a 38 kD protein thought to be an integral part of the insulin secretory granule membrane (29). In the NOD mouse, overt diabetes develops in approximately 80% females and 20% males but insulitis develops in all inbred NOD mice (26). Of BB rats, 60% have diabetes and the majority of those that do not, have evidence of islet cell infiltrates and β cell destruction (30). Disease can be transferred from affected to healthy animals by transferring CD4+ and CD8+ subsets of T-lymphocytes (31, 32). Since the MHC is a major genetic factor responsible for controlling the immune response, it is an obvious candidate for a genetic susceptibility factor. Association and linkage of IDDM to the MHC has been demonstrated in the NOD mouse, BB rat and in humans.

## GENETIC LOCI

### Major Histocompatibility Complex

The major histocompatibility complex (MHC) in humans is located on the short arm of chromosome 6 and spans a region of approximately three million base pairs (see Fig. 9.2). The products from this region were named human leucocyte antigens (HLA) because they were first characterised by the antibody mediated agglutination of leucocytes. MHC gene products present antigens in the form of short peptides to T cells. Such peptides may be derived from intracellular proteins and presented by Class I molecules (HLA A, B and C, found on most nucleated cells) to CD8+ cytotoxic T cells (33, 34) or from exogenous proteins and presented by class II molecules (HLA DP, DQ and DR, restricted to monocytes, macrophages, B cells and activated T cells) to CD4+ helper T cells (35). This presentation is important not only in the generation of an immune response to foreign antigens but also in the shaping of the T cell repertoire during T cell development within the thymus and thus the development of tolerance to the body's own antigens.

Historically, the first evidence for involvement of the MHC in susceptibility to IDDM came from

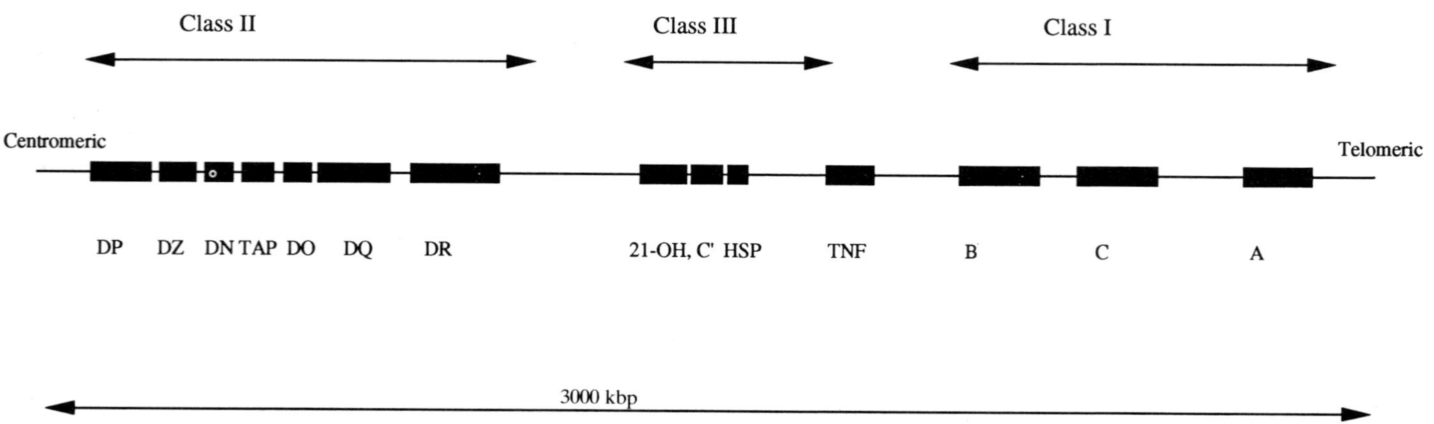


Fig. 9.2. Organisation of human MHC on chromosome 6. Class II region comprises DP DZ DN DO DQ and DR loci as well as transporters associated with antigen presentation (TAP). Class III region contains the genes for 21 hydroxylase (21-OH), complement (C′), heat shock protein (HSP) and tumour necrosis factor (TNF). Class I region comprises A, B, and C loci.

population association studies when it was shown that HLA B8 and B15 were increased in frequency in Caucasian diabetics (36, 37) but subsequently it was found that associations were stronger at the Class II DR locus (38) and the class I associations were attributed to linkage disequilibrium with class II. Approximately 90% of Caucasian IDDM patients carry the DR3 and or DR4 serological specificities, compared to 45% of the general population (1). The risk of IDDM is particularly high for DR3/4 heterozygotes while DR2, and to a lesser extent DR5, have a protective effect. DR1 and DR8 are slightly associated with IDDM. Almost every DR antigen has some effect on IDDM susceptibility (1). As well as the finding of HLA associations, linkage has also been demonstrated by studies within families. The segregation of particular HLA haplotypes with the disease in families has been demonstrated as well as preferential sharing of certain haplotypes amongst affected siblings (1, 5, 39).

There are two types of class II genes: those encoding α polypeptides, and those encoding β polypeptides which together form the functional class II α–β heterodimer (see Fig. 9.3). Not all genes at this locus are expressed, but with the exception of DRA (encoding the DR α chain) which is invariant, those that are expressed exhibit a high degree of polymorphism. HLA gene products are still often referred to on the basis of their associated serological specificities, for example DR3 and DR4, although these provide neither gene specific nor haplotype specific information (see Fig. 9.3).

## The role of DQβ chain genes

With advances in molecular biology, studies of associations between HLA and IDDM could be conducted at the DNA level rather than by serological specificities. Restriction fragment length polymorphisms (RFLP) and studies with subregion specific probes revealed that associations to the DQ locus were stronger than those observed for DR (40–42). For example, in Caucasian DR4-positive haplotypes only those with a DQB1*0302 (DQw8 or DQ3.2) allele are associated with IDDM whereas those with a DQB1*0301 (DQw7 or DQ3.1) allele are not (43). This constitutes another example of linkage disequilibrium and suggested that the 'IDDM locus' was closer to DQ than DR. Studies of the DNA sequence of DRB1, DRB3, DRB4, DQA1 and DQB1 alleles in Caucasians revealed that the strongest correlation with IDDM was with residue 57 of the DQβ chain. Alleles that have an aspartate at this position are found, by and large, on neutral or protective haplotypes, whereas those that have a non-charged amino acid, for example, alanine, serine or valine are found on diabetes associated haplotypes (44). The DQB1*0301 allele found on DR4 haplotypes is Asp 57 positive whereas DQB1*0302 has an alanine in this position (44, 45). This correlation is conserved in the NOD mouse: NOD mice were the only major inbred strain of mice which did not have an aspartate at position 57 of the DQβ mouse homologue, I-Aβ (44). Thus, although there is no unique disease related HLA class II allele, 90% of diabetics are homozygous for non-Asp57 on the β chain of the DQ allele compared with 20% of controls (45).

The fact that multiple alleles exist which differ by only a single residue at position 57 on independent haplotypes suggests that evolutionary selection has been important in selecting this variation in the population on a range of haplotypes. This argues strongly that this position is important in the function of the molecule. Evidence that this residue may be important structurally to the molecule comes from the hypothesis that an aspartate at position 57 of the DQβ chain may allow the formation of a salt bridge with the arginine residue in position 79 of the DQα chain. This could affect the peptide binding capacity of the HLA DQ dimer thus preventing the presentation of islet cell autoantigen to T cells (33, 44). Human T cell clones have been identified which are able to discriminate between the presence or absence of aspartate at position 57 (46, 47).

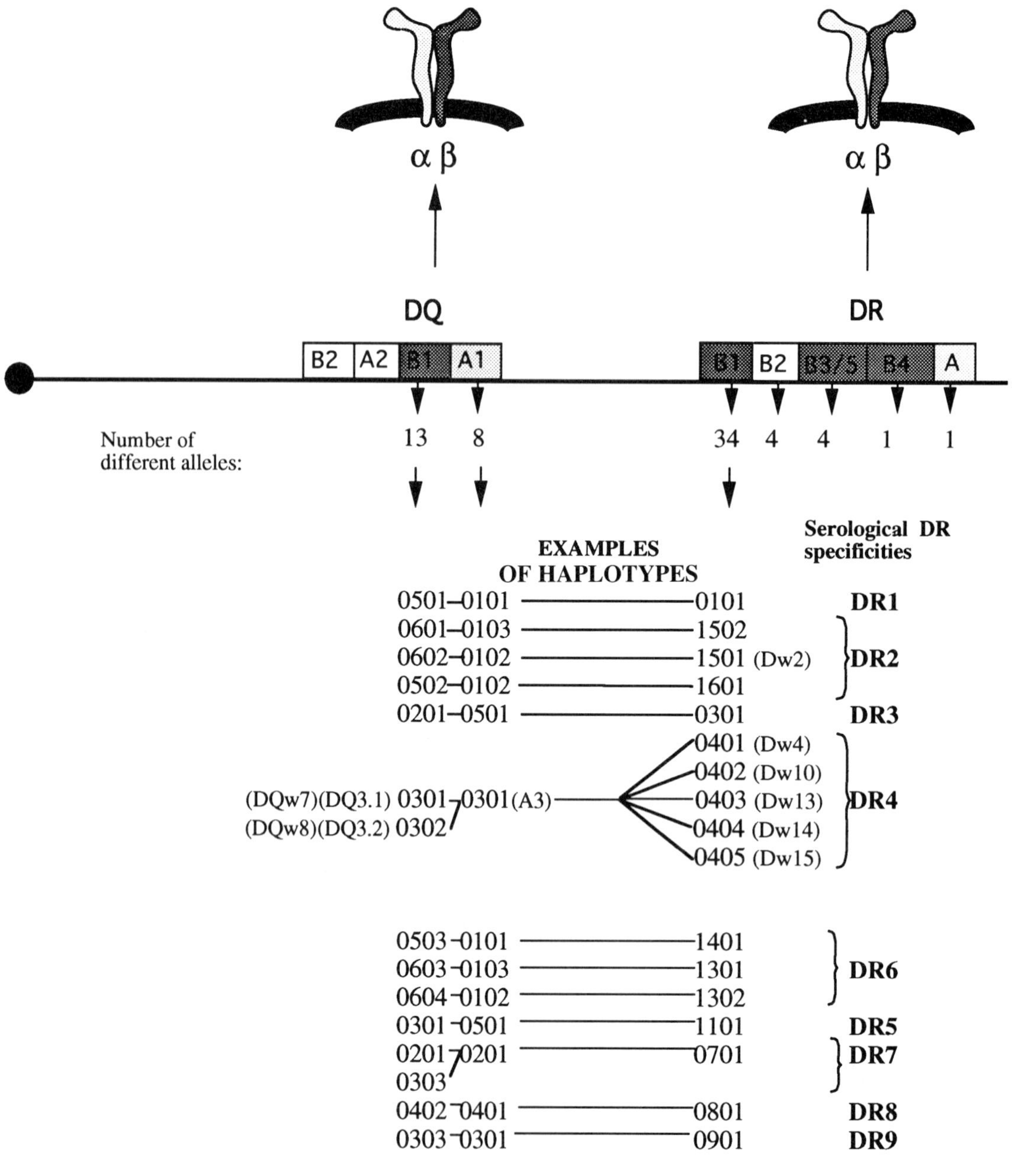


Fig. 9.3. Part of the HLA Class II complex. Expressed genes are shown as ▨ for β chains and ☐ for α chains. The approximate number of allelic variants are given for each gene, and several examples of haplotypes comprising DQB1, DQA1 and DRB1 alleles are shown. (Partly after Ref. 57.)

## Other HLA susceptibility genes

Although strongly correlated with disease, the presence or absence of aspartate at position 57 on the DQβ chain does not alone explain the full extent of HLA associated susceptibility to IDDM. Evidence for this comes from several sources.

1. 2% of Norwegian, 9% of Polish, 22% of Chinese and 56% of Japanese IDDM patients develop the disease despite being homozygous for the protective asp57 allele (48, 49).
2. There is a variation in DR4.DQB1 *0302 haplotype relative risks according to sub-classes at the DRB1 locus. Subtypes DRB1*0401–0405 (Dw4, 10, 13, 14, and 15, respectively) vary in their association with IDDM. For example, one of these sub-types, Dw14, is not associated with IDDM even when DQB1*0302 (non-asp) is on the same haplotype. Dw4 and 10 are highly associated with IDDM whereas 13 and 15 are neutral (50) (see Fig 9.3).

   In DR1/DR4 diabetic heterozygotes, the DR4 haplotype carries the DQB1*0301 allele, not the asp57-negative DQB1*0302 allele. However, there is an increased frequency of DRB1*0401 alleles on the DR4 haplotype (51). Therefore, at least for DR4 haplotypes, high susceptibility to IDDM seems to require a combination of alleles at both DRB1 and DQB1 loci (50) (see Fig. 9.4(*a*))
3. DQB*0201 (DQw2) does not have aspartate at position 57 and is associated with IDDM on the DR3 haplotype but is not associated with IDDM when it occurs on the DR7 haplotype (52). However, *trans*-racial studies have revealed the existence of a DR7 haplotype carrying the DQB*0201 (DQw2) allele that is highly diabetogenic in the Afro-Caribbean population (53) (see Fig. 9.4(*b*)).

### DQA1 alleles

Sequence analysis revealed that the only coding sequence difference between the two DR7 haplotypes in point (**3**) was at the DQA1 locus. In Japanese diabetics, the DQA1 allele, in fact, has the strongest class II association: 96% patients versus 53% controls carry the DQA1*0301 allele (52). DQA1*0301 is associated with IDDM in Caucasians, Afro-Caribbeans and Japanese. However, it is also found on the neutral DR4-DQB1*0301 haplotype in these races and thus it cannot be the sole determinant of susceptibility to IDDM. Furthermore, DR9 haplotypes are neutral in Caucasians, but associated with susceptibility in Afro-Caribbeans and Japanese and all carry the same DQA1 *0301 allele (52).

Since DQα and DQβ chains jointly determine the shape of the peptide binding cleft of DQ molecules, it may be that these molecules interact to confer resistance or protection to IDDM. In a study of Caucasians, Khalil *et al.* found that an arginine at position 52 of the DQα chain confers susceptibility to IDDM while absence of arginine at this position confers protection to IDDM (54). Interaction of different amino acids at these two positions could alter the shape of the antigen binding cleft and thus affect susceptibility to IDDM through different binding of a 'diabetogenic' peptide.

Functional DQ molecules may be expressed on the cell both when encoded by genes in the *cis* (on the same haplotype) and in the *trans* (on different chromosomes) position. This could explain the increased risk observed for IDDM in DR3/4 heterozygotes over DR3 or DR4 homozygotes; *trans* pairing of the DQα allele of the DR3 haplotype (DQA1*0501) with the DQβ allele from the DR4 haplotype (DQB1*0302). DQA1*0501/DQB1*0302 heterodimers have been demonstrated in DR3/4 heterozygotes (55, 56). Again, however, this cannot explain the entire HLA susceptibility, for example, the same DQ molecule should be formed in DR4/5 heterozygotes yet this is a low risk genotype (57).

These examples suggest that there is not one but several class II linked genes that contribute to IDDM susceptibility. The recent discovery of genes within the class II region (situated between DP and DQ (see Fig. 9.2)) involved in endogenous antigen processing and class I assembly provide further potential susceptibility candidates. Transporters associated with antigen presentation (TAP1 and 2) genes (58, 59) are thought to form a complex which is involved in transporting cytoplasmic peptides into the endoplasmic reticulum for interaction with class I molecules (60). However, limited genomic polymorphism appears to exist at these loci: three

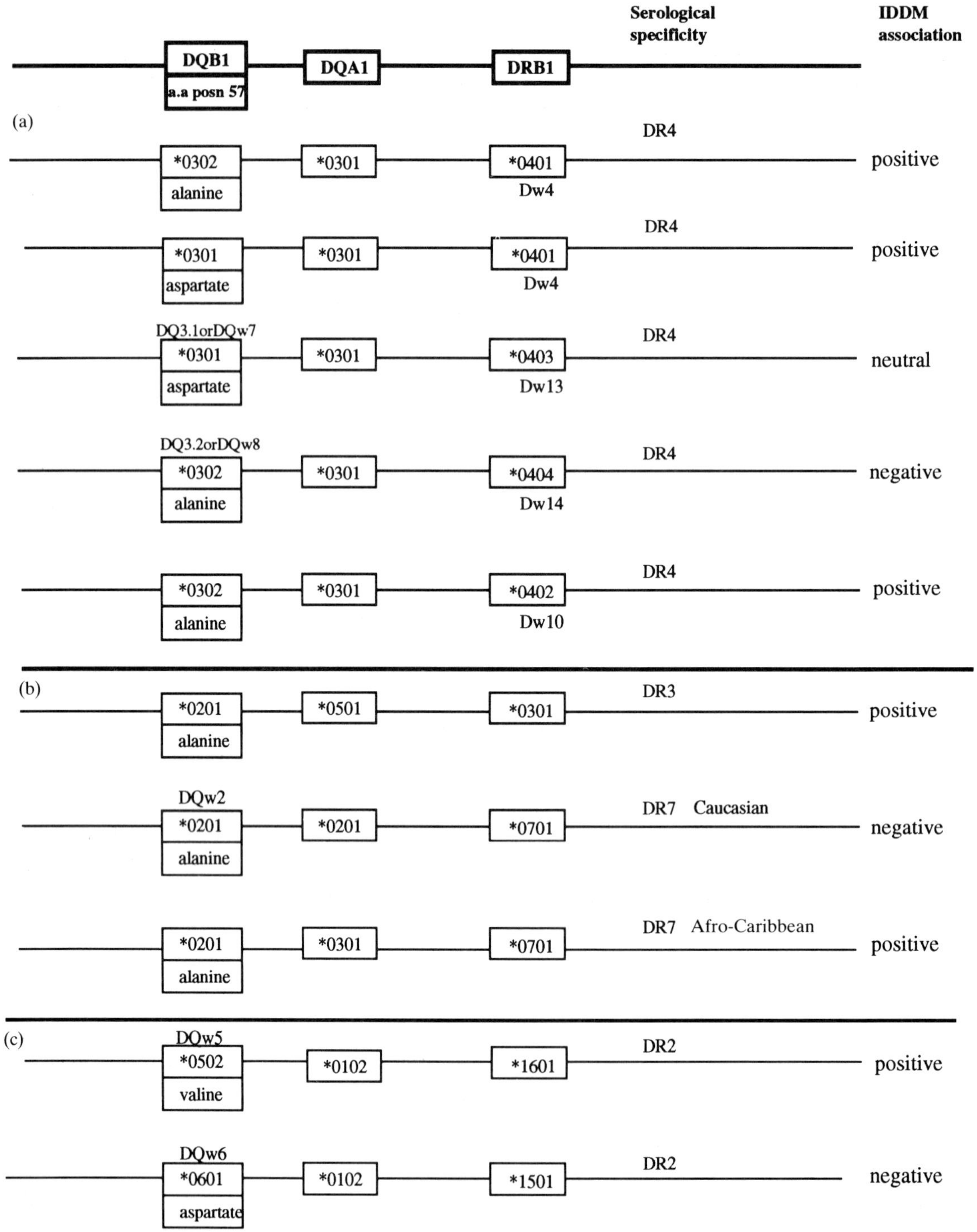


Fig. 9.4. Examples of Class II haplotypes discussed in text. Alleles at DQB1, DQA1 and DRB1 are shown and their associations with IDDM. Associations are in Caucasians unless stated otherwise.

TAP 1 and five TAP 2 alleles have been identified (61, 62). Findings of a population association of TAP alleles to IDDM will need to be confirmed by family studies, to determine whether an independent susceptibility locus is situated in this region rather than linkage disequilibrium with the DQ and DR loci. Indeed, preliminary studies suggest that there is significant linkage disequilibrium between TAP alleles and the HLA-DR region (63).

### Dominant protection

In Caucasians, certain DR2 haplotypes are negatively associated with IDDM. Again, the correlation is strongest at the DQB1 locus: The DQB1* 0602 allele confers protection even if an IDDM susceptibility gene is present on the other haplotype (1, 52). DR2 haplotypes are occasionally observed in IDDM patients but in these cases they carry a non-asp57 DQB1 allele (44, 47, 64, 65) (see Fig 9. 4(c)). Nepom (66) has proposed a model relating the complex genetic interactions associated with susceptibility, to structural properties of the class II molecule: a hierarchy of affinities among different class II molecules for diabetogenic peptides could explain the dominant DR2 effect. The binding of a 'diabetogenic peptide' to, e.g. DQB1*0302 may be competed for by another molecule, e.g. DR2 with higher affinity. Yet other class II molecules may have lower affinities than DQB1*0302 and susceptibility would then ensue. However, this theory does not explain why certain class II molecules are permissive to an autoimmune response yet others binding the same putative diabetogenic peptide fail to elicit an autoimmune response. Furthermore, it assumes that the same peptide can be bound by a range of MHC molecules and thus these should all be potential targets for an auto-immune response. Sheehy (67) has proposed an alternative model: HLA alleles negatively associated with IDDM produce HLA molecules with a high affinity for certain peptides required to establish and maintain tolerance to β cells. Positively associated alleles produce molecules with low affinity for the tolerogenic peptide, or bind the peptide in such a way that tolerance is poorly achieved. Although this theory would receive some support from studies of myelin basic protein in experimental auto-immune encephalomyelitis (68), it is difficult to confirm in IDDM while the nature of the auto-antigen remains unknown and thus class II binding affinities to the tolerogenic peptide cannot be determined.

### Insulin (INS) gene locus

On the basis that there is selective destruction of the pancreatic β cells in IDDM, insulin is a β cell specific product, and antibodies against insulin are detected in IDDM patients, the insulin gene has also been extensively investigated as a potential susceptibility locus in IDDM. The human insulin gene is located on the short arm of chromosome 11, situated between the genes for tyrosine hydroxylase (TH) and insulin-like growth factor 2 (IGF2) (see Fig. 9.5). A highly polymorphic region is located immediately (365 base pairs) upstream from the initiation of transcription for the gene, which provides a useful marker for studies of involvement of the insulin locus in susceptibility (69). The polymorphism arises from a *v*ariable *n*umber of *t*andemly *r*epeated (VNTR) 14 base pair oligonucleotides. Although the VNTR is highly polymorphic in length it can be divided into three broad classes: class I average 570 bp, class II average 1640 bp and class III average 2400 bp. In Caucasians, the intermediate size is rare. Several studies have looked at both associations between the length of VNTR alleles and IDDM, and at linkage of VNTR alleles with IDDM in families (see Table 9.1).

Initial studies focused mainly on associations of the VNTR with non-insulin dependent diabetes and only small numbers of IDDM patients were studied (69, 71). When numbers were increased, a significant association was found between IDDM and class I (small group) of VNTR alleles (72–74, 76). However, scepticism

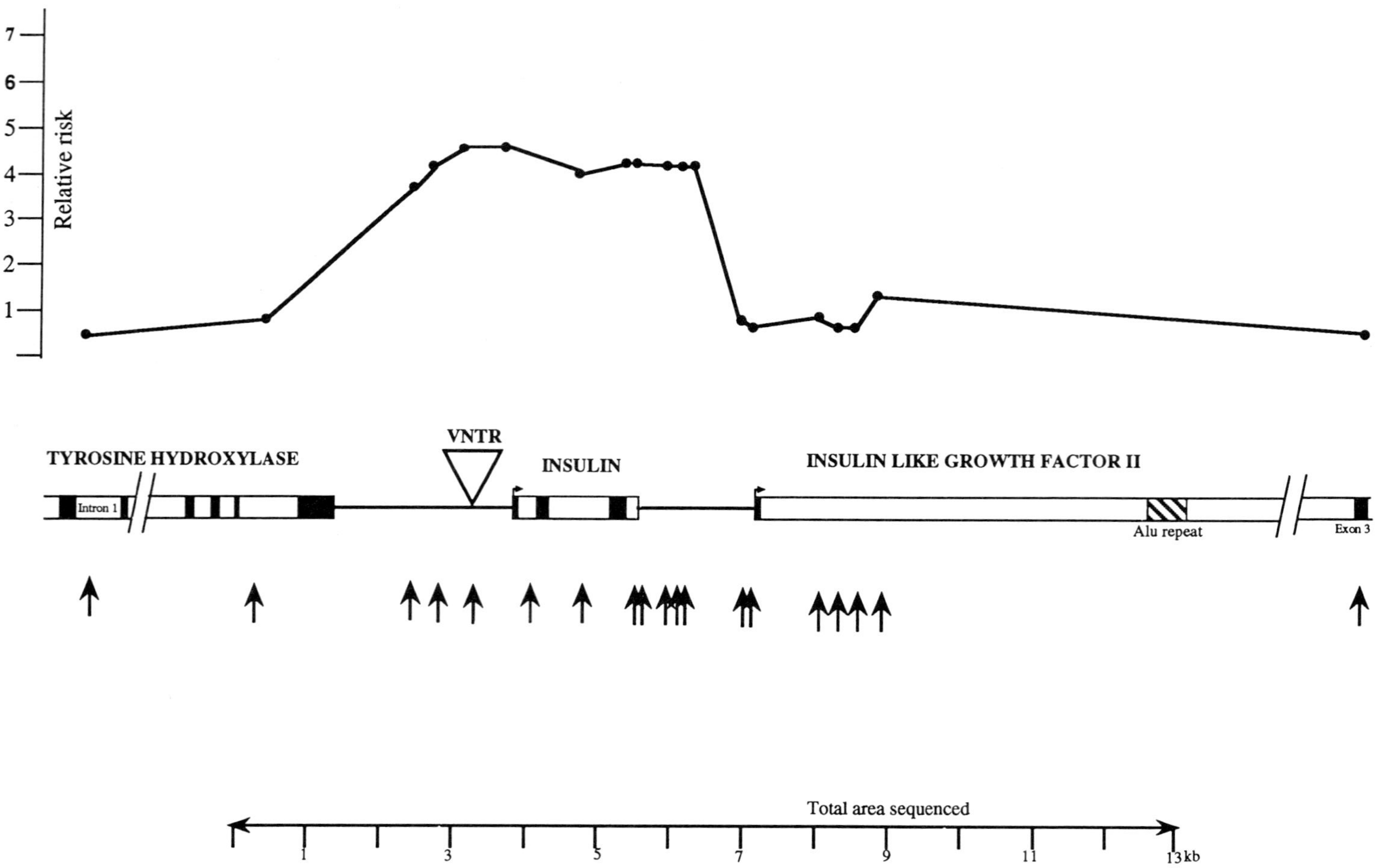


Fig. 9.5. Genomic organisation of INS locus, showing regions sequenced and polymorphisms identified (↑) (see text). Relative risks for IDDM with respect to normal controls are shown for each polymorphism. Black boxes indicate exons, white boxes, introns. (After Ref. 82.)

Table 9.1. *Some of the studies that have examined the INS locus as a susceptibility locus to IDDM in Caucasians.* n=*Numbers of patients and controls studied in population association and ASP families in linkage studies*

| | IDDM *n* | Controls *n* | Association Class I VNTR and IDDM | Family studies *n* | Linkage |
|---|---|---|---|---|---|
| Bell, 1981 (69) | 12 | 28 | No | – | |
| Owerbach, 1982 (70) | 37 | 56 | No | – | |
| Rotwein, 1983 (71) | 17 | 33 | No | | |
| Bell, 1984 (72) | 113 | 83 | Yes $P < 0.0001$ | | |
| Hitman, 1985 (73) | 53 | 88 | Yes $P < 0.00001$ | 17 | No |
| Ferns, 1986 (74) | 44 | 37 | Yes $P < 0.05$ | 14 | No |
| GAW, 1989 (75) | | | | 69 | No |

over the importance of this locus remained due to the inability to demonstrate linkage of the VNTR alleles in families. Several authors examined VNTR alleles in ASP analysis and could demonstrate no deviation from random expectations of allele sharing (73, 74, 77, 78). As numbers of pedigrees were small, an international collaboration was established to collect a large number of IDDM pedigrees and analyse them at the insulin locus. The Fifth Genetic Analysis Workshop (GAW) whose results were published in 1989 collected 94 multiplex families from different centres. Of these families, 64 were informative (parental origin of alleles could be determined), yet no evidence of linkage of the INS VNTR to IDDM was observed (77). Since linkage to HLA could be clearly demonstrated, it was concluded that either there is no susceptibility gene in this region and the population association is due to population stratification, or there is a locus but its effects are too weak to be able to demonstrate linkage.

Recently, this issue has been re-addressed and it has been established that the inability to find linkage is in part attributable to the susceptibility allele being at high frequency in the general population (79, 80). Several new disease-associated polymorphisms were identified at the INS locus which showed strong linkage disequilibrium with the class I VNTR lengths. As class I VNTR lengths occur at high frequency in the general population (approximately 70% in Caucasians), the GAW study had used the fine heterogeneity within class I alleles to increase the number of informative families. However, as these are all in linkage disequilibrium with the same set of candidate disease mutations at the insulin locus, linkage of these to IDDM was masked. By restricting linkage analysis to families where one parent is heterozygous for the disease associated allele, segregation of alleles could be clearly followed and linkage was demonstrated (80). Bain *et al.* have also demonstrated linkage of INS locus polymorphisms to IDDM in families (79). High gene frequency and low penetrance is probably a feature of many susceptibility loci for common polygenic diseases and should be considered before concluding that an association is spurious because linkage is not easily detectable.

## HLA–INS interaction

Several investigators have examined whether these two loci might interact to produce susceptibility. In the French data set (81, 82) INS polymorphisms show a stronger association in diabetics who are HLA-DR4 positive than other HLA-DR subtypes suggesting that there may be an interaction of these two loci in this population. Studies examining this interaction in other populations (79, 83–85) have found no evidence of such an interaction from association data. However, Bain *et al.* (79) do find preferential transmission of INS haplotypes to DR4 positive probands from UK multiplex families. Reanalysis (81) of the genetic analysis workshop data (75) also shows a preferential transmission of INS haplotypes to DR4 positive diabetics. Similarly, evidence for an interaction is seen from linkage studies in the French population (81). Overall therefore, transmission data from family studies indicate a possible INS–DR4 interaction, but population association data in sporadic diabetics show more heterogeneity and this may reflect a variation in INS–DR4 effect between different ethnic groups.

### Nature of INS locus susceptibility

The finding of association and linkage of several alleles in the insulin gene region led us to examine this region in more detail. To identify the exact mutation encoding susceptibility, a systematic analysis of a 14 kilobase region spanning the insulin gene and parts of neighbouring genes, TH and IGF2 was made by sequence comparisons between diabetics and controls (82). Multiple polymorphisms were identified and their association with IDDM studied in 156 random IDDM patients and 96 matched controls (see Fig. 9.5). This allowed identification of a 4 kilobase stretch of DNA containing ten candidate disease mutations which encodes the susceptibility mapped to this region. None of these polymorphisms is located in coding or known regulatory sequence of genes in this region, so that the mechanism of susceptibility remains unclear. Recently, however, repetitive sequences such as those seen in the INS VNTR have been implicated in the pathogenesis of several genetic disorders (86) and it may be that the length of the VNTR correlates with susceptibility, possibly through an effect on insulin regulation.

## T cell receptor

Because IDDM seems, in both humans and animal models to involve T cell recognition of self antigen in the context of particular predisposing HLA antigens, T cell receptor (TCR) loci have also been investigated as susceptibility loci. TCR α and β chains are encoded for by TCRA and B loci located on chromosomes 14q and 7p respectively. Various investigators have addressed the question of T cell receptor involvement in susceptibility to IDDM. As can be seen from Table 9.2, both association and linkage studies have failed to show involvement of the TCRA locus and studies of the TCRB locus have been conflicting. Wilson *et al.* (94) reported very little linkage disequilibrium in the TCRβ complex and suggested therefore that population association findings are more likely to be due to chance association than true genetic causation. Family studies at both loci have failed to show evidence of linkage with TCR, despite linkage to HLA being easily demonstrated in the same families. It is possible that this reflects the different means by which the HLA and TCR molecules achieve antigen binding diversity: HLA molecules achieve diversity by multiple loci and allelic diversity, and TCR molecules by somatic rearrangements during T cell ontogeny.

However, as discussed for the insulin locus, analysis of a small number of families has only the power to detect a major genetic effect and can not detect linkage of alleles at high frequency in the general population. Many of the TCR polymorphisms studied to date are found at high frequency in the population (see Table 9.2). Furthermore, most of the studies have used RFLPs at the TCRA and TCRB loci (which span genomic regions of 1000 and 600 kb, respectively) without demonstrating that these loci are in linkage disequilibrium with polymorphisms of potential functional relevance, so that a role of these loci in IDDM susceptibility cannot be excluded. Several new polymorphisms within coding sequence of both TCRA and TCRB loci have recently been identified in our laboratory (Reyburn and Cornelis, manuscript in preparation) and it will now be possible to examine the role of TCR polymorphisms of functional relevance in IDDM.

Table 9.2. *Summary of various studies investigating the TCRA and B loci. Numbers of IDDM patients (D) and controls (C) are given for association studies and the number of informative affected sibling pairs (ASP) studied for evidence of linkage. Studies are of Caucasians unless stated otherwise*

| | TCRA | | TCRB | |
|---|---|---|---|---|
| | Association | Linkage | Association | Linkage |
| Hoover, 1986 (87) | No<br>D=19, C=15 | | Yes<br>D=105, C=54 | |
| Millward, 1987 (88) | | | Yes<br>D=118, C=126 | |
| Ito, 1988 (89) (*Japanese*) | | | Yes<br>D=50, C=94 | |
| Field, 1988 (90) | | | No<br>D=94, C=72 | |
| Sheehy, 1989 (91) | | No<br>29 ASP | | |
| Hoover, 1989 (87) | | | No<br>D=256, C=74 | |
| Aparicio, 1990 (92) (*Japanese*) | No<br>D=56, C=24 | | No<br>D=24, C=23 | |
| Concannon, 1990 (93) | | No<br>24 ASP | No<br>D=73, C=43 | No<br>40 ASP |

## Immunoglobulin heavy chain (Gm) region

Located on long arm of chromosome 14, this region encodes genes for the constant portions of heavy chains of immunoglobulin IgA, G, M, D, and E. Gm allotypes are serologically defined antigens on the constant portion of the IgG (hence Gm) heavy chain. Many investigators have examined the role of Gm allotypes in susceptibility to IDDM (95–100). None has found evidence of a direct effect either by association or linkage studies. However, various authors have found significant results if diabetics were subdivided according to HLA type implying an interaction between HLA and Gm (101, 102). Field *et al.* (103) also report interactions between Gm and the TCRB locus and Gm and the INS locus. Although polygenic diseases are likely to involve gene interaction or epistatic events (104), if susceptibility to disease is a result of two loci interacting, then it should map to both loci independently (105) and this has not been demonstrated for the Gm locus to date.

## Parental transmission bias

Several authors have reported that diabetic offspring are significantly more likely to inherit diabetes from their father than their mother (106–108). Vadheim *et al.* (107) observed that HLA-DR4+ fathers (diabetic or not) were more likely to transmit this allele to their offspring than were DR4+ mothers. Julier *et al.* (80) showed that diabetic offspring are significantly more likely to inherit the diabetes associated INS haplotype (see above) from their father rather than mother. Possible explanations for these observations include a maternal–foetal interaction (for example, diabetes predisposing alleles in the mother may be tolerised in the fetus), protection through breast-feeding (109), or genomic imprinting (where a chromosome functions differently depending on whether it is inherited paternally or maternally, for review see (110)). However, parental transmission bias may vary between different ethnic groups: no paternal transmission bias is seen in a set of English families (79).

## CONCLUSIONS

IDDM is a multi-factorial disorder with several genes contributing to the genetic susceptibility to this disease. Whilst the MHC provides a large component of this susceptibility and the insulin locus in humans is also a factor, other loci are also likely to be involved. Studies in the mouse have suggested that more than five loci outside the MHC contribute to susceptibility (12). Investigation of human syntenic regions may therefore reveal further genetic loci. However, although animal models provide important insights, they may not specifically mimic the human disease. A study of chromosome 11q (16) with multiple polymorphic probes was undertaken because of the synteny with chromosome 9 in the NOD mouse, where an IDDM susceptibility locus has been mapped (8). This study was able to exclude linkage to IDDM in humans. Although this study did confirm that large-scale mapping in search of areas linked to disease is feasible, it also highlights the fact that allele frequencies and diabetes associations in animal models may be different from humans: important disease susceptibility alleles in the mouse may prove to be relatively minor susceptibility factors in humans simply as a result of different allele frequencies. With progress in the human genome project and the identification of polymorphic markers throughout the genome, a systematic search for genetic susceptibility factors in common diseases such as IDDM will be possible. Characterisation of the genetic components of disease is important to provide all the essential components of the basic mechanism by which the disease occurs. It will also allow identification of high risk individuals, who may then be counselled appropriately and possibly included in future trials of therapeutic agents.

## REFERENCES


1 Thomson G, Robinson WP, Kuhner MK *et al.* Genetic heterogeneity, modes of inheritance, and risk estimates for a joint study of Caucasians with insulin-dependent diabetes mellitus. *Am J Hum Genet* 1988; 43(6): 799–816.

2 Risch N. Assessing the role of HLA-linked and unlinked determinants of disease. *Am J Hum Genet* 1987; 40(1): 1–14.

3 Olmos P, A'Hern R, Heaton DA *et al.* The significance of the concordance rate for type 1 (insulin-dependent) diabetes in identical twins. *Diabetologia* 1988; 31(10): 747–50.

4 Gorusch AN. The immunogenetics of diabetes. *Diabetic Med* 1987; 4: 510–16.

5 Rotter JI, Landaw EM. Measuring the genetic contribution of a single locus to a multilocus disease. *Clin Genet* 1984; 26(6): 529–42.

6 Leiter EH, Prochazka M, Coleman DL. The non-obese diabetic (NOD) mouse. *Am J Pathol* 1987; 128(2): 380–3.

7 Colle E, Ono SJ, Fuks A, Guttmann RD, Seemayer TA. Association of susceptibility to spontaneous diabetes in rat with genes of major histocompatibility complex. *Diabetes* 1988; 37(10): 1438–43.

8 Todd J, Aitman T, Cornall R *et al.* Genetic analysis of auto-immune type 1 diabetes mellitus in mice. *Nature (Lond)* 1991; 351: 542–7.

9 Prochazka M, Leiter EH, Serreze DV, Coleman DL. Three recessive loci required for insulin-dependent diabetes in nonobese diabetic mice. *Science* 1987; 237 (4812): 286–9.

10 Hattori M, Buse JB, Jackson RA *et al.* The NOD mouse: recessive diabetogenic gene in the major histocompatibility complex. *Science* 1986; 231(4739): 733–5.

11 Cornall RJ, Prins JB, Todd JA *et al.* Type 1 diabetes in mice is linked to the interleukin-1 receptor and Lsh/Ity/Bcg genes on chromosome 1. *Nature (Lond)* 1991; 353(6341): 262–5.

12 De Gouyon B, Melanitou E, Richard MF *et al.* Genetic analysis of diabetes and insulinitis in an interspecific cross of the nonobese diabetic mouse with *Mus spretus*. *Proc Natl Acad Sci USA* 1993; 90: 1877–81.

13 Colle E, Fuks A, Poussier P, Edouard P, Guttmann RD. Polygenic nature of spontaneous diabetes in the rat. Permissive MHC haplotype and presence of the lymphopenic trait of the BB rat are not sufficient to produce susceptibility. *Diabetes* 1992; 41(12): 1617–23.

14 Bishop DT, Williamson JA. The power of identity-by-state methods for linkage analysis. *Am J Hum Genet* 1990; 46(2): 254–65.

15 Risch N. Genetics of IDDM: evidence for complex inheritance with HLA. *Genet Epidemiol* 1989; 6(1): 143–8.

16 Hyer RN, Julier C, Buckley JD *et al.* High-resolution linkage mapping for susceptibility genes in human polygenic disease: insulin-dependent diabetes mellitus and chromosome 11q. *Am J Hum Genet* 1991; 48(2): 243–57.

17 Risch N. Linkage strategies for genetically complex traits. II. The power of affected relative pairs. *Am J Hum Genet* 1990; 46(2): 229–41.

18 Risch N. Linkage strategies for genetically complex traits. III. The effect of marker polymorphism on analysis of affected relative pairs. *Am J Hum Genet* 1990; 46(2): 242–53.

19 Bottazzo GF, Dean BM, McNally JM, MacKay EH, Swift PGF, Gamble DRG. *In situ* characterisation of autoimmune phenomena and expression of HLA molecules in the pancreas in diabetic insulinitis. *N Engl J Med* 1985; 313: 353–60.

20 Bottazzo GF, Bosi E, Bonifacio E, Mirakian R, Todd I, Pujol BR. Pathogenesis of type I (insulin-dependent) diabetes: possible mechanisms of autoimmune damage. *Br Med Bull* 1989; 45(1): 37–57.
21 Foulis AK, Liddle CN, Farquharson MA, Richmond JA, Weir RS. The histopathology of the pancreas in type 1 (insulin-dependent) diabetes mellitus: a 25-year review of deaths in patients under 20 years of age in the United Kingdom. *Diabetologia* 1986; 29(5): 267–74.
22 Sibley RK, Sutherland DER, Goetz F, Michael AF. Recurrent diabetes mellitus in the pancreas iso- and allograft. A light and electron microscopic and immunohistochemical analysis of our cases. *Lab Invest* 1985; 53: 132–44.
23 Drell DW, Notkins AL. Multiple immunological abnormalities in patients with type 1 (insulin-dependent) diabetes mellitus. *Diabetologia* 1987; 30(3): 132–43.
24 Faustman D, Eisenbarth G, Daley J, Breitmeyer J. Abnormal T-lymphocyte subsets in type 1 diabetes. *Diabetes* 1989; 38(11): 1462–8.
25 Charles MA, Suzuki M, Waldeck N *et al.* Immune islet killing mechanisms associated with insulin-dependent diabetes: *in vitro* expression of cellular and antibody-mediated islet cell cytotoxicity in humans. *J Immunol* 1983; 130(3): 1189–94.
26 Eisenbarth GS. Type 1 diabetes mellitus. A chronic autoimmune disease. *N Engl J Med* 1986; 314(21): 1360–8.
27 Lernmark A, Li S, Baekkeskov S *et al.* Islet-specific immune mechanisms. *Diabetes Metab Rev* 1987; 3(4): 959–80.
28 Baekkeskov S, Aanstoot HJ, Christgau S *et al.* Identification of the 64K autoantigen in insulin-dependent diabetes as the GABA-synthesizing enzyme glutamic acid decarboxylase. *Nature (Lond)* 1990; 347 (6289): 151–6.
29 Roep BO, Arden SD, de Vries RRP, Hutton JC. T cell clones from a type I diabetes patient respond to insulin secretory granule protein. *Nature (Lond)* 1990; 345: 632–4.
30 Castano L, Eisenbarth GS. Type-I diabetes: a chronic autoimmune disease of human, mouse, and rat. *Annu Rev Immunol* 1990; 8(647): 647–79.
31 Bendelac A, Carnaud C, Boitard C, Bach JF. Syngeneic transfer of autoimmune diabetes from diabetic NOD mice to healthy neonates. Requirement for both L3T4+ and Lyt-2+ T cells. *J Exp Med* 1987; 166(4): 823–32.
32 Miller GG, Hoy JF, Nell LJ, Thomas JW. Antigen processing and the human T cell receptor repertoire for insulin. *J Immunol* 1988; 141(10): 3293–8.
33 Trucco M, Dorman JS. Immunogenetics of insulin-dependent diabetes mellitus in humans. *Crit Rev in Immunol* 1989; 9: 201–45.
34 Bjorkman P, Saper M, Samraoui B, Bennett W, Strominger J, Wiley D. Structure of human class I histocompatibility antigen, HLA-A2. *Nature (Lond)* 1987; 329: 506–11.
35 Kaufman JF, Auffray C, Korman AJ, Shackelford DA, Strominger J. The class II molecules of the human and murine major histocompatibility complex. *Cell* 1984; 36(1): 1–13.
36 Singal DP, Blajchman MA. Histocompatibility (HL-A) antigens, lymphocytotoxic antibodies and tissue antibodies in patients with diabetes mellitus. *Diabetes* 1973; 22: 429–33.
37 Cudworth AG, Woodrow JC. HLA antigens and diabetes mellitus. *Lancet*, 1974; ii: 1153.
38 Svejgaard A, Platz P, Ryder LP. Insulin dependent diabetes mellitus: joint report. Los Angeles: 1980: 638–656. (Terasaki PI, ed. *Histocompatibility testing*; vol UCLA tissue typing laboratory).
39 Payami H, Thomson G, Motro U, Louis EJ, Hudes E. The affected sib method. IV. Sib trios. *Ann Hum Genet* 1985; 49: 303–14.
40 Schreuder G, Tilanus M, Bontrop R *et al.* HLA-DQ polymorphisms associated with resistance to type I diabetes detected with monoclonal antibodies, isoelectric point differences, and restriction fragment length polymorphism. *J Exp Med* 1986; 164: 138–150.
41 Festenstein H, Awad J, Hitman GA *et al.* New HLA DNA polymorphisms associated with autoimmune diseases. *Nature (Lond)* 1986; 322(6074): 64–7.
42 Owerbach D, Gunn S, Ty G, Wible L, Gabbay KH. Oligonucleotide probes for HLA-DQA and DQB genes define susceptibility to type 1 (insulin-dependent) diabetes mellitus. *Diabetologia* 1988; 31(10): 751–7.
43 Nepom GT, Palmer J, Nepom B. Specific HLA class II variants associated with IDDM In: Jaworski M, Molnar GD, Rajotte RV, Singh B, eds. *Immunology of diabetes mellitus*. Elsevier, Amsterdam; 1986: 9–20.
44 Todd J, Bell JI, McDevitt HO. HLA-DQ beta gene contributes to susceptibility and resistance to insulin-dependent diabetes mellitus. *Nature (Lond)* 1987;329 (6140):599–604.
45 Morel PA, Dorman JS, Todd JA, McDevitt HO, Trucco M. Aspartic acid at position 57 of the HLA-DQ beta chain protects against type I diabetes: a family study. *Proc Natl Acad Sci USA* 1988;85(21):8111–5.
46 Mickelson EM, Masewicz SA, Nepom GT, Martin PJ, Hansen JA. Alloreactive T-cell clones identify multiple HLA-DQw3 variants. *Hum Immunol* 1991;30(1): 32–40.
47 Lundin KE, Gaudernack G, Qvigstad E, Sollid LM, Thorsby E. T lymphocyte clones recognizing an HLA-DQw3.2-associated epitope involving residue 57 on the DQ beta chain. *Hum Immunol* 1988;22(4):235–46.
48 Wassmuth R, Lernmark A. The genetics of susceptibility to diabetes. *Clin Immunol Immunopath* 1989;53: 358–99.
49 Yamagata K, Hanafusa T, Nakajima H *et al.* HLA-DQA1*1 contributes to resistance and A1*3 confers susceptibility to type 1 (insulin-dependent) diabetes mellitus in Japanese subjects. *Diabetologia* 1991;34(2):133–6.
50 Sheehy MJ, Scharf SJ, Rowe JR *et al.* A diabetes-susceptible HLA haplotype is best defined by a combination of HLA-DR and -DQ alleles. *J Clin Invest* 1989;83(3):830–5.
51 Erlich HA, Bugawan TL, Scharf S, Nepom GT, Tait B, Griffith RL. HLA-DQ beta sequence polymorphism and genetic susceptibility to IDDM. *Diabetes* 1990; 39(1):96–103.
52 Todd JA. Genetic control of autoimmunity in type 1 diabetes. *Immunol Today* 1990;11(4):122–9.
53 Fletcher J, Mijovic C, Odugbesan O, Jenkins D, Bradwell AR, Barnett AH. Transracial studies implicate HLA-DQ as a component of genetic susceptibility to type 1 (insulin-dependent) diabetes. *Diabetologia* 1988;31(12):864–70.
54 Khalil I, d'Auriol L, Gobet M et al. A combination of HLA-DQ beta Asp57-negative and HLA DQ alpha

Arg52 confers susceptibility to insulin-dependent diabetes mellitus. *J Clin Invest* 1990;85(4):1315–9.
55 Nepom BS, Schwarz D, Palmer JP, Nepom GT. Transcomplementation of HLA genes in IDDM. HLA-DQ alpha- and beta-chains produce hybrid molecules in DR3/4 heterozygotes. *Diabetes* 1987;36(1):114–7.
56 Nepom GT. MHC genes in HLA-associated disease. *Curr Opin Immunol* 1989;2(4): 588–92.
57 Nepom GT, Erlich H. MHC class-II molecules and autoimmunity. *Annu Rev Immunol* 1991; 9(493): 493–525.
58 Spies T, Bresnahan M, Bahram S *et al.* A gene in the human major histocompatibility complex class II region controlling the class I antigen presentation pathway. *Nature (Lond)* 1990; 348(6303): 744–7.
59 Trowsdale J, Hanson I, Mockridge I, Beck S, Townsend A, Kelly A. Sequences encoded in the class II region of the MHC related to the 'ABC' superfamily of transporters. *Nature (Lond)* 1990; 348(6303): 741–4.
60 Trowsdale J. Genomic structure and function in the MHC. *Trends in Genet* 1993; 9(4): 117–22.
61 Colonna M, Bresnahan M, Bahram S, Strominger JL, Spies T. Allelic variants of the human putative peptide transporter involved in antigen processing. *Proc Natl Acad Sci USA* 1992; 89(9): 3932–6.
62 Powis SH, Tonks S, Mockridge I, Kelly A, Bodmer JG, Trowsdale J. Alleles and haplotypes of the MHC encoded ABC transporters TAP1 and TAP2. *Immunogenetics* 1993; 37: 373–380.
63 Van Endert PM, Lopez MT, Patel SD, Monaco JJ, McDevitt HO. Genomic polymorphisms, recombination, and linkage disequilibrium in human major histocompatibility complex-encoded antigen-processing genes. *Proc Natl Acad Sci USA* 1992; 89: 11594–7.
64 Horn GT, Bugawan TL, Long CM, Erlich HA. Allelic sequence variation of the HLA-DQ loci: relationship to serology and to insulin-dependent diabetes susceptibility. *Proc Natl Acad Sci USA* 1988; 85(16): 6012–16.
65 Bach FH, Rich SS, Barbosa J, Segall M. Insulin-dependent diabetes – associated HLA-D region encoded determinants. *Hum Immunol* 1985; 12(2): 59–64.
66 Nepom GT. A unified hypothesis for the complex genetics of HLA associations with IDDM. *Diabetes* 1990; 39(10): 1153–7.
67 Sheehy MJ. HLA and insulin-dependent diabetes. A protective perspective. *Diabetes* 1992; 41(2): 123–9.
68 Wraith DC, Smilek DE, Mitchell DJ, Steinman L, McDevitt HO. Antigen recognition in autoimmune encephalomyelitis and the potential for peptide-mediated immunotherapy. *Cell* 1989; 59(2): 247–55.
69 Bell GI, Karam JH, Rutter WJ. Polymorphic DNA region adjacent to the 5′ end of the human insulin gene. *Proc Natl Acad Sci USA* 1981; 78(9): 5759–63.
70 Owerbach D, Nerup J. Restriction fragment length polymorphism of the insulin gene in diabetes mellitus. *Diabetes* 1982; 31(3): 275–7.
71 Rotwein PS, Chirgwin J, Province M *et al.* Polymorphism in the 5′ flanking region of the human insulin gene: a genetic marker for non-insulin-dependent diabetes. *N Engl J Med* 1983; 308(2): 65–71.
72 Bell GI, Horita S, Karam JH. A polymorphic locus near the human insulin gene is associated with insulin-dependent diabetes mellitus. *Diabetes* 1984; 33(2): 176–83.
73 Hitman GA, Tarn AC, Winter RM *et al.* Type 1 (insulin-dependent) diabetes and a highly variable locus close to the insulin gene on chromosome 11. *Diabetologia* 1985; 28(4): 218–22.
74 Ferns GA, Hitman GA, Trembath R *et al.* DNA polymorphic haplotypes on the short arm of chromosome 11 and the inheritance of type I diabetes mellitus. *J Med Genet* 1986; 23(3): 210–16.
75 Cox NJ, Spielman RS. The insulin gene and susceptibility to IDDM. *Genet Epidemiol* 1989; 6(1): 65–9.
76 Bell GI, Xiang K, Horita S, Sanz N, Karam JH. The molecular genetics of diabetes mellitus. *Ciba Found Symp* 1987; 130(167): 167–83.
77 Cox NJ, Baker L, Spielman RS. Insulin-gene sharing in sib pairs with insulin-dependent diabetes mellitus: no evidence for linkage. *Am J Hum Genet* 1988; 42(1): 167–72.
78 Cox NJ, Gogolin KJ, Horvath VJ *et al.* Restriction fragment polymorphisms of the HLA-DR, HLA-DQ, and insulin gene regions in IDDM: the GAW5 data. *Genet Epidemiol* 1989; 6(1): 21–6.
79 Bain SC, Prins JB, Hearne CM *et al.* Insulin gene region-encoded susceptibility to type 1 diabetes is not restricted to HLA-DR4-positive individuals. *Nature Genet* 1992; 2(3): 212–215.
80 Julier C, Hyer RN, Davies J *et al.* Insulin-IGF2 region on chromosome 11p encodes a gene implicated in HLA-DR4-dependent diabetes susceptibility. *Nature (Lond)* 1991; 354(6349): 155–9.
81 Julier C, Nakamura Y, Lathrop M *et al.* A detailed genetic map of the long arm of chromosome 11. *Genomics* 1990; 7(3): 335–45.
82 Lucassen AM, Julier C, Beressi JP *et al.* Susceptibility to insulin dependent diabetes mellitus maps to a 4.1 Kb segment of DNA spanning the insulin gene and associated VNTR. *Nature Genet* 1993; 4: 305–10.
83 Raffel LJ, Vadheim CM, Klein R *et al.* HLA-DR and the 5′ insulin gene polymorphism in insulin-dependent diabetes. *Metabolism* 1991; 40(12): 1244–8.
84 Donald JA, Barendse W, Cooper DW. Linkage studies of HLA and insulin gene restriction fragment length polymorphisms in families with IDDM. *Genet Epidemiol* 1989; 6(1): 77–81.
85 Field LL. Non-HLA region genes in insulin dependent diabetes mellitus. *Baillières Clin Endocrinol Metab* 1991; 5(3): 413–38.
86 Caskey CT, Pizzuti A, Fu YH, Fenwick RJ, Nelson DL. Triplet repeat mutations in human disease. *Science* 1992; 256(5058): 784–9.
87 Hoover ML, Angelini G, Ball E *et al.* HLA-DQ and T-cell receptor genes in insulin-dependent diabetes mellitus. *Cold Spring Harb Symp Quant Biol* 1986; 2(803): 803–9.
88 Millward BA, Welsh KI, Leslie RD, Pyke DA, Demaine AG. T cell receptor beta chain polymorphisms are associated with insulin-dependent diabetes. *Clin Exp Immunol* 1987; 70(1): 152–7.
89 Ito M, Tanimoto M, Kamura H *et al.* Association of HLA-DR phenotypes and T-lymphocyte-receptor beta-chain-region RFLP with IDDM in Japanese. *Diabetes* 1988; 37(12): 1633–6.
90 Field LL. Insulin-dependent diabetes mellitus: a model for the study of multifactorial disorders. *Am J Hum Genet* 1988; 43(6): 793–8.
91 Sheehy MJ, Meske LM, Emler CA *et al.* Allelic T-cell

receptor α complexes have little or no influence on susceptibility to type 1 diabetes. *Hum Immunol* 1989; 26(4): 261–71.
92 Aparicio JM, Wakisaka A, Takada A, Matsuura N, Yoshiki T. Non-HLA genetic factors and insulin dependent diabetes mellitus in the Japanese: TCRA, TCRB and TCRG, INS, THY1, CD3D and ETS1. *Dis Markers* 1990; 8(5): 283–94.
93 Concannon P, Wright JA, Wright LG, Sylvester DR, Spielman RS. T-cell receptor genes and insulin-dependent diabetes mellitus (IDDM): no evidence for linkage from affected sib pairs. *Am J Hum Genet* 1990; 47(1): 45–52.
94 Wilson RK, Lai E, Concannon P, Barth RK, Hood LE. Structure, organisation and polymorphism of murine and human T-cell receptor alpha and β chain families. *Immunol Rev* 1988; 101: 149–72.
95 Bertrams J, Schoeps L, Baur MP, Luboldt W, van LE. IgG and IgA heavy chain allotypes in Type 1 diabetes. *J Immunogenet* 1983; 10(4): 305–10.
96 Adams YJ, Adams DD, Parkinson R, van LE. Immunoglobulin heavy chain haplotypes in caucasian New Zealanders. *N Z Med J* 1984; 97(752): 178–9.
97 de Jongh B, Bruining GJ, Schreuder GM *et al.* HLA and GM in insulin-dependent diabetes in the Netherlands: report on a combined multiplex family and population study. *Hum Immunol* 1984; 10(1): 5–21.
98 Field LL, Anderson CE, Neiswanger K, Hodge SE, Spence MA, Rotter JI. Interaction of HLA and immunoglobulin antigens in type 1 (insulin-dependent) diabetes. *Diabetologia* 1984; 27(5): 504–8.
99 Dizier MH, Clerget DF, Hochez J. Segregation analysis of two genetic markers in IDDM families under two-locus models. *Genet Epidemiol* 1989; 6(1): 71–5.
100 Easton DF. Linkage analysis and genetic models for IDDM. *Genet Epidemiol* 1989; 6(1): 83–8.
101 Field L, Dizier MH, Anderson CE, Spence MA, Rotter JI. HLA-dependent GM effects in insulin-dependent diabetes: evidence from pairs of affected siblings. *Am J Hum Genet* 1986; 39(5): 640–7.
102 Tait BD, Propert DN, Harrison L, Mandel T, Martin FIR. Interaction between HLA antigens and immunoglobulin (Gm) allotypes in susceptibility to type I diabetes. *Tissue Antigens* 1986; 27: 249–255.
103 Field LL, Stephure DK, McArthur RG. Interaction between T cell receptor beta chain and immunoglobulin heavy chain region genes in susceptibility to insulin-dependent diabetes mellitus. *Am J Hum Genet* 1991; 49(3): 627–34.
104 Ott J. *Analysis of human genetic linkage*. The Johns Hopkins University Press Baltimore, 1985: Chap 1, 8.
105 Bodmer WF. The human genome sequence and the analysis of multifactorial traits. *Ciba Found Symp* 1987; 130(215): 215–28.
106 Warram JH, Krolewski AS, Gottlieb MS, Kahn CR. Differences in risk of insulin-dependent diabetes in offspring of diabetic mothers and diabetic fathers. *N Engl J Med* 1984; 311(3): 149–52.
107 Vadheim CM, Rotter JI, Maclaren NK, Riley WJ, Anderson CE. Preferential transmission of diabetic alleles within the HLA gene complex. Source (Bibliographic Citation): *N Engl J Med* 1986; 315(21): 1314–18.
108 MacDonald MJ, Gottschall J, Hunter JB, Winter KL. HLA-DR4 in insulin-dependent diabetic parents and their diabetic offspring: a clue to dominant inheritance. *Proc Natl Acad Sci USA* 1986; 83(18): 7049–53.
109 Karjalainen J, Martin JM, Knip M *et al.* A bovine albumin peptide as a possible trigger of insulin-dependent diabetes mellitus. *N Engl J Med* 1992; 327(5): 302–7.
110 Hall JG. Genomic imprinting: review and relevance to human diseases. *Am J Hum Genet* 1990; 46(5): 857–73.

# 10 Aetiology of Insulin-dependent Diabetes

R. D. G. Leslie & E. A. M. Gale

## INTRODUCTION

Two major types of diabetes are recognised, insulin-dependent diabetes mellitus (IDDM) and non-insulin dependent diabetes mellitus (NIDDM). Insulin-dependent diabetes is due to destruction of the β-cells of the islets of Langerhans, and is probably caused by environmental factors operating in a genetically susceptible host to initiate a destructive immune process (1). Genetic susceptibility is mediated predominantly by genes in the HLA region of chromosome 6 (2); the environmental event operates over a brief period in early childhood to induce an immune process which destroys the islet β cell (3). β cell destruction in some is chronic and progressive, leading to IDDM, but in others it can remit without diabetes developing. In the months or years before the onset of IDDM clinical, immune and metabolic changes can be detected. The nature, intensity, extent and persistence of these immune changes distinguishes individuals who develop IDDM from those who do not. Immune and metabolic changes may, therefore, be predictive of IDDM. The chronic course of the disease process, before the onset of clinical symptoms, and the potential for predicting the disease has led to attempts to prevent the clinical onset of IDDM (4).

## CHANGES WITHIN POPULATIONS

Ancient texts document the existence of diabetes, though rarely the dramatic clinical features associated with the onset of IDDM. The quality of ancient records was such that it is not possible to conclude that the disease was rare, but it certainly seems to have escaped the attention of many ancient physicians. The disease continues to be extremely rare in primitive hunter–gatherer societies and causal evidence suggests that the incidence rises when such people move to a modern society. It is possible, therefore, that IDDM is predominantly a modern disease. Certainly the disease rate has increased in recent years (see Chapter 8). No country is exempt from IDDM though the incidence of the disease varies considerably from country to country. The incidence of IDDM ranged from 1.7/100 000 person–years in Japan to 29.5/100 000 person–years in Finland between 1978 to 1980 (5). The incidence rates in Western industrialised countries establish IDDM as the second commonest chronic childhood illness after asthma. In other races, such as Asian Indians, Chinese and Black Africans, the prevalence of IDDM is probably low though accurate information is lacking. Several factors could be important in determining the striking variability in disease incidence. IDDM is more common the lower the ambient temperature and the further the population is from the equator (5). The explanation for these geographical differences in disease incidence is unlikely to be simple as there are striking exceptions to the general trend. For example, Sardinia has an incidence (30/100 000 person–years) which approximates to that of Finland, and is substantially higher than that of other Mediterranean countries (6). Both genetic and non-genetic factors may be important in determining these differences.

### Family and twin studies

There are currently 30 or more prospective family studies in progress around the world. These families have usually been recruited by advertising among physicians or through patient organisations, and there is a strong bias in ascertainment. A few groups, notably the Pittsburgh group in the USA, the DiMe study group in Finland, and our own Bart's–Oxford group have attempted to overcome these problems by setting up population-based family studies. The estimated lifetime risk for first-degree relatives of patients with IDDM has been calculated at about 7% for siblings and 5% for children (7). Other family studies have found similar levels of disease risk for siblings, the level varying between 4 and 11% (8–12). Of the reported studies of diabetic twins, most did not categorise diabetes by disease type, confirm monozygosity, or test the unaffected twins; in all but two ascertainment was incomplete. In a Finnish study, which aimed for complete ascertainment, the concordance rates were higher in identical (23% probandwise and 13% pairwise) than non-identical twins (5% probandwise and 3% pairwise) (13). In our own study of identical twins, referred because the index twin was diabetic, the concordance rates for IDDM between identical twins on prospective analysis was 36%; twins who remain non-diabetic more than six years from the diagnosis of their index twin had a low disease risk (<2%) (14). All the studies showed striking agreement in that the majority of identical twins with IDDM have a non-diabetic co-twin irrespective of their country of origin (13–17).

## ROLE OF GENETIC FACTORS

Heritability reflects gene expression or penetrance in a given environment. The best estimate of heritability can be obtained by determining concordance rates of twins. Both identical and non-identical twins share the same environment in childhood but only identical twins share the same genes. In the classic twin method, the difference between the concordance rates for identical and non-identical twins is doubled to give an index of heritability. Estimates of heritability can be obtained from studies in Finland and the University of Southern California; in both the estimates are low (20% and 66%, respectively), the true value may lie somewhere between these values in that the American study preferentially identified concordant pairs, while the Finnish study has just started so concordance rates should increase (13,16). Heritability falls from 66% to 2% according to whether the index twin is diagnosed under 10 years of age or between 15 and 30 years of age, respectively (16).

### MHC genes

Genes encoding HLA molecules and located within the Major Histocompatibility Complex (MHC) on the short arm of chromosome 6 are associated with IDDM (see Chapter 9). The MHC complex is a polymorphic gene complex in that multiple alleles exist for each genetic locus. The MHC is divided into class I (HLA-A, -B, and -C), class II (HLA-DR, -DQ, and -DP), and class III (genes for complement components). The class I and class II proteins coded by the relevant genes are transmembrane cell surface glycoproteins which are critically involved in the presentation of both self- and foreign antigens as short peptides to T lymphocytes. HLA class I glycoprotein is present on all nucleated cells and platelets. It consists of a 'heavy' chain subunit anchored to the cell by a transmembrane hydrophobic tail and an extracellular hydrophilic region with three domains, two of which are polymorphic and show structural determinants specific to the individual. Crystallographic studies show that the two hypervariable $\alpha 1$ and $\alpha 2$ sequences form a groove that serves as the antigen binding site for a processed antigen (18). Class II molecules have a more limited distribution and are found on B lymphocytes, dendritic epithelial cells and activated T lymphocytes. These class II molecules are also composed of transmembrane glycoproteins made up of $\alpha$ and $\beta$ subunits such that the $\alpha 1$ and $\beta 1$ domains determine the hypervariable region and form the antigen binding groove. Crystallographic studies suggest that this class II molecule exists as a dimer, which is, therefore, capable of binding two antigen molecules at any one time (19). Antigen presentation by an antigen presenting cell (APC) in the context of an HLA molecule to a T cell receptor is a pivotal event in the development of an immune response and in the shaping of the T cell repertoire during T cell development in the thymus. Antigenic peptides may be derived from intracellular proteins and presented by class I molecules to CD8+ cytotoxic/suppressor T cells or from exogenous proteins and presented by class II molecules to CD4+ helper/inducer T cells.

## MHC and disease susceptibility

HLA genes are highly polymorphic with a degree of coding region diversity unequalled elsewhere in the genome. Polymorphisms of certain genes probably originated in selection pressures exerted by environmental factors including epidemics, climatic change and availability of food. Non-human somatic studies of the HLA-DQ beta region suggests that this region has been in balanced polymorphism for 10 or more million years. To maintain the extraordinary diversity of HLA types over this time, selection pressures must have been operating; otherwise most alleles would have been lost through genetic drift. It has been proposed that infectious pathogens are the major cause of HLA diversity. The distribution of sequence variation is clustered in nucleotides which code for amino acids composing the antigen binding groove. This implies that natural selection must have acted at this binding site to maintain structural diversity for peptide binding. HLA associations with IDDM may therefore operate through susceptibility to certain undefined infections which could be modern, just as there is an argument that IDDM and other autoimmune diseases are modern diseases.

HLA genes are important in predisposing to a number of autoimmune diseases including IDDM (2). These genes have been shown to be associated with IDDM in both population and family studies (7,20). The evidence is that class II genes are more important than class I genes and that DQ genes are more important than DR genes (21). About 95% of European patients with IDDM have either HLA-DR3 or DR4 as compared with about 60% of the normal population. However, 90% of the DR4 positive diabetic patients have the DQ allele DQB1 0302 and only 10% have the DQB1 0301 while both alleles were equally represented in the normal DR4 positive population. Extended haplotypes identical at the DQB1 loci are associated with very different risks of IDDM, implying that MHC genes outside the DQ region play an important role in determining genetic susceptibility (22). Certain individual residues with the class II region confer a particular susceptibility or protection from disease. Thus, disease susceptibility correlates with expression of a DQ molecule bearing an arginine in the 52 position of the $\alpha$ chain and lacking an aspartate at the 57 position of the $\beta$ chain (2,20). A combination of these changes confers a greater risk for disease than either one alone, as has been shown for DR3 and DR4, implying that two or more genes are important in disease susceptibility. On balance, the evidence suggests that certain amino acid substitutions are important but only within the context of the whole molecule.

### Pattern of inheritance

HLA genes are important if IDDM is to develop. Thus, in families with several affected members, about 95% of the diabetic siblings are HLA identical or haploidentical (7). Nevertheless, most people carrying the susceptibility genes will not develop IDDM and some patients with IDDM do not have HLA susceptibility genes implying that the MHC disease-associated molecules are permissive rather than causative. The pattern of inheritance is complex with a hierarchy of susceptibility so that a given high risk allele may confer different risks within a population as well as between populations. Transracial studies have shown that DR2 protection is more consistent than susceptibility conferred by other alleles (21). In other words, the protective effect of certain alleles is sufficient to counteract co-existing susceptibility alleles, so that protection is dominant. Thus, there is a hierarchy of genetically determined risk to IDDM ranging from susceptibility at one extreme to protection at the other. Even within families the pattern of inheritance can be complex, since children of fathers with IDDM are at higher risk of developing the disease than children of affected mothers (23). This difference may be due, in part, to preferential transmission of diabetic alleles in the HLA complex (24).

### Non-MHC genes

Concordance for IDDM between identical twins has been estimated at about 36% (14) and in HLA identical siblings at about 15–20% (7). This difference could be due to either genes outside the MHC complex or to environmental factors. A number of candidate genes has been examined for their relationship to IDDM but, with the exception of the insulin gene, the results have not shown any consistent association. The insulin gene lies on the short arm of chromosome 11 (25). The major polymorphism for this gene is located 5′ to the transcription region. There are two alleles in populations of European origin which differ in the size of their variable number tandem repeats frequency; the class 1 allele with 40 repeats was found to be increased in some populations though the results were not consistent (25). In a recent study of multiplex families, linkage was confirmed between this allele and IDDM and it was proposed that it might be dependent on an association with HLA-DR4 and a parental origin of the insulin gene (26).

## ROLE FOR NON-GENETIC FACTORS

Population studies are of limited value in determining the role of non-genetic factors as it is often difficult to define genetic differences between populations and how they might influence the disease rate. An alternative method is to assess changes in disease incidence within a population in which the genetic pool is presumed to remain constant. Two such analyses indicate that non-genetic factors are important. A linear increase in risk of IDDM for children under 15 years of age was observed in most of Europe and the Western Pacific but not in North America. The incidence of IDDM in Jewish children of Ashkenazi origin who migrated to Canada is twice that of similar children in Israel (27). The most powerful evidence that IDDM is due to non-genetically determined factors comes from the study of identical twins (14). Differences or discordance between identical twins must be due to non-genetically determined factors. Since most identical twins with IDDM have an unaffected co-twin it is probable that non-genetic factors are important in causing the disease.

## CHARACTERISTICS OF NON-GENETIC FACTORS

Even identical twins can be genetically different for certain genes. For example, genes could undergo random and ordered rearrangement or mutation and may differ between identical twins. In contrast to antibody genes, genes of the

T cell receptor do not appear to undergo somatic hypermutation. If, as is widely believed, T cells are responsible for the immune destruction of islet β cells, it is unlikely that somatic mutations give rise to IDDM. Several other observations argue against somatic mutations causing the disease. It is unlikely that random somatic mutations could explain the almost constant year-on-year disease incidence within different populations without epidemicity (28). In addition, there is no evidence of randomness in either the clinical syndrome or the antigens recognised by antibodies in patients with the disease (29). If a somatic mutation of the immune system caused IDDM, the aberrant immune response would probably be monoclonal and not polyclonal as is the case in IDDM (30). We therefore believe, though we cannot be certain, that the disease is due to environmental agents, not a somatic mutation.

## Characteristics of the environmental factor

Whatever the nature of the environmental factor(s), it is likely to be ubiquitous as is the disease. It is also likely to operate over a brief period. The age-specific pattern of incidence of IDDM is similar worldwide, the disease is extremely rare before 9 months of age, has a peak incidence between 5 and 15 years of age which declines sharply after 15 years of age (31). This decline in disease incidence is a consistent and striking feature and could be due to either a loss of the genetically susceptible pool in a population or a limited period of effect of the environmental agent. We know from twin studies that the majority of genetically susceptible individuals do not develop the disease (14). The decrease in the disease incidence with age is, therefore, likely to be due to a decreased environmental effect. By implication, the environmental effect which causes IDDM must, in the main, operate over a limited period.

## Critical factor operates in early childhood

About 60% of all C-peptide negative cases of diabetes present before the age of 22 (32). About a quarter of childhood cases present before the age of 5, and prospective studies suggest that a child who presents at the age of 13 will typically (but not always) have had detectable circulating levels of islet cell antibodies (ICA) five years or more before onset of the disease. There is, therefore, a strong presumption that the disease process is initiated in early childhood. Other evidence supports this proposal. In man, high titres of insulin autoantibodies (IAA) appear early in childhood and decline rapidly with age (33). Initial seroconversion to ICA positivity usually develops before the age of 5, and our own experience with a sensitive ICA assay suggests that conversion from ICA negativity to ICA positivity is a rare event over the age of 10 (34). If these inferences are correct, the majority of cases of IDDM developing in adolescence or even well into adult life are the end result of a process initiated in infancy. The observation that progression to IDDM slows with increasing age would be consistent with this view (8). Taken together, these observations suggest that the immune process is initiated in early childhood. It is possible, but by no means certain, that the disease process starts at a specific age, perhaps even *in utero*. Three observations suggest that maternal-related events influence the development of IDDM, and that the critical period for the environmental factor could be pre- or peripartum. Children of diabetic mothers are one-third less likely to develop IDDM than children of diabetic fathers (23, 35), this risk is even lower if the mother is already diabetic at conception and if she is more than 25 years old (36). Children who develop IDDM are more likely to have inherited HLA DR3 (a susceptibility gene) from their mother than from their father (24). The extreme rarity of diabetes under 9 months of age would accord with the recognised latency period before the onset of IDDM. Finally, a model of foetal viral infection causing IDDM, namely congenital rubella, is well established (37).

### Exposure or susceptibility to exposure

It is not possible at present to determine whether the decreasing environmental effect with age is due to a lack of exposure to the environmental factor or a change in susceptibility to such a factor. It is difficult to envisage an environmental agent to which only children are exposed. On the other hand, the pattern of disease incidence does resemble that for common viral infections which cause less illness with age as immunity develops. Current evidence favours the latter, as twins can have immune changes, consistent with exposure to an environmental agent, yet not develop IDDM, possibly because exposure induces tolerance to developing diabetes (38). It is not known whether IDDM is initiated by single or multiple exposures during the brief critical period. Diabetes can be produced in animal models using viruses and chemical toxins in combination (39). Cumulative damage, if it were to occur, would probably have to do so over a limited time frame.

### Environment precipitates clinical onset

The association between the clinical onset of IDDM and the seasons, puberty and life events suggests that environmental factors can precipitate the disease presentation though the disease process is likely to have been initiated many months earlier (1,3). The diagnosis of IDDM is made more often in cooler than in warmer months and the peak incidence is consistently associated with the peripubertal years (31). Both immune and metabolic changes have been clearly demonstrated in twins before their pubertal growth spurt and before they developed diabetes (40). Therefore, it is unlikely that the pubertal growth spurt plays a primary role in the pathogenesis of diabetes. At diagnosis of IDDM, 54% of diabetic patients report two or more severe life events (distressing situations) in the preceding three years as compared with 8% of siblings and 8% of neighbourhood controls (41). Stress hormones, like viral infections and puberty, can cause insulin insensitivity which could precipitate clinical diabetes in a metabolically compromised patient.

## VIRUSES AS THE CRITICAL FACTOR

What is the environmental agent responsible for IDDM? Attention has focused on viruses and toxins, including dietary factors. 'Wild' viruses exist which have a specific β cell tropism and a diabetic potential in animals. Viruses with high mutation rates and fast circulation rates such as the single-stranded RNA picornaviruses are particularly prone to produce such variants with pathogenic potential. There are four common human viruses which cause islet lesions in animals: Venezuelan encephalitis virus, Coxsackie B4, reovirus, and rubella virus. A casual relation between viruses and diabetes was suggested last century, and numerous anecdotal reports have recorded the onset of diabetes days or months after viral infections. Viral infections might precipitate the clinical onset of diabetes, but such an acute infection is unlikely to explain the prolonged latent period associated with the disease (3, 42, 43).

Viruses are normally prevented from reaching the islets of Langerhans by the capillary endothelial cells and the basement membrane mechanism of transport of viruses across these structures is unknown, and likely to be a rare event. Viral tropism for the β cell, once it has reached the islets, is mediated by specific viral polypeptides with specific cell receptors on the plasma membrane in a similar way that CD4 is the receptor for the HIV virus (44). Three mechanisms have been proposed for virus-induced diabetes: 1) infection triggering an immune or an autoimmune response which leads to β cell destruction; 2) persistent infection of the β cell causing dysfunction without lysis; 3) acute cytolytic destruction of the β cell.

Viruses could cause diabetes without direct β cell lysis by the induction of an immune response against viral antigens on the cell surface. Expression of novel surface antigens on pancreatic β-cells can result in immune-mediated diabetes. Thus, transgenic mice which express the haemagglutin antigen of the influenza virus, develop hyperglycaemia (45). Viruses could also induce autoimmunity by several mechanisms including polyclonal activation of B lymphocytes, molecular mimicry, anti-idiotypic antibodies and islet β-cell expression of class II antigens or cytokines. The induction of autoimmunity in man by viruses is well established. Antibodies reactive to various cellular constituents in sera have been reported following infection with influenza, rubella and Epstein–Barr virus. Both insulin autoantibodies (IAA) and islet cell antibodies (ICA) can appear following infection with mumps virus and rubella virus (46, 47). Human cytomegalovirus, whose genome has been detected in peripheral lymphocytes of 15% of newly diagnosed diabetic patients (48), can induce islet cell antibodies that react with specific islet cell antigen (49). Expression of class II antigens and interferon are both features of human diabetic islet β-cells (50). In theory, class II expression would enable a β cell specific antigen to be presented to a T-cell receptor, allowing a destructive process to target β-cells. However, in transgenic mice constructed to aberrantly express the class II molecule in their β-cells, such expression does not enable the cell to initiate an immune response against itself (51). On the other hand, expression of interferon without viral infection in the β-cell of a transgeneic mouse induces its destruction by cytotoxic T cells (52). The mechanism whereby interferon recruits cytotoxic T cells is unknown. These observations indicate that a virus or toxin which induces interferon expression in the β-cell might, in theory, be able to induce a destructive immune response against that cell.

The most persuasive evidence that a persistent viral infection can cause human diabetes derives from the studies of patients with congenital rubella syndrome (37.53). Children infected congenitally may show rubella virus in the pancreas with insulitis and β-cell destruction (54). Diabetes is found in about 20% of patients with the congenital rubella syndrome with a latent period of many years and a median age of onset of 13 years (37, 53). Not all cases are dependent on insulin treatment. Antibodies to islet cell cytoplasmic and surface antigens are found in about 70% of those who develop diabetes (37). Those patients with the HLA genetic susceptibility associated with IDDM (HLA DR3 and DR4) tend to develop diabetes and as with IDDM HLA DR2 is apparently protective (53). Rubella-induced diabetes is a rare phenomenon and unlikely to account for the generality of patients with IDDM.

In man, viruses may damage the pancreas either generally, as with mumps pancreatitis, or specifically by only damaging the islets. Damage to the islet cells can be found after fatal viral infections involving Coxsackie B, cytomegalovirus and rubella. Of 250 cases of children succumbing to viral illness, islet cell changes consistent with damage were found in a fraction of those with Coxsackie B, cytomegalovirus and congenital rubella infections (55). More convincing evidence for viral involvement derives from the study of a young boy who died from an overwhelming viral infection and diabetic ketoacidosis (56). A Coxsackie B4 virus was isolated from his pancreas which induced diabetes with islet cell damage in mice susceptible to diabetes.

## TOXINS AS THE CRITICAL FACTOR

A number of structurally diverse agents are diabetogenic in animals and, in some cases, also in man. Toxins could damage the β-cell directly or indirectly, for example, by inducing endogenous viral replication or an immune reaction against a transformed cell. Of toxins, only N-nitroso derivatives are known to induce acute β-cell destruction and diabetic ketoacidosis. Alloxan, one such agent, was originally introduced for its toxicity to renal tubular cells (57). Indeed, most toxic substances damage tissues other than the β-cell and are therefore unlikely candidates to explain the specific β-cell targeting in IDDM.

Both alloxan and a similar compound streptozotocin, when given in large doses, cause diabetes in certain animals by depleting the β-cell of NAD (58). The drug pentamidine can cause diabetes in animals, initially without β-cell destruction (59) by depressing responses to both glucose and arginine and later directly damaging the islets. The rat poison Vacor, a nitrophenylurea, can cause neurotoxicity and diabetes in man, and after fatal poisoning necropsy has shown extensive β-cell damage (60). As with viruses it is unlikely that these or other toxins which cause acute cytolytic damage could account for IDDM with its long latency period. Toxins can, however, damage the β-cell chronically and the best known example in animals is streptozotocin, which produces insulitis and diabetes (61).

### Dietary factors

Evidence that dietary factors are important in the aetiology of IDDM in man derives from a study in Iceland (62) and studies of infant feeding (63). As elsewhere, patients with IDDM in Iceland are more likely to present during the autumn, with a noticeable excess of male diabetic patients born in October (62). It was speculated that this excess was due to parental consumption of smoked, cured mutton, traditionally eaten around the New Year, which is rich in nitrites and N-nitroso compounds. Mice fed with cured mutton had male offspring with increased glucose levels and β-cell destruction (62). The low prevalence of IDDM in primitive societies may be worth noting in the context of toxic food additives. IDDM is also relatively uncommon in Japan, where legal limits for food nitrite content are strict.

The increasing rates of IDDM in certain populations have been attributed to a decline in breast-feeding (63). More recently, attention has focused on early exposure to cow's milk or solid food, rather than lack of breast-feeding, and a consistent but weak relationship has been established. In one American study the attributable risk, that is the proportion of cases that could be prevented by removal of a risk factor from a population, was 8% for cow's milk and 25% for solid foods if these factors were introduced after the age of 3 months or more (64). These observations are consistent with the animal models of spontaneous diabetes in which progression to diabetes is markedly reduced, in the BB rat, if L-amino acids are substituted for protein in their diet (65), and totally prevented, in NOD mice, by hydrolysing the protein content of the diet (66). Particular attention has focused on bovine albumin, a major constituent of cow's milk. Further, analysis of the bovine albumin molecule has identified a 17 amino acid sequence, known as ABBOS, which differs markedly from the equivalent sequence in man and other species, including the mouse and rat (67). Antibodies to bovine serum albumin may be more common in recently diagnosed diabetes than in controls, and cross-react with a β-cell peptide referred to as p69. This peptide is not normally presented at the β-cell membrane but does appear when the cells are exposed *in vitro* to γ interferon, as might occur in response to infection. The 'cow's milk' theory would therefore postulate that individuals genetically susceptible to IDDM can generate antibodies against the ABBOS sequence which cross-react with p69 on the β-cell surface during intercurrent infection (67). This hypothesis fits with the evidence that the immune response leading to IDDM is generated very early in life, but does not explain the rapid rise in incidence of the condition unless commercial processing of cow's milk, or of milk-based food products, has in some way increased their antigenicity.

## DIABETES AS AN AUTOIMMUNE DISEASE

At diagnosis of IDDM, both cellular and humoral immune changes occur in peripheral blood and some islets are heavily infiltrated with lymphocytes (68). Since genetic susceptibility to IDDM operates largely through the HLA region which codes for proteins involved in antigen presentation and recognition, the immune response is probably important in the aetiology of the disease. The rapid destruction of apparently normal β-cells when transplanted from a non-diabetic twin to the diabetic co-twin indicates that the destructive process must be outside the islet, β-cell specific and retain its cytotoxic memory immune system is the most likely candidate for such an extra-islet effect (68). These observations suggest that the destructive process leading to IDDM is probably immune mediated. Autoimmunity is important to the fitness of the organism. Most individuals produce autoantibodies and auto-reactive T-lymphocytes. However, only about 5% of any population develop an autoimmune disease. Control mechanisms must therefore operate to control the development of autoimmune diseases. These control mechanisms remove cytotoxic immune cells in various ways including: clonal deletion, clonal anergy and limiting antigen accessibility to the immune system. Antigen accessibility is limited by being processed for presentation to the immune system or by autoreactive T-lymphocytes circulating in an inert state. Breakdown in these control mechanisms could lead to disease. Diseases associated with autoimmune phenomena tend to distribute themselves within a spectrum of organ specific diseases, such as IDDM and non-organ specific diseases such as systemic lupus erythematosus. There may be clustering of diseases at either end of this spectrum; thus, IDDM is more common in patients with thyroiditis or adrenalitis.

## CHANGES WITHIN INDIVIDUALS

### Islet cells

There are two types of diabetes which *must* be treated with insulin, that is the patients are insulin-dependent. One type is associated with diabetes insipidus, optic atrophy and high-tone deafness (DIDMOAD or Wolfram's syndrome) and is due to malformation of islet β-cells. While the other is Type 1 or insulin-dependent diabetes (IDDM) and is due to destruction of the β-cells. At diagnosis of IDDM about 80% of islets contain no β-cells and the islets may be heavily infiltrated with mononuclear cells (50). These mononuclear cells include macrophages and antigen-specific CD 8-positive T lymphocytes; the T cells show enrichment for certain Vβ T cell receptors (69). An increased expression of intercellular adhesion molecules on vascular endothelium may enhance the accumulation of mononuclear cells in the islets (69). Lymphocyte infiltration is not a consistent feature, and occurs principally in the islets containing insulin-positive β-cells. Not all the insulin secreting β-cells will be destroyed, and even in long-standing diabetic patients about 10% of the islets can have insulin-containing cells. The destructive process does not involve all cells simultaneously, consistent with the chronic nature of the disease process leading to clinical diabetes. Abnormal β-cells at diagnosis tend to be enlarged with either swollen cytoplasm and no granules or enlarged nuclei and reduced granulation. After diagnosis β-cells disappear within 12 months in patients aged less than 7 years, but survive longer in older patients (70). There is no evidence that the exocrine pancreatic cells or the other islet cells secreting glucagon, somatostatin or pancreatic polypeptide are involved in this destructive process. Those residual islets which contain β-cells hyperexpress class I HLA antigens but only the β-cells express class II HLA antigen and contain immunoreactive α-interferon (50). The presence of α-interferon suggests that the cells have been chronically infected with a virus. However, there is no evidence to date that the β-cells contain viral components. Hyperexpression of class I or class II antigens could also result from viral infection, or alternatively it could be secondary to the inflammatory process. More information is required regarding the sequence of changes which characterise the islets during the prediabetic phase before it is possible to interpret the significance of these changes.

Table 10.1. *Antibodies associated with IDDM recognise a variety of structural and functional elements in the islet β-cell*

| | |
|---|---|
| Cytoplasmic islet cell antigens | Carboxypeptidase H |
| Islet cell surface antigens | Glutamic acid decarboxylase |
| Tubulin | Insulin |
| Albumin | Pro-insulin |
| 37/40 kD islet fragments | ?Glucose transporter |

## HLA ANTIGEN PRESENTATION

The pivotal event in the generation of an immune process involves the presentation of antigen in the context of an HLA molecule to a T cell receptor. In considering the role of the HLA molecules, it is important to consider: 1) that most people with the susceptibility genes do not develop IDDM; 2) that individuals without the HLA susceptibility genes can develop the disease, and 3) that the HLA gene associations involve class II genes which are probably important in modulating helper/inducer cellular responses. Two broad mechanisms could account for the HLA association with IDDM. First, the HLA molecule could positively select the T cell repertoire to maintain potentially autoreactive T cells. Alternatively, the structure of the HLA molecule might determine the ability of critical antigens to bind to it or to the T cell receptor or both. Our understanding of these interactions is limited at present. In one model proposed by Nepom HLA susceptibility is determined by the ability of the alleles to bind to a specific peptide or peptides; protective alleles operate by competing for binding of the diabetogenic peptide (71). An alternative model focuses on the protective quality of HLA alleles and the apparent failure of the immune system to maintain tolerance to the islet β-cell (72). Whatever the role of HLA molecules in the aetiology of IDDM, it is likely to be permissive rather than causative for diabetes.

Usually HLA class II molecules are expressed on the surface of antigen presenting cells (APC) such as macrophages or monocytes where they present the antigen to CD4+ T cells inducing T cell proliferation, lymphokine production and subsequent synthesis of immunoglobulin by B lymphocytes. Class II molecules are not normally expressed on endocrine cells but the observation that aberrant expression can occur on a sub-population of β-cells in the islets of patients with IDDM raised the possibility that the insulin-secreting cell itself could present antigen (73). Whilst there is evidence that a thyroid cell can aberrantly express class II antigens and act as an APC the evidence is less clear in IDDM (74). Cells which contain insulin and class II molecules may be macrophages which have engulfed β-cells and not simply β-cells (75). In transgenic mice whose β-cells aberrantly express class II molecules, cell destruction does not ensue (51). It is possible, therefore, that class II expression on β-cells is an epiphenomenon or that, if real, it need not result in either cytokine release or β-cell destruction.

## ANTIGEN TARGETS OF AUTOIMMUNITY

In distinguishing between self and non-self, the organism's most efficient approach is to identify features (antigens) conserved within a species and not features unique to a sub-type of that species. Therefore, conserved elements, both structural and functional, are obvious targets for immunity (Table 10.1). Organ specific diseases tend to target functional elements such as enzymes, e.g. thyroid peroxidase (Hashimoto's thyroiditis) whilst non-organ specific diseases target structural elements, e.g. histones and DNA (systemic lupus erythematosus). The 'luxury function' of all endocrine cells is to recognise a signal (glucose for the β-cell) and produce and secrete a hormone (insulin and insulin precursors). Whilst IDDM patients can have antibodies which interfere with β-cell glucose transport, hormone secretion systems may be more important antigen targets and include enzymes (carboxypeptidase H and glutamic acid decarboxylase) and insulin and proinsulin. One of the striking features of antigens associated with IDDM is the sheer number of them. The existence of so many antigens obfuscates efforts to identify the single antigen which reductionism tells us must be critical. At the same time, it raises the possibility that many or all of the antigens are mere epiphenomena.

### Islet cell antibodies

These antibodies are detected by indirect immunofluorescence in about 80% of newly diagnosed patients with IDDM and only 0.8 to 4% of the normal community (76). The antibodies are IgG, polyclonal and usually restricted to the IgG1 isotype (30). They recognise antigens on islet β cells but also other non-beta-islet cells. The nature of the antigen remains unclear but in polyendocrine patients it appears to be the enzyme glutamic acid decarboxylase (GAD) and in patients with IDDM it may be, in part, a glycolipid (77).

### Insulin autoantibodies

Insulin autoantibodies (IAA) can be detected using a radiobinding assay or an enzyme-linked immunoabsorbent assay (ELISA). Antibodies detected by the radiobinding assay are more closely associated with IDDM than IAA detected by ELISA (78, 79). IAA are not specific for IDDM and can also be found in other autoimmune diseases, in drug-induced autoimmunity and following viral infections. Newly diagnosed diabetic patients have IAA but the frequency of IAA, unlike ICA, varies inversely with age being found in up to 100% of diabetic children aged less than five years but as little as 4% of adult diabetic patients (77).

### Autoantibodies to a 64K islet protein

The 64K antigen was originally detected as a major radiolabelled protein immunoprecipitated from detergent extracts of metabolically labelled islet by circulating autoantibodies in the sera of IDDM patients (80). Antibodies to 64K were also detected in two animal models of diabetes – the BB rat and the NOD mouse. The protein is typically resolved as two components of $M_r$-64 000 and 67 000 by SDS polyacrylamide gel electrophoresis and may therefore represent a complex of more than one polypeptide chain. At least part of the antigen complex has more recently been identified as glutamic acid decarboxylase (GAD) (81). Evidence that the 64K antigen is GAD, derived from studies of a rare and severe neurological disease called stiff-man syndrome. Most patients with this syndrome have autoantibodies to GAD (82). These patients have an increased incidence of IDDM, and those patients with IDDM and stiff-man syndrome not only had GAD antibodies but also ICA. The evidence is that ICA in these patients is predominantly, maybe entirely, composed of antibodies to GAD. Patients with polyendocrine diseases including IDDM also tend to have serum ICA which persists for many years and, in them, the predominant antigen also appears to be GAD (unpublished observations). GAD is the enzyme responsible for the synthesis of the neurotransmitter, gamma-amino butyric acid (GABA) in the GABA-ergic neurons of the central nervous system. In addition to the central nervous system and pancreatic beta-cells, GAD and GABA have also been detected in several other tissues including kidney, liver, adrenal gland, ovary and testis. Within the pancreatic islet, GAD and GABA expression have been shown to be restricted to the beta-cells where GABA synthesis and secretion may be involved with paracrine regulation of glucagon and somatostatin secretion (83). There is evidence that GAD exists as multiple isoforms. In mammalian brain, two forms of GAD (GAD 65K and GAD 67K) have been distinguished on the basis of antigenicity and intraneuronal distribution, and three others on their chemical characteristics (84). Both GAD 65K and GAD 67K have been detected in pancreatic islets, and both forms are recognised by diabetes-associated antibodies.

Both GAD 65K and GAD 67K derive from a single separate gene localised to chromosome 10 and chromosome 2, respectively (84). These genes code for polypeptides of 585 and 594 amino acids respectively and there is considerable sequence homology (65%) between the two genes and also between these genes and their counterparts in rats, cats and the fruit fly. These extensive sequence homologies suggest that GAD structure has been subject to intense selective pressure during phylogeny.

### Antibodies to a 37K antigen

Tryptic proteolysis of purified 64K antigen reveals several major fragments which are themselves antigenic, including fragments of molecular weights 50K, 40K and 37K (85). Such trypsin digestion might either reveal hidden or distinct epitopes. The evidence is that two distinct antibody specificities are associated with the 64K antigen, one specificity associated with the 50K fragment which retains GAD activity, and another specificity associated with the 37K and 40K fragments which do not have GAD activity (86). These 37K and 40K antigens might be part of GAD or, as now seems more likely, separate polypeptides complexed with GAD in the 64K antigen. Approximately 93% of patients recently diagnosed with IDDM have at least one of these two distinct antibody specificities; that is 81% had antibodies to the 50K fragment and 78% had antibodies to the 37K or 40K fragment but only 7% did not have antibodies to either antibody specificities (85); these antibodies are rare in controls. The nature and function of the 37K and 40K antigens remain unknown.

### 38K antigen

Immunoprecipitation of radiolabelled islet proteins by antibodies in sera of IDDM subjects identified a 38K antigen (80). Autoantibodies to this 38K protein are found in about 30% of recently diagnosed patients. The protein has been partially purified from the insulin secretory granule and is also found in neuroendocrine secretory cells. This antigen has been shown to generate T cell lines from the peripheral blood of 8 of 10 IDDM patients but not from two control subjects (86). In separate studies, mice immunised with human cytomegalovirus (CMV) developed antibodies which also recognised a 38K antigen in human islets (49). These observations raise the possibility that CMV infection could generate antibodies to a 38K antigen either by induction of a neoantigen or through molecular mimicry.

### Antibodies to carboxypeptidase H

This enzyme is involved in the cleavage of proinsulin to insulin in the insulin secretory granule, where it is one of the major constituent proteins. It was initially identified as an antigen in screening an islet cDNA library with diabetic sera. Subsequently, it was shown to react with sera from 5 of 20 non-diabetic subjects with ICA but none of 14 control subjects (87).

### Antibodies to ICA512

Using a human islet cell cDNA library and screening diabetic sera, two clones were identified (88). Proteins expressed by these λ phages reacted specifically with antibodies in the sera of newly diagnosed diabetic children. Antibodies to ICA512 but not ICA12 could be identified in the sera of prediabetic twins (personal unpublished observation); further analysis is in progress.

### Antibodies to a glucose transporter

An immunoglobulin (IgG) from the sera of recent-onset patients with IDDM has been found to specifically inhibit glucose uptake by rat islet cells (89). Since these cells express the GLUT-2 transporter, the antibodies might recognise GLUT-2 or a component of intracellular glucose transport.

## T CELL RESPONSE TO ANTIGEN

The T cell receptor is composed of two polypeptide chains and linked by disulphide bonds. Each chain is about 40 and 50K in size and contains both constant and variable regions. These α and β chains undergo rearrangement of germline sequences, similar to those of immunoglobulin genes, to generate the diversity of combining sites required to recognise many different antigens. It is proposed that the highly polymorphic variable region contacts antigenic peptide in the HLA antigen binding-groove, an interaction which probably evolved to allow recognition of foreign peptides associated with self HLA so that infected cells could be destroyed. The nature of the T cell repertoire in IDDM is not known, and studies of the T cell antigen specific response are at a very early stage. It is known, however, that an increased T cell response can occur to both GAD and to the 38K antigen in patients with IDDM or at risk of developing IDDM (86, 90). It has been recently shown that high T cell proliferation to recombinant GAD in relatives of patients with IDDM is associated with low concentrations of autoantibodies to GAD (91). It was proposed that sensitisation to GAD is more likely to lead to IDDM when the immune response deviates towards an expansion of autoreactive T cells, rather than towards the generation of autoantibodies (91).

## EXPOSURE NEED NOT LEAD TO IDDM

The immune changes associated with IDDM do not always lead on to the disease (38). Increased levels of activated T lymphocytes have been detected in the majority of non-diabetic identical twins of recently diagnosed diabetic patients who were then followed for up to 10 years without developing diabetes themselves (92); further analysis of these cells indicates that it is the CD4+ (helper/inducer) cells which are activated. Autoantibodies to islet cells, insulin, GAD and tryptic fragments of the 64K islet antigen have also been detected in non-diabetic twins and siblings of diabetic patients who, we calculate, are unlikely now to develop diabetes (29, 92–94). In both twin and population-based studies, ICA can remit without progression to diabetes (92,95). As identical twins can be discordant for these immune changes, namely the production of ICA, GAD antibodies and activation of T lymphocytes, the changes probably reflect exposure to an environmental event (29, 92). By implication, exposure to the critical environmental event which causes these immune changes need not lead on to IDDM. This observation is consistent with the known association with HLA related gene polymorphisms and the relative protection from IDDM afforded by other HLA genes. If the disease process was inevitably cytopathic, there could be no selection of genetic polymorphisms, since everyone exposed to the process would develop the disease.

Evidence now suggests that the islet β-cells can be damaged without progression to IDDM. Impaired glucose tolerance was observed in five of 41 identical twins of patients with IDDM, none of whom developed diabetes themselves, and all of whom now have normal glucose tolerance (96). Some of these non-diabetic twins also had a decreased insulin response to intravenous glucose and an altered insulin to glucose dose–response relationship (97). Finally, increased peripheral blood levels of proinsulin, the precursor of insulin, have been found in twins and siblings of diabetic patients many years after the diagnosis of the index case, and when they themselves are unlikely to develop IDDM (98–100). It should be noted that the changes in proinsulin secretion were detected in non-HLA identical siblings; this observation raises the possibility that β-cell damage, in contrast to β-cell destruction, is not HLA restricted (100). We have known for some years that immune changes in organ-orientated diseases such as thyroiditis need not lead to destruction of the target cells. It now looks as if the disease process associated with IDDM also encompasses a wide spectrum including immune and metabolic changes which do not lead on to diabetes.

## EXPOSURE COULD LEAD TO NIDDM

Since there is clear evidence that the islet β cells can be damaged without IDDM developing, it is reasonable to anticipate that in some individuals the damage may be sufficient to cause impaired glucose tolerance, even diabetes, without absolute insulin deficiency. Until more is known of those immune features which clearly define the process associated with IDDM this argument will remain hypothetical. There is, however, evidence that in some of those patients, who present with non-insulin dependent diabetes and later become frankly insulin dependent, the pathogenesis is similar to that of IDDM. In families with a Type 2 non-insulin dependent diabetic parent and an IDDM child, shared genetic factors linked to HLA-DR4 seem to be important determinants of disease (101). About 30% of patients who develop IDDM do so after the age of 35 years. In addition, up to 1% of patients with NIDDM each year become insulin deficient. These patients have many features of IDDM including low or normal body weight, ICA, antibodies to GAD and high rates of HLA-DR3 and DR4 (102).

## EXPOSURE CAN LEAD TO IDDM

A destructive immune process, once initiated, can pursue a chronic progressive course of β cell destruction. Changes can be detected up to 14 years before the onset of diabetes during which period immune, metabolic and clinical changes may herald the onset of clinical diabetes (15, 40, 103).

### Cellular changes

Activation of T-lymphocytes with increased expression of the HLA-DR antigen can be detected in prediabetic individuals when first ascertained irrespective of the time before they develop diabetes (103). T cell activation was increased in both the CD4 (helper/inducer) and CD8 (cytotoxic/suppressor) population, and the changes persisted until the clinical onset months, even years, later without any consistent alteration in their level (103).

### Cytokine changes

Activated lymphocytes and macrophages should produce cytokines. The detection of α interferon in islet β-cells at diagnosis of IDDM suggests that cytokines are involved in the immune response associated with disease and is important evidence that β-cells have been exposed to a virus (50). Cytokines may be responsible for the aberrant expression of Class II glycoproteins on islet β-cells, and may themselves cause islet β cell destruction. In preliminary prospective studies of non-diabetic twins of IDDM patients, circulating levels of tumour necrosis factor (TNF)-α, interleukin-1α and interferon-γ were estimated; TNF and interleukin-1 levels were elevated above the normal range in about 70% of samples of those twins who developed IDDM subsequently, in contrast to twins who remained non-diabetic who had elevated levels in less than 15% of samples (104).

### Humoral changes

Antigens recognised by serum antibodies in the prediabetic period include: islet cell cytoplasmic antigens (ICA), insulin, GAD, a 64K antigen which incorporates GAD, trypsin derived fragments of this 64K antigen including 37K, 40K and 50K fragments (29)(Table 10.2). If autoantibodies did cause IDDM, they should fulfil the following criteria which, to date, they do not: 1) specificity for the β-cell and in particular its membrane; 2) destructive potential; 3) presence in all patients with IDDM and in all individuals who subsequently develop IDDM; 4) ability to transfer disease from IDDM patients to healthy individuals or animal models. Autoantibodies could therefore be beneficial scavengers of antigen debris or result from a T cell dependent cyto-

Table 10.2. *Frequency of antibodies in 58 non-diabetic identical twins of diabetic patients who later developed IDDM* (n=12) *or remain non-diabetic* (n=46)

| | Prediabetic twins | Non-diabetic twins |
|---|---|---|
| GAD | 67% | 13% |
| 50 kD | 75% | 15% |
| 37/40 kD | 67% | 2% |
| ICA (>4 JDF units) | 75% | 11% |
| IAA | 25% | 4% |

37/40 kD antibodies had the highest positive predictive value (29).

toxic response. Since the levels of both ICA and activated T lymphocytes persist up to the onset of the disease, at least in twins who develop IDDM, but decrease thereafter with the destruction of the target (the β-cell), it is likely that these immune changes are antigen dependent and antigen driven (103).

In summary, the immune response during the prediabetic period involves both cellular and humoral changes probably initiated by an environmental factor and maintained by islet cell antigens. This response persists over a prolonged period up to diagnosis, indicating that the process associated with it is not intermittent but continuous.

## METABOLIC CHANGES BEFORE IDDM

Metabolic changes can precede the onset of IDDM by many months, and include changes in both glucose metabolism and β-cell function.

### Qualitative changes in β-cell function

Possibly the earliest abnormalities are an increase in the fasting proinsulin level even when the fasting glucose and insulin levels are normal (99) and a loss of the regular oscillatory insulin pulses (105). The nature of the increased proinsulin is unclear; it could be due to an excess release of the precursors, including partially processed forms of proinsulin from the secretory pathway, or to release of the intact hormone from the non-secretory pathway proinsulin assays which have been used do not distinguish between intact proinsulin and proinsulin intermediates (99). The increased proinsulin secretion could result from an inherited susceptibility to IDDM or, alternatively, it could be secondary to β-cell damage. Studies of baboons confirm that β-cell damage which leads to insulin-dependent diabetes can cause an increase in fasting proinsulin levels (106). The β-cell normally secretes insulin as regular oscillatory pulses which can be detected in the peripheral circulation as basal insulin oscillations with a mean period of 13 minutes. A group of siblings of patients with IDDM who also had ICA were tested to establish whether they showed oscillatory insulin secretion (105). They did, though regular oscillatory activity was generally absent even when the insulin response to intravenous glucose was in the normal range. Insulin secretion responds to increasing intravenous glucose loads in a step-wise fashion (97). The increasing response to glucose provides a dose–response relationship which shows a high degree of fit in a non-linear logarithmic curve fitting programme. We found that twins tested up to 10 months before the onset of IDDM did not demonstrate such a step-wise increase in their insulin responses (97). The loss of normal glucose to insulin relationship in prediabetic twins is consistent with a qualitative β-cell defect before the onset of IDDM.

Sites on the cell membrane that could provide specific targets for β-cell destruction include the glucose recognition system and those systems responsible for insulin secretion. If the glucose recognition system is involved early in the disease, then it should be possible to demonstrate differential sensitivity of the β-cell to glucose as compared to other insulin secretagogues. Prediabetic patients can show an absent response to intravenous glucose when the response to glucagon or arginine is present but greatly reduced (107, 108). One reason for the rapid disappearance of the insulin response to glucose could be the attendant hyperglycaemia (109). Usually, however, glucose and glucagon recognition decline in parallel before the onset of clinical diabetes (108). The differential response, whilst it can occur, is not a characteristic feature of the prediabetic period.

### Quantitative changes in β-cell function

During the prediabetic period, the insulin response to intravenous glucose may be decreased (15, 97); the insulin response can decline over a number of years even when it is the normal range (15). This decreased insulin response could be due either to decreased sensitivity to glucose or to decreased islet β-cell secretory capacity. The evidence is that prediabetic twins have a decreased maximum insulin secretory response to intravenous glucose (97), and that the insulin response can decline, though not always in a linear fashion (15).

### Changes in glucose metabolism

Impairment of glucose tolerance and glucose clearance and an increase in random blood glucose levels have been observed many months before the onset of diabetes and before changes in fasting glucose (96, 107). Impaired glucose tolerance can occur without changes in either other intermediary metabolites or insulin. However, glucose tolerance can improve with time in some twins who do not develop diabetes (96). In our experience, the two-hour glucose level after an oral glucose load starts to increase above the control range as early as three years before the diagnosis of diabetes, while the fasting glucose remains normal (107). In the final stage, glucose tolerance deteriorates rapidly; fasting glucose increases gradually over the last 18 months before the clinical onset of IDDM but only increases dramatically at the time of diagnosis (110).

## CLINICAL CHANGES BEFORE IDDM

Changes in growth can occur before the onset of IDDM. Twins usually grow at the same rate and to the same final height. However, at diagnosis of diabetes, a diabetic twin aged 9 years or more is often shorter than his unaffected co-twin, consistent with growth delay being prevalent in the prediabetic period (111). In a group of young non-diabetic twins of patients with IDDM, there was indeed a significant tendency for growth to fall below the third percentile compared with their diabetic twins (40). These changes were predominantly detected in twins who developed IDDM, and rarely in twins who remained non-diabetic. Growth delay occurred many months before the diagnosis of diabetes. Subtle changes in glucose tolerance and sex hormones at growth nadir raised the possibility that either metabolic or hormonal disturbances accounted for the growth delay (40). Family studies confirm the tendency for chidren aged more than 10 years at diagnosis to be shorter than their unaffected siblings. Interestingly, no such difference was noted in younger diabetic patients (112). However, young diabetic patients and their siblings are taller than normal. These patients, especially boys, are taller than expected, up to 5 years before the diagnosis of IDDM (113). Quite how a tendency to be tall predisposes to IDDM remains unclear. The evidence suggests that, once the disease process is estabished, the prediabetic patients may then experience transient growth delay.

## PREDICTION OF IDDM

It is clear that both immune and metabolic changes can precede the onset of IDDM and that there are distinct differences in the nature of these changes between those individuals who subsequently develop diabetes and those who do not. Those observations raise the important question as to whether certain immune and metabolic changes can predict the onset of IDDM. The predictive values of any change can be calculated by studying that change in a cohort of individuals, some of whom subsequently develop IDDM. The positive predictive value is determined by calculating the number of individuals in the cohort with an abnormality who develop IDDM as a percentage of the overall number of individuals with that abnormality. Highly specific prediction is now becoming feasible in relatives of diabetic patients, so it is important to recognise certain limitations of the approach to be outlined. One such limitation is that prediction works best close to the onset of diabetes, and therefore, by definition, at a time when there is least scope for β-cell salvage. Secondly, increased specificity implies reduced sensitivity; in other words, we must pass over many individuals at lower degrees of risk to arrive at a subset in whom early onset of diabetes appears almost inevitable. Finally, predictive values for immune or metabolic changes will be different in twin, family or population studies. This latter point is of considerable importance since only about 1 in 10 children who develop diabetes have an affected first-degree relative which means that, for intervention strategies to have a significant impact on the overall incidence of IDDM, the disease must be predicted and prevented in the general population (4). Familial and non-familial IDDM appear to be the same disease. In fact, there is no direct evidence that familial cases of IDDM differ from sporadic cases (114). At the same time, genetic and immune markers of susceptibility may prove to have a different significance within families as compared with the general population.

## Genetic markers

Since genetic markers of susceptibility have relatively low specificity, their principal value in prediction of IDDM within the general population is likely to be identification of high risk groups. Oligonucleotide probes to HLA-DR and -DQ alleles have the potential to identify individuals in a general population who have a similar risk to that for siblings of a child with IDDM. Thus, a Finnish study found that a panel of four sequence-specific oligonucleotide probes which detected alleles conferring susceptibility to, and protection against, IDDM identified subjects with a lifetime absolute risk (for a Finnish population) of 14%, considerably greater than the risk to an unselected sibling (115). Genetic markers could therefore define risk in individuals identified with immune changes in the general population, such a strategy is outlined below.

## Humoral immune changes

ICA are detectable in 5–8% of first-degree relatives, provided a sensitive assay is used (7). Within a group of relatives, the majority of future cases of IDDM will come from the ICA positive subgroup. The positive predictive value of ICA varies from 90% to 3% in twins and siblings of patients with IDDM respectively depending on the titre of the antibody (34,93). Some 5% of relatives with ICA in the range 4–19 JDF units, and 35% of those with ICA $\geqslant$ 20 JDF units will develop insulin requiring diabetes within 5 years (34). There is still some controversy concerning the predictive value of ICA within the general population, although it is clear that ICA are associated with increased risk of IDDM in children with no family history of diabetes. Studies of ICA in school children have found a prevalence varying between 0.3 and 4% (116–118). In a study in The Netherlands, at least 10 years follow-up was available on 2805 children with no family history of diabetes. 8/2805 (0.3%) were found to have ICA and 4 (50%) of these developed IDDM compared with 3/2797 (0.1%) without ICA (119). ICA could constitute a useful predictor of IDDM in the general population. In our own study, in the Oxford region, we have obtained an indirect estimate of the positive predictive value of ICA by combining data from family studies with those obtained by screening 2925 schoolchildren (120). The prevalence of ICA > 4 JDF units in the schoolchildren was 2.8% compared with 6.6% in 274 siblings of children with IDDM living in the same area. The siblings' calculated risk of developing IDDM between the ages of 10 and 20 was 2.8%, whilst the cumulative incidence of IDDM in the general population was only 0.21%. These data imply that ICA would be expected to have a positive predictive value some 6–7 times lower in the general population than that observed in family studies. Recent research efforts have been directed mainly towards refinement of prediction based on this single marker, and we have described a decision tree approach which can allow a complex and evolving body of data to be integrated and analysed within a relatively simple format (4). ICA appear to carry widely differing predictive values according to the population in which they are measured. Heterogeneity within ICA positive individuals has also been recognised. Some ICA stain β-cells predominantly and are associated with a lower risk of progression than ICA that stain all types of islet cells (121–123). These β-cell selective antibodies may account for 25% of all ICA positive first-degree relatives (122).

The two other autoantibodies of major importance in diabetes prediction are autoantibodies to insulin (IAA) (124) and the islet 64K antigen identified as the enzyme GAD (81). IAA probably have little predictive value in the absence of ICA, provided a sensitive ICA assay is used, but the combination, present in around 50% of those who develop IDDM, is highly predictive (125,126). IAA are inversely related to age (33), as is risk of progression to IDDM in ICA positive individuals, so these variables might not be independent. It remains possible that IAA, estimated using a radioligand assay, are more predictive in children aged less than 5 years than are ICA.

Antibodies to the 64K antigen were detected in samples from 34 of 42 patients tested up to 91 months before the onset of IDDM (127, 128). However, the predictive value of 64K antibodies may be limited as they have been detected in individuals who remain non-diabetic for up to 6 years without any deterioration in their β cell function (129). Antibodies to GAD, which comprise some or all of the 64K antigen, appear in some 80% of high risk relatives before diagnosis, but their prognostic value also appears limited (29). In contrast, tryptic fragments of the 64K antigen, notably the 37K moiety, correlate well with whole islet ICA, appear in only 2% of twins who remain non-diabetic, and are absent in ICA positive polyendocrine patients who have not developed diabetes (29, 130). Thus, distinct antibodies to 64K antigen confer different risks for IDDM, the highest risk being associated with the 37K antigen. A combined analysis of risk in 101 ICA positive first-degree relatives was performed using ICA titre and staining pattern in addition to IAA, GAD, 37K and 40K tryptic fragments (131). No single 'marker of choice' emerged from this analysis. Instead, risk mounted according to the number of antibody species present, from 6% for ICA alone (≥10 JDF units) to 86% for cases with three or more antibodies. This confirms evidence from a study of 56 non-diabetic twins in whom 10 of 12 prediabetic twins had two or more antibody specificities as compared with only 2 of 46 twins who remained non-diabetic (29). This approach promises to enhance prediction of diabetes without loss of sensitivity (4). Population screening could use different sets of antibodies to provide maximum sensitivity or maximum specificity for disease prediction.

## Cellular immune changes

The extent and persistence of immune changes is important (103). In a 10-year prospective study of a cohort of 20 non-diabetic twins, 10 of whom developed IDDM, increased levels of activated T lymphocytes and either ICA or insulin autoantibodies were strongly predictive of diabetes (103). Furthermore, the presence of both cellular and humoral immune changes throughout the prediabetic period emerged as one feature which distinguished twins who developed IDDM.

### Metabolic markers

A logical extension of the approach outlined above would be to assess the extent of target organ damage. Differences in method coupled with poor reproducibility of insulin responses have limited comparisons between centres and individuals, although a new international standard for these tests has been agreed (132). The first phase insulin response to intravenous glucose does fall well before the onset of diabetes in most individuals. ICA-positive relatives with insulin responses below the first centile developed diabetes faster (0.48 per subject–year) than those with higher insulin response (0.05 per subject–year) (108). A predictive model combining IAA and first phase insulin response predicted progression to IDDM within 4 years in about 90% of high risk subjects (133). This model needs to be validated. A decrease in first phase insulin response in a group of twins of patients with IDDM, gave a positive predictive value of 58% (97). Impaired glucose tolerance has a limited positive predictive value being only 33%, even in twin studies (96).

## POTENTIAL PREDICTIVE STRATEGIES

Screening and intervention in the population at large must be our goal. Strategies for disease prevention will involve identification of high risk individuals using the immune and metabolic changes associated with the disease. One such strategy might include a two-test and two-sample approach. Thus, an initial test of high sensitivity (for example, selecting genetically susceptible individuals) can be coupled with ICA testing, and more specific tests could be repeated after an undefined period. The practical value of screening healthy populations for markers of susceptibility could be enormously enhanced by changes in intervention strategy. If very safe preventive measures become available, use of sensitive but non-specific screening tests would then become equally appropriate, since these could also be given to large numbers of children who may not otherwise develop diabetes. A family study is a form of screening, carried out within a population that is by definition already at high risk, well informed and highly motivated. What happens when the screening process is extended to a low risk, relatively ill-informed population? One major consequence must be to generate anxiety where none existed. Worse still, much of this anxiety will be unfounded if the screening test results in a large number of false positive predictions. In the longer term, increased public awareness of the possibility of predicting IDDM would awaken the possibility that predictive tests, however inaccurate, might be used to the disadvantage of the individual with regard to employment, health insurance, and so forth. Screening should not be undertaken lightly, and should always be carried out with appropriate counselling and the potential for review. The observations outlined in this chapter indicate just how far we have progressed in the last decade in identifying high risk individuals through their immune response to islet antigens. These developments could now introduce a new era of multicentre intervention trials with the express aim of preventing, even curing, this potentially devastating disease.

## REFERENCES

1 Leslie RDG, Elliott RB. Perspectives in Diabetes. Early environmental events as a cause of IDDM. Evidence and implications. *Diabetes* 1994; 43: 843–50.
2 Todd JA, Bell JI, McDevitt HO. HLA DQ beta gene contributes to susceptibility and resistance to insulin-dependent diabetes mellitus. *Nature* (*Lond*) 1987; 329: 599–604.
3 Lo SSS, Tun RYM, Leslie RDG. Non-genetic factors causing Type 1 diabetes. *Diabetic Med* 1991; 8: 609–18.
4 Bingley PJ, Bonifacio E, Gale EAM. Can we really predict IDDM? *Diabetes* 1993; 42:213–20.
5 Diabetes Epidemiology Research International Group. Geographical patterns of childhood insulin-dependent diabetes mellitus. *Diabetes* 1988; 37: 1113–19.
6 Green A, Gale EAM, Patterson CC for the EURODIAB ACE Study Group. Incidence of childhood-onset insulin-dependent diabetes mellitus: the EURODIAB ACE study. *Lancet* 1992; 339: 905–9.
7 Tarn AC, Thomas JM, Dean BM *et al.* Predicting insulin-dependent diabetes. *Lancet* 1988; i: 845–50.
8 Riley WJ, Maclaren NK, Krischer J *et al.* A prospective study of the development of diabetes in relatives of patients with insulin-dependent diabetes. *N Engl J Med* 1990; 323: 1167–72.

9 Cavender DE, Wagener DK, Rabin BS *et al.* The Pittsburgh insulin-dependent diabetes mellitus (IDDM) study. HLA antigens and haplotypes as risk factors for the development of IDDM in IDDM patients and their siblings. *J Chronic Dis* 1984; 37:555–68.

10 Deschamps I, Boitard C, Hors J *et al.* Life table analysis of the risk of Type 1(insulin-dependent) diabetes in siblngs according to islet cell antibodies and HLA markers. *Diabetologia* 1992; 35:951–7.

11 Tillil H, Kobberling J. Age-corrected empirical genetic risk estimates for first degree relatives of IDDM patients. *Diabetes* 1987; 36:93–9.

12 Schatz DA, Schwartz S, Malone J *et al.* A prospective study of the development of diabetes in relatives of patients with insulin-dependent diabetes. *N Engl J Med* 1990; 323: 1167–72.

13 Kaprio J, Tuomilehto J, Koskenvuo M, Romanov K *et al.* Concordance for Type 1 (insulin-dependent) diabetes mellitus in a population-based cohort of twins in Finland. *Diabetologia* 1992; 35: 1060–7.

14 Olmos P, A'Hern R, Heaton DA *et al.* Significance of the concordance rate for Type 1 (insulin-dependent) diabetes in identical twins. *Diabetologia* 1988; 31: 747–50.

15 Srikanta S, Ganda OP, Jackson RA *et al.* Type 1 diabetes mellitus in monozygotic twins: chronic progressive β cell dysfunction. *Ann Int Med* 1983; 99: 320–6.

16 Kumar D, Gemayel NS, Mack TM. Significance of age at onset of insulin-dependent diabetes mellitus and disease concordance in monozygotic and dizygotic twins. *Diabetes* 1992 41: Suppl 1; 129A.

17 Committee of Diabetic Twins, Japan Diabetes Society. Diabetes Mellitus in twins: a cooperative study in Japan. *Diabetes Res Clin Pract* 1988; 5: 271–80.

18 Bjorkman PJ, Saper MA, Samraoui B, Bennett WS, Strominger JL, Wiley DC. Structure of the human class 1 histocompatibility antigen, HLA-A2. *Nature* (*Lond*) 1987; 12: 329–506.

19 Brown JH, Jardetzky TS, Corga JC *et al.* Three-dimensional structure of the human class II histocompatibility antigen HLA-DR1. Nature (*Lond*) 1993; 364: 33–9.

20 Khalil I, d'Auriol L, Gobet M *et al.* A combination of HLA-DQB Asp 57-negative and HLA DQA Arg 52 confers susceptibility to Insulin-dependent diabetes mellitus. *J Clin Invest* 1990; 85: 1315–19.

21 Todd JA, Mijovic C, Fletcher J, Jenkins D, Bradwell AR, Barnett AH. Identification of susceptibility loci for insulin dependent diabetes mellitus by trans-racial gene mapping. *Nature* (*Lond*) 1989; 338: 587–9.

22 Tienari PJ, Tuomilehto-Wolf E, Tuomilehto J, Peltonen L, The DIME Study Group. HLA haplotypes in Type 1 (insulin-dependent) diabetes mellitus: molecular analysis of the HLA-DQ locus. *Diabetologia* 1992; 35: 254–60.

23 Warram JH, Krolewski AS, Gottlieb MS, Kahn CR. Differences in risk of insulin dependent diabetes in offspring of diabetic mothers and diabetic fathers. *N Engl J Med* 1984; ii: 299–302.

24 Vadheim CM, Rotter JI, Maclaren NK, Riley WJ, Anderson CE. Preferential transmission of diabetic alleles within the HLA gene complex. *N Engl J Med* 1986; 315: 1314–18.

25 Bell GI, Horita S, Karam JH. A polymorphic locus near the insulin gene is associated with insulin-dependent diabetes mellitus. *Diabetes* 1984; 33: 176–83.

26 Julier C, Hyer RN, Davies J *et al.* Insulin-IGF2 region on chromosome 11p encodes a gene implicated in HLA-DR4 dependent diabetes susceptibility. *Nature* (*Lond*) 1991; 354: 155–9.

27 Siemiatycki J, Colle E, Campbell S, Dewar R, Aubert D, Belmonte MM. Incidence of IDDM in Montreal by ethnic group and by social class and comparisons with ethnic groups living elsewhere. *Diabetes* 1988; 37: 1096–102.

28 Diabetes Epidemiology Research International Group. Secular trends in incidence of childhood IDDM in 10 countries. *Diabetes* 1990; 39: 858–64.

29 Christie MR, Tun RYM, Lo SSS *et al.* Antibodies to glutamate acid decarboxylase as markers for the development of insulin-dependent diabetes. Studies with identical twins. *Diabetes* 1992; 41: 782–7.

30 Millward BA, Hussain MJ, Peakman M, Pyke DA, Leslie RDG, Vergani D. Characterization of islet cell antibody in insulin-dependent diabetes: evidence for IgG1 subclass restriction and polyclonality. *J Clin Exp Immunol* 1988; 71: 353–6.

31 Christau B, Kromann H, Ortved Anderson O *et al.* Incidence, seasonal and geographical patterns of juvenile-onset insulin-dependent diabetes mellitus in Denmark. *Diabetologia* 1977; 13: 281–4.

32 Laakso M, Pyorala K. Age of onset and type of diabetes. *Diabetes Care* 1985; 8: 114–17.

33 Vardi P, Ziegler AG, Mathews JH *et al.* Concentration of insulin autoantibodies at onset of Type 1 diabetes. Inverse log-linear corrrelation with age. *Diabetes Care* 1988; 11: 736–9.

34 Bonifacio E, Bingley PJ, Dean BM *et al.* Quantification of islet-cell antibodies and prediction of insulin-dependent diabetes. *Lancet* 1990; 335: 147–9.

35 Warram JH, Krolewski AS, Kahn R. Determinants of Type 1 diabetes and perinatal mortality in children of diabetic mothers. *Diabetes* 1988; 37: 1328–4.

36 Warram JH, Martin BC, Krolewski AS. Risk of IDDM in children of diabetic mothers decreased with increasing maternal age at pregnancy. *Diabetes* 1991; 40: 1679–84.

37 Ginsberg-Fellner, Witt ME, Yaagihasi S *et al.* Congenital rubella syndrome as model for Type 1 (insulin-dependent) diabetes mellitus: increased prevelance of islet cell surface antibodies. *Diabetologia* 1984; 27(Suppl): 87–9.

38 Leslie RDG, Pyke DA. Escaping insulin dependent diabetes. *Br Med J* 1991; 302: 1103–4.

39 Toniolo A, Onodera T, Yoon JW, Notkins AL. Induction of diabetes by cumulative environmental insults from viruses and chemicals. *Nature* (*Lond*) 1980; 288: 383–5.

40 Leslie RDG, Lo S, Millward BA, Honour J, Pyke DA. Decreased growth velocity before IDDM onset. *Diabetes* 1991; 40: 211–16.

41 Robinson N, Fuller JH. Role of life events and difficulties in the onset of diabetes mellitus. *J Psychosomatic Res* 1985; 29: 583–91.

42 Gamble DR. Taylor KW, Cumming H. Coxsackie B viruses and diabetes. *Br Med J* 1973; 4: 260–2.

43 Banatvala JE, Schernthaner G, Schober E *et al.* Coxsackie B, mumps, rubella and cytomegalovirus specific IgM responses in patients with juvenile-onset

insulin-dependent diabetes in Britain, Austria and Australia. *Lancet* 1985; i: 1409–12.
44 Dalgleish AG, Beverley PCL, Clapham PR, Crawford DH, Greaves MF, Weiss RA. CD4 (T4) antigen is an essential component of the receptor for the AIDS retrovirus. *Nature (Lond)* 1984; 312: 763–7.
45 Roman LM, Simons LF, Hammer RE, Sambrook JF, Gething MJH. The expression of influenza virus hemagglutinin in the pancreatic B-cells of transgenic mice results in autoimmune diabetes. *Cell* 1990; 61: 383–6.
46 Bodansky HJ, Grant PJ, Dean BM *et al.* Islet cell antibodies and insulin autoantibodies in association with common viral infections. *Lancet* 1986; ii: 1351–3.
47 Federlin K, Otten A, Helmke K. Islet cell antibodies and viral infections. *Exp Clin Endocrinol* 1987; 89: 368–74.
48 Pak CY, Eun HM, McArthur RG, Yoon JW. Association of cytomegalovirus infection with autoimmune type 1 diabetes. *Lancet* 1988; ii: 1–4.
49 Pak CY, Cha CY, Rajotte RV, McArthur RG, Yoon JW. Human pancreatic islet cell specific 38 kilodalton autoantigen identified by cytomegalovirus-induced monoclonal islet cell autoantibody. *Diabetologia* 1990; 33: 569–72.
50 Foulis AK, Farquharson MA, Meager A. Immunoreactive alpha-interferon in insulin-secreting beta cells on Type 1 diabetes mellitus. *Lancet* 1987; ii: 1423–7.
51 Bohme J, Haskins K, Stecha P *et al.* Transgenic mice with I-A are normal glycaemic but immunologically intolerant. *Science* 1989; 244: 1179–83.
52 Sarvetnick N, Shizuru J, Liggit D *et al.* Loss of pancreatic islet tolerance induced by B-cell expression of interferon. *Nature (Lond)* 1990; 346: 844–7.
53 Rubinstein P, Walker ME, Fedun N, Witt ME, Cooper LZ, Ginsberg-Fellner F. HLA system in congenital rubella patients with and without diabetes. *Diabetes* 1982; 31: 1088–91.
54 Patterson K, Chandra RS, Jenson AB. Congenital rubella, insulitis, and diabetes mellitus in an infant. *Lancet* 1981; i: 1048–9.
55 Jenson AB, Rosenberg HS, Notkins AL. Pancreatic islet cell damage in children with fatal viral infections. *Lancet* 1980; ii: 354–8.
56 Yoon JW, Austin M, Onodera T, Notkins AL. Virus-induced diabetes mellitus: isolation of a virus from the pancreas of a child with diabetic ketoacidosis. *N Engl J Med* 1979; 300: 1173–9.
57 Dunn JS, McLetchie NGB. Experimental alloxan diabetes in the rat. *Lancet* 1943; ii: 384–6.
58 Wilson GL, Hartig PC, Patton NJ, LeDoux SP. Mechanisms of nitrosourea-induced beta-cell damage. Activation of poly(ADP-ribose) synthetase and cellular distribution. *Diabetes* 1989; 37: 213–16.
59 Sai P, Boillot D, Boitard Ch, Debray-Sachs M, Reach G, Assan R. Pentamidine, a new diabetogenic drug in laboratory rodents. *Diabetologia* 1983; 25: 418–23.
60 Karam JH, Lewitt PA, Young CW *et al.* Insulinopenic diabetes after rodenticide (Vacor) ingestion. A unique model of acquired diabetes in man. *Diabetes* 1980; 29: 971–80.
61 Like AA, Rossini AA. Streptozotocin-induced pancreatic insulitis: new model of diabetes mellitus. *Science* 1976; 193: 415–17.
62 Helgason T, Ewen SWB, Ross IS, Stowers JM. Diabetes produced in mice by smoked/cured mutton. *Lancet* 1982; ii: 1017–24.
63 Borch-Johnsen K, Joner G, Mandrup-Poulsen T *et al.* Relation between breast-feeding and incidence rates of insulin-dependent diabetes mellitus: a hypothesis. *Lancet* 1984; ii: 1083–86.
64 Kostraba JN, Cruickshanks KJ, Lawler-Heavner J *et al.* Early exposure to cow's milk and solid foods ininfancy, genetic predisposition, and risk of IDDM. *Diabetes* 1993; 42: 288–95.
65 Elliott RB, Martin JM. Dietary protein: a trigger of insulin-dependent diabetes in the BB rat? *Diabetologia* 1984; 26:297–9.
66 Coleman DL, Kuzava JE, Leiter EH. Effect of diet on incidence of diabetes in nonobese diabetic mice. *Diabetes* 1990; 39:432–6.
67 Karjalainen J, Martin JM, Knip M. A bovine serum albumen peptide as a possible trigger of insulin-dependent diabetes mellitus. *N Engl J Med* 1992; 327: 302–7.
68 Sutherland DE, Sibley R, Yu X-Z *et al.* Twin-to-twin pancreas transplantation: reversal and reenactment of the pathogenesis of Type 1 diabetes. *Trans Assoc Am Phys* 1984; 97:80–7.
69 Hanninen A, Jalkanen S, Salmi M *et al.* Macrophages, T cell receptor usage, and endothelial cell activation in the pancreas at the onset of insulin-dependent diabetes mellitus. *J Clin Invest* 1992; 90:1901–10.
70 Pipeleers D, Ling Z. Pancreatic beta cells in insulin-dependent diabetes. *Diabetes/Metab Rev* 1992; 8: 209–227.
71 Nepom GT. A unified hypothesis for the complex genetics of HLA associations with IDDM. *Diabetes* 1990; 39:1153–7.
72 Sheehy MJ. HLA and insulin-dependent diabetes: a protective perspective. *Diabetes* 1992; 41: 123–9.
73 Foulis AK, Stewart JA. The pancreas in recent-onset Type 1 (insulin-dependent) diabetes mellitus: insulin content of islets, insulitis and associated changes in the exocrine acinar tissue. *Diabetologia* 1984; 26:456–61.
74 Londei M, Bottazzo GF, Feldmann M. Human T-cell clones from thyroid autoimmune thyroid glands: specific recognition of autologous thyroid cells. *Science* 1985; 228: 85–9.
75 In't Veld PA, Pipeleers D. *In situ* analysis of pancreatic islets in rats developing diabetes: appearance of nonendocrine cells with surface MHC class II antigens and cytoplasmic insulin immunoreactivity. *J Clin Invest* 1988; 82: 1123–8.
76 Bottazzo GF, Dean B, Gorsuch AN, Cudworth AG, Doniach D. Complement-fixing islet cell antibodies in Type I diabetes: possible monitors of active beta cell damage. *Lancet* 1980; i: 668–72.
77 Ziegler AG, Herskowitz RD, Jackson RA, Soeldner JS, Eisenbarth GS. Predicting Type 1 diabetes. *Diabetes Care* 1990; 13: 762–75.
78 Ziegler AF, Zeigler R, Vardi P *et al.* Life-table analysis of progression to diabetes of anti-insulin autoantibody-positive relative of individuals with type 1 diabetes. *Diabetes* 1989; 38: 1320–5.
79 Wilkin T, Hoskins PJ, Armitage M, *et al.* Value of insulin autoantibodies as serum markers for insulin dependent diabetes mellitus. *Lancet* 1985; i: 480–2.
80 Baekkeskov S, Neilson JH, Marner B, Bilde T, Ludvigs-

son J, Lernmark A. Autoantibodies in newly diagnosed diabetic children immunoprecipitate human pancreatic islet cell proteins. *Nature (Lond)* 1982; 298: 167–9.
81 Baekkeskov S, Aanstoot H-K, Christgau S *et al.* Identification of the 64k autoantigen in insulin-dependent diabetes as the GABA-synthesizing enzyme glutamic acid decarboxylase. *Nature (Lond)* 1990; 347: 151–6.
82 Solimena M, Folli F, Aparisi R, Pozza G, De Camilli PN. Autoantibodies to GABA-ergic neurones and pancreatic beta cells in Stiff-syndrome. *N Engl J Med* 1990; 322: 1555–60.
83 Rorsman P, Berggren P-O, Bokvist K *et al.* Glucose inhibition of glucagon secretion involves activation of GAGA-A receptor chloride channels. *Nature (Lond)* 1989; 341: 233–6.
84 Bu D-F, Erlander MG, Hitz BC *et al.* Two human glutamate decarboxylases, 65 kDa GAD and 67 kDa GAD, are each encoded by a single gene. *Proc Natl Acad Sci USA* 1992; 89: 2115–19.
85 Christie MR, Vohra G, Champagne P, Daneman D, Delovitch TL. Distinct antibody specificities to a 64 kD islet cell antigen in type 1 diabetes as revealed by trypsin treatment. *J Exp Med* 1990; 172: 789–94.
86 Christie MR, Brown TJ, Cassidy D. Binding of antibodies in sera from Type 1 (insulin-dependent) diabetic patients to glutamate decarboxylase from rat tissues. Evidence for antigenic and non-antigenic forms of the enzyme. *Diabetologia* 1992; 35: 380–4.
86 Roep BO, Kallan AA, Hazenbos WW *et al.* T-cell reactivity to 38 kD insulin-secretory granule protein in patients with recent onset type 1 diabetes. *Lancet* 1991; 337: 1439–41.
87 Castano L, Russo R, Zhou L *et al.* Identification and cloning of a granule autoantigen (carboxypeptidatc H) associated with type 1 diabetes. *J Clin Endocrinol Metab* 1991; 73: 1197–201.
88 Rabin DU, Pleasic SM, Palmer-Crocker R, Shapiro JA. Cloning and expression of IDDM-specific human autoantigens. *Diabetes* 1992; 41: 183–6.
89 Johnson JH, Crider BP, McCorkle K, Alford M, Unger RH. Inhibition of glucose transport into rat islet cells by immunoglobulins from patients with new-onset insulin-dependent diabetes mellitus. *N Engl J Med* 1990; 322: 653–9.
90 Atkinson MA, Kaufman DL, Campbell L *et al.* Response of peripheral blood mononuclear cells to glutamate decarboxylase in insulin-dependent diabetes. *Lancet* 1992; 339: 458–9.
91 Harrison LC, Honeyman MC, Deaizpurua HJ *et al.* Inverse relation between humoral and cellular immunity to glutamic acid decarboxylase in subjects at risk of insulin-dependent diabetes. *Lancet* 1993; 341: 1365–9.
92 Millward BA, Alviggi L, Hoskins PJ *et al.* Immune changes associated with insulin dependent diabetes may remit without causing diabetes: a study in identical twins. *Br Med J* 1986; 292: 793–6.
93 Johnston C, Millward BA, Hoskins P, Leslie RDG, Bottazzo GF. Islet cell antibodies as predictors of the later development of Type 1 (insulin-dependent) diabetes. *Diabetologia* 1989; 32: 382–6.
94 Riley WJ, Maclaren NK, Krischer J *et al.* A prospective study of the development of diabetes in relatives of patients with insulin-dependent diabetes. *N Engl J Med* 1990; 323: 1167–72.
95 Notsu K, Oka N, Note S, Nabeya N, Kuno S, Sakurami T. Islet cell antibodies in the Japanese population and subjects with Type 1 (insulin-dependent) diabetes. *Diabetologia* 1985; 28: 660–2.
96 Beer SF, Heaton DA, Alberti KGMM, Pyke DA, Leslie RDG. Impaired glucose tolerance precedes but does not predict insulin-dependent diabetes mellitus: a study of identical twins. *Diabetologia* 1990; 33: 497–502.
97 Lo SSS, Hawa M, Beer SF, Pyke DA, Leslie RDG. Altered islet Beta-cell function before the onset of Type 1 (insulin-dependent) diabetes mellitus. *Diabetologia* 1992; 35: 277–82.
98 Heaton DA, Millward BA, Gray IP *et al.* Evidence of beta cell dysfunction which does not lead on to diabetes: a study of identical twins of insulin dependent diabetics. *Br Med J* 1987; 294: 145–6.
99 Heaton DA, Millward BA, Gray IP *et al.* Increased proinsulin levels as an early indicator of beta cell dysfunction in non-diabetic twins of Type 1 (insulin-dependent) diabetic patients. *Diabetologia* 1988; 31: 182–4.
100 Hartling SG, Lindgren F, Dahlqvist G, Persson B, Binder C. Elevated proinsulin in healthy siblings of IDDM patients independent of HLA identity. *Diabetes* 1989; 38: 1271–4.
101 Rich SS, French LR, Sprafka JM *et al.* HLA-associated suceptibility to Type 2 (non-insulin-dependent) diabetes mellitus: the Wadena City Health Study. *Diabetologia* 1993; 36: 234–8.
102 Groop L, Miettinen A, Groop PH *et al.* Organ-specific autoimmunityand HLA-DR antigens as markers for beta cell destruction in patients with type II diabetes. *Diabetes* 1988; 37: 99–103.
103 Tun RYM, Peakman M, Alviggi L *et al.* The importance of persistent cellular and humoral immune changes in the pre-diabetic period. A prospective identical twin study. *Br Med J* 1994; 308: 1063–8.
104 Hussain MJ, Peakman M, Lo SSS, Leslie RDG, Vergani D. Elevated levels of tumour necrosis factor-alpha and interleukin-1 alpha presage the onset of type 1 (insulin-dependent) diabetes. *Diabetologia* 1991; 34 (Suppl 2) A191: 760.
105 Bingley PJ, Matthews DR, Williams AJK, Bottazzo GF, Gale EAM. Loss of regular oscillatory insulin secretion in islet cell antibody positive non-diabetic subjects. *Diabetologia* 1992; 35: 32–8.
106 Kahn SE, McCulloch DK, Schwartz W, Palmer JP, Porte D Jr. Effect of insulin resistance and hyperglycaemia on proinsulin release in a primate model of diabetes mellitus. *J Clin Endocr Metab* 1992; 74: 192–7.
107 Heaton DA, Lazarus NR, Pyke DA, Leslie RDG. B-cell responses to IV glucose and glucagon in non-diabetic twins of patients with Type 1 (insulin-dependent) diabetes mellitus. *Diabetologia* 1989; 32: 814–17.
108 Vialettes B, Zevaco-Mattei C, Thirion X *et al.* Acute insulin response to glucose and glucagon in subjects at risk of developing Type 1 diabetes. *Diabetes Care* 1993; 16: 973–77.
109 Leahy JL, Cooper HE, Deal DA, Weir GG. Chronic hyperglycaemia is associated with impaired glucose influence on insulin secretion. *J Clin Invest* 1986; 77: 908–15.
110 Vardi P, Crisa L, Jackson RA *et al.* Predictive value of intravenous glucose tolerance test insulin secretion less

than or greater than the first percentile in islet cell antibody positive relatives of Type 1 (insulin-dependent) diabetic patients. *Diabetologia* 1991; 34: 93–102.

111 Hoskins PJ, Leslie RDG, Pyke DA. Height at diagnosis of diabetes in children: a study in identical twins. *Br Med* J 1985; 290: 278–80.

112 Sanger TJ, LaPort RE, Tajima N *et al.* Height at diagnosis of insulin-dependent diabetes inpatients and their non-diabetic family members. *Br Med J* 1986; 292: 1419–22.

113 Blom L, Persson LA, Dahlquist. A high linear growth is associated with an increased risk of childhood diabetes mellitus. *Diabetologia* 1992; 35: 528–33.

114 Anderson CE, Hodge SE, Rubin R *et al.* A search for heterogeneity in insulin dependent diabetes mellitus (IDDM): HLA and autoimmune studies in simplex, multiplex and multigenerational families. *Metabolism* 1983; 32: 471–7.

115 Reijonen H, Ilonen J, Knip M, Akerblom HK. HLA-DQB1 alleles and absence of Asp 57 as susceptibility factors of IDDM in Finland. *Diabetes* 1991; 40: 1640–4.

116 Maclaren NK, Horne G, Spillar RP, Barbour H, Harrison D, Duncan J. Islet cell antibodies (ICA) in US school children. *Diabetes* 1985; 34 (suppl. 1): 84A.

117 Bergua M, Sole J, Marion G *et al.* Prevalence of islet cell antibodies, insulin antibodies and hyperglycaemia in 2291 schoolchildren. *Diabetologia* 1987; 30: 724–6.

118 Karjalainen J. Islet cell antibodies as predictive markers for IDDM in children with high background incidence of disease. *Diabetes* 1990; 39: 1144–50.

119 Bruining GJ, Molenaar JL, Grobbee DE *et al.* Ten-year follow-up study of islet cell antibodies and childhood diabetes mellitus. *Lancet* 1989; i: 1100–3.

120 Bingley PJ, Bonifacio E, Shattock M *et al.* Can islet cell antibodies predict IDDM in the general population? *Diabetes Care* 1993; 16: 45–50.

121 Genovese S, Bonifacio E, Dean BM *et al.* Distinct cytoplasmic islet cell antibodies with different risks for Type 1 (insulin-dependent) diabetes mellitus. *Diabetologia* 1992; 35: 385–8.

122 Gianini R, Pugliese A, Bonner-Weir S *et al.* Prognostically significant heterogeneity of cytoplasmic islet cell antibodies in relatives of patients with Type 1 diabetes. *Diabetes* 1992; 41: 347–53.

123 Timsit J, Caillat-Zucman S, Blondel H, Chedin P, Bach JF, Boitard C. Islet cell antibody heterogeneity among Type 1 (insulin-dependent) diabetic patients. *Diabetologia* 1992; 35: 792–5.

124 Palmer JP, Asplin CM, Clemons P *et al.* Insulin antibodies in insulin-dependent diabetes before insulin treatment. *Science* 1983; 222: 1337–9.

125 Ziegler AG, Ziegler R, Vardi P, Jackson RA, Soeldner JS, Eisenbarth GS. Life-table analysis of progression to diabetes of anti-insulin autoantibody-positive relatives of individuals with Type 1 diabetes. *Diabetes* 1989; 38: 1320–5.

126 Atkinson MA, Maclaren NK, Riley WJ, Winter WE, Fisk DD, Spillar RP. Are insulin autoantibodies markers for insulin-dependent diabetes mellitus? *Diabetes* 1986; 35: 894–8.

127 Baekkeskov S, Landin M, Kristensen JK *et al.* Antibodies to a 64,000 Mr human islet cell antigen precede the clinical onset of insulin-dependent diabetes. *J Clin Invest* 1987; 79: 926–34.

128 Atkinson MA, Maclaren NK, Scharp DW, Lacy PE, Riley WJ. 64,000 Mr autoantibodies to predictors of insulin-dependent diabetes. *Lancet* 1990; 335: 1357–60.

129 Barmeirer H, McCulloch DK, Neifing JL *et al.* Risk for developing Type 1 (insulin-dependent) diabetes mellitus and the presence of islet 64K antibodies. *Diabetologia* 1991; 34: 727–33.

130 Genovese S, Cassidy D, Bonifacio E, Bottazzo GF, Christie MR. Antibodies to 37/40 kD tryptic fragments of 64 kD antigen are markers of rapid progression to Type 1 insulin-dependent diabetes (abstract). *Diabetes Res Clin Pract* 1991; 14 (Suppl 1): S11.

131 Bingley PJ, Christie MR, Bonfanti R *et al.* Combined analysis of autoantibodies enhances prediction of IDDM in islet cell antibody (ICA) positive relatives. *Diabetic Med* 1993; in press:

132 Bingley PJ, Colman PG, Eisenbarth GS *et al.* Standardization of IVGTT to predict IDDM. *Diabetes Care* 1992; 15: 93–102.

133 Colman PG, Eisenbarth GS. Immunology of Type 1 diabetes – 1987. In: Alberti KGGM, Krall LP, eds. *Diabetes Annual/4*. Elsevier, Amsterdam, 1988; 17–45.

## Additional references added in proof

Lohmann, T, Leslie RDG, Hawa M, Geysen M, Rodda S, Londei M. Immunodominant epitopes of glutamic acid decarboxylase 65 and 67 in insulin-dependent diabetes mellitus. *Lancet* 1994; 343: 1607–8.

Schatz D, Krischer J, Horne G *et al.* Islet cell antibodies predict insulin-dependent diabetes in United States school age children as powerfully as in unaffected relatives. *J Clin Invest* 1994; 93: 2403–7.

Tuomilehto J, Zimmet P, Mackay IR *et al.* Antibodies to glutamic acid decarboxylase as predictors of insulin-dependent diabetes mellitus before clinical onset of disease. *Lancet* 1994; 343: 1383–5.

# 11 Epidemiology of Non-insulin-dependent Diabetes

William H. Herman & Linda S. Geiss

## INTRODUCTION

Diabetes mellitus is not a single disorder but a group of disorders with different genetic and environmental risk factors, pathophysiologies, and clinical presentations. All types of diabetes are characterised by hyperglycaemia and abnormalities of protein and fat metabolism. In addition, all types of overt diabetes are associated with specific microvascular complications including retinal, renal, and neurological disease, and an increased risk of atherosclerotic cardiovascular disease.

Both the National Diabetes Data Group (1) and World Health Organisation (2) classification systems recognise two major types of overt diabetes: insulin dependent or Type I diabetes mellitus (IDDM) and non-insulin dependent or Type II diabetes mellitus (NIDDM). People with IDDM have an absolute deficiency of insulin, are ketosis prone under basal conditions, and are dependent on exogenous insulin for life. IDDM probably represents an idiopathic autoimmune disease or an autoimmune disease triggered by an environmental insult in genetically predisposed individuals. In contrast, people with NIDDM have a relative deficiency of insulin, and are not ketosis prone under basal conditions. Current thinking is that NIDDM arises as a result of two defects, impaired insulin secretion and insulin resistance.

Diabetes may be diagnosed in non-pregnant adults with classical symptoms of diabetes and unequivocal elevations of plasma glucose (random plasma glucose ≥200 mg/dl) and in those with fasting glucose levels ≥140 mg/dl. Diabetes may also be diagnosed on the basis of sustained elevations of plasma glucose after a 75 gram oral glucose load. For oral glucose tolerance testing, subjects must be otherwise healthy, ambulatory, and must have at least 3 days of unrestricted diet and physical activity. The test should be performed in the morning, and subjects must be fasting and remain seated and non-smoking. In clinical practice, such testing is performed only when there is a clinical suspicion of diabetes, but fasting glucose levels are consistently <140 mg/dl.

Because people with NIDDM are not dependent on exogenous insulin for life, and may have levels of hyperglycaemia insufficient to cause symptoms, there is incomplete ascertainment of the disease. Ascertainment is a function of both access to care and standards of care in a community. In western societies, it is estimated that about half of persons with diabetes have not been diagnosed (3). Studies performed in areas with better access to care and standards of care, and those which involve population screening and active case finding, are likely to report higher rates of NIDDM. Studies which report on clinically diagnosed patients, particularly those performed in areas with limited resources and poor access to care, are likely to report lower rates and potentially greater severity of disease. Obviously, these limitations have major effects on both the data and their interpretation.

In this chapter, we synthesise and interpret data on the epidemiology of NIDDM. Specifically, we discuss the incidence of, and risk factors for, the development of NIDDM, the prevalence of NIDDM, and the mortality of NIDDM including causes and risk factors. Wherever possible, we have relied on data from sources providing periodic and representative surveys of the population. Data are presented for the United States and, whenever possible, for other areas of the world.

## INCIDENCE OF NIDDM

Incidence refers to the number of new cases of NIDDM diagnosed in a population during a period of time, or the rate of new cases per 100 population per year. The incidence of NIDDM can only be calculated by monitoring a population prospectively. As a result, few studies of the incidence of NIDDM have been reported. Because 97% of incident cases of diabetes are NIDDM (4), most researchers have equated incidence of diabetes mellitus in population surveys with that of NIDDM.

US surveillance data based on self-report of diabetes show that, during the 1980s, the incidence of diabetes increased and then levelled off (5). In 1990, there were 607 000 new cases of diabetes in the US (6). In 1990, the incidence of diabetes was 0.24 per 100 population per year. The lowest age-specific incidence occurred among persons younger than 45 (0.12 per 100 population per year), and the highest age-specific incidence occurred among persons 45 to 64 (0.60 per 100 population per year). The incidence in the population 65 years of age and older was 0.41 per 100 population per year. In general, females had higher incidence rates than males (0.29 vs. 0.20). Among white females, the incidence of diabetes was 0.28 per 100 population per year and among white males, the incidence was 0.20 per 100 population per year. In the US, incidence rates of diabetes have not been reported among representative samples of blacks.

Smaller population-based surveys conducted in white populations in the north–central US have reported the incidence of NIDDM to be 0.12 (7) to 0.16 per 100 population per year (4).

In the San Antonio Heart Study, a population-based study of diabetes and cardiovascular disease in Mexican Americans and non-Hispanic whites, the 8-year incidence of NIDDM was 6.5% in Mexican Americans and 2.0% in non-Hispanic whites who were 25 to 64 years of age and free of diabetes at baseline (8). The ethnic odds ratio adjusted for age and sex was 4.5 in Mexican Americans compared to non-Hispanic Whites. After 8 years, 5.9% of Mexican American men and 6.9% of Mexican American women developed diabetes in comparison to 0.8% of non-Hispanic white men and 2.8% of non-Hispanic white women. In all gender and ethnic groups, diabetes incidence tended to increase with age, and Mexican Americans had a higher incidence of diabetes than non-Hispanic whites at all ages. The magnitude of the relative risk associated with Mexican–American ethnicity was, however, greater among the younger age groups than among the older age groups.

Among the Pima Indians, an American Indian group with the highest known rates of NIDDM, the incidence of NIDDM diagnosed by oral glucose tolerance testing was 1.76 per 100 population per year between 1965 and 1990 (9). During the 25 years of the Pima Indian study, the incidence of NIDDM has increased in most age groups (10).

In a population-based study of diabetes conducted between 1983 and 1987 in Laxa, Sweden, a rural community with approximately 8000 inhabitants, the mean annual incidence of

NIDDM was 0.39% per year in men and 0.41% per year in women (11). In the Paris Prospective Study, the incidence of NIDDM among male civil servants aged 43–54 years at baseline was 0.54% per year (12). Among the Nauruans of Micronesia, the incidence of NIDDM was reported to be 1.6 per 100 person–years in subjects aged 20 years and older (13).

Women with histories of glucose intolerance during pregnancy, that is, women with histories of gestational diabetes mellitus (GDM), have long been recognised as being at increased risk for the subsequent development of NIDDM. In a prospective follow-up study of 615 women with former GDM diagnosed by the criteria of O'Sullivan and Mahan (14) and 328 women with normal glucose tolerance tests during pregnancy, O'Sullivan found that, after up to 28 years, the incidence of diabetes by WHO criteria was 36.4% in women with former GDM and 5.5% in control women (15). In a recent review of 12 world-wide studies of diabetes among former GDM patients, a wide range of incidence rates was reported (16). Observed variability was due, at least in part, to the use of different criteria to diagnose GDM, failure to exclude overt diabetes initially discovered during pregnancy, and failure to require a return to normal glucose tolerance after pregnancy. Nevertheless, GDM clearly appears to predict future NIDDM.

Impaired glucose tolerance (IGT) has also been recognised as a risk factor for NIDDM. IGT is a diagnostic category based on oral glucose tolerance test criteria that is intermediate between normal glucose tolerance and NIDDM (1, 2). Subjects in this range do not have diabetes and do not develop the microvascular complications of diabetes, but are at increased risk for cardiovascular disease and for developing diabetes. IGT has an unpredictable course. Some subjects appear to have a transient abnormality of glucose tolerance, others have persistent IGT, and still others progress to frank diabetes. Studies reported from the United Kingdom (17, 18), Japan (19), and the Micronesian population of Nauru (20) all suggest that the risk of diabetes in subjects with IGT is approximately 4% per year. After controlling for the effects of age, the risk of subsequent diabetes for subjects with IGT is approximately four-fold higher than for subjects with normal glucose tolerance (20).

When considered as continuous variables, higher fasting levels of both glucose and insulin have also been recognised as risk factors for NIDDM. In the Paris Prospective Study, a 3-year follow-up study of 5042 middle-aged white men without diabetes, plasma glucose concentration in the years before the occurrence of disease was a major risk factor for NIDDM (21). In an 8-year follow-up study of Mexican Americans in San Antonio, both fasting glucose (odds ratio = 5.8) and insulin (odds ratio = 3.1) were significantly related to conversion to diabetes (22).

In addition to its associated glucose intolerance, the incidence of NIDDM is associated with potentially modifiable risk factors including obesity, lack of physical activity, and, in some studies, dietary fat consumption.

In an 8-year follow-up study of US women aged 30–55 years at baseline, the relative risk of NIDDM among women with body mass indices (BMI) 23–23.9 kg/m$^2$ was 3.6 times that of women with BMI <22 kg/m$^2$ and increased with further increases in BMI (23). In this study, weight gain after age 18 was a major determinant of risk. In a recent prospective study of 1972 men enrolled in the Department of Veterans Affairs Normative Aging Study in the greater Boston area, men in the top tertile for BMI had a 1.3-fold greater risk of diabetes than did men in the lowest tertile, even after adjusting for age, the ratio of abdominal circumference to hip breadth, and cigarette smoking (24). In another prospective study of 2322 men in Uppsala, Sweden, aged 47 to 53 at baseline, BMI was an independent predictor of NIDDM. After adjusting for measures of glucose, insulin, systolic blood pressure, and antihypertensive drug therapy, those with BMI ⩾28.2 kg/m$^2$ were 1.4 times as likely to develop NIDDM than those with BMI <28.2 kg/m$^2$ (25). Studies among the Pima Indians have demonstrated that the incidence of NIDDM is almost 7-fold higher among the most obese group (BMI >40 $kg/m^2$) compared to the least obese group (BMI <25 $kg/m^2$) (10). A recent study among the Pima Indians has demonstrated that duration of obesity, defined as the time since BMI was first known to be at least 30 $kg/m^2$, is associated with the incidence of diabetes adjusted for age, sex, and current BMI (26). The adjusted incidence of NIDDM was 24.8 per 1000 person years of obesity for people with less than 5 years of obesity, 35.2 for those with 5 to 10 years of obesity, and 59.8 for those with at least 10 years of obesity. There was no apparent excess risk of diabetes for people who had a BMI of at least 30 $kg/m^2$ and then lost weight (26).

Unfavourable body fat distribution, that is, android, upper body, or centralised distribution of adipose tissue, has also been demonstrated to be an important risk factor for the incidence of NIDDM. In a 12-year study of women in Gothenburg, Sweden, correlations were studied between adiposity and adipose tissue distribution and the incidence of diabetes. In multivariate analysis, body mass index, sum of two skinfolds, and waist-to-hip ratio were all positively and significantly associated with incidence of diabetes (27, 28). In the follow-up study of Mexican Americans in San Antonio, central obesity, measured as the ratio of subscapular to triceps skinfold thickness, was associated with the 8-year incidence of NIDDM, even after adjustment for overall adiposity as measured by BMI (29). Women in the highest tertile of centrality had a 10.7-fold higher risk of NIDDM than women in the lowest tertile and those in the middle tertile had an 8.6-fold higher risk than those in the lowest tertile. Men in the highest tertile of centrality had a 3.7-fold higher risk of NIDDM than men in the lowest tertile and those in the middle tertile had an 1.4-fold higher risk than those in the lowest tertile. In a recent prospective study of 1972 men enrolled in the Department of Veterans Affairs Normative Aging Study in the greater Boston area, men in the top tertile for the ratio of abdominal circumference to hip breadth had a 2.4-fold greater risk of diabetes than did men in the lowest tertile, even after adjusting for age, body mass index, and cigarette smoking (24).

In a retrospective study of female former college athletes, the relative risk of diabetes in non-athletes versus athletes was 3.4. Former athletes were leaner and more likely to exercise than non-athletes (30). Among male college alumni at risk for NIDDM (e.g. those with family history of diabetes, BMI >25 $kg/m^2$, or history of hypertension), the incidence of NIDDM was almost 1.5 fold higher in those who were least physically active (physical activity index <500 kcal/week) compared to those who were most physically active (physical activity index >2000 kcal/week) (31). In an 8-year prospective study of 87 253 US women aged 34–59 years who were free of diabetes at baseline, the age- and BMI-adjusted relative risk of NIDDM was 0.8 for women who engaged in vigorous exercise at least once per week compared to those who did not exercise weekly (32). Among women who exercised at least once per week, there was no clear dose–response gradient according to frequency of exercise. In a 5-year prospective study of 21 271 US male physicians aged 40 to 84 years and free of diabetes baseline, the age-adjusted relative risk of NIDDM decreased with increasing frequency of exercise (33). After adjusting for both age and BMI, those who exercised at least once per week were 0.7 times less likely to develop NIDDM than those who exercised less than once a week. The inverse relation of exercise to risk of NIDDM was particularly pronounced among overweight men.

In some, but not all studies, dietary fat consumption has been independently associated with risk of NIDDM. One prospective study failed to show an association between nutrient consumption and the risk of NIDDM (27, 28) and another demonstrated a weak association between saturated fat consumption and NIDDM (34). A recent cross-sectional study demonstrated that a high-fat, low-carbohydrate diet as assessed by 24-hour diet recall was associated with both IGT and previously undiagnosed NIDDM (35). In the latter study, the adjusted odds ratio relating a 40 g/day increase in total fat consumption to NIDDM was 1.51. The effect of a high-fat, low-carbohydrate diet on glucose tolerance was greatest in persons with low levels of physical activity.

One hypothesis to explain the extremely high incidence of NIDDM in populations that have experienced rapid modernisation is the 'thrifty genotype hypothesis' (36). Originally proposed by Neel in 1962, this hypothesis holds that a thrifty genotype has offered a survival advantage by favouring fat deposition during periods of abundance in individuals in hunter–gatherer and early agrarian societies who were subject to cyclical food deprivation (37). In modern times, when physical activity decreased and a surfeit of calories were readily available, the genotype has favoured the development of obesity and NIDDM.

Twin studies of NIDDM (38–40), population studies (41, 42) and migrant studies of populations undergoing lifestyle changes in developed countries (43–47) all suggest a strong genetic component to NIDDM.

In recent years, great advances have been made in the search for the gene or genes responsible for NIDDM. It is unlikely that a single genetic defect is responsible for all NIDDM, rather polygenic causation resulting in a number of phenotypically similar syndromes appears to be a more likely explanation. Recent studies focusing on mutations to key enzymes in maturity onset diabetes of the young (MODY), an uncommon form of NIDDM with autosomal dominant inheritance, have demonstrated mutations to the glucokinase gene (48). Glucokinase is the major enzyme that phosphorylates glucose upon entry into liver and islet β-cells. A defect in glucokinase might account for defective glucose sensing, resulting in a higher set point for glucose induced insulin release. This defect is clearly associated with some, but not all, MODY pedigrees. Recent studies of NIDDM in whites and American blacks have suggested that mutations in the glucokinase gene are a rare cause of NIDDM (48).

## PREVALENCE OF NIDDM

Prevalence refers to the number of persons with NIDDM in the population at a given point in time or the rate per 100 population. In any population, prevalence estimates depend on both incidence and survival. Because at least 92% of prevalent cases of diabetes are NIDDM, most researchers have equated the prevalence of diabetes mellitus with that of NIDDM.

Surveillance data based on self-report of diabetes in household interviews show that, in 1990, there were 6.5 million persons with known diabetes in the United States (6). This represented about 2.6% of the US population. The lowest age-specific prevalence occurred among persons younger than 45 (0.68 per 100 population), and the highest age-specific prevalence occurred among persons 65 to 74 years of age (9.6 per 100 population). The prevalence in the population 45 to 64 years of age was 5.4 per 100 population and the prevalence in the population 75 years of age and older was 8.3 per 100 population. The prevalence of NIDDM has increased in the United States since 1959, but in recent years the rate of increase has slowed and levelled off. From 1959 to 1966, prevalence increased by 67%, from 1966 to 1973 it increased by 41%, from 1973 to 1980 it increased by 21%, and from 1980 to 1990 it increased by 2% (6). Since diabetes becomes more prevalent with advancing age, differences in the age structure of different populations can lead to misleading comparisons, unless rates are standardised. In specific race and gender groups, the prevalence of diabetes (and the age-adjusted prevalence of diabetes) were as follows: white males 2.2% (2.3%), white females 2.8% (2.4%), black males 2.9% (4.1%), black females 4.0% (4.6%) (6).

In 1982–84, the prevalence of self-reported diabetes among Cuban Americans in Florida was slightly higher than that for non-Hispanic whites, but among Puerto Ricans in the New York City area and Mexican Americans in the southwest, the prevalence was approximately two-fold higher than for non-Hispanic whites. Among Cuban Americans, the prevalence was 3.6%, among Puerto Ricans 5.5%, and among Mexican Americans, 5.4% (49). In men and women 45–74 years of age, the prevalence of previously diagnosed diabetes was highest: 5.9% among Cuban Americans and 14.3% among both Puerto Ricans and Mexican Americans (50).

In 1987, a review of outpatient records from the Indian Health Service indicated that 8.9% of American Indians aged ≥15 yr were seen at least once for diabetes (51). There was wide variation in the prevalence of known diabetes according to Tribe (52) and region (51) with a low of 2.0% in Alaska and a high of 15.4% in Tucson, Arizona. Among Native Americans, susceptibility to NIDDM is proportional to Native American genetic admixture, with subjects of mixed ethnicity having a risk of NIDDM intermediate between that of full-blood Native Americans and Caucasians (53, 54). In 1981, the prevalence of NIDDM among Pima Indians ≥35 years of age was approximately 50% (9). In men and women 55 to 64 years of age, the prevalence of diabetes was the highest: 69% in men and 86% in women.

In the US, the prevalence of undiagnosed NIDDM has also been investigated among whites, blacks, and Hispanics aged 20–74 years of age using national surveys and 75 g 2 h oral glucose tolerance tests. In general, for each person with diagnosed diabetes, there is another person with undiagnosed diabetes. In 1976–80, NHANES II found that 3.4% of whites and 4.7% of blacks 20 to 74 years of age had undiagnosed NIDDM by WHO criteria (3). In 1982–84, HHANES found that 5.4% of Cuban Americans, 5.4% of Puerto Rican Americans, and 4.2% of Mexican Americans 20 to 74 years of age had undiagnosed NIDDM (49). In general, rates of undiagnosed diabetes increased with age. Among whites and blacks, women were more likely than men to have undiagnosed diabetes. Among the Hispanic groups, men were more likely than women to have undiagnosed diabetes.

King, Rewers, and the WHO *Ad Hoc* Diabetes Reporting Group have recently reported standardised estimates for the prevalence of diabetes mellitus for 75 communities in 32 countries (55). The report was limited to population-based investigations conducted during 1976–91 that used WHO criteria for diagnosis and classification of diabetes. Age-specific prevalence was reported for selected populations and prevalence for the truncated age range of 30–64 yr was adjusted to the standard world population. The highest age-standardised prevalence was found in the Pima/Papago Indians (50%) and the Nauruans (41%). Some Arab, migrant Asian Indian, Chinese, and Hispanic American populations were at high risk with prevalence of 14–20%. In European populations, the prevalence varied from 3% to 10%. Diabetes was absent or rare (<3%) in some traditional communities in developing countries. The prevalence of diabetes rose with age in all populations in which age-specific data were examined. This trend was most pronounced in those at moderate to high risk. The ratio of prevalence of diabetes in men versus women varied markedly between populations with little discernible trend. In most communities, at least 20% of diabetes cases were unknown before the survey, and in many communities, >50% were previously undiagnosed.

## MORTALITY OF NIDDM

Diabetes mortality has been reported from population-based cohorts of diabetic persons and from analyses of vital records (death certificates). Although generally small, population-based surveys provide excellent follow-up and accurate assessments of mortality and causes of death among diabetic persons. Death certificates are designed to capture causes of death, not to describe prevalent conditions at death. Consequently, vital records may not accurately describe mortality among diabetic persons. Data from population-based surveys indicate that 95% of diabetic deaths are among persons with NIDDM.

In a follow-up study of a national sample of white respondents aged 40 to 77 years at baseline with self-reported diabetes, the age-adjusted death rate was 64.5 per 1000 person–years among diabetic men and 32.3 per 1000 person–years among diabetic women (56). After adjustment for age, blood pressure, cholesterol, body mass index, and smoking, the relative risk of death was 2.3 for diabetic men compared to non-diabetic men and 2.0 for diabetic women compared to non-diabetic women (56). Mortality rates have not been reported among representative samples of blacks.

In a population-based investigation among the residents of Rochester, Minnesota, the age-adjusted diabetes mortality rate was 9.3 per 100 000 person–years with diabetes as the underlying cause of death, 35.9 per 100 000 person–years with diabetes as an underlying or contributory cause, and 94.6 per 100 000 person–years if all deaths among diabetic individuals were counted (57). In another study of diabetes mortality conducted in three cities in Minnesota, the crude mortality rate per 100 000 was 14.0 for diabetes as underlying cause, 54.7 for diabetes as underlying or contributing cause, and 112.2 for all subjects with diabetes (7). The age-adjusted diabetes mortality rate was 63.3 per 100 000 for men and 80.0 per 100 000 for women, and the overall age- and sex-adjusted diabetes mortality rate was 72.1 (7). Among Pima Indians with NIDDM studied between 1975 and 1984, all-cause mortality was 1970 per 100 000 person–years (58). The rate for women with NIDDM was 1530 per 100 000 person–years and for men with NIDDM was 2430 per 100 000 person–years (58).

Cardiovascular disease, including both cardiac and cerebrovascular disease, is the leading cause of death among persons with NIDDM. In a follow-up study of a national sample of white diabetic respondents aged 40 to 77 years at baseline with self-reported diabetes, about 61% of deaths among men and 55% of deaths among women were due to cardiovascular disease (56). Seventy-five per cent of the excess mortality among diabetic men and 57% of that among diabetic women was attributable to cardiovascular disease deaths (56). In Rochester, Minnesota, 49% of all diabetic deaths were attributed to cardiovascular disease (57). In the Minnesota three cities study, 62% of deaths were associated with cardiovascular disease (7). In the Wisconsin Epidemiologic Study of Diabetic Retinopathy, 58% of deaths among older-onset subjects were attributed to cardiovascular disease (59). In Pima Indians with NIDDM, cardiovascular disease (including ischaemic heart disease and stroke) is the leading cause of death by disease, but the proportion of deaths associated with CVD (16% of deaths) is lower than among whites (58). Among Pima Indians, diabetic nephropathy is a more important cause of death (13% of deaths). A partial explanation for this disparity is that onset of NIDDM occurs at a much younger age in Pimas (approximately 36 years of age) than in US whites (approximately 60 years of age), resulting in diabetic nephropathy and death at an age when the risk of ischaemic heart disease is still quite low (58).

In a 12-year prospective study of mortality among the London cohort of the WHO Multinational Study of Vascular Disease in Diabetics, the age-adjusted mortality rate was 22.6 per 1000 person–years in males with NIDDM and 9.1 per 1000 person–years in females with NIDDM who were 35–54 years of age at baseline (60). Cardiovascular disease accounted for 63% of deaths among males and 61% of deaths among females. Other studies of diabetes mortality in the United Kingdom have found that atherosclerotic cardiovascular disease is the major cause of death in NIDDM. In a multiple-cause of death analysis for England and Wales, circulatory diseases were the underlying cause of death in just over 50% of death certificates mentioning diabetes (61). In the WHO Multinational Study of Vascular Disease in Diabetics, all-cause mortality rates in males with NIDDM varied about three-fold among the ten participating centres (62). The highest rates occurred in Warsaw and Havana (28.7 and 26.1 per 1000 person–years at risk) and the lowest rates occurred in Tokyo and Zagreb (6.6 and 8.9, respectively). All-cause mortality rates for females varied about four-fold, with the highest rates in Oklahoma and the lowest rates in Tokyo.

Data from vital statistics are readily available, but consistently underestimate mortality among persons with diabetes. Several US-based studies have demonstrated that death certificates identify only about 40% of people who have diabetes at the time of death, and only about one-quarter of death certificates listing diabetes list it as the underlying cause of death (57, 63). Under-reporting of diabetes on death certificates is remarkably similar for US whites (61%), blacks (64%), and Native Americans (63%), although under-reporting of Native American heritage presents an additional problem in interpreting mortality data among Native Americans (64). Broad differences in coding practices for diabetes mortality have been demonstrated among European countries (65).

The frequency of recording of diabetes on death certificates is strongly related to age, duration of diabetes, and co-morbidities (63). Thus, diabetes is less likely to be recorded in the population with NIDDM (e.g. older people with shorter duration of diabetes dying with ischaemic heart disease) than in those with IDDM (e.g. younger people with longer duration of diabetes dying with renal disease). Coding of diabetes is lower still for deaths related to accidents and cancers as underlying cause, compared to circulatory disease (61). Some groups have used these studies of under-reporting to correct vital statistics data to better assess diabetes mortality. These estimates have provided numbers of the same order of magnitude as those obtained when age- and sex-adjusted mortality rates from population-based cohorts have been applied to national populations (66).

Using vital statistics data, diabetes is recognized as the seventh leading cause of death in the United States and the thirteenth leading cause of years of potential life lost before age 65 (5). In 1989, 46 833 deaths were reported with diabetes as the underlying cause and 160 848 deaths were reported with diabetes as any listed cause. In 1989, mortality was 19.0 per 100 000 population for diabetes as the underlying cause of death and 65.2 per 100 000 population for diabetes as any listed cause. In the US, mortality rates for diabetes increase dramatically with age, with the highest rates occurring among those aged 85 and older. Among persons aged 85 and older, 1989 mortality was 252.6 per 100 000 population for diabetes as the underlying cause of death and 904.4 per 100 000 population for diabetes as any listed cause.

In the United States, there are minor differences in diabetes mortality between men and women, but rates are higher in blacks, Hispanic–Americans, and Native Americans than in whites. In 1989, the age-adjusted mortality rate for diabetes as underlying cause of death was 16.9 per 100 000 population for white males, 15.1 per 100 000 population for white females, 33.3 per 100 000 population for black males, and 36.3 per 100 000 population for black females (6). In 1983–87, the age-adjusted mortality rate for diabetes as underlying cause of death was 25.3 in Hispanic white males in New Mexico and 33.3 in Hispanic white females in New Mexico (67). In 1984–86, the age-adjusted mortality rate for diabetes as the underlying cause of death was 96 per 1000 000 population for Native Americans (63). The corresponding age-adjusted mortality rates for diabetes as any listed cause were 63.8 per 100 000 for white males, 50.5 per 100 000 for white females, 99.6 per 100 000 for black males, 104.6 per 100 000 for black females (6), and 264 per 100 000 for Native Americans (64). Thus, in the United States, age-adjusted mortality is approximately 2-fold higher in blacks and Hispanics and 4-fold higher in Native Americans than in whites.

Between 1980 and 1988, the age-standardized

mortality rates for diabetes as an underlying cause of death remained relatively constant for white males and white females, but increased by 18% and 4% in black males and black females respectively (5). In 1989, mortality for diabetes as an underlying cause increased 14% (6). This increase corresponded with the implementation of the revised 1989 US Standard Certificate of Death. Results of a CDC analysis suggest that this finding is, at least in part, related to reporting factors including an increase in the number of lines on which to report causes of death, and the provision of more detailed instructions on the certificate (including instructions that use diabetes as an example of a contributing cause of death to illustrate the proper completion of a death certificate).

Between 1980 and 1989, the age-standardized mortality rates for diabetes as any listed cause of death remained relatively constant for white males and white females, but increased by 28% and 11% in black males and black females, respectively. In the 30-year period between 1958 and 1987, the age-adjusted diabetes mortality rates among New Mexico Hispanics and Native Americans increased dramatically: 140% and 112% in Hispanic males and females, and 249% and 550% in Native American males and females respectively (67).

In England and Wales in 1985–86, the crude diabetes death rate per 100 000 population per year was 44.2 among men and 49.4 among women (68). Among those 45 years of age and older, rates were 179.1 among men and 122.9 among women. In the United Kingdom, diabetes mortality has been reported by country of birth for persons born in the Indian subcontinent (India, Pakistan, Bangladesh, and Sri Lanka) (Asians) and those born in the African and Caribbean Commonwealths (Afro-Caribbeans). Age-standardised rate ratios for mortality were 289 among Asian men, 260 among Asian women, 251 among Afro-Caribbean men, and 248 among Afro-Caribbean women (69). Between 1975 and 76 and 1985 and 86 there was a fall in diabetes-related mortality of 12% in women and a rise of 3% in men of all ages.

Although limited by systematic underreporting, general population rates provide a measure of the mortality of diabetes in the population and are useful to compare the mortality of diabetes with that of other diseases and conditions. These rates are affected, however, by differences in diabetes prevalence among different age, sex, or race groups (see above). For that reason, it is useful to calculate rates using estimates of the number of persons known to have diabetes as the denominators. These calculations are especially useful for comparing mortality rates among subgroups of people with diabetes. Many of the apparent differences in mortality among sex–race groups (especially among minority populations) are due to differences in diabetes prevalence and age distributions among the population groups.

In the US in 1989, mortality was 731.5 per 100 000 diabetic population for diabetes as the underlying cause of death and 2512.3 per 100 000 diabetic population for diabetes as any listed cause (6). Among persons aged 75 and older, mortality was 2005.0 per 100 000 diabetic population for diabetes as the underlying cause of death and 7292.6 per 100 000 diabetic population for diabetes as any listed cause. In 1989, the age-adjusted mortality rate for diabetes as the underlying cause of death was 731.1 per 100 000 diabetic population for white males, 674.0 per 100 000 diabetic population for white females, 801.5 per 100 000 diabetic population for black males and 720.6 per 100 000 diabetic population for black females. The corresponding age-adjusted mortality rates for diabetes as any listed cause were 2751.0, 2259.8, 2378.9, and 2075.1 per 100 000 diabetic population. Between 1980 and 1988, the age-standardised mortality rates for diabetes as an underlying cause of death decreased for white males, black males, and black females. White females were the only group whose rates were higher in 1988 than in 1980. All groups experienced an increase in 1989 such that 1989 rates were higher than

1980 rates for all groups except black females.

The major risk factors associated with mortality in the general population operate in the population with NIDDM. In NIDDM, age, male gender, current smoking, hypertension, hypercholesterolaemia, and non-leisure physical inactivity are risk factors for mortality (69). Studies have also identified diabetic kidney disease as an important risk factor for mortality in NIDDM. In some studies, use of diuretics has also been associated with mortality.

A number of retrospective studies have shown an association between microalbuminuria and all-cause, chiefly cardiovascular, mortality (70–72). A recent prospective study of 36 patients with microalbuminuria (urinary albumin excretion 20–200 micrograms/min) and NIDDM and 105 patients with normal (<20 micrograms/min) urinary albumin excretion and NIDDM demonstrated significantly excess mortality among those with microalbuminuria (73). In univariate survival analysis, significant predictors of all-cause mortality included microalbuminuria, hypercholesterolaemia, hypertriglyceridaemia, and pre-existing coronary heart disease. After adjustment for age and the effects of the other major risk factors, microalbuminuria was the only significant risk factor for mortality in NIDDM. Those with NIDDM and microalbuminuria were four times as likely to have died as those without microalbuminuria (73).

In another multiple regression analysis of risk factors associated with all-cause mortality in patients with NIDDM, serum cholesterol, proteinuria, and plasma creatinine were associated with mortality risk. Current smoking and proteinuria were associated with cardiovascular mortality in NIDDM and diabetes duration was associated with non-cardiovascular mortality (60, 74). Two recent studies have also reported an association between use of diuretics and mortality in NIDDM (75, 76). A recent study also demonstrated that lack of cardiorespiratory fitness is associated with age-adjusted mortality in NIDDM. In an 8-year prospective study of men classified as fit or non-fit on the basis of a maximal-exercise treadmill testing, unfit men with NIDDM experienced an age-adjusted death rate of 82.5 per 10 000 person–years of follow-up, and fit men experienced a rate of 45.9 (77).

## CONCLUSIONS

The disease burden of NIDDM is large and will grow as societies 'modernise', as access to care and disease detection improve, and as populations age. Twin studies, family studies, and studies of ancestral admixture all suggest a strong genetic contribution to NIDDM. As identified in this review, important modifiable environmental risk factors associated with 'modernisation' also contribute to NIDDM. These include obesity, sedentary lifestyle, and perhaps increased fat consumption. Although detection of diabetes appears to be relatively good in a number of industrialised, urban communities, approximately 50% of persons with NIDDM in North America and Western Europe are undiagnosed, and 75% to almost 100% are undiagnosed in certain Pacific populations. Since the prevalence of NIDDM increases with age in all populations, changing population demographics will profoundly affect the world-wide burden of NIDDM. Based upon careful observations in migrant populations, some Pacific Island, Asian, Arab, and African populations appear to be at particularly high risk for NIDDM. The younger age-at-onset of diabetes, the higher prevalence, and the higher rates of mortality, and the association between duration of diabetes and its complications, all suggest that the burden of NIDDM may be greater in populations beginning to experience 'modernisation' than it has been in the majority populations of North America and Western Europe.

Effective prevention and intervention strategies are urgently needed to prevent NIDDM and reduce its current and potential disease burden, especially in high-risk populations. Primary prevention strategies that address the environmental risk factors for NIDDM, particularly obesity and sedentary lifestyle must be developed, tested, and widely implemented, and efforts to address cardiovascular risk factors and risk factors for mortality including cigarette smoking, uncontrolled hypertension, and hyperlipidaemia must be intensified in persons with NIDDM.

## REFERENCES


1 National Diabetes Data Group. Classification and diagnosis of diabetes mellitus and other categories of glucose intolerance. *Diabetes* 1979; 28: 1039–57.
2 WHO Expert Committee. Second report on diabetes mellitus. WHO Technical Report Series, No. 646, Geneva, World Health Organization, 1980.
3 Harris MI, Hadden WC, Knowler WC, Bennett PH. Prevalence of diabetes and impaired glucose tolerance and plasma glucose levels in US population aged 20–74 yr. *Diabetes* 1987; 36: 523–34.
4 Melton JS, Palumbo PJ, Chu C. Incidence of diabetes mellitus by clinical type. *Diabetes Care* 1983; 6: 75–86.
5 Centers for Disease Control. Diabetes Surveillance, 1991. Atlanta, GA, US Department of Health and Human Services, Public Health Service, 1992.
6 Centers for Disease Control and Prevention. Diabetes Surveillance, 1993. Atlanta, GA, US Department of Health and Human Services, Public Health Service, 1993.
7 Bender AP, Sprafka JM, Jagger HG, Muckala KH, Martin CP, Edwards TR. Incidence, prevalence, and mortality of diabetes mellitus in Wadena, Marshall and Grand Rapids, Minnesota: the Three-City Study. *Diabetes Care* 1986; 9: 343–50.
8 Haffner SM, Hazuda HP, Mitchell BD, Patterson JK, Stern MP. Increased incidence of Type II diabetes mellitus in Mexican Americans. *Diabetes Care* 1991*a*; 14: 102–8.
9 Knowler WC, Saad MF, Pettitt DJ, Nelson RG, Bennett PH. Determinants of Diabetes Mellitus in the Pima Indians. *Diabetes Care* 1993; 16: Suppl 1, 216–27.
10 Knowler WC, Pettitt, DJ, Lillioja S, Nelson RG. Genetic and environmental factors in the development of diabetes mellitus in Pima Indians. In: Smith U, Eriksson S, Lindgarde F, ed. *Genetic susceptibility to environmental factors – a challenge for public intervention.* Almqvist & Wiksell International Stockholm, 1988; 67–74.
11 Andersson DK, Svardsudd K, Tibblin G. Prevalence and incidence of diabetes in a Swedish Community 1972–1987. *Diabetic Med* 1991; 8: 428–34.
12 Papoz L, Eschwege E, Warnet J, Richard J, Claude J. Incidence and risk factors of diabetes in the Paris prospective study. In: Eschwege E, ed. *Adv Diabetes Epidemiol, INSERM 22,* Elsevier Biomedical Press BV; 113–122.
13 Balkau B, King H, Zimmet P, Raper LR. Factors associated with the development of diabetes in the Micronesian Population of Nauru. *Am J Epidemiol* 1985; 122: 594–605.
14 Mahan CM, O'Sullivan JR. Criteria for the oral glucose tolerance test in pregnancy. *Diabetes* 1964; 13: 278–85.
15 O'Sullivan JB. The Boston gestational diabetes studies: reviews and perspectives. In: Pearson DWM, Stowers JM, Sutherland HW, eds. *Carbohydrate metabolism in pregnancy and the newborn.* Springer-Verlag, London, 1989; 4: 287–294.
16 O'Sullivan JB. Diabetes Mellitus after GDM. *Diabetes* 1991; 40, Suppl 2: 131–5.
17 Jarrett RJ, Keen H, Fuller JH, McCartney M. Worsening diabetes in men with impaired glucose tolerance ('borderline diabetes'). *Diabetologia* 1979; 16: 25–30.
18 Keen H, Jarrett RJ, McCartney P. The ten-year follow-up of the Bedford survey (1962–1972): glucose tolerance and diabetes. *Diabetologia* 1982; 22: 73–8.
19 Sasaki A, Suzuki T, Horiuchi N. Development of diabetes in Japanese subjects with impaired glucose tolerance: a seven-year follow-up study. *Diabetologia* 1982; 22: 154–7.
20 King H, Zimmet P, Raper LR, Balkau B. The natural history of impaired glucose tolerance in the micronesian population of Naura: a six year follow-up study. *Diabetologia* 1984; 26; 39–43.
21 Charles MA, Fontbonne A, Thibult N, Warnet JM, Rosselin GE, Eschwege E. Risk factors for NIDDM in white population: Paris prospective study. *Diabetes* 1991; 40: 796–9.
22 Haffner, SM, Stern MP, Mitchell BD, Hazuda HP, Patterson JK. Incidence of Type II diabetes in Mexican Americans predicted by fasting insulin and glucose levels, obesity, and body-fat distribution. *Diabetes* 1990; 39: 283–8.
23 Colditz GA, Willet WC, Stampfer MJ, Manson JE, Hennekens CH, Arky RA. Weight as a risk factor for clinical diabetes in women. *Am J Epidemiol* 1990; 132: 501–13.
24 Cassano PA, Rosner B, Vokonas PS, Weiss ST. Obesity and body fat distribution in relation to the incidence of non-insulin-dependent diabetes mellitus. *Am J Epidemiol* 1992; 136: 1474–86.
25 Skarfors ET, Selinus KI, Lithell HO. Risk factors for developing non-insulin-dependent diabetes: a 10-year follow-up of men in Uppsala. *Br Med J* 1991; 303: 755–60.
26 Everhart JE, Pettitt DJ, Bennett PH, Knowler WC. Duration of obesity increases the incidence of NIDDM. *Diabetes* 1992; 41: 235–40.
27 Lundgren H, Bengtsson C, Blohme G. *et al.* Dietary habits and incidence of non-insulin-dependent diabetes mellitus in a population study of women in Gothenburg, Sweden. *Am J Clin Nutrit* 1989; 49: 708–12.
27 Lundgren H, Bengtsson C, Blohme G, Lapidus L, Sjostrom L. Adiposity and adipose tissue distribution in relation to incidence of diabetes in women: results from a prospective population study in Gothenburg, Sweden. *Int J Obesity* 1989; 13: 413–23.
28 Haffner SM, Mitchell BD, Hazuda HP, Stern MP. Greater influence of central distribution of adipose tissue on incidence of non-insulin-dependent diabetes in women than men. *Am J Clin Nutrit* 1991; 53: 1312–17.
29 Frisch RE, Wyshak G, Albright TE, Albright NL, Schiff I. Lower prevalence of diabetes in female former college athletes compared with nonathletes. *Diabetes* 1986; 35: 1101–5.
30 Helmrich SP, Ragland DR, Leung RW, Paffenbarger RS

Jr. Physical activity and reduced occurrence of non-insulin-dependent diabetes mellitus. *N Engl J Med* 1991; 325: 147–52.
31 Manson JE, Rimm EB, Stampfer MJ *et al*. Physical activity and incidence of non-insulin-dependent diabetes mellitus in women. *Lancet* 1991; 338: 774–8.
32 Manson JE, Nathan DM, Krolewski AS, Stampfer MJ, Willett WC, Hennekens CH. A prospective study of exercise and incidence of diabetes among US male physicians *J Am Med Assoc* 1992; 268: 63–7.
34 Feskens EJ, Kromhout D. Habitual dietary intake and glucose tolerance in euglycaemic men: the Zutphen study. *Int J Epidemiol* 1990; 19: 953–9.
35 Marshall JA, Hamman RF, Baxter J. High-fat, low-carbohydrate diet and the etiology of non-insulin-dependent diabetes mellitus: the San Luis Valley Diabetes Study. *Am J Epidemiol* 1991; 134: 590–603.
36 Wendorf M, Goldfine ID. Perspectives in diabetes: archaeology of NIDDM excavation of the 'thrifty' genotype. *Diabetes* 1991; 40: 161–5.
37 Neel JV. Diabetes mellitus: a 'thifty' genotype rendered detrimental by 'progress'. *Am J Human Genet* 1962; 14: 353–62.
38 Newman B, Selby JV, King MC, Slemenda C, Fabsitz R, Friedman GD. Concordance for type 2 (non-insulin-dependent) diabetes mellitus in male twins. *Diabetologia* 1987; 30: 763–8.
39 Committee on Diabetic Twins. Japan Diabetes Society. Diabetes Mellitus in Twins: a cooperative study in Japan. *Diabetes Res Clin Pract* 1988; 5: 271–80.
40 Lo SSS, Tun RYM, Hawa M, Leslie RDG. Studies of diabetic twins. *Diabetes Metab Rev* 1991; 7: 223–8.
41 Hanis CL, Hewett-Emmett D, Bertin TK, Schull WJ. Origins of US Hispanics. Implications for diabetes. *Diabetes Care* 1991; 14: 618–27.
42 Simmons D, Williams DR, Powell MJ. The Conventry Diabetes Study: prevalence of diabetes and impaired glucose tolerance in Europids and Asians. *Quart J Med* 1991; 81; 1021–30.
43 Taylor R, Bennett P, Uili R *et al*. Diabetes in Wallis Polynesians: a comparison of residents of Wallis Island and first generation migrants to Noumea, New Caledonia. *Diabetes Res Clin Pract* 1985; 1: 169–78.
44 Cohen MP, Stern E, Rusecki Y, Zeidler A. High prevalence of diabetes in young adult Ethiopian immigrants to Israel. *Diabetes* 1988; 37: 824–8.
45 Ostbye T, Welby TJ, Prior IA, Salmond CE, Stokes YM. Type 2 (non-insulin-dependent) diabetes mellitus, migration and westernization: the Tokelau Island Migrant Study. *Diabetologia* 1989; 32: 585–90.
46 Fujimoto WY. The growing prevalence of non-insulin-dependent diabetes in migrant Asian populations and its implications for Asia. *Diabetes Res Clin Pract* 1992; 15: 167–83.
47 Stern MP, Gonzalez, C, Mitchell BD, Villalpando E, Haffner SM, Hazuda HP. Genetic and environmental determinants of type II diabetes in Mexico City and San Antonio. *Diabetes* 1992; 41: 484–92.
48 Permutt MA, Chiu KC, Tanizawa Y. Perspectives in diabetes: glucokinase and NIDDM a candidate gene that paid off. *Diabetes* 1992; 41: 1367–72.
49 National Center for Health Statistics, Centers for Disease Control and Prevention, unpublished data.
50 Flegal KM, Ezzati TM, Harris MI *et al*. Prevalence of diabetes in Mexican Americans, Cubans and Puerto Ricans from the Hispanic health and nutrition examination survey 1982–1984. *Diabetes Care* 1991; 14, Suppl 3: 628–38.
51 Gohdes D, Kaufman S, Valway S. Diabetes in American Indians. *Diabetes Care* 1993; 16, Suppl 1: 239–24.
52 Stahn RM, Gohdes D, Valway SE. Diabetes and its complications among selected tribes in North Dakota, South Dakota and Nebraska. *Diabetes Care* 1993; 16, Suppl 1: 244–7.
53 Gardner LI Jr, Stern MP, Haffner SM *et al*. Prevalence of diabetes in Mexican Americans. Relationship to percent of gene pool derived from native American sources. *Diabetes* 1984; 33: 86–92.
54 Farrell MA, Quiggins PA, Eller JD *et al*. Prevalence of diabetes and its complications in the Eastern band of Cherokee Indians. *Diabetes Care* 1993; 16, Suppl 1: 253–6.
55 King H, Rewers M. Global estimates for prevalence of diabetes mellitus and impaired glucose tolerance in adults. *Diabetes Care* 1993; 16: 157–77.
56 Kleinman JC, Donahue RP, Harris MI, Finucane FF, Madans JH, Brock DB. Mortality among diabetics in a national sample. *Am J Epidemiol* 1988; 128: 389–401.
57 Ochi JW, Melton LJ, Palumbo PJ, Chu CP. A population-based study of diabetes mortality. *Diabetes Care* 1985; 8: 224–9.
58 Sievers ML, Nelson RG, Knowler WC, Bennett PH. Impact of NIDDM on mortality and causes of death in Pima Indians. *Diabetes Care* 1992; 15: 1541–9.
59 Moss SE, Klein R, Klein BEK. Cause-specific mortality in a population-based study of diabetes. *Am J Public Health* 1991; 81: 1158–62.
60 Morrish NJ, Stevens LK, Head J, Fuller JH, Jarrett RJ, Keen H. A prospective study of mortality among middle-aged diabetic patients (the London Cohort of the WHO Multinational Study of Vascular Disease in Diabetics) I: Causes and death rates. *Diabetologia* 1990*a*; 33: 538.
61 Fuller JH, Elford J, Goldblatt P, Adelstein AM. Diabetes mortality: new light on an underestimated public health problem. *Diabetologia* 1983; 24: 336–41.
62 Head J, Fuller JH. International variations in mortality among diabetic patients: the WHO Multinational Study of Vascular Disease in Diabetics. *Diabetologia* 1990; 33: 477–81.
63 Bild DE, Stevenson JM. Frequency of recording of diabetes on US death certificates: analysis of the 1986 National Followback Survey. *J Clin Epidemiol* 1992; 45: 275–81.
64 Newman JM, DeStefano F, Valway SE, German RR, Muneta B. Diabetes-associated mortality in native Americans. *Diabetes Care* 1993; 16, Suppl: 297–305.
65 Jougla E, Papoz L, Balkau B, Manguin P, Hatton F. Death certificate coding practices related to diabetes in European countries – the 'Eurodiab Subarea C' Study. *Int J Epidemiol* 1992; 21: 343–51.
66 Herman WH, Sinnock P, Brenner E. An epidemiologic model for diabetes mellitus: incidence, prevalence, and mortality. *Diabetes Care* 1984; 7: 367–71.
67 Carter JS, Wiggins CL, Becker TM, Key CR. Diabetes mortality among New Mexico's American Indian, Hispanic, and non-Hispanic white population, 1958–1987. *Diabetes Care* 1993; 16, Suppl 1: 306–9.

68 Stephenson J, Swerdlow AJ, Devis T, Fuller JH. Recent trends in diabetes mortality in England and Wales. *Diabetic Med* 1992; 9: 417–21.
69 Ford ES, DeStefano F. Risk factors for mortality from all causes and from coronary heart disease among persons with diabetes. *Am J Epidemiol* 1991; 133: 1220–30.
70 Jarrett RJ, Viberti GC, Argyropoulos A, Hill RD, Mahmud U, Murrells TJ. Microalbuminuria predicts mortality in non-insulin-dependent diabetics. *Diabetic Med* 1984; 1: 17–19.
71 Mogensen CE. Microalbuminuria predicts clinical proteinuria and early mortality in maturity-onset diabetes. *N Eng J Med* 1984; 310: 356–60.
72 Schmitz A. Microalbuminuria and mortality in non-insulin-dependent diabetes. In: Mogensen CE, ed. *The kidney and hypertension in diabetes mellitus*. Martinus, Nijhoff, Boston, 1988; 65–70.
73 Mattock MB, Morrish NJ, Viberti G, Keen H, Fitzgerald AP, Jackson G. Prospective study of microalbuminuria as predictor of mortality in NIDDM. *Diabetes* 1992; 41: 736–41.
74 Morrish NJ, Stevens LK, Head J, Fuller JH, Jarrett RJ, Keen H. A prospective study of mortality among middle-aged diabetic patients (the London Cohort of the WHO Multinational Study of Vascular Disease in Diabetics) II: associated risk factors. *Diabetologia* 1990*b*; 33: 542–8.
75 Warram JH, Laffel LMD, Valsania P, Christleib AR, Krolewski AS. Excess mortality associated with diuretic therapy in diabetes mellitus. *Arch Internal Med* 1991; 151: 1350–6.
76 Klein BEK, Moss SE, Klein R. Use of cardiovascular disease medications and mortality in people with older onset diabetes. *Am J Public Health* 1992; 82: 1142–4.
77 Kohl HW, Gordon NF, Villegas JA, Blair SN. Cardiorespiratory fitness glycemic status, and mortality risk in men. *Diabetes Care* 1992; 15: 184–92.

# 12 Genetic Basis of the Aetiology of Non-insulin-dependent Diabetes

Kwame Osei

## INTRODUCTION

The World Health Organisation (WHO) and The International Diabetes Federation (IDF) have recently reported that the prevalence and the incidence of NIDDM are increasing world-wide. The current estimate is that there are approximately 100 million diabetics world-wide. The rate of increase is predominantly in the hitherto agrarian cultures of the third world and developing countries where approximately three-quarters of the world's 6 billion population reside. In these countries, recent epidemiological studies have suggested that there are 40 million diabetics, and this figure is expected to increase to 65 million by the turn of the century. Similarly, in the developed countries in the western world, the incidence of the disease is estimated at 7% annually. Furthermore, diabetes probably accounts for, or significantly contributes to, a third of deaths in the USA. The economic costs of the disease have progressively increased, reaching 20 billion dollars in 1987 with a projected estimate of 100 billion dollars at the turn of the century in United States alone. In the third world and developing countries, the increasing prevalence of the disease with its associated morbidity and mortality could rapidly replace infections as the leading or primary cause of deaths. Thus, without national coordination and planning, the increasing incidence and prevalence of diabetes could put a tremendous strain on the limited economic resources in the third world and developing countries.

Although, there are several forms of diabetes as defined by the WHO (1) and the National Diabetes Data Group Criteria (2), idiopathic NIDDM remains the commonest form of diabetes in the world. Nevertheless, there are ethnic, racial and geographical differences in the prevalence of NIDDM in the world's population (3–8). For example, the Pima Indians living in the Arizona, USA, have the highest rate of NIDDM in the world (4). Similarly, the African–Americans, Mexican–Americans, Micronesians, South Eastern Asians as well as Australian Aborigines have extraordinary propensity to develop NIDDM when compared to the Caucasians (3–8). Whether the aetiology of the disease is similar in different populations remains uncertain. However, it is clear that the disease is heterogeneous with strong genetic and familial components (9–13). Regarding the genetics, previous studies have demonstrated that the concordance rate for monozygotic NIDDM patients approaches 90–100% in the western countries (11, 12), in contrast with the 50% found in the monozygotic patients with IDDM (9–12). Similar data are not available in the monozygotic twins with NIDDM in the third world and developing countries. Note however, that the prevalence of NIDDM in these countries remains very low, less than 1–2%, when compared to 3–6% in several western countries (14).

In order to understand further the primary aetiology of NIDDM, several approaches and experimental techniques have been adopted in various laboratories world-wide. This has become necessary since the results of numerous studies evaluating genetic marker(s) of the disease have failed to identify any specific genetic defect(s) and have remained elusive. This is ironic since the disease has a strong genetic component. Moreover, highly sophisticated and advanced genetic and molecular biological techniques have been employed in these studies. In this regard, the commonest and, perhaps, the simplest approach is to investigate persons with greater risk for the disease such as the siblings, first-degree relatives and offspring of patients with NIDDM. In the same vein, studies in people from ethnic and racial groups with higher prevalence of the disease have been performed. Typically, such studies have focused on potential genetic markers and/or metabolic abnormalities in the selected and well-characterized study populations. In all these studies, the basic premises are that genetic markers and/or metabolic abnormalities that predispose patients to NIDDM cluster and co-segregate together and thus, would be more prevalent in these selected populations.

The main objectives of this review are: 1) to discuss the genetic basis of the aetiological factors of NIDDM and 2) to compare and contrast different aspects of the multiple aetiological factors underlying the disease in different racial, ethnic and geographical populations. For the sake of clarity, we have opted to discuss this review under specific subheadings, namely: 1) beta cell dysfunction, 2) hepatic glucose overproduction, 3) insulin-mediated glucose disposal, and 4) non-insulin-dependent glucose disposal. Although alterations in these four parameters commonly determine the hyperglycaemic state, it should be noted that, in a given patient or population, one or more of these factors would tend to dominate; however, there are tremendous interplay and interactions between these metabolic variables.

## AETIOLOGY OF BETA CELL DYSFUNCTION IN NIDDM

Patients with NIDDM are often characterized by either normal, decreased or increased serum insulin concentrations when compared to the healthy non-diabetic subjects as shown in Fig. 12.1 and Table 12.1. Although the cause for this variability in the insulin secretion, as assessed by both serum insulin and c-peptide, remains uncertain, this could be ascribed to the heterogeneous nature of the disease. It is equally possible, however, that the beta cell secretory responses reflect inherited and genetic traits in a given race, ethnic group and family (3, 4, 6, 8, 15–26). Previous studies in the monozygotic twins tend to indicate that this is the case. Note, however, that, even in the presence of higher

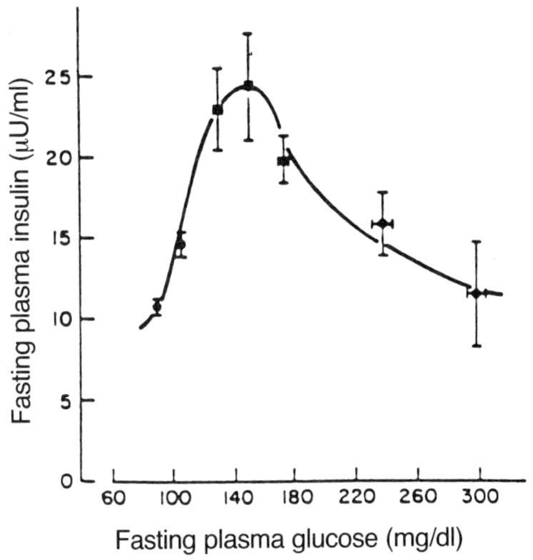


Fig. 12.1. Fasting plasma glucose and insulin concentrations in healthy subjects, and patients with impaired glucose tolerance and diabetes. (Adapted with permission from the American Diabetes Association.)

Table 12.1. *Comparison of common biochemical abnormalities in first-degree relatives with and without impaired glucose tolerance and patients with type 2 diabetes*

| | Glucose-tolerant relatives | Impaired glucose-tolerant relatives | Type 2 diabetics |
|---|---|---|---|
| *OGTT glucose (mg/dl)* | | | |
| Fasting | → | → | ↑ ↑ |
| 2 h PP | → | ↑ | ↑ ↑ |
| *IVGTT insulin (μU/ml)* | | | |
| 1st phase | →↑ | ↓ | ↓ ↓ |
| 2nd phase | →↑ | → | ↓ ↓ |
| *Insulin-mediated glucose disposal* | | | |
| Total | ↓ | ↓ | ↓ ↓ |
| Oxidative | → | → | →↓ |
| Non-oxidative | ↓ | ↓ | ↓ ↓ |
| *Non-insulin-dependent disposal* | → | →↓ | ↓ ↓ |
| *Hepatic glucose production* | | | |
| Basal | → | ↑ | ↑ |
| % Post-prandial suppression | → | ↓ | ↓ ↓ |
| *Lipid metabolism* | | | |
| Basal FFA | → | → | ↑ ↑ |
| FFA fluxes | → | → | ↑ ↑ |
| Lipid oxidation | → | → | ↑ ↑ |
| % Lipid suppression | →↑ | →↓ | ↓ ↓ |

Normal=→, decreased= ↓ , increased= ↑ , PP=post-prandial, FFA=free fatty acid markedly increased= ↑ ↑ , markedly decreased= ↓ ↓ .

immunoreactive insulin (IRI) levels in the patients with NIDDM, it is clear that this is inappropriately low in the face of the severe hyperglycaemia (27). Moreover, comparison of beta cell function and secretory capacity among patients living in diverse environments should be made under extreme caution and with caveats.

The evidence for the genetic basis of the beta cell dysfunction also stems from several population studies. In this regard, non-diabetic first-degree relatives and offspring of patients living in the western world (e.g. Pima Indians, African–Americans, Mexican–Americans, etc.) and Australian Aborigines as well as Micronesian Nauruans and several populations with extraordinary propensity to develop diabetes manifest both fasting and post-stimulation hyperinsulinaemia (15–21). In contrast, the recent evidence from native African populations has indicated that first-degree relatives of Nigerian NIDDM patients have rather lower insulin secretion (28). Furthermore, Shire *et al.* (29) and Rubenstein *et al.* (30) have reported that black Southern Africans living in Johannesburg have markedly lower insulin concentrations when compared to the whites, irrespective of the obesity indices. Furthermore, a recent report in Japanese patients with non-insulin-dependent diabetes who maintain normal ideal body weight have markedly reduced plasma insulin levels (31). Thus, clearly, there are obvious ethnic and racial differences in the circulating insulin concentrations and the beta cell insulin secretion in different populations living in diverse environments.

The beta cell dysfunction in patients with NIDDM is manifested as the loss or blunting of the acute first-phase and early insulin release to glucose stimulation (Fig. 12.2). This aberration

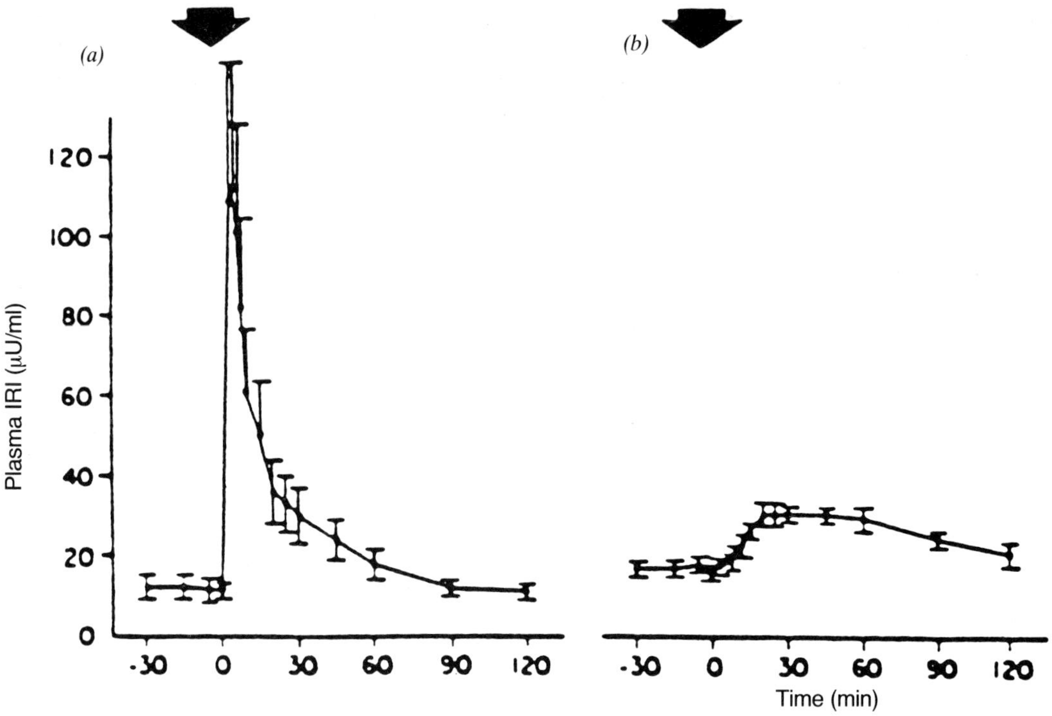


Fig. 12.2. Beta cell insulin responses to intravenous glucose challenge in (*a*) healthy subjects and (*b*) in patients with NIDDM. The arrow represents the time of intravenous glucose administration. Note the loss of the acute first phase insulin release (*t*=0–5 min) in the NIDDM patients. (Adapted with the permission from American Diabetes Association.)

appears to be specific for glucose-dependent or glucose-mediated insulin release, but not to non-glucose stimuli such as arginine, glucagon, tolbutamide, etc. The mechanism of the glucose unresponsiveness by the beta cells in the patients with idiopathic NIDDM is unknown. However, several recent studies have linked the abnormality to the transport and subsequent metabolism of intracellular glucose by the beta cells (32–36). The glucokinase (GCK) enzyme is the rate-limiting step that catalyses the ATP-dependent phosphorylation of glucose to glucose-6-phosphate. The latter is an important substrate that initiates the glycolytic process. In this regard, the glucokinase (GCK) enzyme is now considered the potential candidate for the putative intracellular beta cell glucose sensor. The GCK gene is reported to be located on chromosome 7b in different populations (32, 35, 36). Although to date, abnormalities in the glucokinase activity and genetic mutations have been identified in only a few patients with idiopathic late- or adult-onset NIDDM, recent studies in patients with maturity onset diabetes of the youth (MODY), or the early-onset NIDDM, have identified genetic mutations in the glucokinase gene in some patients (32–34). These studies have also demonstrated that the acute first or early phase insulin release is often decreased in patients with glucokinase gene mutation than the first-degree relatives without the GCK gene defect. Note that there are several genetic defects (nonsense and missense mutations and deletions) in the glucokinase gene in different patients and siblings from the same ethnic group, families and race (32, 34). Velho *et al.* (33) reported that nine patients with

MODY from four kindreds had mutant GCK. Similarly, in the study by Froguel *et al.* (32), 16 mutations were identified in the 18 of the 32 families with MODY, but none was found in the families with late-onset NIDDM. In contrast, Katagiri *et al.* (34) found five NIDDM in their Japanese pedigree with nonsense mutation of the GCK gene. Note, however, that in many family pedigree studies, not all the siblings with identifiable genetic mutations in GCK gene manifest defective insulin secretion and diabetes. Whether such individuals would eventually develop beta cell decompensation in later life remains to be elucidated in long-term prospective studies. It is worthy also to note that several studies have failed to identify any GCK gene mutations in Caucasian patients with idiopathic NIDDM (38). Finally, in the Mauritian Creoles, Chiu *et al.* (37) have reported a higher frequency of the Z + 2 allele of the GCK gene in patients with NIDDM. However, the frequency of the Z allele which is very common in the Creoles was lower in the diabetic patients. Of interest is that, in the Mauritian Indians, no differences in the frequency of the individual alleles were observed in the diabetic and non-diabetic populations (36). In addition, Chiu *et al.* (36) have indicated that the Z + 4 allele confers greater risk for NIDDM in the American blacks. However, in a recent report (37) these investigators were unable to identify any structural abnormalities of GCK in the American blacks. Although, these studies indicate that the alterations in glucokinase gene may be important in the pathogenesis of early onset NIDDM or MODY, this may be racially and ethnically dependent. Moreover, its role in idiopathic adult-onset NIDDM remains debatable.

Because of the difficulty in identifying genetic markers of NIDDM, several investigators have resorted to investigating early insulin secretory changes in an attempt to identify individuals at risk for developing idiopathic NIDDM (15–25). These studies are usually performed in the offspring, siblings and the first-degree relatives of patients with NIDDM as well as ethnic groups with extraordinary propensity to develop the disease. The experimental approaches for these metabolic studies have varied considerably in different laboratories ranging from simple oral glucose tolerance test to euglycaemic or hyperglycaemic hyperinsulinaemic clamp technique (39) as well as the minimal model method described by Bergman and his colleagues (40, 41). In the western world, the general consensus is that first-degree relatives of patients with NIDDM manifest both fasting and/or stimulated hyperinsulinaemia as well as insulin insensitivity when compared to the healthy controls (15–25). These findings tend to argue against the lower acute and early insulin release found in the patients with impaired glucose tolerance (IGT), MODY and NIDDM as the earliest and primary lesions that result in the genesis of the disease. However, it is clear that these healthy, first-degree relatives will eventually develop beta cell secretory dysfunction in the later life prior to clinical disease. This would be consistent with the exhaustion theory of the pancreatic beta cells (42–47). In the study by Warram *et al.* (21), only 25 of 156 offspring who had fasting and post-glucose hyperinsulinaemia developed the disease during 6–25 yr follow-up.

Recently, several investigators have reported that the immunoreactive insulin (IRI) concentrations measured in patients with NIDDM is not true insulin since the current radioimmunoassays, substantially, cross-react with pro-insulin (PI) and its intermediate split products (48–55). The PI and its split products have less biological action in the peripheral tissues when compared to true insulin. Most importantly, recent reports have shown that the component of the PI in the IRI is elevated in the patients with NIDDM (50–52, 54, 55). However, the alterations in the PI are not evident in non-diabetic, first-degree relatives (51) and remain controversial in patients with impaired glucose tolerance test (51, 54, 55). Thus, it appears that the elevation in the PI is secondary to the persistent hyperglycaemia, but not to the insulin resistant state *per se* (53, 54).

Nevertheless, it remains to be determined whether the disproportionate elevation in the PI/IRI ratios in family members could represent a beta cell marker for future development of NIDDM. Furthermore, in patients with MODY and the rare patients with NIDDM due to mutant GCK gene, it would be of great interest to examine the PI/IRI ratios.

Previous histological findings in pancreata of patients with NIDDM have demonstrated an increased content of amyloid that could not be attributed to age alone. Recently, several investigators have demonstrated amyloid-like peptide, amylin, in the pancreata of both human and animal NIDDM models (56–64). The cloning of amylin gene with subsequent synthesis of amylin has confirmed the pancreatic source on this protein (56, 57). Moreover, the peptide is found in the circulation of healthy subjects and patients with NIDDM (56, 58, 60, 61). Of interest is that amylin is co-segregated in the beta cell as well as co-secreted with insulin, c-peptide and PI by similar secretagogues (58–60). This has raised considerable interest in its potential role in the pathogenesis of the disease (57, 62, 63). In the *in vitro* and experimental animal studies, amylin has been demonstrated to impair beta cell insulin release as well as glucose uptake (62, 63). However, this initial enthusiasm has not been substantiated in several studies in humans (64). Thus, the role of amylin in the genesis of hyperglycaemia in humans remains to be defined in future studies. In a recent report, the mRNA content of the amylin gene was similar in the diabetic and non-diabetic Pima Indians (56). Thus, altered genetic mutation appears to be an unlikely cause of the increased amylin in the NIDDM patients. Furthermore, the amylin concentrations in the *in vivo* studies, in which peripheral insulin resistance has been demonstrated, were in the supraphysiological and/or pharmacological ranges.

Beta cell insulin release occurs in pulsatile manner in humans and experimental animals (65–67). The pulsatility is considered as a necessary prerequisite for the expression of the full biological actions of insulin (68, 69). Several previous studies have shown that pancreatic insulin release entrains the glucose output by the liver. In patients with NIDDM, it is now well established that this pulsatility of insulin release as well as the temporal relations with glucose are disorganised, while the peaks and amplitudes are blunted (66). Polonsky *et al.* (66) have also reported decreased ultradian insulin release in the NIDDM patients when compared to the healthy control subjects as shown in Fig. 12.3. O'Rahilly *et al.* (67), have also reported that impaired glucose-tolerant, first-degree relatives of patients with NIDDM have blunted insulin pulsatility. The mechanism for the impaired insulin pulsatility in the patients with IGT and NIDDM remains unknown. Whether this is genetically inherited or reflects predisposition to future diabetes remains to be investigated. In this light, it has been previously demonstrated that the insulin secretion in monozygotic twins tends to be identical. Indeed, the first-degree relatives of Caucasian and African–American NIDDM patients have consistently demonstrated greater insulin concentrations than the healthy controls (14, 15, 17, 19–24). Furthermore, recent evidence indicates racial differences in the insulin secretion and metabolism in African–Americans (22–25), Pima Indians (17) and Afro-Caribbeans (8), manifesting greater insulin levels when compared to the Caucasians. Although, these studies support the role of genetic inheritance in the alterations of beta cell insulin release, other factors such as diet and physical activity contribute significantly to the insulin secretion and glucose homeostasis. In this regard, a preliminary study from our laboratory has demonstrated that first-degree relatives of native African NIDDM patients residing in Nigeria manifest lower serum insulin concentrations when compared to the healthy control subjects without positive family history of diabetes (28). Furthermore, metabolic studies in the obese southern African blacks have demonstrated markedly lower serum insulin and c-peptide levels when compared to whites (29, 30).

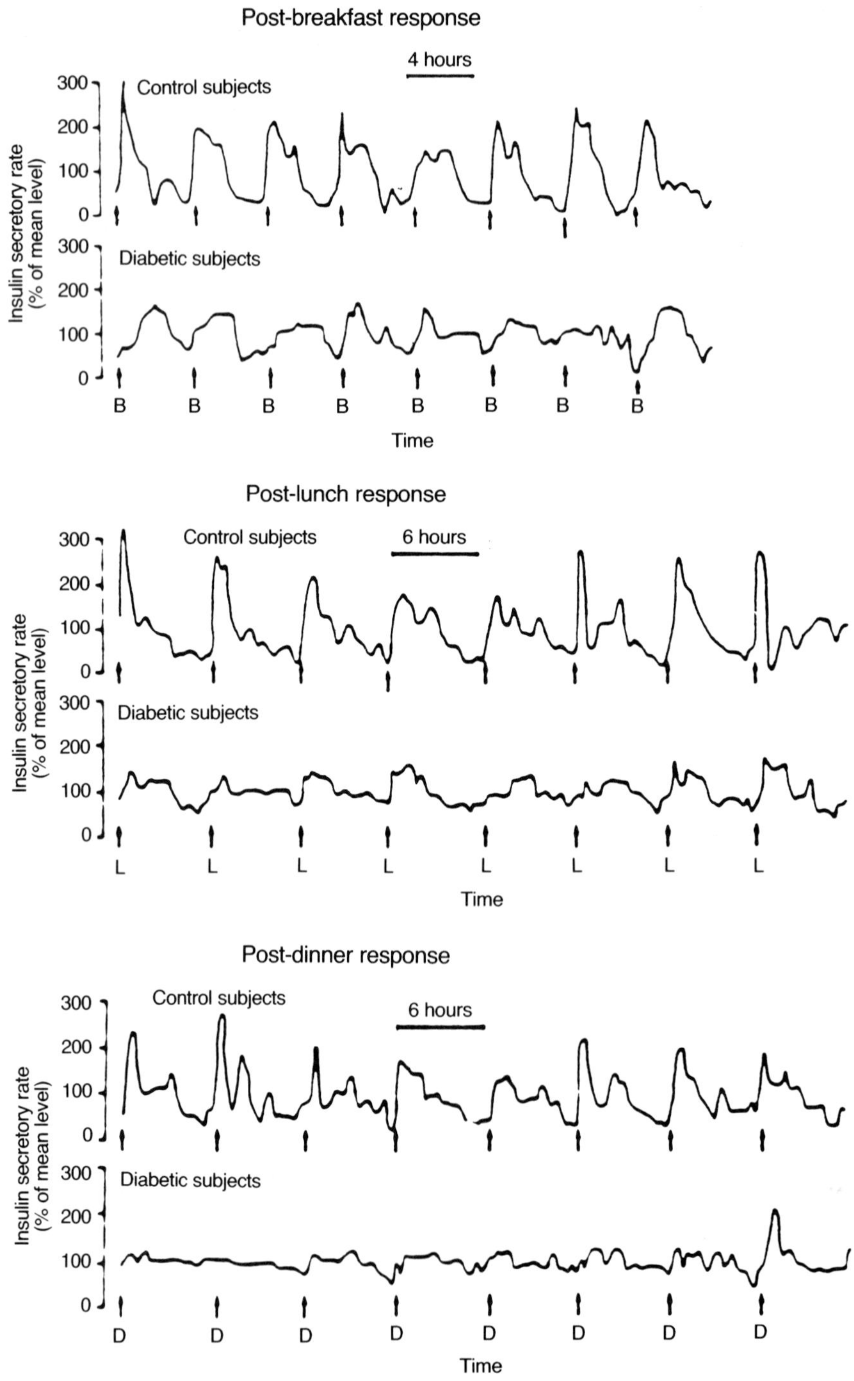


Fig. 12.3. Pulsatile insulin release in NIDDM patients and healthy control subjects. (Adapted with permission of *New England Journal of Medicine*.)

These findings in the native Africans are in contrast to those of African–Americans and Afro-Caribbeans living in the western countries. The reason for this discrepant and disparate beta cell secretion remains unknown in different races but deserves to be elucidated in future studies.

## AETIOLOGY OF HEPATIC GLUCOSE PRODUCTION IN THE NIDDM

The liver plays an essential and critical role in the pathogenesis of the basal and post-prandial hyperglycaemia in patients with NIDDM (70–75). The basal hepatic glucose production is considered as a major determinant of fasting hyperglycaemia in patients with NIDDM (75). As shown in Fig. 12.4, the basal HGP correlates positively with the fasting plasma glucose. Several factors contribute to the increased hepatic glucose over-production. There is increasing evidence to indicate that the insulin- and/or glucose-mediated suppression of hepatic glucose production is impaired in the patients with NIDDM (73–78). However, because of methodo-

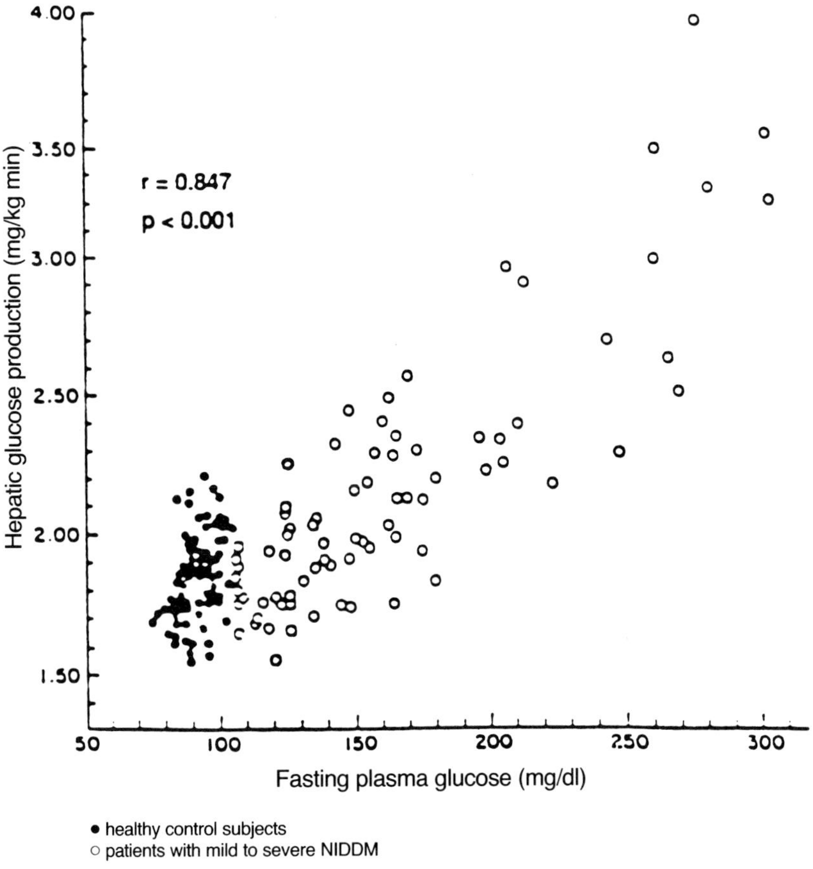


Fig. 12.4. Relationships between basal hepatic glucose production and fasting plasma glucose level in healthy control subjects (closed circles) and in patients with mild to severe NIDDM (open circles). (Adapted with permission from American Diabetes Association.)

Table 12.2. *Summary of genetic and environmental factors affecting beta cell function*

| Genetic | Environmental |
|---|---|
| 1. Glucose transporter 2 defect | 1. Chemical toxins, e.g. alcohol, vacor, etc. |
| 2. Decreased glucokinase activity | 2. Malnutrition-related |
| 3. Glucokinase gene mutation | 3. Chronic pancreatitis |
| 4. Defects in intracellular calcium and potassium metabolism | 4. Amylin accumulation |
| 5. Defects in phosphoinositol | 5. Intrauterine environment |
| 6. Defects in enteroinsular axis, e.g. decreased GIP, GLP-1, CCK | 6. Drugs, e.g. thiazide, beta blockers generation |

GIP=Gastric inhibitory polypeptide; GLP-1=glucagon-like peptide-1, CCK=cholecystokinin.

logical differences, the extent of hepatic glucose suppressibility has remained controversial. Using superphysiological and/or supraphysiological levels of serum insulin concentrations during the euglycaemic clamp, it has been argued that the hepatic glucose suppression is intact in patients with NIDDM when compared to healthy control subjects (72–74). However, using low physiological insulin levels Groop *et al.* (77) and Efendic *et al.* (78) have reported that the suppression of HGP is impaired even in these patients with mild disease. Indeed, several investigators have reported that, an enhanced hepatic glucose production with increased rate of glucose appearance is the major determinant of postprandial hyperglycaemia even in patients with impaired glucose tolerance. Note that the total rate of glucose disappearance is often increased in patients with hyperglycaemia due to the mass action effect, while the metabolic clearance rate of glucose (MCR) is decreased or similar to that of the healthy controls.

The mechanism(s) for the impaired hepatic glucose production or dysregulation in the NIDDM remains debatable but appears to be multifactorial (72–79). Some of the factors responsible for the excess hepatic glucose production are shown in Table 12.3. In patients with NIDDM, the basal serum glucagon levels are often elevated in the face of inappropriately decreased portal insulin resulting in an increased intrahepatic glucagon/insulin ratio. This could contribute to the excess HGP by stimulating the gluconeogenic mechanism. Secondly, free fatty acid (FFA), lactic acid, arginine, glycerol, etc., levels which constitute the major gluconeogenic precursors are often increased in patients with NIDDM (80–82). Thirdly, the hepatic insulin receptor number may be decreased in the hepatocytes of patients and experimental models of NIDDM (83, 84). The latter can result in alterations in the hepatic extraction of insulin which may be important for the hepatic action of insulin. Fourthly, the beta cells share the same GCK as the hepatocytes. Thus, it is possible that a simultaneous mutation in the hepatic GCK gene could co-exist with beta cell GCK gene mutation in some patients with NIDDM. This could alter the conversion of glucose to G-6-P, a critical step in the subsequent glucose metabolism. Finally, the Glut-2 glucose transporter number, activity and intracytoplasmic translocation to the plasma membrane may be defective in the hepatocytes in patients with NIDDM (85, 86). Alcolado *et al.* (85) found that the allele frequency for the Taq 1 restriction fragment length polymorphism (RFLP) for GluT-2 is increased in 60 unrelated Caucasian NIDDM patients when compared to those of racially matched 122 subjects with no family history of the disease. However, the EcoR1 RFLP for the GluT-2 in the liver/islet was not associated with NIDDM in the Caucasians in the study by Elbein *et al.* (86).

The hepatic glucose metabolism depends on the efficient uptake of glucose into the hepatocyte, a non-insulin-dependent process. Intrahepatic glucose can undergo active glycolysis, resulting in 3-carbon atom moieties, which eventually enter the Kreb's cycle or are diverted into the non-oxidative pathway in the form of glycogen storage or the synthesis of lipids and lipoproteins. A key metabolic substrate in the glycolytic pathway is the fructo 2,6 bisphosphate (F2,6P) (87–91). This substrate is an important co-factor for the rate-limiting enzyme, 6-phosphofructo-1-kinase, for the glycolytic pathway (87). Furthermore, F2,6P suppresses gluconeogenesis in the liver by inhibiting fructo 1,6 phosphatase (87). The content of the hepatic F2,6P is modulated by several hormones and substrates. While insulin and glucose increase the F2,6P in the liver, glucagon and epinephrine decrease the hepatic content of this substrate (89–91). Previous studies have shown that the content of this substrate is markedly decreased in the liver of experimental diabetic animals when compared with non-diabetic animals (91). Despite the critical role of this substrate in the hepatic glucose metabolism, it has not been extensively evaluated in the hepatocytes of patients with NIDDM due to ethical reasons. Thus, whether F2,6P plays any significant role in human diabetes remains to be elucidated. Pilkis *et al.* (88) have extensively reviewed this topic in their recent publications.

## AETIOLOGY OF INSULIN RESISTANCE IN NIDDM

The role of insulin resistance in the aetiology of the hyperglycaemia in patients with NIDDM is now very well established (39, 40, 70–78). The insulin resistance is found predominantly in the insulin sensitive tissues, namely the liver, adipose tissue and the skeletal muscles (69–72). As shown in Fig. 12.5, the latter appears to be the most important quantitatively, since the skeletal muscles are responsible for at least 40% of the total body glucose disposal after meal stimulation (70–72). Although the causes of the insulin resistance remain controversial, recent studies have identified several potential mechanisms as

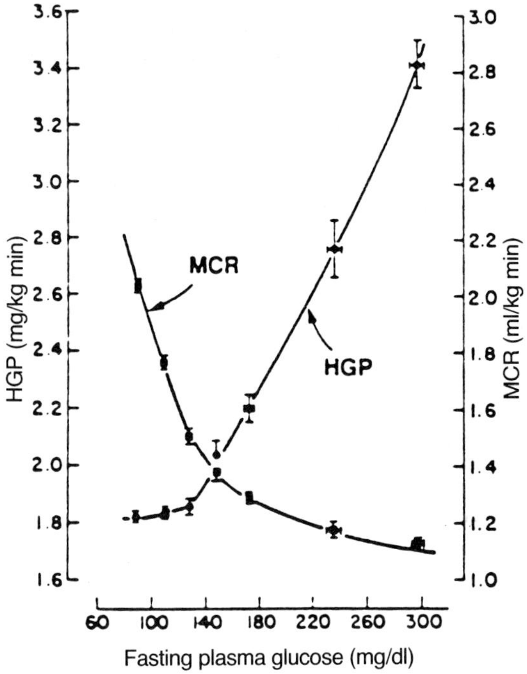


Fig. 12.5. Relationships between basal hepatic glucose production (HGP), fasting serum glucose (FSG) and metabolic clearance rate of glucose (MCR) in patients with NIDDM and healthy control subjects. (Adapted with permission from the American Diabetes Association.)

shown in Table 12.3. In this regard, most patients with idiopathic NIDDM have predominantly postreceptor insulin abnormalities that are responsible for the alterations in glucose disposal in various NIDDM models (70–78), although few patients with insulin receptor defect due to mutant genes have been reported (92). First, the insulin receptor tyrosine kinase activity has been demonstrated to be decreased in the skeletal muscle (93) and adipose tissues (94) of patients with NIDDM and experimental diabetic models, respectively. Secondly, several recent studies have shown a diminished insulin-stimulated glycogen synthase activity in the skeletal muscles of healthy, first-degree relatives of patients with NIDDM as well as patients with clinical diabetes and obesity (95–99). The glycogen synthase is responsible for the glycogen syn-

Table 12.3. *Summary of potential genetic and environmental factors affecting hepatic glucose production*

| Genetic | Environmental |
|---|---|
| 1. Hepatic insulin receptor defect | 1. Decreased intrahepatic insulin |
| 2. Decreased hepatic insulin extraction | 2. Increased intrahepatic glucagon |
| 3. Decreased glucokinase activity | 3. Increased free fatty acid |
| 4. Glucokinase gene mutation | 4. Increased gluconeogenic precursors, e.g. alanine, glycerol |
| 5. GluT-2 glucose transporter defect | 5. Enhanced hepatic responsiveness to stress hormones |
| 6. Defective hepatic fructo 2,6 bisphosphate content? | 6. Altered intrahepatic innervation? |
| 7. Defective hepatic autoregulation? | |

thesis and glucose storage in man, both processes are markedly decreased in the patients with NIDDM (97, 98). Thirdly, the phosphorylase phosphatase activity is also impaired in these patients (97, 99).

Despite these important recent observations regarding insulin resistance in patients with NIDDM, the actual genetic defect(s) remains unknown. However, the genetic basis of the insulin resistance is indirectly supported by several lines of evidence (96, 97, 100–104). Recently, Vaag *et al.* (96) have reported that the non-diabetic and non-obese first-degree relatives of patients with NIDDM manifest decreased insulin-mediated glycogen synthase activity which appears to antecede the development of the disease by decades. Similarly, Schalin-Janti *et al.* (97) have reported that the glycogen synthase and phosphorylase phosphatase activities are reduced in first-degree relatives of patients with NIDDM. Furthermore, Wells *et al.* (103) have demonstrated impaired activation of glycogen synthesis and thymidine incorporation in fibroblasts of non-diabetic first-degree relatives of NIDDM patients.

The most important evidence for the genetic basis of insulin resistance is derived from metabolic studies in first-degree relatives (siblings, offspring) of patients with NIDDM. Several previous reports have demonstrated that both fasting and/or post-stimulation hyperinsulinaemia, an indirect evidence of insulin resistance, exist in the first-degree relatives of NIDDM patients who reside in the western world, especially the Caucasians, Mexican–Americans, African–Americans and native American Indians (15–25). Thus, it has been argued that the insulin resistance is the primary lesion underlying the disease and that the beta cell secretory defects are secondary phenomena or epiphenomena associated with the former (15–25). Indeed, Warram *et al.* (21) and Martin *et al.* (22) have demonstrated that the glucose decay constant ($K_G$) as well as insulin sensitivity index ($S_I$) are decreased in the first-degree relatives and offspring of patients with NIDDM while the acute phase insulin release remain intact decades prior to developing the disease. Furthermore, the insulin resistance and hyperinsulinaemia are regarded as important predictors for future development of NIDDM in the first-degree relatives and offspring of patients with NIDDM in the western world (6, 21, 22). Finally, note that the hyperinsulinaemia *per se* could worsen the insulin resistance by down-regulating the tissue insulin receptors (105–108). A summary of the comparison of common biochemical abnormalities in persons at risk for NIDDM and patients with established disease is shown in Table 12.1.

Another potential mechanism of the insulin resistance in NIDDM has been ascribed to the alterations in the glucose transporter activity and protein content in skeletal muscles (109–110). The alterations in GluT-4 isoform of the glucose transporter which is found mainly in the skeletal muscles is viewed as the major candidate for the insulin resistance especially during insulin stimulation (109). Note that, in the basal state, the glucose transport and disposal is by the non-insulin-dependent mechanism via the GluT-1 transporters in humans and experimental animals. Recent studies have suggested that the major abnormality in the GluT-4 glucose transporters is not the transporter protein content or the mRNA, but the translocation of the intracellular glucose transporter pool to the surface membrane, a process which is both insulin responsive and sensitive. It is of interest to note that some investigators have reported a positive relation between the total body glucose disposal with the GluT-4 transporter content in healthy subjects and patients with NIDDM, but others did not. It is worth noting that Eriksson *et al.* (110) have demonstrated that, in the insulin resistant first-degree relatives of NIDDM patients, the GluT-4 transporter protein content and mRNA are reported to be similar to that of the healthy control subjects without family history of diabetes. Thus, further studies are clearly needed to define the mechanism of GluT-4 transporter activity in the overall peripheral glucose uptake in humans.

Several substrates are also known to interfere with glucose metabolism. In this regard free fatty acid has received the most attention (80–82, 111, 112). This has been attributed to the classic report by Randle *et al.* (111) in 1963 which demonstrated that FFA inhibits glucose oxidation in the isolated heart and diaphragm muscles from rats. This process has been termed glucose-free fatty acid cycle. Several human studies have suggested that FFA could inhibit the glucose oxidation and disposal, but the clinical and physiological significances have been conflicting since most of these studies employed supraphysiological and non-physiological concentrations of FFA (112, 113). Thus, whether physiological FFA levels would impair glucose disposal and oxidation remains uncertain. Note that Fulcher *et al.* (113) have demonstrated that reduction in FFA levels by acipomox decreases hepatic glucose production as well as increases peripheral and hepatic sensitivities to insulin action in patients with NIDDM. Of great interest is that alterations in FFA metabolism could occur simultaneously with those of glucose metabolism in the glucose-tolerant, first-degree relatives and offspring of patients with NIDDM (114–116). The study by Gulli and his coworkers (115) in the offspring and first-degree relatives of non-diabetic Mexican–American NIDDM is somewhat similar to that reported by Osei *et al.* (116) in Caucasians, but at odds with that of Eriksson *et al.* (117). However, when taken together, we are tempted to conclude that the glucose-tolerant, first-degree relatives of Caucasian patients with NIDDM manifest multiple metabolic defects in insulin action that antecede the development of clinical diabetes by decades. Whether these multiple defects are co-inherited remains to be proven in different ethnic and racial populations.

Obesity is common in patients with NIDDM and occurs in 90% of patients with NIDDM in the western world (1–6). Obesity *per se* without association with positive family history of diabetes is often associated with hyperinsulinaemia and insulin resistance (118). Thus, obesity (body mass index greater than 27 kg/m$^2$) tends to aggravate the insulin resistance found in patients with NIDDM. Indeed, a significant weight reduction in obese patients with NIDDM often results in decreased insulin resistance and normalisation or improvement in glucose homeostasis (119). For decades, the pattern of body fat distribution has been recognised as an important risk factor for several diseases. Since the original description by Vague J. (120), the upper body fat distribution pattern has been shown to be associated with alterations in glucose homeostasis, hyperlipidaemia and cardiovascular risk factors in patients with NIDDM and non-diabetic individuals (120–123). Furthermore, the upper body obesity is associated with increased intra-abdominal lipolysis and perhaps an enhanced FFA delivery to the liver and subsequently, the peripheral tissues (121). In this light, it has been argued that the increased body fat content, insulin resistance and hyperinsulinaemia may be co-inherited in individuals who are susceptible to develop NIDDM and other cardiovascular diseases in later life (15, 124–126). Although the available evidence implicates obesity in the aetiology of insulin resistance and hyperinsulinaemia in patients with NIDDM and their first-degree relatives, note that the latter can occur in the absence of obesity.

## AETIOLOGY OF ALTERED GLUCOSE-DEPENDENT GLUCOSE TRANSPORT IN NIDDM

The glucose transport and disposal are determined by two main mechanisms in humans and experimental animals, namely the insulin-mediated and non-insulin-mediated components. Although the latter could be demonstrated *in vitro*, the measurement of the glucose-dependent glucose disposal in the absence of insulin *in vivo* is physiologically untenable and has been difficult to study in the past in humans. Recently, the introduction of the Bergman's minimal model method (16, 22, 40, 41, 127) has provided a means of quantifying the glucose-dependent glucose disposal parameters in humans and experimental animals with and without alterations in glucose and insulin metabolism, although this mathematical model remains controversial. The non-insulin-dependent glucose disposal, also referred to as glucose effectiveness ($S_G$), is reported to be normal in most first-degree relatives of patients with NIDDM (15) and individuals with obesity (41). However, in the diabetic state with hyperglycaemia, the $S_G$ is reported to be markedly decreased in conjunction with the reduced insulin sensitivity index ($S_I$) (127). This is in contrast with a previous report by Baron *et al.* (128) in which the non-insulin-dependent glucose uptake (NIMGU) was assessed using euglycaemic clamp technique. Furthermore, Taniguchi *et al.* (31), employing the insulin-modified frequent sampling intravenous glucose tolerance test (127), have demonstrated that, in non-obese Japanese NIDDM patients with mild disease, the $S_G$ is markedly reduced while the $S_I$ remains normal. In addition, experimental studies by Kahn *et al.* (129) have demonstrated that s.c. injection of octreotide resulted in a reduced insulin secretion and mild hyperglycaemia in healthy subjects in their study. While insulin sensitivity ($S_I$) remained normal, the $S_G$ was markedly reduced. Similarly, Tobin *et al.* (130) have reported that in non-diabetic pancreatic autotransplanted rats, the decreased plasma insulin levels resulted in a reduced $S_G$ while the $S_I$ remained normal. Furthermore, Page *et al.* (131) have reported that patients with Cushing's syndrome and impaired glucose tolerance have a reduction in both $S_I$ and $S_G$. While the $S_I$ improves, following normalisation of plasma cortisol, the $S_G$ remains decreased. These recent studies have provided important data on the role of $S_G$ in the pathogenesis of altered glucose homeostasis in several disease states. However, whether the reduced $S_G$ is genetically inherited or acquired has been controversial. We have previously reported that the $S_G$ is normal while $S_I$ is reduced by 45% in first-degree relatives of NIDDM patients in a cross-sectional study (16). In this regard, the recent report by Martin *et al.* (22) in a retrospective analyses of their metabolic data, demonstrated that offspring of two diabetic parents with the lower quintile for $S_G$ (albeit within normal limits) and $S_I$ have 76% cumulative risk of developing future NIDDM in a 25 year follow-up study (Fig. 12.6). This latter study has, for the first time, clearly demonstrated that both insulin- and glucose-tissue resistance are necessary prerequisites for the development of NIDDM, and tend to antecede the disease by decades. If this study is further confirmed by other investigators, it will be also necessary to search, not only for the insulin resistance genes, but also those for the tissue glucose resistance. Whether concomitant alterations in both $S_I$ and/or $S_G$ serve as risk factors for the disease in other non-white ethnic populations remain to be investigated.

In summary, the aetiology of NIDDM is complex and involves the interplay of both genetic and non-genetic factors (e.g. diet, physical

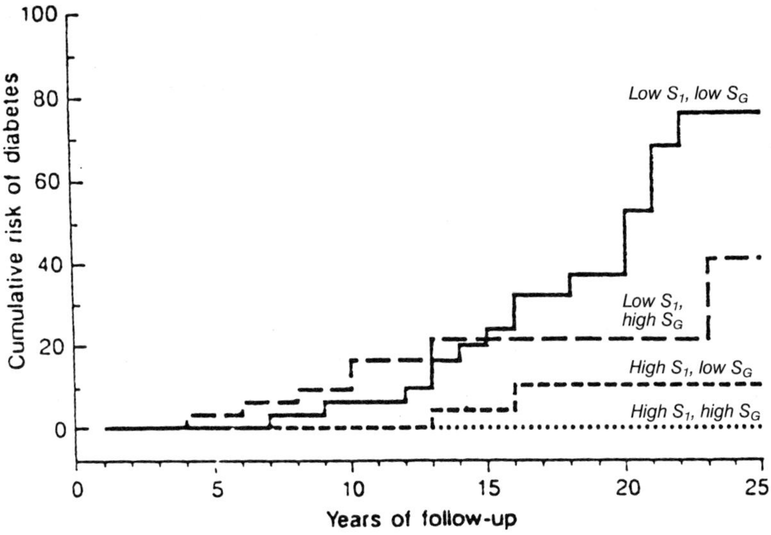


Fig. 12.6. Per cent cumulative risk of developing NIDDM based on the quintiles of both $S_I$ and $S_G$ in the offspring of two parent diabetic patients. (Adapted with the permission from *Lancet*.)

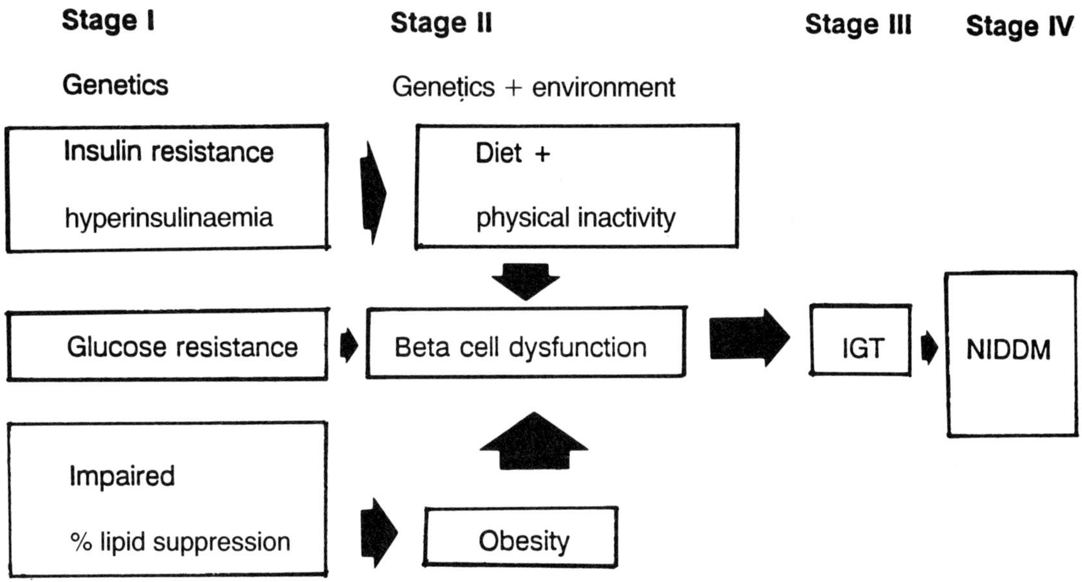


Fig. 12.7. Hypothetical stages for the development of NIDDM in humans.

Table 12.4. *Summary of common factors affecting insulin sensitivity in patients with NIDDM*

| Genetic | Environmental |
|---|---|
| 1. Polygenetic inheritance | 1. Dietary |
| 2. Decreased glycogen synthase activity | 2. Physical activity |
| 3. Glycogen synthase gene mutation | 3. Hyperinsulinaemia |
| 4. Defective tyrosine kinase activity | 4. Hyperglycaemia |
| 5. Defective protein kinase C activity | 5. Drugs, e.g. prednisone |
| 6. Race | 6. Obesity |
| 7. Obesity | 7. Intramuscular blood flow |
| 8. Decreased GluT-4 glucose transporter activity | |
| 9. Defective insulin receptor function, e.g. genetic mutation | |

activity, socioeconomic status, etc.) which evolve over decades as depicted in the hypothetical schema shown in Fig. 12.7 and Table 12.4. There are clearly racial, ethnic and geographic differences in the prevalence and incidence of the disease world-wide, although the specific aetological factors in each race remain to be elucidated. Despite the intense ongoing and promising research to identify the putative diabetic genes, this has failed to identify any specific *diabetogenic genes*, although several linkages and RFLP have been described. Based on the available evidence in the literature, it appears that the inheritance of NIDDM is polygenic with variable penetrance. Therefore, future studies should focus on the isolation of individual genes that control beta cell insulin secretion, as well as tissue insulin- and glucose-sensitivity in humans and genetic animal models of NIDDM. In the absence of specific genetic markers, however, ongoing metabolic studies in persons at greater risk for the disease could provide the necessary aetiological link between genetic and clinical manifestation of NIDDM. The understanding of these various risk factors in well-characterised populations could provide insights into the evolution and pathogenesis of the development as well as the prevention of NIDDM in humans.

## ACKNOWLEDGEMENT

We wish to thank Elizabeth Robinson for her secretarial assistance in preparing the manuscript.

## REFERENCES

1 World Health Organization. *Diabetes mellitus report of a WHO study group*. World Health Organization Geneva, 1985 (Tech Rep Ser No 727).
2 National Diabetes Criteria Data Groups. Classification and diagnosis of diabetes mellitus and other categories of glucose intolerance. *Diabetes* 1979; 28: 1039–57.
3 Zimmet P. Type 2 (non-insulin-dependent) diabetes, an epidemiological overview. *Diabetologia* 1982; 22: 399–41.
4 Bennet PH, Burch TA, Miller M. The high prevalence of diabetes in the Pima Indians of Arizona (USA). *Amsterdam, Excerpta Medical (International Congress Series)* 1970; 221: 33–9.
5 Harris MI *et al.* Prevalence of diabetes and impaired glucose tolerance and plasma glucose levels in US population aged 20–74. *Diabetes* 1987; 36: 523–4.
6 Haffner SM, *et al.* Incidence of type II diabetes in Mexican Americans predicted by fasting insulin and glucose levels, obesity and body fat distribution. *Diabetes* 1989; 39: 283–8.
7 Zimmet P, Whitehouse S, Kiss J. Ethic variability in the plasma insulin response to oral glucose in Polynesian and Micronesian subjects. *Diabetes* 1979; 28: 624–8.
8 Cruickshank JK *et al.* Ethnic differences in fasting plasma c-peptide and insulin in relation to glucose tolerance and blood pressure. *Lancet* 1991; ii: 824–7.
9 Tattersal RB, Fajans SS. A differences between the inheritance of classical juvenile-onset and maturity-onset diabetes in young people. *Diabetes* 1975; 24: 44–53.
10 Barnett AH *et al.* Diabetes in identical twins: a study of 200 pairs. *Diabetologia* 1981; 20: 87–93.
11 Tattersal RB, Fajans SS. Prevalence of diabetes and glucose intolerance in 199 offspring of 37 conjugal diabetic parents. *Diabetes* 1975; 24: 452–62.
12 Newman B, Selby JV, King MC, Slemenda C, Fabsitz R, Friedman GD. Concordance for type 2 (non-insulin-dependent) diabetes mellitus in male twins. *Diabetologia* 1987; 30: 763–8.
13 Kobberling J, Tillil H, Lorenz HJ. Genetics of type 2A and 2B diabetes mellitus [Abstract]. *Diabetes Res Clin Pract* 1983; suppl 1: 5311.
14 McLarty DG. Prevalence of diabetes and impaired glucose tolerance in rural Tanzania. *Lancet* 1989; i: 871–5.
15 Leslie RDG *et al.* Metabolic abnormalities in children of

noninsulin-dependent diabetes. *Br Med J* 1986; 394: 840–2.
16 Osei K, Cottrell DA, Orabella MM. Insulin sensitivity, glucose effectiveness and body fat distribution pattern in nondiabetic offspring of patients with NIDDM. *Diabetes Care* 1991; 14: 890–6.
17 Aronoff SL *et al.* Unexplained hyperinsulinemia in normal and prediabetic Pima Indians compared with normal Caucasians. An example of racial differences in insulin secretion. *Diabetes* 1977; 26: 827–40.
18 Erikson J *et al.* Early metabolic defects in persons at increased risk for noninsulin-dependent diabetes mellitus. *N Engl J Med* 1989; 321: 337–43.
19 Haffner SM *et al.* Increased insulin concentrations in nondiabetic offspring of diabetic patients. *N Engl J Med* 1988; 319: 1297–1301.
20 Leslie RDG *et al.* Insensitivity of insulin in offspring of noninsulin-dependent diabetic patients. *Diab Nutr Metab* 1989; 3: 235–7.
21 Warram JH *et al.* Slow glucose removal rate and hyperinsulinemia precede the development of type II diabetes in the offspring of diabetic patients. *Ann Int Med* 1990; 113: 909–15.
22 Martin BC *et al.* Role of glucose and insulin resistance in development of type II diabetes mellitus: results of a 25-year follow-up. *Lancet* 1992; i: 925–9.
23 Freedman DS *et al.* Relation of body fat distribution to hyperinsulinemia in children and adolescents. The Bogalusa Heart Study. *Am J Clin Nutr* 1987; 46: 403–10.
24 Newman WP *et al.* Relations of serum lipoprotein levels and systolic blood pressure to early atherosclerosis: The Bogalusa Heart Study. *Diabetes* 1986; 314: 138–44.
25 Svec F *et al.* Black-white contrasts in insulin levels during pubertal developments: The Bogalusa Heart Study. *Diabetes* 1992; 41: 314–17.
26 Osei K, Cottrell DA, Harris B. Differences in basal and post-stimulation glucose homeostasis in nondiabetic first-degree relatives of black and white patients with type 2 diabetes mellitus. *J Clin Endocrinol Metab* 1992; 75: 82–6.
27 Reaven GM *et al.* Nonketotic diabetes mellitus: insulin deficiency or insulin resistance. *Am J Med* 1976; 60: 80–8.
28 Ezenwaka CE *et al.* Glucose and insulin response to intravenous glucose challenge in relatives of Nigerian patients with noninsulin-dependent diabetes mellitus. *Diab Res Clin Pract* 1993; (in press).
29 Shires R, Joffe BL, Seftel HC. Maximal pancreatic beta-cell stimulation and the counter-regulatory hormonal responses in South African black and white obese subjects. *S Afr Med J* 1985; 67: 845–7.
30 Rubenstein AH *et al.* Metabolic response to oral glucose in healthy South African white, Indian and African subjects. *Br Med J* 1969; 1: 748–51.
31 Taniguchi A *et al.* Pathogenic factors responsible for glucose intolerance in patients with NIDDM. *Diabetes* 1992; 41: 1540–6.
32 Froguel P *et al.* Familial hyperglycemia due to mutations in glucokinase definition of a subtype of diabetes mellitus. *N Engl J Med* 1983 328: 697–702.
33 Velho C Primary pancreatic beta cell secretory defect caused by mutations in glucokinase gene in kindred of maturity onset diabetes of young. *Lancet* 1992; 340: 632–8.
34 Katagiri H *et al.* Nonsense mutation of glucokinase gene in late-onset non-insulin-dependent diabetes. *Lancet* 1992; 340: 1316–17.
35 Bell GI *et al.* Gene for noninsulin-dependent diabetes mellitus (maturity-onset diabetes of the young subtype) is linked to DNA polymorphism on chromosome 20q. *Proc Natl Acad Sci USA* 1990; 88: 1484–8.
36 Chiu KC, Tanizawa Y, Permutt MA. Glucokinase gene variants in the common form of NIDDM. *Diabetes* 1993; 42: 579–82.
37 Chiu KC *et al.* A genetic marker at the glucokinase gene locus for type 2 (non-insulin-dependent) diabetes mellitus in Mauritian creols. *Diabetologia* 1992; 35: 632–38.
38 Hattersley AT *et al.* Linkage analysis of glucokinase gene with NIDDM in Caucasian pedigrees. *Diabetes* 1992; 41: 1496–9.
39 DeFronzo R, Simonson D, Ferrannini E. Hepatic and peripheral insulin resistance: a common feature of type 2 (non-insulin dependent) and type 1 diabetes mellitus. *Diabetologia* 1982; 23; 313–19.
40 Bergman RN. Toward physiological understanding of glucose tolerance. Minimal-model approach. *Diabetes* 1989; 38; 1512–27.
41 Bergman RN *et al.* Equivalence of the insulin sensitivity index in man derived by the minimal model method and the euglycaemic glucose clamp. *J Clin Invest* 1987; 79: 790–800.
42 Saad MF *et al.* A two-step model for development of noninsulin-dependent diabetes. *Am J Med* 1991; 90: 229–35.
43 Hansen BC, Bodkin ML. Heterogeneity of insulin responses: phases leading to type 2 (non-insulin-dependent) diabetes mellitus in the rhesus monkey. *Diabetologia* 1986; 29: 713–19.
44 Joffe BI *et al.* Pathogenesis of noninsulin-dependent diabetes mellitus in the black population of Southern Africa. *Lancet* 1992; II: 460–2.
45 Saad MF *et al.* Sequential changes in serum insulin concentration during development of non-insulin dependent diabetes. *Lancet* 1989; i: 1356–8.
46 Saad MF *et al.* The natural history of impaired glucose tolerance in the Pima Indians. *N Engl J Med* 1988; 319, 1500–6.
47 O'Rahilly SP *et al.* Beta-cell dysfunction, fate than insulin insensitivity, is the primary defect in familial type 2 diabetes. *Lancet* 1986; I: 360–4.
48 Porte D Jr, Kahn SE. Hyperproinsulinemia and amyloid in NIDDM: Clues to etiology of B-cell dysfunction? *Diabetes* 1989; 38: 133–6.
49 Temple RC *et al.* Insulin deficiency in non-insulin-dependent diabetes. *Lancet* 1989; I: 293–5.
50 Temple RC *et al.* Radioimmunoassay may overestimate insulin in non-insulin-dependent diabetics. *Clin Endocrinol* 1990; 32: 689–93.
51 Saad MF *et al.* Disproportionately elevated pro-insulin in Pima Indians with noninsulin-dependent diabetes mellitus. *J Clin Endocrinol Metab* 1990; 70: 1247–53.
52 Davis SN *et al.* Pro-insulin and insulin concentrations following intravenous glucose challenges in normal, obese, and non-insulin-dependent diabetic subjects. *Metabolism* 1993; 42: 30–5.
53 Prigeon RL *et al.* Effect of experimental insulin resistance on pro-insulin and insulin release in the elderly with B-cell dysfunction [abstract]. *Clin Res* 1991; 39:254A.
54 Ward WK *et al.* Disproportionate elevation of immuno-

reactive pro-insulin in type 2 (non-insulin-dependent) diabetes mellitus in an experimental insulin resistance. *Diabetologia* 1987; 30: 698–72.
55 Yoskioka N *et al.* Serum pro-insulin levels at fasting and after oral glucose load in patients with type 2 (non-insulin-dependent) diabetes mellitus. *Diabetologia* 1988; 31: 335–60.
56 Nishi M, Bell GI, Steiner DF. Islet amyloid polypeptide (amylin); no evidence of an abnormal precursor sequence in 25 type 2 (non-insulin-dependent) diabetic patients. *Diabetologia* 1990; 33: 628–30.
57 Cooper GJS *et al.* Purification and characterization of a peptide from amyloid-rich pancreas of type 2 diabetic patients. *Proc Natl Acad Sci USA* 1987; 84: 8628–32.
58 Sanke T *et al.* Plasma islet amyloid polypeptide (Amylin) levels and their responses to oral glucose in type 2 (noninsulin-dependent) diabetic patients. *Diabetologia* 1990; 34: 129–32.
59 Kahn SE *et al.* Evidence of cosecretion of islet amyloid polypeptide and insulin by B-cells. *Diabetes* 1990; 39: 634–8.
60 Butler PC *et al.* Effects of meal ingestion on plasma ameslan concentration in NIDDM and nondiabetic humans. *Diabetes* 1990; 39: 752–6.
61 Clark A *et al.* Islet amyloid in diabetic and nondiabetic Pima Indians. *Diabetologia* 1990; 33: 295–9.
62 Clark A *et al.* Islet amyloid formed from diabetes-associated peptide may be pathogenetic in type 2 diabetes. *Lancet* 1987; ii: 231–4.
63 Sowa R *et al.* Islet amyloid polypeptide amide causes peripheral insulin resistance *in vivo* in dogs. *Diabetologia* 1990; 33: 118–20.
64 Bretherton-Watt D *et al.* Failure to establish islet amyloid polypeptide (amylin) as a circulating beta cell inhibiting hormone in man. *Diabetologia* 1990; 33: 115–17.
65 Jaspan JB *et al.* *In vivo* pulsatility of pancreatic islet peptides. *Am J Physiol* 1986; 251: E215–26.
66 Polonsky KS *et al.* Abnormal patterns of insulin secretion in non-insulin-dependent diabetes mellitus. *N Engl J Med* 1988; 318: 1231–9.
67 O'Rahilly S, Turner RC & Mathews DR. Impaired pulsatile secretion of insulin in relatives of patients with noninsulin-dependent diabetes mellitus. *N Engl J Med* 1988; 318: 1225–30.
68 Mathews DR *et al.* Pulsatile insulin has greater hypoglycemic effect than continuous delivery. *Diabetes* 1983; 32: 617–21.
69 Ward GM *et al.* Effects of prolonged pulsatile hyperinsulinemia in humans; enhancements of insulin sensitivity. *Diabetes* 1990; 39: 601–7.
70 Reaven GM, Moore J, Greenfield M. Quantification of insulin secretion and *in vivo* insulin action in nonobese and moderately obese individuals with hormonal glucose tolerance. *Diabetes* 1983; 32: 600–4.
71 Ginsberg H *et al.* Demonstration of insulin resistance in untreated adult diabetic subjects with fasting hyperglycemia. *J Clin Invest* 1975; 55: 454–61.
72 DeFronzo RA, Ferrannini E, Koivisto V. New concepts in the pathogenesis and treatment of noninsulin-dependent diabetes mellitus. *Am J Med* 1983; 74(suppl 1A): 52–81.
73 Kolterman OG *et al.* Receptor and postreceptor defect contribute to the insulin resistance in noninsulin-dependent diabetes mellitus. *J Clin Invest* 1981; 68: 957–63.
74 Bogardus C *et al.* Relationships between insulin secretion, insulin action and fasting plasma glucose concentration in nondiabetic and noninsulin-dependent diabetic subjects. *J Clin Invest* 1984; 74: 1238–46.
75 DeFronzo RA. Lilly Lecture 1987. The triumvirate B cell muscle liver: a collusion responsible for NIDDM. *Diabetes* 1988; 37: 667–87.
76 Magnusson I *et al.* Increased rate of gluconeogenesis in type II diabetes mellitus: A $^{13}C$ nuclear magnetic resonance study. *J Clin Invest* 1992; 90: 1323–27.
77 Groop L *et al.* Glucose and free fatty acid metabolism in noninsulin dependent diabetes mellitus: evidence for multiple sites of insulin resistance. *J Clin Invest* 1989; 84: 205–13.
78 Efendic S, Karlander S, Vranic M. Mild type II diabetes markedly increases glucose cycling in the postabsorptive state and during glucose infusion irrespective of obesity. *J Clin Invest* 1988; 81: 1953–61.
79 Jackson RA *et al.* Impact of glucose ingestion on hepatic and peripheral glucose metabolism in man: an analysis based on simultaneous use of the forearm and double isotope techniques. *J Clin Endocrinol Metab* 1986; 63: 541–9.
80 Bevilacqua S *et al.* Acute elevation in free fatty acid levels leads to hepatic glucose resistance in obese subjects. *Metabolism* 1987; 36: 502–7.
81 Ferrannini E *et al.* Effect of fatty acids on glucose production and utilization in man. *J Clin Invest* 1983; 72: 1737–47.
82 Golay A *et al.* Relationships between plasma free fatty acid concentration, endogenous glucose production and fasting hyperglycemia in normal and non-insulin-dependent diabetic individuals. *Metab Clin Exp* 1987; 36: 692–6.
83 Caro JF *et al.* Studies on the mechanism of insulin resistance in the liver from humans with noninsulin-dependent diabetes. *J Clin Invest* 1986; 78: 249–58.
84 Arner P *et al.* Studies of the human liver insulin receptor in noninsulin dependent diabetes mellitus. *J Clin Invest* 1986; 77: 1716–18.
85 Alcolado JC, Baroni MG, Li SL. Association between a restriction fragment length polymorphism at the liver/islet cell (GLUT 2) glucose transporter and familial type (non-insulin-dependent) diabetes mellitus. *Diabetologia* 1991; 34: 734–6.
86 Elbein SC *et al.* Linkage analysis of GLUT 1 (Hep G2) and GLUT 2 (liver/islet) genes in familial NIDDM. *Diabetes* 1992; 41: 1660–7.
87 El-Maghrabi MR *et al.* Cyclic AMP-dependent phosphorylation of rat liver 6-phosphofructo 2-kinase/fructo 2, 6-bisphosphate. *Biochem Biophys Res Commun* 1982; 106: 794–802.
88 Pilkis JJ, El-Maghrabi MR, Claus TH. Fructose-2 6-bisphosphate in control of hepatic gluconeogenesis: from metabolites to molecular genetics. *Diabetics Care* 1990; 13: 582–99.
89 Neely PK *et al.* Effect of diabetes, insulin, starvation and refeeding on the level of rat hepatic fructose, 2, 6-bisphosphate. *Diabetes* 1981; 30: 1062–4.
90 Claus TH *et al.* The role of Fru-2, 6-P in the regulation

of hepatic carbohydrate metabolism. *Curr Top Cell Regul* 1984; 23: 57–86.
91 Hue L, Blackmore P, Exton JH. Fructose 2, 6 bisphosphate; hormonal regulation and mechanism of its formation in liver. *J Biol Chem* 1981; 256: 8900–5.
92 Taylor SI. Molecular mechanisms of insulin resistance: lesions from patients with mutations in the insulin-receptor gene. *Diabetes* 1992; 41: 1473–90.
93 Nyomba BL *et al.* Insulin sensitivity and tyrosine kinase activity changes in parallel with plasma insulin and glucose concentrations in humans. *J Clin Endocrinol Metab* 1991; 72: 1212–19.
94 Ortmeyer HK, Bodkin NL, Hansen BC. Adipose tissue glycogen synthase activation by *in vivo* insulin in spontaneously insulin-resistant and type 2 (non-insulin-dependent) diabetic rhesus monkeys. *Diabetologia* 1993; 36: 200–6.
95 Bogardus C *et al.* Correlation between muscle glycogen synthase activity and *in vivo* insulin action in man. *J Clin Invest* 1984; 73: 1185–90.
96 Vaag A, Henriksen JE, Beck-Nielsen H. Decreased insulin activation of glycogen synthase in skeletal muscles in young non-obese Caucasian first-degree relatives of patients with non-insulin-dependent diabetes mellitus. *J Clin Invest* 1988; 89: 782–8.
97 Schalin-Janti C, Harkonen M, Groop LC. Impaired activation of glycogen synthase in people at increased risk for developing NIDDM. *Diabetes* 1992; 41: 598–604.
98 Johnson AB *et al.* Impaired activation of skeletal muscle glycogen synthase in non-insulin-dependent diabetes mellitus is unrelated to the degree of obesity. *Metabolism* 1991; 40: 252–60.
99 Rothman DL Shulman RG, Shulman GI. $^{31}$P nuclear magnetic resonance measurements of muscle glucose-6-phosphate. Evidence for reduced insulin-dependent muscle glucose transport or phosphorylation activity in non-insulin-dependent diabetes mellitus. *J Clin Invest* 1992; 89: 1069–75.
100 Haring HU, Mehnert H. Pathogenesis of type 2 (non-insulin-dependent) diabetes mellitus: candidates for a signal transmitter defect causing insulin resistance of the skeletal muscle. *Diabetologia* 1993; 36: 176–82.
101 Wing JR. Changes in glucose disposal and cellular insulin binding in obese black southern African patients with type 2 diabetes mellitus before and after sulfonylurea therapy. *Diabetic Med* 1993; 10: 50–5.
102 Groop LC *et al.* Association between polymorphism of the glycogen synthase gene and non-insulin-dependent diabetes mellitus. *N Engl J Med* 1993; 328: 10–14.
103 Wells AM *et al.* Abnormal activation of glycogen synthesis in fibroblasts from NIDDM subjects: evidence for an abnormality specific to glucose metabolism. *Diabetes* 1993; 42: 583–9.
104 Kida Y *et al.* Defective insulin response of phosphonylase phosphatase in insulin-resistant humans. *J Clin Invest* 1992; 89: 610–17.
105 Olefsky JM, Reaven GM. Insulin binding in diabetes. Relationship with plasma insulin levels and insulin sensitivity. *Diabetes* 1977; 26: 680–8.
106 Gavin J *et al.* Insulin dependent regulation of insulin receptor concentrations – a direct demonstration in cell culture. *Proc Natl Acad Sci USA* 1974; 71: 84–8.
107 Rizza R *et al.* Production of insulin resistance by hyperinsulinemia in man. *Diabetologia* 1985; 28: 70–5.
108 Marangou AG *et al.* Metabolic consequences of prolonged hyperinsulinemia in humans: evidence of induction of insulin insensitivity. *Diabetes* 1986; 35: 1383–9.
109 Buse JB *et al.* Human Glut 4/muscle-fat glucose-transporter gene; characterization and genetic variation. *Diabetes* 1992; 41: 1436–45.
110 Eriksson J *et al.* Insulin resistance in type 2 (non-insulin-dependent) diabetic patients and their relatives is not associated with a defect in the expression of the insulin-responsive glucose transporter (GLUT-4) gene in human skeletal muscle. *Diabetologia* 1992; 35: 143–7.
111 Randle PJ *et al.* The glucose fatty acid cycle: its role in insulin sensitivity and the metabolic disturbances of diabetes. *Lancet* 1963; 1: 785–9.
112 Chen Y-I *et al.* Resistance to insulin suppression of plasma free fatty acid concentrations and insulin stimulation of glucose uptake in non-insulin-dependent diabetes mellitus. *J Clin Endocr Metab* 1987; 64: 17–21.
113 Fulcher GR *et al.* Metabolic effects of suppression of nonessential free fatty acid levels with acipimox in obese NIDDM subjects. *Diabetes* 1992; 41: 1400–7.
114 Laws, A, Stefanick, ML, Reaven GM. Insulin resistance and hypertriglyceridemia in nondiabetic relatives of patients with noninsulin-dependent diabetes mellitus. *J Clin Endocrinol Metab* 1989; 69: 343–7.
115 Gulli G *et al.* The metabolic profile is fully established in glucose-tolerant offspring of two Mexican–American NIDDM patients. *Diabetes* 1992; 41: 1575–86.
116 Osei K. The effects of superphysiologic hyperinsulinemia on glucose and lipid metabolism in glucose tolerant offspring of patients with noninsulin-dependent diabetes mellitus (NIDDM). *Diabetes Res Clin Pract* 1992; 17: 169–82.
117 Eriksson J *et al.* Nonesterified fatty acids do not contribute to insulin resistance in persons at increased risk of developing type 2 (non-insulin-dependent) diabetes mellitus. *Diabetologia* 1991; 34: 192–7.
118 Polonsky KS, Given BD, VanCouter E. Twenty-four-hour profiles and pulsatile patterns of insulin secretion in normal and obese subjects. *J Clin Invest* 1988; 81: 441–8.
119 Friedman JE *et al.* Restoration of insulin responsiveness in skeletal muscle of morbidly obese patients after weight loss. *J Clin Invest* 1992; 89: 701–5.
120 Vague J. The degree of masculine differentiation of obesities: a factor in determining predisposition of diabetes, atherosclerosis, gout and uric acid calculus disease. *Am J Clin Nutr* 1956; 4: 20–32.
121 Kissebah AH *et al.* Relation of body fat distribution to metabolic complications of obesity. *J Clin Endocrinol Metab* 1982; 54: 254–60.
122 Evans, DJ *et al.* Relationship of body fat topography to insulin sensitivity and metabolic profiles in premenopausal women. *Metabolism* 1984; 3: 68–75.
123 Peiris AN *et al.* Relative contribution of obesity and body fat distribution to alterations in glucose and insulin homeostasis: predictive values of selected indices in premenopausal women. *Am J Clin Nutr* 1989; 49, 758–64.
124 Poehlman ET *et al.* Genotype-controlled changes in

body composition and fat morphology following overfeeding in twins. *Am J Clin Nutr* 1986; 43: 723–31.
125 Bouchard C *et al.* Inheritance of the amount and distribution of human body fat. *Int J Obesity* 1988; 12: 205–15.
126 Laskarzewski PM *et al.* Familial obesity and leanness. *Int J Obesity* 1983; 7: 505–27.
127 Welch S *et al.* Minimal model analysis of intravenous glucose tolerance test-derived insulin sensitivity in diabetic subjects. *J Clin Endocrinol Metab* 1990; 71: 1508–18.
128 Baron AD *et al.* Rates of noninsulin-mediated glucose uptake are elevated in type II diabetic subjects. *J Clin Invest* 1985; 76: 1782–88.
129 Kahn SE *et al.* Treatment with a somatostatin analogue decreases pancreatic B-cell and whole body sensitivity to glucose. *J Clin Endocrinol Metab* 1990; 71: 994–1002.
130 Tobin BW *et al.* Markedly reduced beta cell function does not result in insulin-resistance in islet autografted dogs. *Diabetes* 1992; 41: 1172–81.
131 Page R *et al.* Insulin secretion, insulin sensitivity and glucose-mediated disposal in Cushing's disease: a minimal model analysis. *Clinic Endocrinol* 1991; 35: 509–17.

# 13 Islet Amyloid Polypeptide and Amyloid in the Islets of Langerhans

Per Westermark

Occurrence of islet amyloid (hyalin) has been known since the turn of the century. To understand why so little interest was shown in islet amyloid until recently is probably to comprehend our previous lack of knowledge of amyloid in general. Amyloid was long believed to be a non-specific degenerative product similar to fibrosis, telling us very little of importance about the disorder behind its deposition. When the nature of different types of amyloid began to be clarified at the beginning of the 1970s, modern analytical methods were also applied to islet amyloid. Electron microscopy showed that the hyalin stroma in insulinomas and in human pancreatic islets has a fine fibrillar structure similar to other amyloid forms, and after Congo red staining, a green birefringence, characteristic of all types of amyloid, was obtained (1–3). Since it was shown that the fibrils in several different forms of systemic amyloid consist of aggregated small proteins (4), one could suspect the same to be true also for islet amyloid. The fibrils in insulinomas and in islet amyloid are topographically closely related to tumour cells and β cells, respectively, and therefore it was natural to suspect that the amyloid was derived from insulin or its precursor, especially since it was known that insulin can form amyloid-like fibrils *in vitro*. However, when amino acid sequence analysis was performed on the main component of the amyloid which was first purified from an insulinoma (5) and, subsequently, also from human, cat and cougar islets (6–8), it turned out to be a previously undescribed putative polypeptide hormone, now known as islet amyloid polypeptide (IAPP) or 'amylin'. Later, it was shown that insulin also really does form islet amyloid, not in humans but in the little hystricomorph South American rodent Degu (9).

## ISLET AMYLOID POLYPEPTIDE AND ITS BIOLOGICAL ACTIVITY

### Islet amyloid polypeptide and its gene

IAPP is a 37 amino acid long, C-terminally amidated polypeptide. IAPP has 43–46% identity to the two calcitonin gene-related peptides (CGRP) (6, 7) and is expressed in man as a 89 amino acid prepropolypeptide, from which a 22 amino acid signal peptide is split off yielding a 67 amino acid precursor (10–12) (Fig. 13.1). In this propeptide, IAPP constitutes a central segment flanked by two short propeptides, which are cleaved at double basic amino acid residues by a proprotein convertase to yield the mature molecule in the same way as pro-insulin and many other polypeptide hormone precursors. While

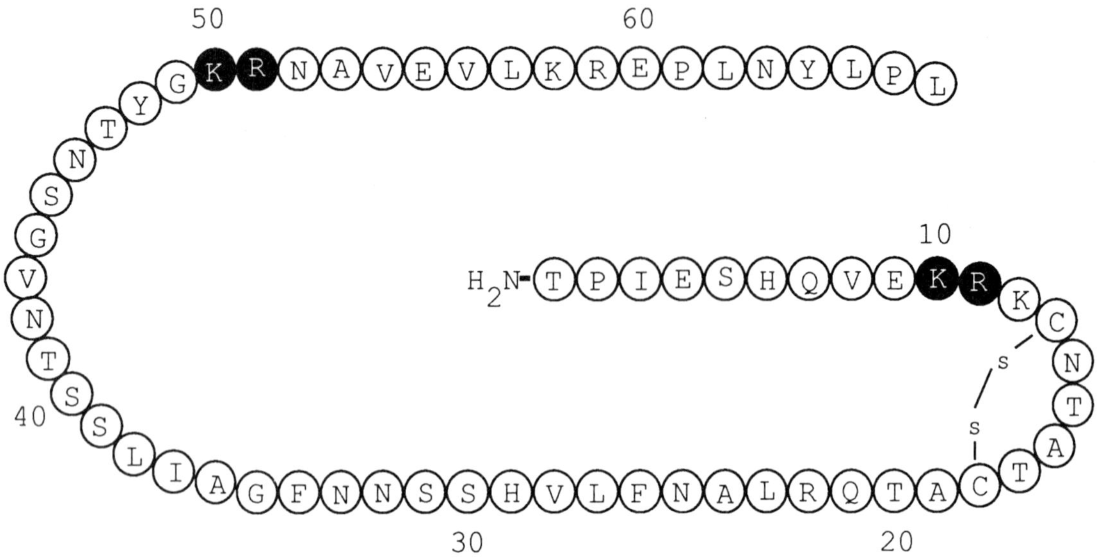


Fig. 13.1. The primary structure of pro-IAPP. Pro-IAPP is processed by cleavage at double basic amino acid residues (black) similar to pro-insulin. The C-terminal glycine residue serves as an amidation signal. The removed short propeptides do not seem to have any biological function. (From Westermark *et al.*, *Diabetologia* 1992; 35: 297.)

| | |
|---|---|
| Human | KCNTATCATQRLANFLVHSSNNFGAILSSTNVGSNTY-$NH_2$ |
| Macaque | -----------------R------T------------$NH_2$ |
| Cat | ----------------IR----L-----P---------$NH_2$ |
| Rat | -----------------R----L-PV-PP---------$NH_2$ |
| Hamster | -------------------N--L-PV--P---------$NH_2$ |

Fig. 13.2. The primary structures of islet amyloid polypeptide of five mammalian species. The N- and C-terminal segments are conserved while the central segment, which is of special importance for the amyloid fibril formation, shows considerable variation.

IAPP is highly conserved between mammalian and at least one avian species (Fig. 13.2), the sequences of the flanking peptides are varying, indicating that they do not have biological activity (13). The human IAPP gene is on the short arm of chromosome 12 while the insulin and CGRP genes are situated on the evolutionary related chromosome 11. The regulation of IAPP is at present unknown and although the degree of expression of insulin and IAPP usually are parallel, there is no certain indication that the IAPP and insulin genes are co-regulated. However, similarities in some regulatory element areas of these genes have been suggested. The intracellular events and trafficking giving rise to the mature IAPP have not been clarified but IAPP is stored together with insulin in the secretory granules and is released with this hormone at exocytosis (14, 15). While insulin constitutes the electron dense core of the β-cell secretory granules, IAPP most probably is located in the translucent halo together with the C-peptide or on the surface of the insulin core.

IAPP is a difficult molecule to study and to measure owing to its ability to stick to surfaces. Human, but not rat, IAPP also has a strong tendency to self-aggregate to amyloid-like fibrils. Furthermore, direct assay of IAPP in plasma is difficult due to interference with other, not identified plasma components. Therefore, the reported plasma concentrations of IAPP have varied in different studies but have usually been found to be approximately 2–3% of the insulin levels (16). The human plasma level of IAPP at fasting is usually reported to be around 8 pmol/l with an increase to 15–20 pmol/l after a glucose load. Studies on plasma and pancreatic extracts (in rats, mice and humans) have shown that the ratio between insulin and IAPP concentration seems to be fairly constant at normal conditions, both at fasting and after a glucose load.

In humans, IAPP is almost exclusively expressed by the islet β cells but in the mouse, IAPP-immunoreactivity has been seen also in δ-cells. A very low degree of production is also seen in the gastrointestinal tract and dorsal root ganglia (17). In these latter organs, the IAPP-expressing cells have not been fully characterized but no concomitant insulin production occurs.

## Function of IAPP

In the search for a function of IAPP, the partial sequence identity with a known regulatory protein (CGRP) and the production of IAPP concentrated to the islet β cells made it natural to look primarily for influences on glucose metabolism. Indeed, such effects were soon found in the skeletal muscle and liver. Furthermore, autocrine or paracrine functions of IAPP have also been suggested and to certain degree supported. However, the normal function(s) of IAPP is still not fully established.

Several studies have been devoted to find a specific IAPP receptor. To date, no definite such receptor has been identified in any tissue and it has been commonly assumed that the IAPP effects are generated through the CGRP receptors of which both high affinity and low affinity forms have been found (18). Since higher concentration of IAPP has to be used as compared with CGRP for comparable response in some systems, there have been doubts as to whether the obtained IAPP effects really reflect physiological events. However, recently biological effects of IAPP at concentrations lower than 0.5 nmol/l have been reported (3). It is still possible that specific IAPP receptors do exist.

### Skeletal muscle and liver

In looking for a normal function of IAPP, much interest has focused on skeletal muscle and liver. It has been found that IAPP inhibits basal and insulin-stimulated glycogen synthesis in the skeletal muscle (19), both of human and animal origin. This might be the result of the influence of IAPP at several post-receptor levels. Thus, inhibition of glucose transport and of glycogen synthase has been demonstrated in several experiments as well as promotion of the formation of lactate (19). These effects of IAPP have been confirmed by several research groups and seem to be well established. However, fairly high (>1 nmol/l) concentrations of IAPP have to be used to achieve these results so that the effects can be characterised as pharmacological rather than physiological. Similar effects have also been obtained with CGRP (3). Exactly how IAPP acts on the muscle cell is not known but there is no indication that IAPP interferes directly with the insulin receptor or with the binding of insulin to the receptor.

The studies on the action of IAPP on the liver have given somewhat more variable results. Several studies have failed to show an insulin-antagonising effect by IAPP on perfused liver or on liver cells (2). In contrast, in one study on rats, IAPP antagonised insulin resulting in an increase of hepatic glucose output and the liver was found to be more sensitive to IAPP than skeletal muscle (20). There are also other studies indicating that IAPP promotes hepatic gluconeogenesis (21, 22) and glycogenolysis independently of insulin. On isolated, perfused rat livers, IAPP increased the glucagon-sensitive glycogen pool. Interestingly, small elevations of the concentration of IAPP in the 1–10 pmol/l range have recently been shown to stimulate glycogenolysis and gluconeogenesis in liver cells *in vitro* (21). Since the basal plasma concentration of IAPP in human is within this range (and close to the lower limits of the assay methods), small variations of the IAPP production, perhaps not detectable with the available assay systems, might be of importance for glucose homeostasis. However, the efficiency of IAPP in such low molar concentration has to be confirmed and further studies are needed. There seems to be general agreement that the metabolism by adipose tissue is not affected by IAPP.

### Effects on islet cells

IAPP might also act in an autocrine or paracrine fashion with inhibition of insulin and glucagon secretion. In several experiments with isolated rat islets and perfused rat pancreata, IAPP has been demonstrated to inhibit insulin release (23). However, in other studies no effects on insulin release or production have been found (2). Thus, somewhat contradictory results have been also obtained in this area, and there is at present no definite consensus regarding the biological effect of IAPP on islet β-cells. IAPP has also been reported to inhibit glucagon release in mice, both *in vitro* and *in vivo* (24). To get these effects, high concentration of IAPP has been used but, in contrast to peripheral plasma, a high local concentration of IAPP probably occurs normally in the islets. The possible influence of IAPP on α-cells is especially interesting since the blood flow in the pancreatic islets is from the β cells towards the α-cells. Although more studies are needed to settle the importance of IAPP in islet auto-regulation, autocrine and/or paracrine effects seem probable. The small amounts of IAPP produced in the gastrointestinal tract may also have a paracrine effect.

### Anorectic effects

In experimental animals, IAPP has also been shown to decrease the appetite. These effects have been obtained both by direct injection of IAPP in the hypothalamus and by intravenous infusion (25). Interestingly, when IAPP was infused intravenously over weeks in rats, these rats showed initially a significantly reduced food intake and slower weight gain than control animals but this effect tended to disappear after one week of treatment (Arnelo *et al.*, unpublished observations). Whether IAPP is a physiological regulator of appetite is still unknown, but it is tempting to speculate that the severe weight loss seen in most patients with pancreatic carcinoma can depend partially on the high plasma IAPP levels often seen in this disease (see below).

### Calcium metabolism

IAPP has a calcitonin-like effect on the calcium metabolism (26). The effect is, however, much weaker than that obtained with calcitonin and, most presumably, it depends on binding of IAPP to the calcitonin receptor (2). Whether this rather weak calcitonin-like effect is of any practical importance in humans is unknown.

## ISLET AMYLOID

### Prevalence of islet amyloid

Amyloid is recognised by its tinctorial properties. Staining with Congo red is most commonly used and gives a quite specific green birefringence. If a good technique is not used, even fairly large deposits can easily be missed and this is probably the reason why different studies vary so much in reporting the prevalence of amyloid.

### Islet amyloid in diabetic individuals

The prevalence of islet amyloid in diabetic persons has been estimated in several series. In our studies, we have found some degree of islet amyloidosis in 95% of NIDDM individuals (Fig. 13.3). In some earlier studies, there is no distinction made between IDDM and NIDDM diabetes and, since islet amyloid is not seen in the former, the prevalence is slightly underestimated due to that reason. Even if islet amyloid is typical of NIDDM, there are occasional reports on its occurrence in juvenile diabetic individuals. Thus Opie (27), Ahronheim (28) and Ogilvie (29), each report one such case. In none of these cases, has it been possible to analyse the type of amyloid and it is not known as to whether these patients had typical insulin dependent diabetes (IDDM).

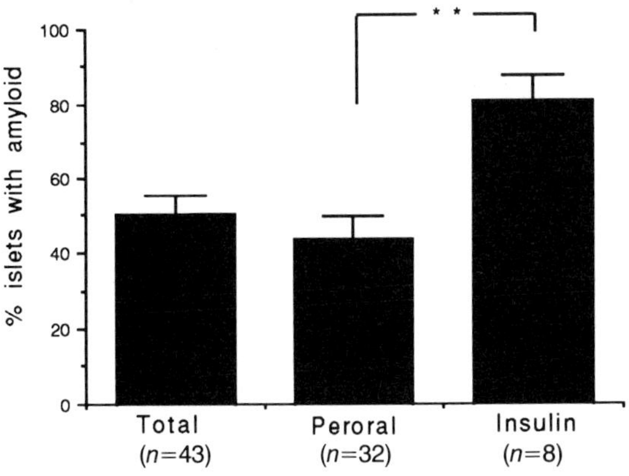


Fig. 13.3. The percentage (mean ±SEM) of islets containing amyloid deposits in a pancreatic material from NIDDM diabetic individuals. There was a significantly higher frequency of amyloidotic islets in patients who had received insulin owing to secondary failure of peroral treatment.

### Islet amyloid in non-diabetic individuals

There were several reports from early 1900s in which islet amyloid was found in non-diabetic individuals. Bell, in his report on islet amyloid in diabetes (30), claimed that these patients represent individuals with undiagnosed diabetes mellitus and believed that islet amyloid, although of no pathogenic importance, is specific for diabetes. Several later studies have shown that small amyloid deposits affecting a few islets occur so frequently in non-diabetic individuals that it is unlikely that they are simply a sign of prediabetes.

## Composition of islet amyloid

In all types of amyloid, the fibrils consist of small proteins, arranged in anti-parallel cross β structure (4). This arrangement is believed to explain the important properties of the amyloid, including resistance to degradation. Each amyloid type is characterised by its own protein and several highly divergent proteins are known to form amyloid fibrils in human. The main component of islet amyloid is full-length IAPP (5).

## Other components in islet amyloid

Immunohistochemically and immunocytochemically, some minor components have been demonstrated in human islet amyloid. Thus, a small amount of insulin B-chain and proIAPP seems to be present. Furthermore, amyloid P-component, known from virtually all types of amyloid, and heparan sulphate proteoglycan, can also be demonstrated. It is not presently known whether or not these minor components have any role in the formation or persistence of the amyloid or alternatively whether they are absorbed to the amyloid fibrils. It is of interest to note that early islet amyloid appears in close contact with the heparan sulphate proteoglycan-rich basement membrane (see below). Deposition of calcium is commonly encountered in islet amyloid but is probably a secondary phenomenon.

## Properties of islet amyloid

The islet amyloid has typical amyloid properties such as fibrillar ultrastructure, affinity for Congo red stain and green birefringence after such staining. It is extremely resistant to most solvents and to enzymatic cleavage. In contrast to most other amyloids, it is not soluble in guanidine. HCl or urea but is soluble after treatment with strong acids. In this respect islet amyloid resembles the amyloid of the neuritic plaques in Alzheimer's disease.

## Localisation of islet amyloid and its formation

Islet amyloid is strictly limited to the islets and not found in other parts of the pancreas or in other organs. The presence of amyloid in islets parallels that of β-cells and the highest prevalence is within the tail and the body, while the pancreatic head (31), especially the PP-rich lobe (32) has a significantly lower percentage of amyloid-containing islets. Processus uncinatus contains no or very little islet amyloid. When present in small amounts, amyloid often delineates the outer borders of the islets and capillaries within the islet. Sometimes, small nodules or star-shaped corpuscles are found. Typically, many small depositions are found within an islet. The distribution of amyloid-containing islets is not necessarily even throughout a pancreatic region. Quite often small clusters of islets with amyloid are found, indicating that unknown local factors are of importance for the formation of amyloid.

The question about the exact localisation of islet amyloid formation is not simply academic as knowledge of this may give insight to the pathological mechanism behind islet amyloids' connection to NIDDM. Electron microscopic studies have shown that early amyloid deposits are found in close connection to the basement membrane of the β-cells (33) (Figs. 13.4 and 13.5) and with bundles of fibrils running perpendicularly from pockets in β-cells through the basement membrane. These studies indicate that in human islets the amyloid is formed in close connection to the β-cell membranes but probably extracellularly. An alternative proposition for the mode of formation, based on studies of insulinomas and of islets of diabetic monkeys, is that the polymerisation of IAPP to amyloid takes place in lysosomes intracellularly and larger amyloid masses develop through fusion of such deposits when islet β-cells degenerate (34). According to this hypothetical model, excessive granules are internally degraded in lysosomes (crinophagia). The possible high concentration of IAPP combined with an acidic milieu might facilitate polymerisation of IAPP into enzyme-resistant amyloid fibrils while insulin is decomposed. In human islets, this idea is contradicted by the findings (see above) that the earliest amyloid is along the external surface of the epithelial cell cords without intracellular amyloid. At present, several laboratories have developed transgenic mice carrying the human IAPP gene. These mice over-express IAPP significantly, but so far there are no reports of development of islet amyloid or abnormal glucose metabolism in these animals (35). It is possible, however, that the transgenic mice carrying the human IAPP gene may serve as a useful model for the detailed study of islet amyloid formation.

## Pathogenesis of islet amyloid

Experimental studies with purified and synthetic human IAPP, as well as with some other amyloid fibril proteins, have shown that they have an intrinsic potential for creating amyloid-like fibrils *in vitro* without other components being present. In IAPP, a limited and central segment (Gly-Ala-Ile-Leu-Ser) (Fig. 13.2) seems to be responsible for that property (36). Interestingly, this segment is within a small region (20–29) that is highly divergent between species (13, 37). Variations within this segment of IAPP seem to explain why only certain mammalian species can develop islet amyloid. Thus, an amyloidogenic sequence is present in man, monkey and cat (species with islet amyloid) while rodent species, without IAPP-derived islet amyloid, have other sequence characteristics. Although an amyloidogenic sequence is a prerequisite for the development of islet amyloid it is not the

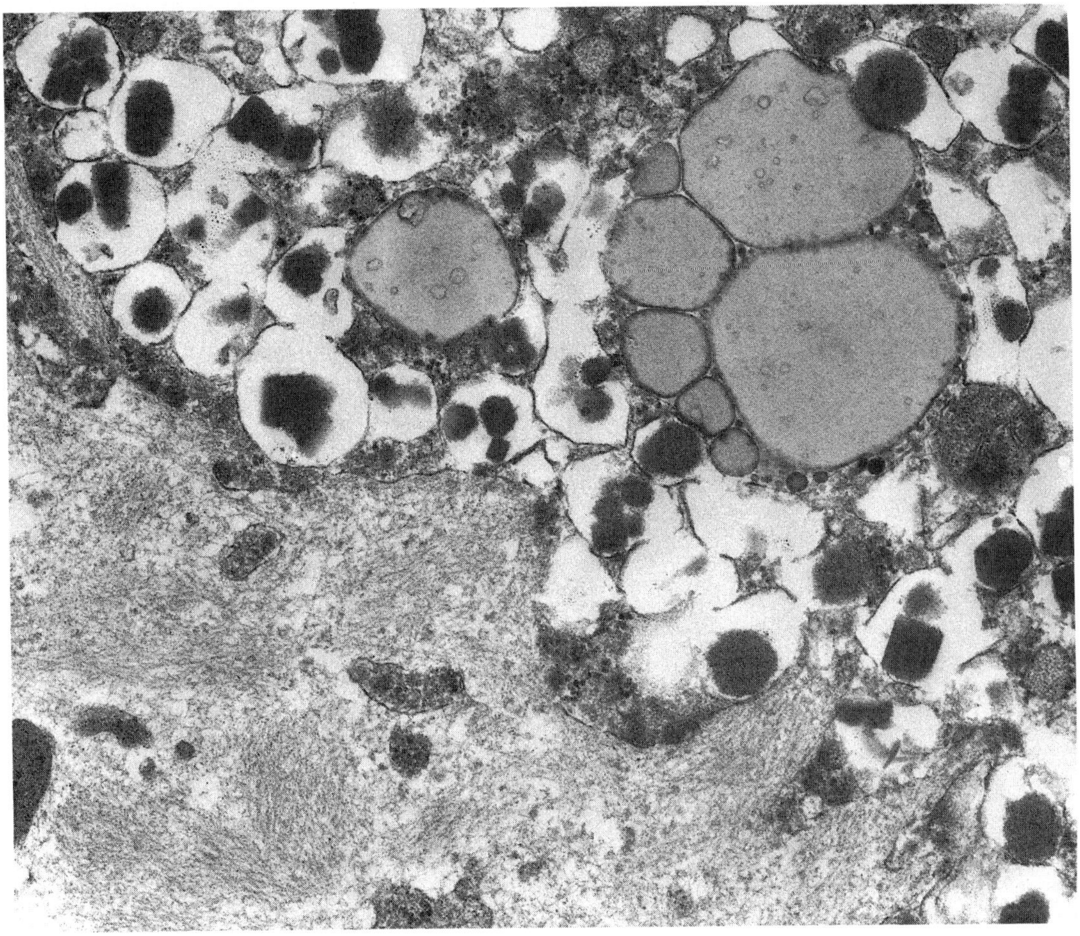

Fig. 13.4. Electron microscopic picture of an outer part of an islet β-cell in close contact with islet amyloid. The amyloid runs in deep pockets into (or from) the cell.

only component in the amyloidogenesis since not all individuals develop deposits. Moreover, some animal species, such as the dog and rabbit, have amyloidogenic sequences but never show islet amyloidosis.

A possible second factor in the development of islet amyloid could be oversecretion of IAPP. Most studies have failed to demonstrate significantly higher plasma IAPP values in NIDDM patients compared to matched controls. There is, however, a small increase of plasma IAPP concentration in obese NIDDM patients and relatives of NIDDM patients (16, 38). Furthermore, glucose-intolerant but not yet diabetic cats have increased content of IAPP in their β cells which might be due to increased IAPP-production. Paradoxically, humans with NIDDM and diabetic cats with islet amyloid have greatly reduced IAPP-content in those β cells which are not degranulated (39, 40). *In situ* hybridisation studies on human pancreatic tissues from patients with and without NIDDM indicate that this lack of IAPP-storage is not due to lack of IAPP-synthesis in islets that are IAPP-negative immunohistochemically, but that synthesised IAPP is

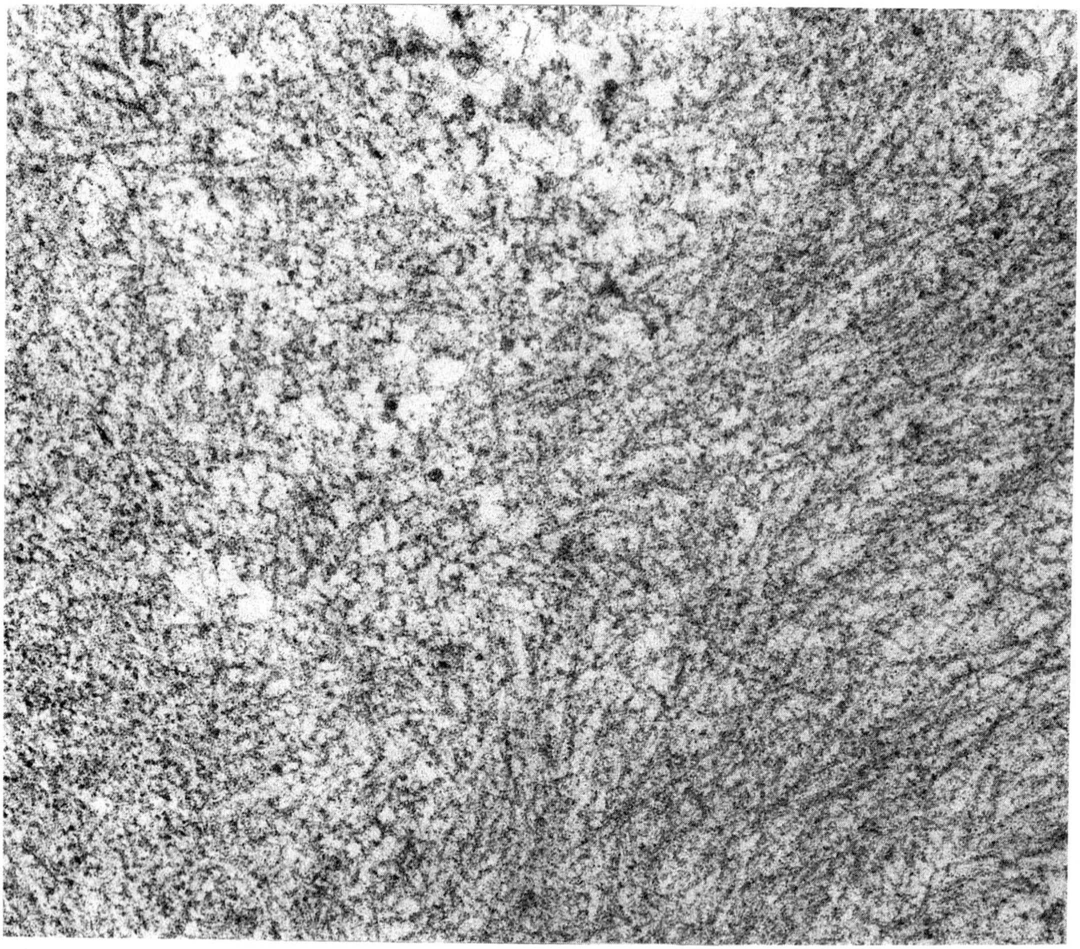

Fig. 13.5. Islet amyloid in higher magnification. The amyloid consists of fibrils approximately 10 nm thick, which are polymers of islet amyloid polypeptide.

not stored normally in the secretory granules (41). The reason for this is unknown but a more rapid IAPP secretion is a possible explanation. This may play a key role in the formation of fibrils from IAPP but the question about the possible roles of aberrations in synthesis, storage or release of IAPP in amyloidogenesis is not resolved.

## ISLET AMYLOID POLYPEPTIDE AND ITS IMPORTANCE IN DIABETES

### Has islet amyloid any impact on the islet cell function?

There are several studies showing that the islet cell mass is diminished in NIDDM and that this is mainly due to a reduction in the number of β-cells (42, 43). Thus, the β-cell mass has been estimated to about 50% of the normal in pancreata of NIDDM individuals. However, in contrast to IDDM, the reduction of β-cell mass *per se* is not large enough to explain the diabetic state.

There are quite a few autopsy studies on the frequency of islet amyloidosis in which the percentage of islets with amyloid deposits has been estimated or the percentage of persons with islet amyloid has been determined. However, there are very few quantitative investigations on the effect of islet amyloid on the islet volume or on the masses of different islet cells. Westermark and Wilander (42), when studying pancreata from 12 individuals with NIDDM of 1–12 years duration, found that islet amyloid constituted 11.9% of the total islet area while Clark *et al.* found 6.5% of islet tissue consisted of amyloid in a similar study (43). Therefore, in a majority of patients, the total amount of amyloid is not large enough to explain the loss of β-cell function. However, the islet amyloid is usually widely spread in affected islets and due to its interposition between endocrine cells and capillaries, it may act as a diffusion barrier although no studies on this problem have been performed. Furthermore, β cells in contact with amyloid appear more or less injured with bundles of amyloid fibrils penetrating the basement and cell membranes creating a morphological poration. With the assumption that amyloid-containing islets only contain injured β cells, it was estimated that in NIDDM, only 25% of morphologically normal β-cell mass remains (42). There is, however, a huge inter-individual variation since in a few individuals with NIDDM, no islet amyloid at all is found while in some other patients, virtually no amyloid-free islets remain. Obviously, infiltration with amyloid offers no uniform explanation for the islet cell dysfunction in NIDDM. However, assuming that the deposition is long-lasting or perhaps even a continuous process, it may well contribute to the secondary β-cell failure. This assumption is supported by the finding of a more advanced islet amyloidosis in NIDDM patients who have needed insulin-treatment as compared to patients who only need drug treatment (Fig. 13.3) (44; Westermark, unpublished observations).

## IAPP and insulin resistance in NIDDM

Interestingly, a glucose intolerant state, similar to what is seen in NIDDM, can be induced experimentally in animals by intravenous infusion of IAPP. However, glucose intolerance has been obtained only with doses of IAPP, much in excess of what can be produced endogenously and, at present, it is uncertain whether these effects of IAPP occur in man. A higher than normal IAPP plasma concentration has been found in obese humans with and without NIDDM, but the increase has only been moderate (16, 45). As compared to controls, a moderate but statistically significant increase in the plasma concentration of IAPP has also been seen in first-degree relatives of NIDDM individuals (38). However, compared to the plasma concentrations needed for *in vivo* effects of IAPP experimentally, the IAPP levels measured in human plasma have been comparably low.

Pancreatic carcinoma is commonly associated with impaired glucose tolerance or diabetes. This cancer-related form of diabetes resembles NIDDM in that it is usually mild and associated with signs of both β-cell defect and peripheral insulin resistance (46). Fasting plasma IAPP values up to five times the normal have been demonstrated. Interestingly, after resection of the tumour, patients with pancreatic carcinoma-associated diabetes often recover from their diabetes as the IAPP-values in plasma normalise, and this in spite of a markedly diminished insulin response to glucose load. However, it is still an open question as to whether IAPP is involved in the pathogenesis of the cancer-associated diabetes form.

To summarize, experimental effects have been obtained with IAPP that resemble several of the characteristic features of NIDDM. However, as yet it has not been shown convincingly that IAPP is of importance for the development of any of these abnormalities in humans. Therefore, although attractive, the hypothesis that over-production of IAPP is a major cause of insulin resistance in NIDDM is unproved and more studies are needed.

## IAPP IN IDDM

In IDDM, there is an almost total lack of β cells with an absolute insulin deficiency. Since IAPP is almost exclusively produced by the β cells, it is natural that low plasma values of IAPP are seen in this form of diabetes. As to whether this IAPP deficiency has any pathophysiological impact is not known but it has been proposed that it may lead to an abnormal insulin sensitivity in some individuals. Another speculation concerns the possibility that lack of IAPP co-operates with the lack of insulin in the pathogenesis of the late complications seen in some diabetic patients. The proposed possibilities are of putative importance but there are not yet any data supporting these speculations.

## REFERENCES


1 Johnson KH, O'Brien TD, Betsholtz C, Westermark P. Islet amyloid, Islet amyloid polypeptide, and diabetes mellitus. *New Engl J Med* 1989; 321: 513–18.

2 Westermark P, Johnson KH, O'Brien TD, Betsholtz C. Islet amyloid polypeptide – a novel controversy in diabetes research. *Diabetologia* 1992; 35: 297–303.

3 Johnson KH, O'Brien TD, Betsholtz C, Westermark P. Islet amyloid polypeptide: mechanisms of amyloidogenesis in the pancreatic islets and potential roles in diabetes mellitus. *Lab Invest* 1992; 66: 522–35.

4 Glenner GG. Amyloid deposits and amyloidosis. The β-fibrilloses. *New Engl J Med* 1980; 302: 1283–92, 1333–43.

5 Westermark P, Wernstedt C, Wilander E, Sletten K. A novel peptide in the calcitonin gene related peptide family as an amyloid fibril protein in the endocrine pancreas. *Biochem Biophys Res Commun* 1986; 140: 827–31.

6 Westermark P, Wernstedt C, Wilander E, Hayden DW, O'Brien TD, Johnson KH. Amyloid fibrils in human insulinoma and islets of Langerhans of the diabetic cat are derived from a neuropeptide-like protein also present in normal islet cells. *Proc Natl Acad Sci USA* 1987; 84: 3881–8.

7 Cooper GJS, Willis AC, Clark A, Turner RC, Sim RB, Reid KBM. Purification and characterization of a peptide from amyloid-rich pancreases of type 2 diabetic patients. *Proc Natl Acad Sci USA* 1987; 84: 8628–32.

8 Johnson KH, Wernstedt C, O'Brien TD, Westermark P. Amyloid in the pancreatic islets of the cougar (*Felis concolor*) is derived from islet amyloid polypeptide (IAPP). *Comp Biochem Physiol* 1991; 98B: 115–19.

9 Hellman U, Wernstedt C, Westermark P, O'Brien TD, Rathbun WB, Johnson KH. Amino acid sequence from degu islet amyloid-derived insulin shows unique sequence characteristics. *Biochem Biophys Res Commun* 1990; 169: 571–7.

10 Sanke T, Bell GI, Sample C, Rubenstein AH, Steiner DF. An islet amyloid peptide is derived from an 89-amino acid precursor by proteolytic processing. *J Biol Chem* 1988; 263: 17243–6.

11 Betsholtz C, Svensson V, Rorsman F *et al.* Islet amyloid polypeptide (IAPP): cDNA cloning and identification of an amyloidogenic region associated with the species-specific occurrence of age-related diabetes mellitus. *Exp Cell Res* 1989; 183: 484–93.

12 Mosselman S, Höppener JWM, Lips CJM, Jansz HS. The complete islet amyloid polypeptide precursor is encoded by two exons. *FEBS Lett* 1989; 247: 154–8.

13 Nishi M, Chan SJ, Nagamatsu S, Bell GI, Steiner DF. Conservation of the sequence of islet amyloid polypeptide in five mammals is consistent with its putative role as an islet hormone. *Proc Natl Acad Sci USA* 1989; 86: 5738–42.

14 Lukinius A, Wilander E, Westermark GT, Engström U, Westermark P. Co-localization of islet amyloid polypeptide and insulin in the B cell secretory granules of the human pancreatic islets. *Diabetologia* 1989; 32: 240–4.

15 Clark A, Edwards CA, Ostle LR *et al.* Localization of islet amyloid polypeptide in lipofuscin bodies and secretory granules of human B-cells and in islets of type-2 diabetic subjects. *Cell Tissue Res* 1989; 257: 179–85.

16 Sanke T, Hanabusa T, Nakano Y *et al.* Plasma islet amyloid polypeptide (amylin) levels and their responses to oral glucose in Type 2 (non-insulin-dependent) diabetic patients. *Diabetologia* 1991; 34: 129–32.

17 Ferrier GJM, Pierson AM, Jones PM, Bloom SR, Girgis SI, Legon S. Expression of the rat amylin (IAPP/DAP) gene. *J Endocrinol* 1989; 3: R1–4.

18 Galeuzza MT, O'Brien TD, Johnson KH, Seybold KS. Islet amyloid polypeptide (IAPP) competes for two binding sites of CGRP. *Peptides* 1991; 12: 585–91.

19 Leighton B, Foot E. The effects of amylin on carbohydrate metabolism in skeletal muscle *in vitro* and *in vivo*. *Biochem J* 1990; 269: 19–23.

20 Koopmans SJ, van Mansfeld ADM, Jansz HS *et al.* Amylin-induced *in vivo* insulin resistance in conscious rats: the liver is more sensitive to amylin than peripheral tissues. *Diabetologia* 1991; 34:218–24.

21 Ciaraldi TP, Goldberg M, Odom R, Stolpe M. *In vitro* effects of amylin on carbohydrate metabolism in liver cells. *Diabetes* 1992; 41:975–81.

22 Roden M, Leiner K, Furnsinn C *et al.* Effects of islet amyloid polypeptide on hepatic insulin resistance and glucose production in the isolated perfused rat liver. *Diabetologia* 1992; 35:116–20.

23 Wang Z-L, Bennet WM, Ghatei MA, Byfield PGH, Smith DM, Bloom SR. Influence of islet amyloid polypeptide and the 8–37 fragment of islet amyloid polypeptide on insulin release from perifused rat islets. *Diabetes* 1993 42:330–5.

24 Panagiotidis G, Salehi AA, Westermark P, Lundquist I. Homologous islet amyloid polypeptide: effects on

plasma levels of glucagon, insulin and glucose in the mouse. *Diab Res Clin Pract* 1992; 18:167–71.

25 Chance WT, Balasubramaniam A, Zhang FS, Wimalawansa SJ, Fischer JE. Anorexia following the intrahypothalamic administration of amylin. *Brain Res* 1991; 539: 352–4.

26 Datta HK, Zaidi M, Wimalawansa SJ, Ghatei MA, Beacham JL, Bloom SR, MacIntyre I. *In vivo* and *in vitro* effects of amylin and amylin-amide on calcium metabolism in the rat and rabbit. *Biochem Biophys Res Commun* 1989; 162:876–81.

27 Opie EL. On the relation of chronic interstitial pancreatitis to the islands of Langerhans and to diabetes mellitus. *J Exp Med* 1901; 5:397–428.

28 Ahronheim JH. The nature of the hyaline material in the pancreatic islands in diabetes mellitus. *Am J Pathol* 1943; 19:873–82.

29 Ogilvie RF. The endocrine pancreas in human and experimental diabetes. In: Cameron MP and O'Conner M, eds. Aetiology of diabetes mellitus and its complications, Ciba Foundation Colloqia on Endocrinology, Little, Brown & Company, Boston, 1964; 49–66.

30 Bell ET. Hyalinization of the islets of Langerhans in diabetes mellitus. *Diabetes* 1952; 1:341–4.

31 Westermark P. Quantitative studies of amyloid in the islets of Langerhans. *Upsala J Med Sci* 1972; 77:91–4.

32 Clark A, Holman RR, Mathews DR, Hockaday TDR, Turner RC. Non-uniform distribution of islet amyloid in the pancreas of maturity-onset diabetic patients. *Diabetologia* 1984; 27:527–8.

33 Westermark P. Fine structure of islets of Langerhans in insular amyloidosis. *Virchows Arch A* 1973; 359: 1–18.

34 Clark A, Morris JF, Scott LA *et al.* Intracellular formation of amyloid fibrils in B-cells of human insulinom and pre-diabetic monkey islets. In: Natvig JB *et al.*, eds. *Amyloid and amyloidosis*. Kluwer, Dordrecht, 1990: 453–56.

35 Fox N, Schrementi J, Nishi M *et al.* Human islet amyloid polypeptide transgenic mice as a model of non-insulin-dependent diabetes mellitus (NIDDM). *FEBS Lett* 1993; 323:40–44.

36 Westermark P, Engström U, Johnson KH, Westermark GT, Betsholtz C. Islet amyloid polypeptide: pinpointing amino acid residues linked to amyloid fibril formation. *Proc Natl Acad Sci USA* 1990; 87:5036–40.

37 Betsholtz C, Christmanson, L, Engström U *et al.* Sequence divergence in a specific region of islet amyloid polypeptide (IAPP) explains differences in islet amyloid formation between species. *FEBS Lett* 1989; 251: 261–4.

38 Eriksson J, Nakazato M, Miyazato M, Shiomi K, Matsukura S, Groop L. Islet amyloid polypeptide plasma concentrations in individuals at increased risk of developing Type 2 (non-insulin-dependent) diabetes mellitus. *Diabetologia* 1992; 35: 291–3.

39 Westermark P, Wilander E, Westermark GT, Johnson KH. Islet amyloid polypeptide-like immunoreactivity in the islet B cells of Type 2 (non-insulin-dependent) diabetic and non-diabetic individuals. *Diabetologia* 1987; 30: 887–92.

40 Johnson KH, O'Brien TD, Jordan K, Westermark P. Impaired glucose tolerance is associated with increased islet amyloid polypeptide (IAPP) immunoreactivity in pancreatic beta cells. *Am J Pathol* 1989; 135: 245–50.

41 Westermark GT, Christmanson L, Terenghi G *et al.* Islet amyloid polypeptide: demonstration of mRNA in human pancreatic islets by *in situ* hybridization in islets with and without amyloid deposits. *Diabetologia* 1993; 36: 323–8.

42 Westermark P, Wilander E. The influence of islet amyloid deposits on the islet volume in maturity onset diabetes mellitus. *Diabetologia* 1978; 15: 417–21.

43 Clark A, Wells CA, Buley ID. Islet amyloid, increased A-cells, reduced B-cells and exocrine fibrosis: quantitative changes in the pancreas in type 2 diabetes. *Diabetes Res* 1988; 9: 151–9.

44 Maloy AL, Longnecker DS, Greenberg ER. The relation of islet amyloid to the clinical type of diabetes. *Human Path* 1981; 12: 917–22.

45 Enoki S, Mitsukawa T, Takemura J *et al.* Plasma islet amyloid polypeptide levels in obesity, impaired glucose tolerance and non-insulin-dependent diabetes mellitus. *Diabetes Res Clin Pract* 1992; 15: 97–102.

46 Permert J, Adrian TE, Jacobsson P, Jorfeldt L, Fruin AB, Larsson J. Is profound peripheral insulin resistance in patients with pancreatic cancer caused by a tumour-associated factor? *Am J Surg* 1993; 165: 61–7.

# 14 Primary Insulin Resistance: A Risk Syndrome

E. Ferrannini & M. P. Stern

## INTRODUCTION

Syndrome X is the term coined by G. M. Reaven in 1988 (1) to indicate the association of glucose intolerance, dyslipidaemia, hypertension, and insulin resistance. An individual presenting impaired glucose tolerance (IGT) or overt non-insulin-dependent (Type 2) diabetes (NIDDM) (as fasting hyperglycaemia or excessive glycaemic excursions on the oral glucose tolerance test), high serum triglyceride concentrations coupled with abnormally low high-density-lipoprotein(HDL)-cholesterol levels, and hypertension (as arterial blood pressure values above the norm by conventional criteria, or current antihypertensive treatment) would be the carrier of a syndrome of unknown (hence 'X') aetiology, in which insulin resistance is the common pathophysiological element and, putatively, the cause.

Syndrome X is also the name previously (in 1967) introduced by Kemp *et al.* (2) to indicate the association of chest pain with typical electrocardiographical evidence of myocardial ischaemia but angiographically normal epicardial coronary arteries. Patients with this syndrome are often middle age women, frequently with clear-cut or borderline hypertension, variable degrees of glucose intolerance or family history of either diabetes or hypertension. The definition is broad enough to include patients with chest pain at rest or with angina on effort, with or without myocardial dysfunction on echocardiography, reduced vasodilatory capacity, or abnormal motility of coronary microvessels (3). Cardiological syndrome X is also called microvascular angina (4) on the grounds that the ST segment depression and chest pain in these patients are thought to originate from smaller myocardial vessels than can be visualised by angiography.

A recent study (5) has reported the presence of hyperinsulinaemia (i.e. the manifestation of insulin resistance) in a group of patients with the cardiological syndrome X. This has led Reaven (6) to defend the continued use of the term syndrome X to indicate either the metabolic or the cardiological variant, with the implicit understanding that they are likely to be one and the same syndrome. This possibility cannot currently be tested, in conformity with the philosophical dictum that what is gratuitously asserted may be gratuitously denied. However, cardiological syndrome X is a heterogeneous condition. When patients are selected to exclude those with diabetes, hyperlipidaemia, hypertension, mitral valve prolapse, or other cardiac or extracardiac disease, no classical sign of myocardial ischaemia (e.g. net lactate release into the coronary sinus) is found during pacing stress despite the emergence of angina and ST segment depression (7). Furthermore, in this selected subgroup of patients with angina and normal angiograms we found no clear evidence of insulin resistance on the euglycaemic insulin clamp (Ferrannini E *et al.* unpublished observations). Thus, it would appear that any insulin resistance found in patients with the cardiological syndrome X may be due to the associated diabetes, hypertension, or hypertriglyceridaemia. Also important is that the long-term prognosis of patients with cardiological syndrome X is quite good (8) whereas metabolic syndrome X is thought to be an atherogenic condition (as will be discussed later). For these reasons, it seems more practical to avoid the name of syndrome X for both the cardiological and the metabolic variant.

That IGT, hypertension, and dyslipidaemia tend to occur in the same patient, more often than chance dictates, is a relatively old clinical notion. This association *per se* would not deserve the name of syndrome, which implies a shared, unknown aetiology. Recently, however, hyperinsulinaemia and/or insulin resistance have consistently been shown to be part of the association, and there is strong argument in favour of a causal role for insulin in the genesis of the whole problem. Thus, an insulin resistance syndrome (IRS) claims a place in the inventory of human diseases.

In this chapter, we shall attempt to define and characterise IRS, and to indicate its clinical relevance and potential pathogenetic implications.

## HYPERINSULINAEMIA

### General

In recent years, plasma insulin concentration has been repeatedly measured in populations. In the San Antonio Heart Study (SAHS), a population-based survey of Southwestern US involving about 3000 individuals, both fasting and post-glucose (2 hours after a standard oral glucose load) plasma insulin concentrations show a skewed distribution (Fig. 14.1), similar to those of serum cholesterol and blood pressure. Unlike the latter, plasma insulin is only weakly age related. Logarithmic transformation of plasma insulin values yields a distribution that does not appreciably deviate from a unimodal, normal distribution. Of note is that, in this biethnic population sample (consisting of 60% Mexican–Americans and 40% non-Hispanic whites), plasma glucose concentrations do show a bimodal distribution on account of the high prevalence of diabetes and IGT among Mexican–Americans (9). Bimodality of a trait is evidence that one mutant allele of a major gene has been injected into the population. Conversely, a strong environmental pressure can shift a trait without altering its distribution, i.e., it can change the trait by the same amount in every subject. According to this scheme, the skew in the distribution of insulin levels suggests that the population is enriched with individuals with a relatively high plasma insulin concentration that expresses both genetic and acquired influences.

### Clinical definition

An issue of practical relevance is the clinical definition of hyperinsulinaemia. The cut-off between normal and high insulin levels could be set on a purely statistical basis. In any population sample of large enough size, the top 2.5% of the normalised (i.e. logarithmically transformed) distribution of fasting insulin levels will, by definition, contain all subjects with fasting insulin more than two standard deviations above the population mean value. This segment will contain more than 2.5% of the whole sample because of the skewed distribution of the untransformed insulin values. Different percentiles may be chosen depending on the ratio of sensitivity to specificity that is needed for the particular purpose of such an analysis. In general, however, these exercises may prove futile until a hard endpoint is at hand. Thus, in a population in which plasma insulin is an independent

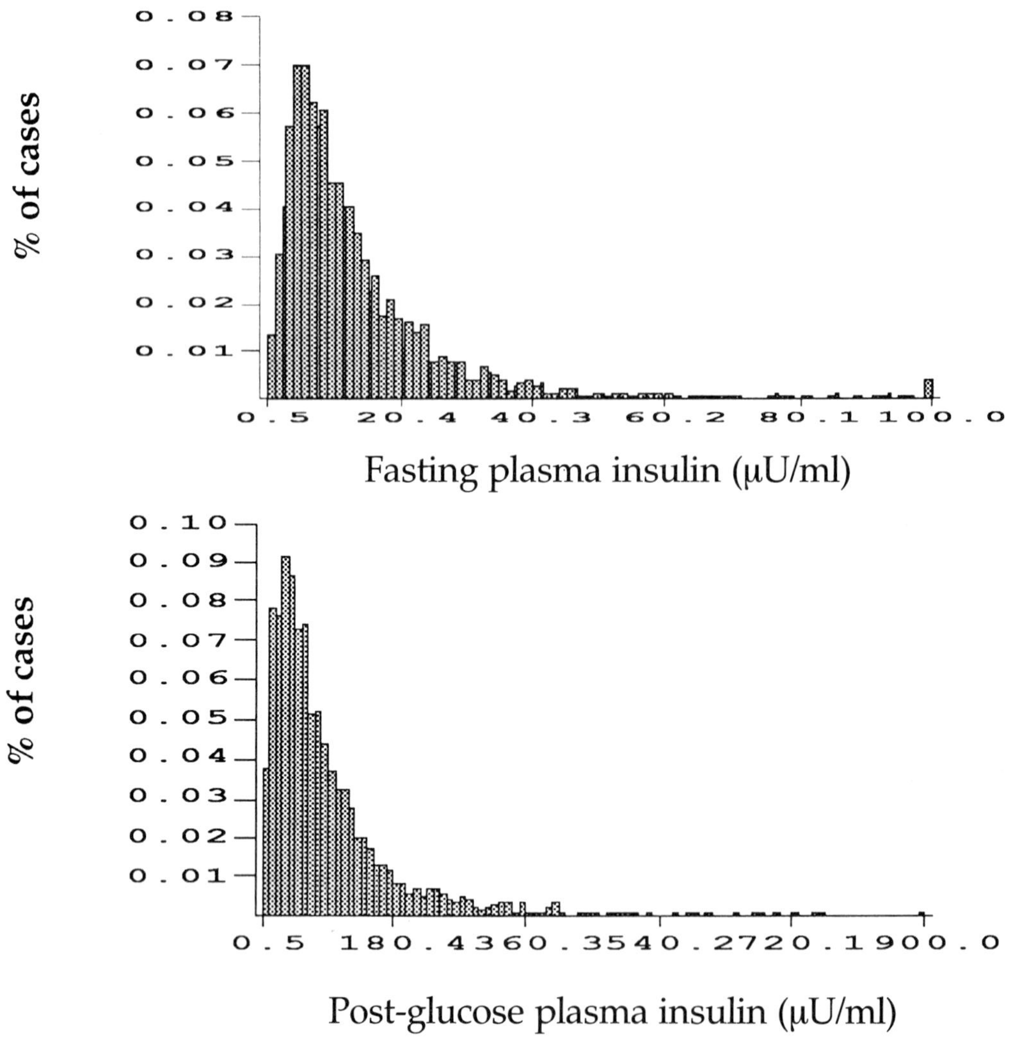


Fig. 14.1. Frequency distribution plot of fasting (top) and post-glucose (bottom) plasma insulin concentrations in a population-based survey of 2930 individuals (the San Antonio Heart Study, SAHS).

predictor of cardiovascular mortality, the boundary of hyperinsulinaemia can be set as the lowest insulin level that is associated with a statistically increased probability of cardiovascular disease. This is analogous to studies of arterial blood pressure or serum ch lesterol, and, like the latter, is subject to shifts as more information is acquired.

## Obesity

The strongest acquired factor that impacts on the circulating concentration of insulin is obesity. Fig. 14.2 shows the relationship between the body mass index (BMI, weight divided by the square of height) and fasting and post-glucose insulin levels in men and women in the SAHS. It is obvious that both measures of insulin concentration increase steeply with body mass, reaching a plateau only at BMI levels (>40 kg/m$^2$) describing massive obesity. Interestingly,

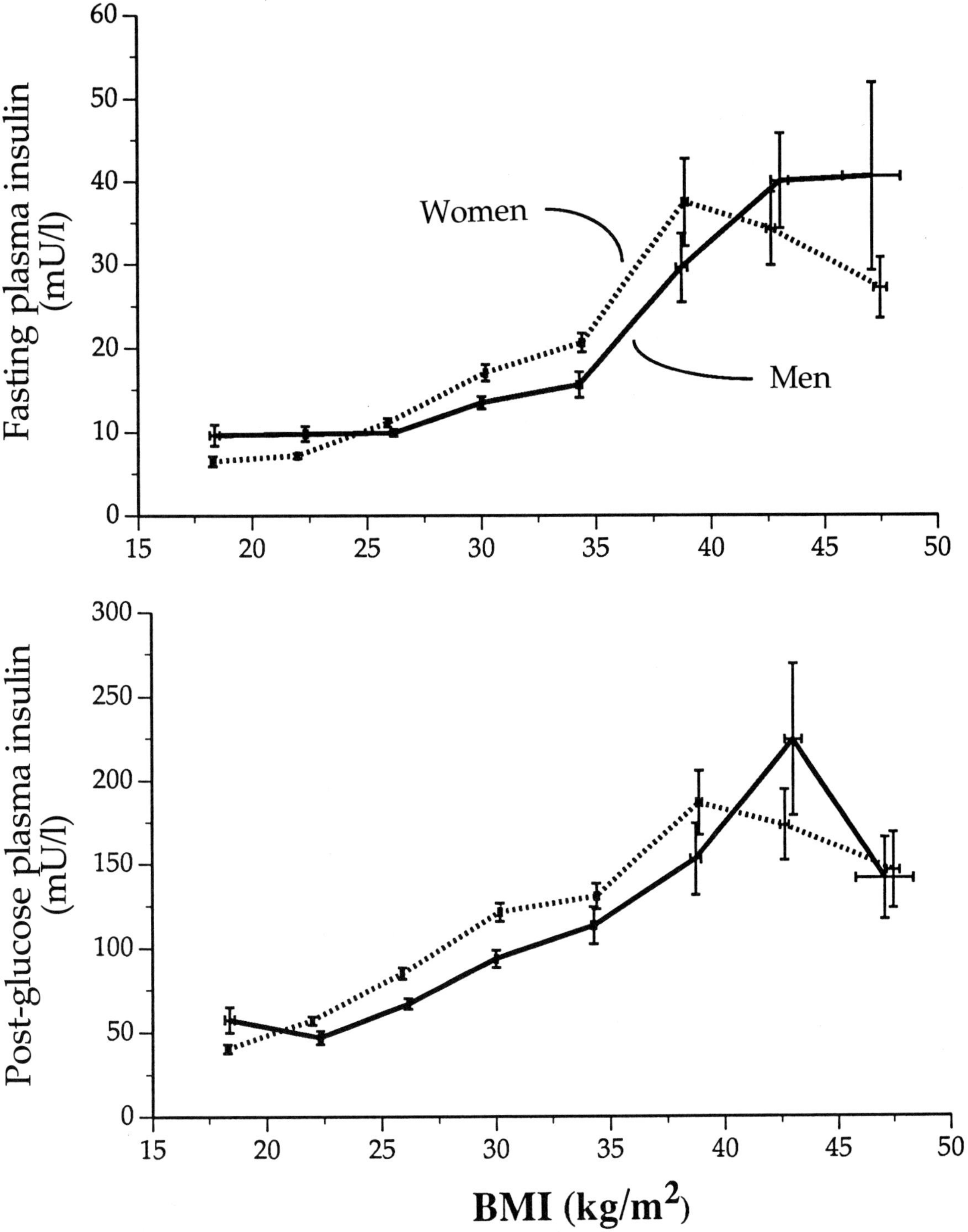


Fig. 14.2. Fasting (top) and post-glucose (bottom) plasma insulin concentrations by octiles of body mass index (BMI) in men and women in the SAHS. Data are mean and SEM values.

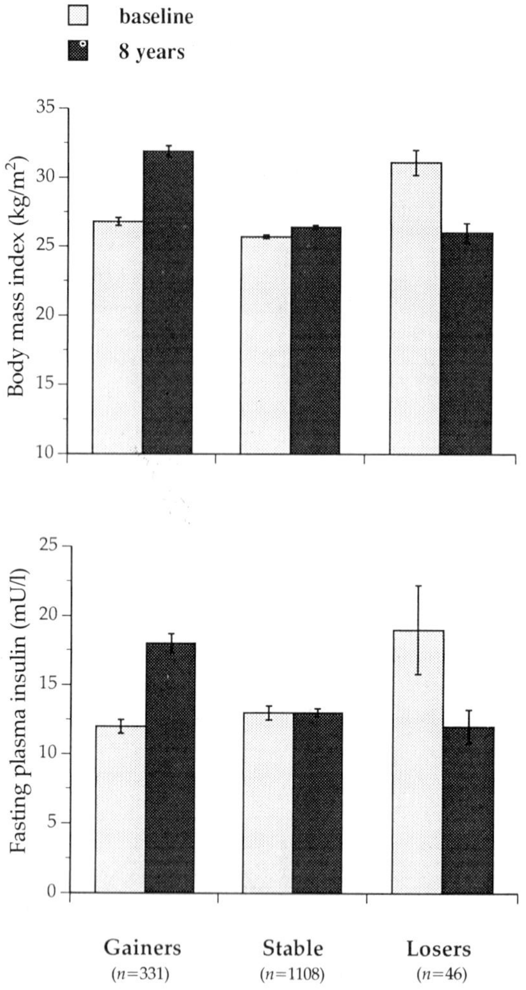


Fig. 14.3. Body mass index (top) and fasting plasma insulin concentrations (bottom) in 1485 subjects screened in the SAHS at baseline and 8 years later. 'Gainers' are those individuals who gained >3 units of BMI over the 8-year period of time; 'stable' identifies those who maintained their weight within 3 BMI units of baseline, 'losers' those who lost >3 BMI units.

among lean persons (BMI <23 kg/m$^2$) men are relatively hyperinsulinaemic compared to women, while the opposite is seen as weight increases.

There is substantial evidence that, in humans as well as in animal, gaining weight raises, and losing weight decreases, plasma insulin. For example, among 1485 subjects screened in the SAHS and followed up for 8 years, 22% gained more than 3 units of BMI (~8 kg), the majority maintained their body weight within 3 BMI units, and a few lost weight. Fasting plasma insulin closely paralleled BMI changes in all three groups (Fig. 14.3).

Upper body (or android) rather than lower body (or gynaecoid) accumulation of fat has itself been convincingly associated with hyperinsulinaemia (10). The relative proportion of adipose mass that is found on the trunk rather than in the extremities is most commonly expressed as the waist-to-hip circumference ratio (WHR). In the SAHS database, both in women and in men, plasma insulin concentrations are related to the WHR independently of BMI in the obese but not in the lean population (Fig. 14.4). This indicates an interaction between obesity and body fat distribution, such that, in the overweight individual, a higher WHR signals the presence of further insulin resistance. The WHR is a constitutive feature, with marked sexual dimorphism. The hormonal background against which preferential routing of fat to the abdominal region occurs is not fully characterised,

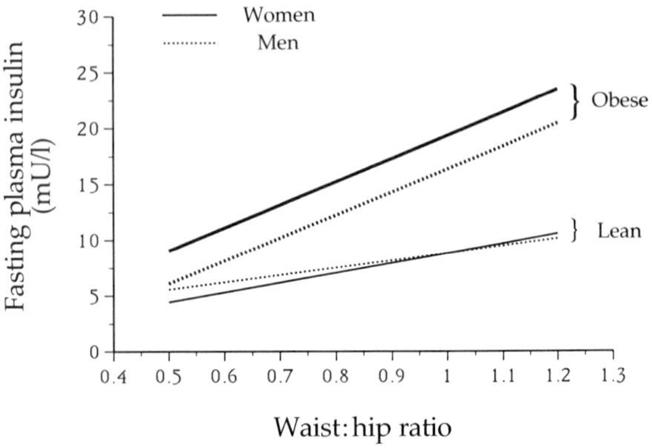


Fig. 14.4. Relationship between fasting plasma insulin levels and the waist : hip ratio (an index of upper body fat distribution) in men and women in the SAHS. Subjects were classified as obese if their BMI exceeded 27 kg$^2$ (men) or 26 kg/m$^2$ (women). The regression lines are adjusted for BMI. The slopes of the regression lines for the lean groups are not significantly different from zero, those for the obese groups are significantly greater than zero (P<0.0001 for both).

although steroid hormones (cortisol, androgens, oestrogen) seem to play a dominant role (11). The extent to which homing of adipose mass to the subcutaneous and visceral depots is also affected by other environmental factors, such as stress, diet, and physical activity, has yet to be studied in detail (12). The latter factors have an established influence on plasma insulin levels regardless of any effect on body fat distribution. Thus, physical training reduces (13), and a diet disproportionately rich in carbohydrates increases (14), plasma insulin concentrations in humans. Smoking, an iterative stimulus for the sympathetic nervous system, may raise plasma insulin (15).

In summary (Fig. 14.5), the circulating plasma insulin concentration in any given individual is the integrated result of (a) current or past overeating, (b) a hormonal mode favouring accumulation of excess fat in the trunk, (c) a sedentary lifestyle, and (d) chronically stressful circumstances, regardless of the driving forces (genetic and behavioural) and interconnections of these factors.

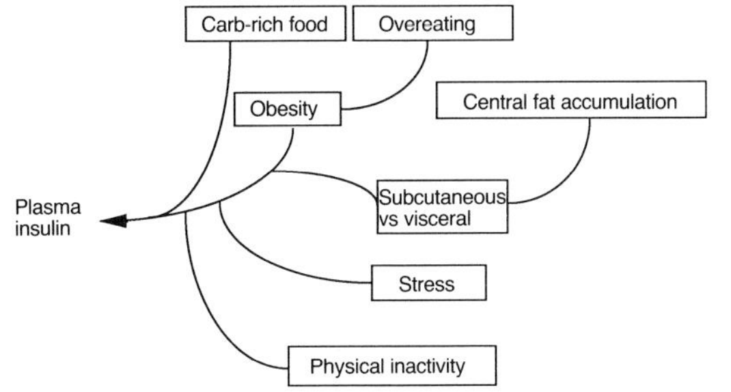


Fig. 14.5. Major environmental factors that influence plasma insulin concentration.

## Inheritance

Despite powerful environmental effects on fasting plasma insulin concentration evidence indicates that it is subject, to some extent, to genetic control. For example, in over 200 family members of patients with NIDDM (16) fasting insulin levels segregate as an autosomal recessive allele, with a frequency of 0.25. Clearly, this kind of estimate is somewhat uncertain, for it depends on the number and quality of pedigrees available for analysis, and ultimately represents only the best statistical fit of the data from a range of compatible models of segregation analysis. It should also be mentioned that the fasting insulin concentration often seems to convey more information (in terms of associations with other variables) than stimulated insulin levels, which are more strictly dependent on glucose tolerance. However, fasting insulin is measured with less precision than stimulated insulin, i.e. with coefficients of variation of 5–15%. Furthermore, proinsulin and split proinsulins make up a greater percentage of fasting than stimulated insulin concentrations (17). These peptides may carry their own message as markers for cardiovascular risk factors, as recently suggested [18]. None the less, it is possible to conclude that the fasting insulin concentration has been identified as a moderately inheritable trait in any individual, subject to modulation by a relatively small number of quantifiable external factors.

## Plasma glucose

In the SAHS database, plasma insulin is also directly associated with plasma glucose (both fasting and post-glucose), with serum triglyceride and HDL-cholesterol levels, and with arterial blood pressure (Fig. 14.6). The relationship with plasma glucose is expected, except that in

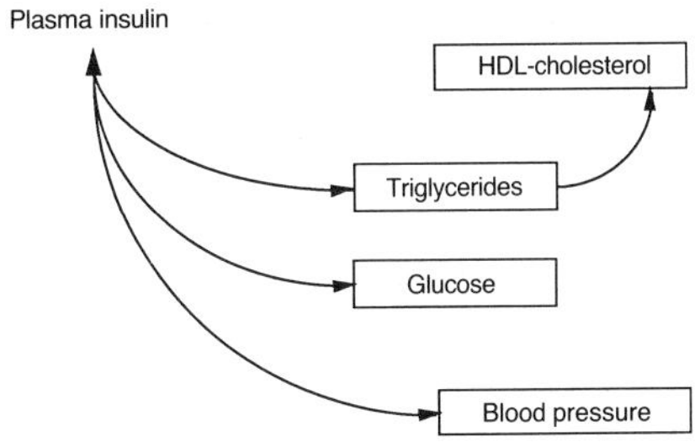


Fig. 14.6. Statistically significant associations between plasma insulin concentration and plasma glucose, triglycerides, and HDL-cholesterol levels, and blood pressure in the SAHS. The direction of the arrows has no particular meaning in this scheme.

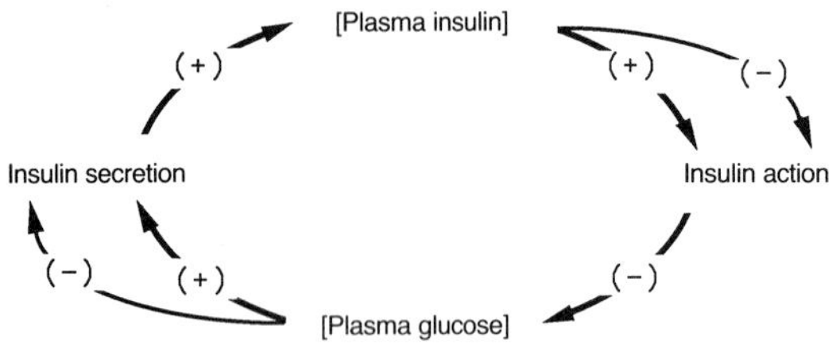


Fig. 14.7. Feed-back loops between plasma glucose and plasma insulin concentration via insulin secretion and action. (+) = stimulation; (−) = inhibition. Thick lines = acute effects; thinner lines = chronic effects. See text for explanation.

severely diabetic individuals (i.e. in a few per cent of the population), higher glucose is invariably coupled with higher insulin. This association is the expression of the glucose–insulin homeostatic system. With reference to Fig.14.7, suppose a pulse of glucose (e.g. from feeding) reaches the systemic circulation: if the rise in insulin secretion elicited by the corresponding rise in plasma glucose were able to return glucose immediately and exactly to the starting level, this in turn would bring insulin secretion back to baseline. The homeostatic couple would oscillate closely around typical values under all circumstances. However, whereas insulin secretion responds to changes in glucose concentration very rapidly (within seconds), and while plasma insulin kinetics are fast and relatively constant under physiological conditions (19), insulin action introduces a significant delay (in the order of minutes) between the increase in plasma insulin and the decrease in plasma glucose. Thus, before the initial perturbation has been quenched through this arm of the feedback, another pulse of glucose may come in. The result will be a resetting of the homeostatic couple at higher values for some time. Furthermore, chronic elevation of plasma insulin concentrations down-regulates insulin action, one of the earliest and best-documented modulating effects on insulin binding to its membrane receptors (20). Consequently, the ability of any given level of plasma insulin to lower plasma glucose will be dampened on a long-term basis, thereby amplifying the shift in the homeostatic couple. On the other hand, chronically higher plasma glucose levels are thought to down-regulate glucose-induced insulin secretion, one of the manifestations of the glucose toxicity phenomenon (21). The overall output of this homeostatic system and its loops is such that, even in the absence of external factors acting upon insulin action or secretion, the two variables, plasma insulin and plasma glucose, will always vary in direct proportion to one another (unless insulin secretion fails).

### Lipids

The direct link between plasma insulin and triglycerides, and the inverse association of the latter (and insulin itself) with HDL-cholesterol concentrations, also are the output of another, more complex homeostatic system, involving plasma free fatty acid (FFA) levels, hepatic secretion of very-low-density (VLDL)-triglycerides and VLDL-cholesterol, delipidation and removal of lipoproteins. Description of this system is beyond the scope of this chapter, but in this case too insulin concentrations and insulin action play a prominent role, at multiple levels and with several secondary loops.

### Blood pressure

Finally, the direct relationship between plasma insulin and blood pressure is the most recent (and least understood) association, one that has called attention to the connections between metabolic and circulatory events. This association was well evident in the SAHS database, in which it was found in the whole population sample as well as in the healthy (non-obese, non-diabetic, normotensive, and normolipidaemic) segment of the population, and resisted adjustment for age, gender, BMI, and WHR (22). In several other epidemiological studies, a similar relationship between some measure of arterial blood pressure (systolic, diastolic, mean, or pulse pressure) and some measure of plasma insulin (fasting, single post-glucose value, or sum of post-glucose values) has been

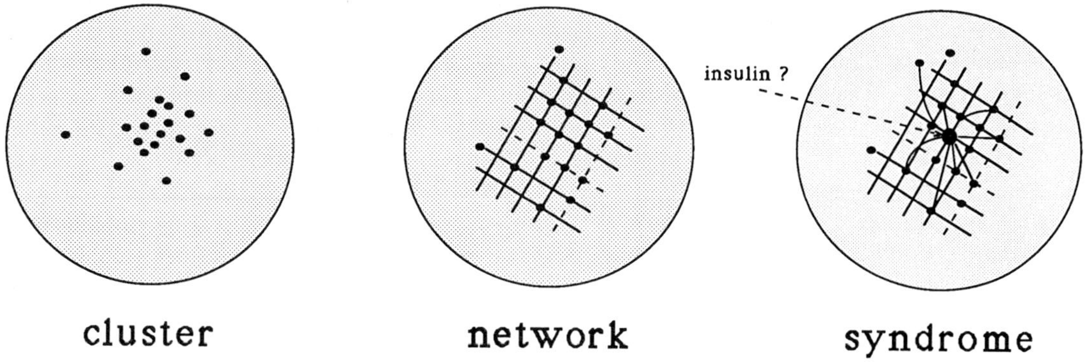


Fig. 14.8. Conceptualisation of the terms cluster, network, and syndrome. See text for further explanation.

reported, often with adjustment for age, gender, or BMI. The association, however, has generally been rather weak, and this may explain why some surveys have yielded negative results. Inter-ethnic variability, which is evident in the SAHS (23), also must contribute to this relative inconsistency. The physiological structure of the link between insulin and blood pressure is still unknown. It seems that high blood pressure *per se* does not beget hyperinsulinaemia because secondary forms of hypertension are not conspicuously associated with elevated plasma insulin. Hyperinsulinaemia, on the other hand, has the potential of raising blood pressure through a variety of mechanisms (stimulation of renal sodium reabsorption, activation of the adrenergic nervous system, stimulation of smooth muscle cell growth, alteration of transmembrane ion traffic) (24). Which mechanism, in what time frame, and under what circumstances operates to determine the association between hyperinsulinaemia and blood pressure is a complex issue that falls outside the scope of the present discussion.

## TOWARDS A SYNDROME

### Terminology

If the information so far reviewed (and schematised in Figs. 14.5 and 14.6) is considered as a whole, the result is a set of associations that have the following general features: (a) they surface as statistically significant correlations in surveys of human populations; (b) they often have a sound physiological substrate; and (c) they are centred around insulin. This 'insulinocentric' view, however, should not obscure the fact that many significant relations also exist between other variables of the set, for example between BMI and triglycerides, WHR and HDL-cholesterol, BMI and blood pressure. It could therefore be argued that placing insulin, rather than BMI or WHR or lipids or blood pressure, at the core of the set reflects the investigator's bias rather than a necessary key to interpret the whole.

For the sake of the following discussion, it is useful to first clarify our terminology. As sketched in Fig. 14.8, a cluster is a group of variables that lump closer to one another than to a large number of other parameters. The interrelation is merely one of co-variance, or consensuality, of parameters among individuals in a population as well as within the same subject in response to perturbations (e.g., diet). In a network, on the other hand, the variables in the cluster are connected by mechanisms (or multiple cause–effect relationships), which are the basis for the observed co-variance. These mechanisms operate under physiological circumstances and are testable by experiment, and their malfunction produces a disease state. In a syndrome, one knot in the network stands out as being the prime mover, or the most powerful force, which drags most other variables along. In this case, the network is structured as a hierarchy; in case of malfunction, the dominant element accounts for the aetiology of the corresponding disease(s).

How far can we take insulin in this sequence? The answer is tantamount to assessing the role of insulin as a cause of disease. For most hormones both excess and deficiency lead to a pathological state (e.g., hypo- and hyperthyroidism). Insulin stands apart because (a) it is a phylogenetically ancient peptide, which during evolution has accumulated both acute effects on intermediary metabolism and chronic actions on tissue growth and differentiation; (b) it is potentially lethal by virtue of its tight control of plasma glucose, and, thereupon, brain function; (c) it is not known to be directly regulated by any *ad hoc* pituitary or hypothalamic hormone (like TSH or TRH for thyroxin), i.e., it lacks central integration; and (d) its action is antagonised by many other hormones (GH, cortisol, glucagon, catecholamines, thyroid hormones, sex steroids), which together form the redundant counter-system that is typical of vital functions. Insulin lack produces IDDM diabetes, but we are still short of understanding what disease is caused by insulin excess. Since persistent insulin excess is incompatible with life, insulin resistance must have evolved as a means to blunt the effects of hyperinsulinism.

## The cluster

When dealing with a relatively large number of inter-related variables, ordinary techniques of multivariate analysis, such as multiple regression, may prove unsatisfactory because they require that the dependent variable be chosen *a priori*. This choice is the angle under which the information carried by the data is viewed, and can bias the interpretation. An unbiased way of compacting the available numerical information in its entirety is to use principal component analysis. With this technique, variables are ranked along two or more hidden components according to their complete correlation matrix. On the SAHS database, this analysis gave the results shown in Fig. 14.9, in which the loadings of 12 different parameters on three hidden components are plotted in three dimensions. It is clear that, despite the fact that each variable was correlated with all the others, there were distinct lumps: one for glucose (fasting and post-glucose plasma glucose concentrations), one for insulin (fasting and post-glucose levels), one for BMI, triglycerides, and HDL-cholesterol, and one for blood pressure (systolic and diastolic values), whereas age, WHR, and serum low-density-lipoprotein (LDL)-cholesterol concentrations fell close to the blood pressure domain but were the least correlated of all parameters. In general, the metabolic variables proper (glucose, insulin, BMI, triglycerides, and HDL-cholesterol) formed a separate subcluster from the constitutional (age, WHR, and LDL-cholesterol) and haemodynamic variables (blood pressure). This analysis thus recovers in numerical form the qualitative information reviewed in section B. Insulin occupies a central position between glucose and lipid parameters, with obesity very close to it. Age and body fat distribution, on the other hand, cluster together with blood pressure (the latter rises drastically with age and is higher in men (who have a higher WHR) than in women).

## The network

We have already mentioned the complex physiological mechanisms that underlie the associations between plasma insulin and glucose, lipid or blood pressure. Although knowledge is incomplete in some areas (e.g., plasma insulin and blood pressure), there is little doubt that a network of cause–effect relationships do exist. Indeed, on the basis of physiology it is possible to predict where many other parameters, had they been measured, would fall within the network. Thus, if an estimate of physical activity were available, it would join the glucose/insulin complex; if daily caloric intake had been

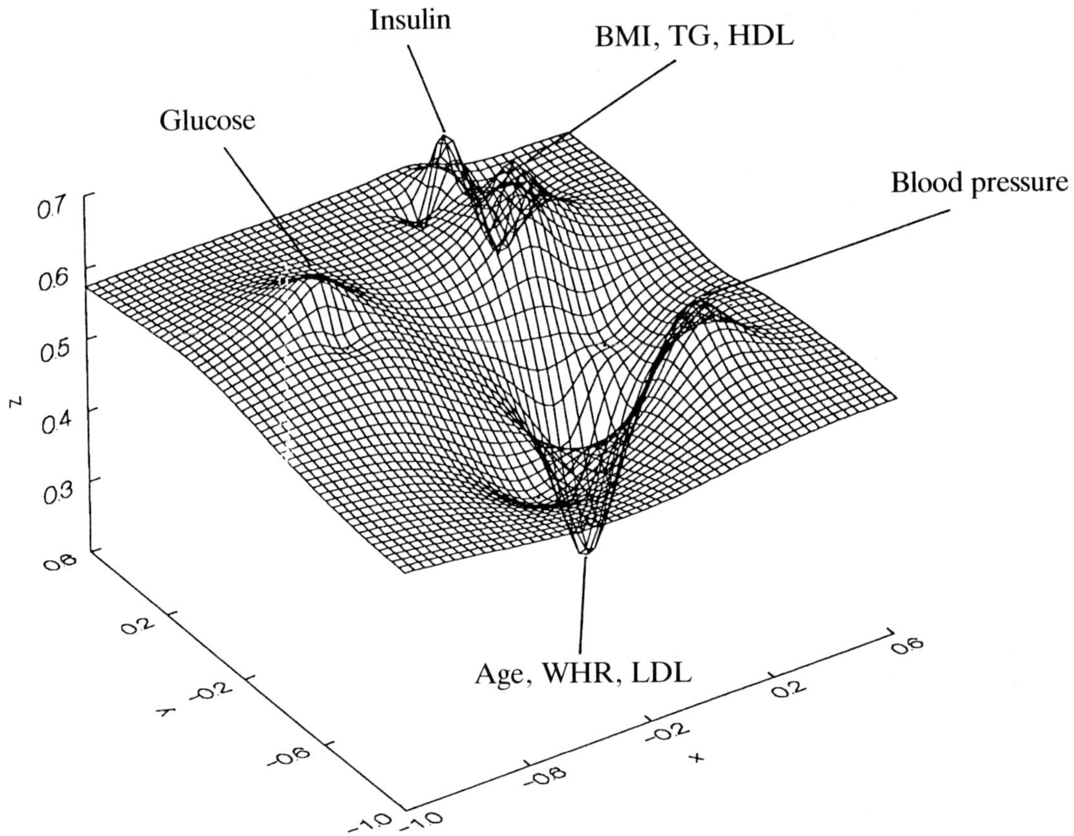


Fig. 14.9. Principal component analysis of the SAHS database. Twelve variables (age, waist : hip ratio (WHR), LDL- and HDL-cholesterol, systolic and diastolic blood pressure, fasting and post-glucose plasma insulin and glucose concentrations, body mass index (BMI), and serum triglycerides (TG) are plotted in a three-dimensional space according to the their loadings on three principal components (*x*, *y*, and *z*) identified from the complete correlation (Pearson) matrix. The percentages of the total variance explained are 31, 12, and 11% for the three components.

quantified with any degree of accuracy, the measure would probably fit in the obesity peak just as a measure of salt intake would gravitate around blood pressure. This predictability at the same time validates the network and diminishes its interest insofar as nothing new is learned. However, a broad perspective is gained, and unexpected results are always possible. It is the unexpected or the counter-intuitive finding that stimulates research.

One important issue at this point is the role of obesity. Since plasma insulin and overweight are so closely bound together, is it possible that the entire network simply is an updated version of the pathophysiology of obesity? Indeed, one can read Fig. 14.9 as an illustration of the physiological consequences of overweight on metabolism and haemodynamics. For that matter, principal component analysis is meant not to be partial to any of several compatible views. Furthermore, obesity is the most prevalent disease state in westernised populations (e.g., 54% in the SAHS), and it would therefore not be surprising if the main attractor of the cluster was in fact obesity *through* insulin.

One approach to this issue is to restrict analysis to the non-obese population. In the SAHS, when the principal component analysis was performed on the lean segment of the population (i.e., BMI < 27 kg/m$^2$ in men and < 26 in women), insulin still retained its relations to most metabolic and haemodynamic parameters. The emerging pattern (Fig. 14.10) resembled that of the whole sample, although, perhaps not surprisingly, the insulin peak was less prominent, and BMI had now divorced itself to a degree from both lipids and insulin. By a different approach, Zavaroni and colleagues obtained an analogous result: among 100 *non-obese*, healthy Italian factory workers, the 25 subjects with relatively higher plasma insulin concentrations also presented higher plasma glucose, triglyceride, and blood pressure, and lower HDL-cholesterol, values than the 75 normo-insulinaemic individuals (25). These findings clearly indicate that the network, while amplified in the obese, can also be found in the lean. Obesity strains the network probably in more ways than by just causing hyperinsulinaemia (e.g., by raising blood pressure by purely haemodynamic mechanisms (26)), and can be regarded as the most frequent cause of the constellation

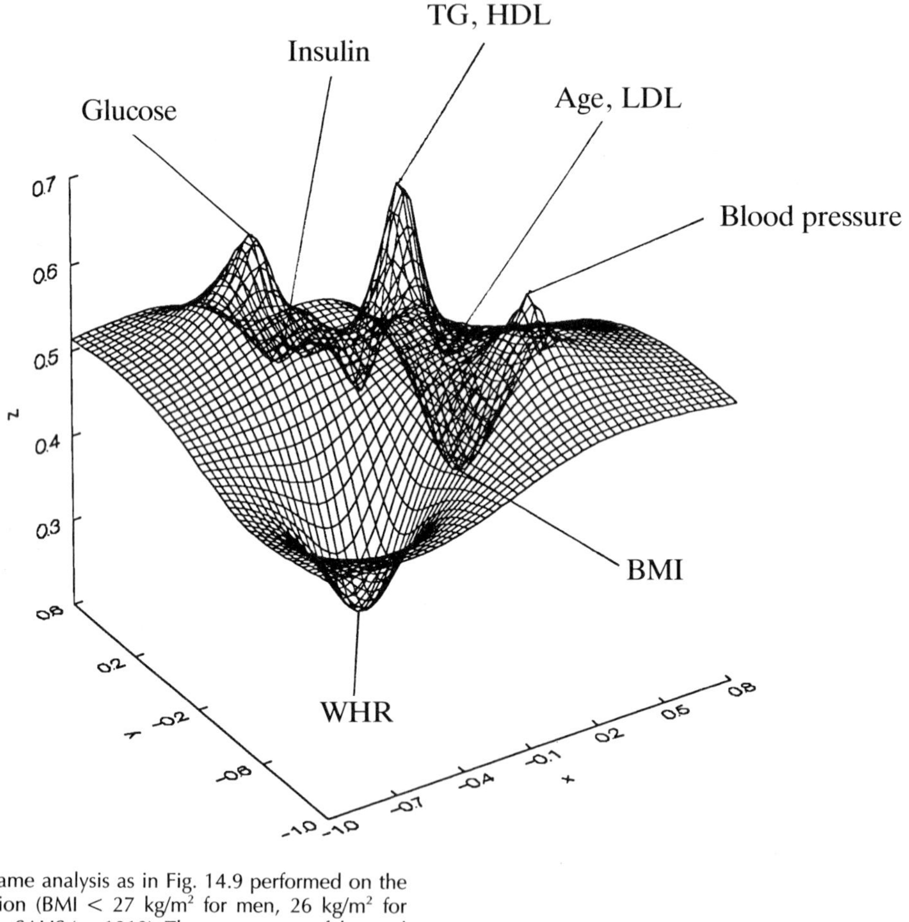


Fig. 14.10. Same analysis as in Fig. 14.9 performed on the lean population (BMI < 27 kg/m$^2$ for men, 26 kg/m$^2$ for women) of the SAHS ($n$=1219). The percentages of the total variance explained are 26, 12, and 10% for the three components.

of changes here discussed. However, as Reaven originally proposed (1), the network itself is not an exclusive prerogative of obesity.

## INSULIN RESISTANCE

So far, discussion has been based on insulin as the circulating plasma concentration of the hormone. As already mentioned (Fig. 14.7), insulin action modulates insulin secretion by setting the demand for insulin by the body tissues. It is therefore not surprising that, when both insulin secretion (expressed as the plasma insulin response to oral glucose loading) and insulin sensitivity (measured as whole-body glucose disposal under conditions of stable euglycaemic hyperinsulinaemia, e.g. with the use of the insulin clamp) have been determined in the same subjects, an inverse relationship has uniformly been found. However, as schematically depicted in Fig. 14.11, the scatter around the regression line is wide, such that at any level of insulin sensitivity insulin levels can vary over a wide range, and, conversely, each level of plasma insulin can be associated with very different levels of insulin sensitivity. This association depends not only on the precision of the two measurements (and on the kinetics of plasma insulin disappearance) but also on individual set-points of the homeostatic couple. When insulin secretion is abnormally low, as in the case of insulin-dependent diabetes (IDDM) and severe NIDDM, but insulin action is impaired, the points will fall off to the left and below the regression line (Fig. 14.11). Thus, although in general hyperinsulinaemia can be viewed as a compensatory adaptation to insulin resistance, the underlying physiological state spans from normal insulin sensitivity associated with true insulin hypersecretion to abnormal insulin sensitivity with normal or low insulin levels. For this reason, insulin secretion and insulin sensitivity should be measured by separate tests in the same subject rather than inferring one from the other.

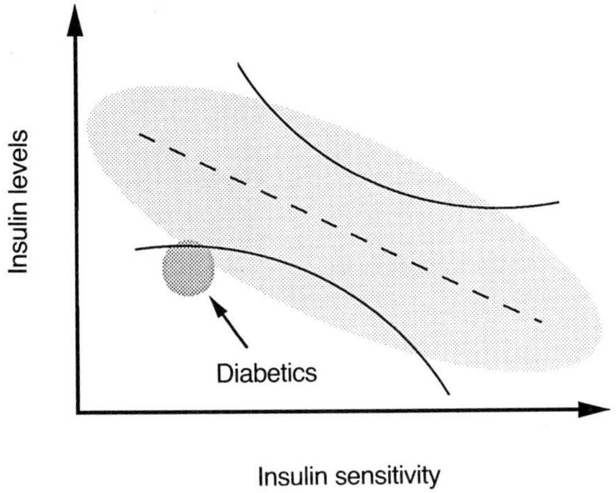


Fig. 14.11. Schematic representation of the inverse relationship between insulin sensitivity and insulin secretion (expressed as plasma insulin concentration). The scheme shows the dispersion of the data around the regression line (with hypothetical confidence intervals). It also shows the position on the plot of patients with severe hyperglycaemia, in whom insulin sensitivity is generally reduced as is the plasma insulin response to glucose stimulation.

Unfortunately, insulin sensitivity is laborious to measure (27), and has therefore not been determined at the population level. Information is none the less available. A preliminary point is the distinction between *primary* and *secondary insulin resistance*. For example, the insulin resistance that accompanies stress of any kind (e.g., surgery, trauma) clearly has the function of sparing plasma glucose at times when supply and assimilation of exogenous nutrients are jeopardised. As the stress subsides, insulin sensitivity is fully restored. Likewise, the insulin resistance of puberty reflects the need for more insulin to sustain accelerated tissue growth without the dangers of hypoglycaemia. These physiological instances of insulin resistance are mediated by a transient, timed surge of insulin-antagonistic hormones. Experimentally, the infusion of anti-insulin hormones mimics all the features of stress-induced or puberty-related insulin resistance. In other conditions, such as liver cirrhosis or chronic renal insufficiency, the presence of insulin resistance can be easily explained on the basis of the organ failure with the attendant toxic state. In general, the forms of insulin resistance that are explained, experimentally reproducible, and reversible can be termed secondary. *Primary insulin resistance, then, is of unknown origin, only partially reproducible experimentally, and essentially irreversible.*

Insulin affects carbohydrate, lipid, protein, ion, nuclei acid and energy metabolism by virtue of a system of multiple intracellular signalling. Several messengers, so far tentatively identified, are generated or triggered following insulin-induced phosphorylation of the insulin receptor (28). Defects in insulin binding to its receptor are known to cause clinically detectable insulin resistance. For example, in the syndrome of insulin resistance and *Acanthosis nigricans* type B, a rare inherited condition in which endogenous antibodies are raised against the insulin receptor, the resulting insulin resistance is profound and probably complete (28). Experimentally, injection of anti-insulin antibodies *in vivo* impairs all aspects of insulin action. However, the great majority of insulin resistant states, whether primary or secondary, have been characterised as post-receptor defects, with pathway-specific changes in hormone action. The common element of all cases of insulin resistance is a reduced ability of the hormone, endogenous or exogenous, to stimulate glucose uptake. It has therefore become customary to refer to resistance of glucose uptake to insulin stimulation as insulin resistance *tout court*.

## PRIMARY INSULIN RESISTANCE

### Healthy subjects

In Pima Indians, insulin-stimulated glucose uptake (as measured by the insulin clamp at submaximal insulin levels), appears to have a trimodal distribution (29) and aggregates in the family (30). In the offspring of two NIDDM parents, insulin sensitivity also shows familial clustering, and the data are compatible with the trait being under the control of a few major genes operating in combination with multiple loci (31). Hyperinsulinaemia has also been found in non-diabetic Mexican–Americans in the SAHS, a population at high risk of NIDDM (32).

In healthy volunteers with normal glucose tolerance, insulin sensitivity (at high physiological plasma insulin levels, ~400 pM) varies over a three–fourfold range. Thus, some individuals in perfectly good health are insulin resistant. In case-control studies, insulin resistance (or weight-adjusted hyperinsulinaemia) has also been found in non-obese offspring of diabetic parents (33, 34), in whom the full spectrum of metabolic changes of NIDDM is already present at a time when their glucose metabolism is still normal (35).

### Non-insulin dependent

Primary insulin resistance is present in the majority of NIDDM patients (lean or obese) (1). Most importantly, in longitudinal studies insulin resistance (or its proxy, hyperinsulinaemia) has been shown to precede and predict the appearance of diagnostic hyperglycemia in non-diabetic subjects (36–38) and in normoglycaemic offspring of NIDDM parents (39).

The insulin resistance of NIDDM is multiple in site, usually severe in degree (40), and only partially reversible (41).

### Essential hypertension

Primary insulin resistance is found in a significant proportion of patients with essential hypertension (42). Interestingly, this finding, unlike the results obtained with plasma insulin measurements, has so far been entirely consistent (43–46). The insulin resistance of essential hypertension is predominantly located in skeletal muscle, and specifically involves glucose conversion to glycogen (42, 44) independent of forearm blood flow (45), while hepatic glucose metabolism is unaffected (46). The degree of insulin resistance is roughly related to the severity of hypertension (42, 43). The relationship between plasma insulin (23) or insulin sensitivity (47) and blood pressure shows distinct ethnic variability. Altered insulin sensitivity is found in young black men with borderline hypertension (a frequent antecedent of established hypertension) (48) and in normotensive, lean young subjects with a hypertensive parent (49). In follow-up investigations, relatively high baseline insulin concentrations are a significant predictor of subsequent development of hypertension in both non-diabetic (50) and diabetic subjects (51, 52).

### Dyslipidaemia

While it has long been known that endogenous hypertriglyceridaemia is associated with hyperinsulinaemia (53), more recent evidence shows that insulin sensitivity is reduced in hypercholesterolaemia with high triglycerides (familial combined hyperlipoproteinaemia) but is fully preserved in true familial hypercholesterolaemia (54). Thus, isolated increments in LDL-cholesterol are not associated with insulin resistance, in accord with the position of LDL-cholesterol in the cluster (Figs. 14.9 and 14.10). Plasma insulin has also been found to predict the appearance of both hypertriglyceridaemia and low HDL-cholesterol in non-diabetic subjects in the SAHS (55).

### Interactions

As documented by cross-sectional studies, NIDDM patients with essential hypertension (56) or hypertriglyceridaemia (57) are more resistant than diabetic patients without either. In familial dyslipidaemic hypertension (58), a condition in which high blood pressure and dyslipidaemia are associated in multiple members of families, plasma insulin levels are elevated more than can be accounted for by obesity, and male twins tend to be concordant for the condition (59). Parental history of diabetes is associated with higher triglycerides, lower HDL-cholesterol, higher blood pressure and higher plasma glucose levels in the offspring (60). Already in children, plasma glucose and insulin concentrations, and blood pressure levels are significantly associated with one another (61).

With regard to longitudinal observations, in lean pre-hypertensive subjects the association of insulin levels with future hypertension clusters with higher triglyceride and total cholesterol, and lower HDL-cholesterol, concentrations (50). Furthermore, subjects with NIDDM at baseline have an increased incidence of hypertension at follow-up relative to subjects with normal glucose tolerance (17 *vs* 8%) (50). Fasting hyperinsulinaemia simultaneously predicts NIDDM, hypertension, and dyslipidaemia in the SAHS (55). In the general population, higher blood pressure and serum cholesterol levels are significant predictors of NIDDM (62). Conversely, in non-diabetic subjects a higher plasma glucose response to oral glucose predicts development of hypertension over a period of 18 years (63).

## A PRIMARY INSULIN RESISTANCE SYNDROME?

In summary: (a) insulin sensitivity is detectably under genetic control; (b) insulin resistance is present in NIDDM, essential hypertension, and dyslipidaemia independent of obesity; (c) insulin sensitivity is consistently found in groups of healthy individuals at risk of NIDDM or hypertension (relatives of dyslipidaemic patients have not been studied in this respect); (d) insulin resistance (or weight-adjusted hyperinsulinaemia) precedes and predicts the development of NIDDM, dyslipidaemia and, albeit more weakly, hypertension; and (e) the presence (in probands or their families) of one condition, NIDDM or hypertension, predicts the appearance of the other over time (less is known for dyslipidaemia); in the population at large, plasma glucose, blood pressure and, possibly, plasma insulin behave as 'co-tracking' variables from childhood onwards.

On the grounds of independence (of obesity), antecedence (of the actual diseases), and cross-predictivity, it seems logical to conclude that there exists a situation in which primary (genetic?) insulin resistance is the substrate from which the clinical triad of disordered glucose, lipid, and blood pressure homeostasis evolves later in life. It is important to specify that insulin resistance is often but not always found in diabetes, hypertension or dyslipidaemia, all of which are heterogeneous conditions. Furthermore, even when insulin resistance is present, it appears to anticipate or precipitate, but not directly cause, full-blown diabetes, hypertension or dyslipidaemia. Thus, according to our terminology (Fig. 14.8), this state of affairs still falls short of a true insulin resistance syndrome. The name, IRS, could be maintained with the proviso that it is a 'risk syndrome' rather than a *de facto* pathological state (like Cushing's syndrome). Possibly, as the present gaps of information or understanding are filled, one might come closer to identifying insulin resistance as a slow-acting cause of disease. It is, however, also possible that some other factor behind or beyond insulin will be discovered. With regard to this, it is relevant to recall that insulin resistance and hyperinsulinaemia very often co-exist, and there might be pathological consequences to one, the other, or both.

It is also worth emphasising that IRS can be secondary to obesity but obesity does not necessarily follow insulin resistance. In fact, available evidence indicates that better, rather than worse, insulin sensitivity (in Pima Indians (64)), or lower plasma insulin concentrations (in the SAHS (65)), predict weight gain. To the extent that obesity itself is under genetic control (66), the respective genes of insulin sensitivity and body weight homeostasis should not be in linkage dysequilibrium (as can be hypothesised for the genes of insulin sensitivity and those of diabetes, hypertension, and dyslipidaemia). Whether primary and secondary IRS carry the same pathogenic potential remains to be established.

## NEW ELEMENTS

Other associations of plasma insulin or insulin action have emerged in recent years, which may be related to other non-classical actions of insulin of potential significance as disease mechanisms.

### Ionic abnormalities

A high rate of sodium/lithium counter-transport activity (Na/Li CT), a marker related to hypertension heritability as a monogenic trait (67), is associated with insulin resistance in non-diabetic hypertensive patients (68). Furthermore, high Na/Li CT identifies a subgroup of IDDM patients who are predisposed to hypertension and diabetic nephropathy (69), and segregates with insulin resistance, lipid disturbances and microalbuminuria in hypertensive patients with NIDDM (70). In red blood cells, insulin increases both the $K_m$ and the $V_{max}$ of Na/Li CT (71) and, via this change, might promote cell growth (72).

High intracellular calcium concentrations have been described in adipocytes of obese, insulin resistant subjects (73). Conversely, low intracellular magnesium levels have been found in circulating cells of patients with insulin resistance (74). These findings have led to the concept that opposite changes in the free cytosolic levels of calcium and magnesium are possible mediators of insulin action in insulin resistant states (75).

### Microalbuminuria

In patients with IDDM, microalbuminuria is the best predictor of the progression of diabetic nephropathy toward end-stage renal failure (76). Whether high blood pressure may precede, and actually anticipate rather than follow, nephropathy is somewhat controversial. A family history of hypertension (77) and a high rate of Na/Li CT activity in red cells of IDDM patients (78) appear to have prognostic value for diabetic nephropathy. On the other hand, essential hypertension in non-diabetic individuals also is associated with an increased rate of urinary albumin excretion (79). Furthermore, in normotensive patients with proven pancreatic diabetes (secondary to chronic pancreatitis) urinary albumin excretion rates show the same distribution as in IDDM patients with matched duration of diabetes, degree of hyperglycaemia, and daily insulin dose. These findings suggests that, in the absence of the genetic background of IDDM both high blood pressure and hyperglycaemia itself may cause albumin leakage into the urine.

Diabetic nephropathy with proteinuria occurs half as often in NIDDM as in IDDM, and renal failure is relatively uncommon (5–10%) in NIDDM patients. Whether a family history of hypertension, abnormalities in ion exchange across plasma membranes, or other factors predispose NIDDM patients to nephropathy is not clear; nor is it understood what circumstances protect these patients from progressing to renal failure despite degrees of hyperglycaemia and rates of hypertension similar to (or higher than) those of IDDM patients. A major ethnic factor appears to be at play, since in native Americans, Hispanics, and blacks the frequency of end-stage renal failure due to diabetic nephropathy approaches that in IDDM.

It should be mentioned at this point that, despite widely diverse aetiologies, IDDM and NIDDM are not totally separate conditions in the population. Thus, although the overall frequency of hypertension in the families of IDDM probands is only slightly higher than in the non-diabetic population, there is definitely more NIDDM in parents (13%) and siblings (7%) of IDDM patients than among their spouses (2%) or in the general population (~2%) (80, 81).

Finally, microalbuminuria has recently been found to be significantly associated with hyperinsulinaemia and higher serum triglycerides in non-diabetic subjects both with and without hypertension (82). Thus, microalbuminuria attracts its own subcluster with hyperinsulinaemia, hyperglycaemia, and blood pressure.

### Fibrinolysis

Increased plasma concentrations of plasminogen activator inhibitor 1 (PAI-1) have been described in obesity (particularly central obesity), NIDDM, essential hypertension, hypertriglyceridaemia, and in patients with coronary heart disease (83), i.e., in conditions of insulin resistance. Modulating insulin sensitivity by diet, physical activity, or metformin induces consensual changes in PAI-1 levels (83). Although *in vitro* insulin stimulates PAI-1 secretion by cultured liver cells (84), *in vivo* acute insulin administration does not change circulating PAI-1 levels. Defective fibrinolysis caused by excess PAI-1 has been hypothesised to mediate the atherogenic effects of insulin.

### Hyperuricaemia

Clinically, hyperuricaemia is often associated with glucose intolerance, obesity, diabetes, and hypertension. In healthy subjects, serum uric acid concentrations are inversely related to insulin sensitivity, while uric acid clearance, a determinant of uricaemia, is directly related to insulin sensitivity (85). Insulin resistance has therefore been thought to underlie the known association between hyperuricaemia and coronary heart disease.

### Birthweight

A low weight at birth has been linked with development of hypertension (86) and glucose intolerance (87) in adult life. Indeed, several components of IRS have been traced back to low birthweight both in Caucasians (88) and in the bi-ethnic population of the SAHS (89). Reduced foetal growth has therefore been proposed as a general antecedent of the syndrome. Compatible with this hypothesis is the observation that, in normal mothers relative hyperinsulinaemia during the third trimester of pregnancy is associated with a lower weight of the newborn (90). Thus, material insulin resistance might be passed on to progeny also through intrauterine influences.

## CLINICAL SIGNIFICANCE

The concept of an IRS calls attention to the deep inter-relationships among diabetes, essential

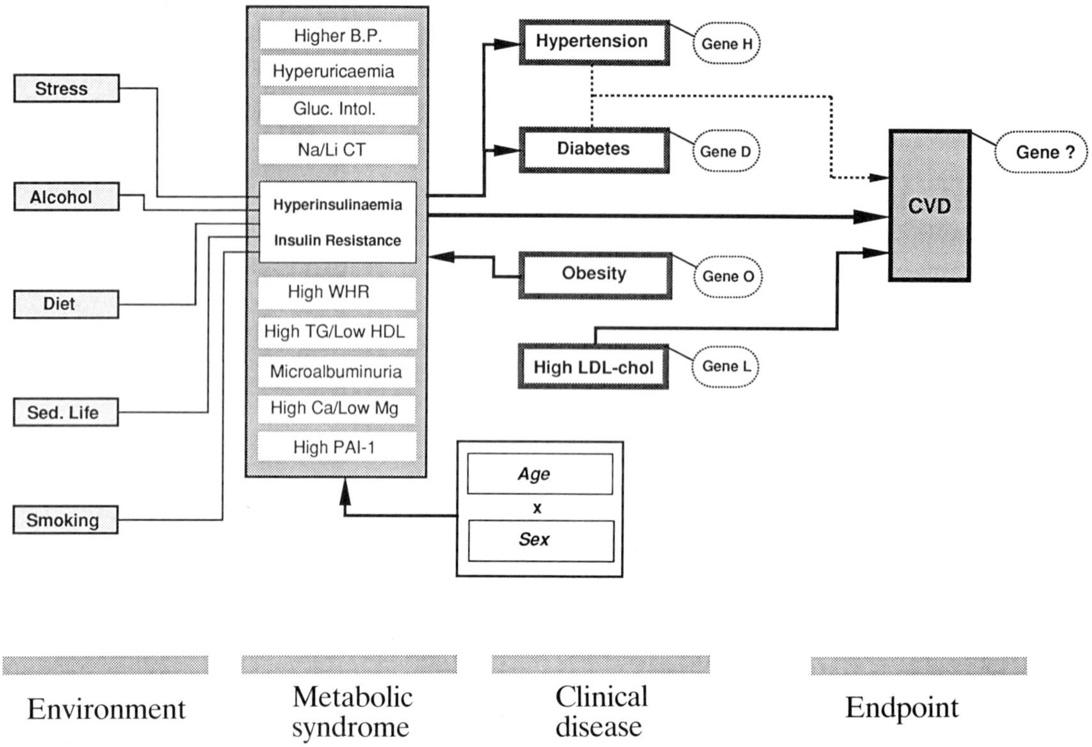


Fig. 14.12. Summary of the metabolic syndrome, here represented as a group of changes in functions that are linked with one another by physiological mechanisms, and centred around insulin resistance and hyperinsulinaemia. Age and gender (particularly in interaction with each other), the chief environmental influences (stress, alcohol, diet, physical inactivity, and smoking), and obesity convey their impact on morbidity through the syndrome, which is a distant predecessor of both Type 2 diabetes and hypertension. Atherosclerotic cardiovascular disease (CVD) is envisioned as the endpoint of the metabolic syndrome, with a separate contribution from high LDL-cholesterol levels (not part of the syndrome). The dotted line connecting diabetes and hypertension directly to CVD alludes to the fact that the two diseases can contribute to CVD by additional mechanisms (e.g., cardiac hypertrophy, microvascular dysfunction, severe chronic hyperglycaemia) initially not part of the syndrome. Mention is also made of the fact that the clinical disorders (diabetes, hypertension, obesity, hypercholesterolaemia, and, possibly, CVD itself are under genetic control. Thus, the metabolic syndrome is a risk complex rather than the direct cause of disease.

hypertension, and some dyslipidaemias. Traditionally regarded as overlapping but separate diseases, the insulin angle offers proof of the inherent kinship of these conditions.

The concept gains further momentum when considering atherosclerotic cardiovascular diseases (CVD) as the endpoint. Several elements in IRS have been shown to be, in isolation, risk factors for CVD: classically higher glucose and blood pressure values, but also high triglycerides/low HDL-cholesterol, high PAI-1 levels, high WHR, hyperuricaemia, microalbuminuria, low birthweight. For example, microalbuminuria has emerged as an independent predictor of CVD in both non-diabetic (91) and diabetic individuals (92, 93), while Barker and colleagues have associated a low birthweight with CVD mortality (94). Of interest is that, in a large prospective survey carried out in Sweden (the Malmö Study), several of the independent risk factors for the development of overt NIDDM (or IGT) in normoglycaemic individuals over 6 years are also recognised risk factors for CVD (i.e. obesity, a sedentary lifestyle, higher fasting and

2-hour plasma glucose concentrations, family history of diabetes, treatment for hypertension) (95). This provides a logical explanation for the finding (96) that in a 24-year follow-up examination cardiovascular mortality in men and women with NIDDM was already higher than in the non-diabetic population 3 years after diagnosis. Similar conclusions have been reached from the analysis of cardiovascular risk factors in confirmed pre-diabetic individuals (97), leading to the idea that the clock for CVD starts ticking long before the onset of clinical diabetes.

Plasma insulin concentration itself has emerged as an independent risk factor for CVD in three longitudinal studies (98–100), although more recent findings have failed to confirm this association.

In conclusion (Fig. 14.12), IRS can be viewed as an ensemble of metabolic, constitutional, and haemodynamic changes (many under genetic influence) more or less tightly connected with insulin resistance and/or hyperinsulinaemia by cause–effect relationships. IRS can be the predecessor of diseases (diabetes and hypertension) leading to accelerated atherosclerosis and CVD. IRS is the extension of normal relationships into the pathological domain. It appears to work as a relay station for environmental influences on their route to disease. In the latter sense, it may also transduce the atherogenic potential of obesity. IRS is likely to present different patterns in different ethnic groups according to their genetic make-up and environmental pressure.

To test whether insulin resistance carries more pathogenic weight than just hyperinsulinaemia requires measuring this trait in large population samples. However, to prove that insulin resistance (or hyperinsulinaemia) is a *unique* atherogenic factor in humans may ultimately be impossible: any single factor is liable to surrender its independent association with CVD in multivariate analysis as the crowd of risk factors and markers grows. The natural history of IRS may actually illustrate how multifactorial disorders like CVD originate from a whole present at the very beginning rather than by accruing unrelated factors along the way. Some compounded index of IRS may well prove to be a clinically useful predictor of atherogenesis and a point of physiological or pharmacological intervention.

## REFERENCES


1 Reaven GM. Role of insulin resistance in human disease. *Diabetes* 1988; 37: 1595–607.

2 Kemp HG. Left ventricular function in patients with the anginal syndrome and normal coronary arteriograms. *Am J Cardiol* 1973; 32: 257–63.

3 Conti CR. What is syndrome X? *Clin Cardiol* 1993; 16: 1–3.

4 Cannon RO III, Epstein SE. 'Microvascular angina' as a cause of chest pain with angiographically normal coronary arteries. *Am J Cardiol* 1988; 61: 1338–43.

5 Dean JD, Jones CJ, Hutchison SJ, Peters JR, Henderson AH. Hyperinsulinaemia and microvascular angina ('syndrome X'). *Lancet* 1991; 337: 456–7.

6 Reaven GM. A syndrome of resistance to insulin-stimulated glucose uptake (Syndrome X): definition and implications. *Cardiovasc Risk Fact* 1993; 3: 2–11.

7 Camici PG, Marraccini P, Lorenzoni R *et al.* Coronary hemodynamics and myocardial metabolism in patients with Syndrome X: response to pacing stress. *JACC* 1991; 17: 1461–1.

8 Opherk D, Schuler G, Wetterauer K, Manthey J, Schwartz F, Kübler W. Four-year follow-up study in patients with angina pectoris and normal coronary arteriograms ('Syndrome X'). *Circulation* 1989; 80: 1610–16.

9 Haffner SM, Hazuda HP, Mitchell BD, Patterson JK, Stern MP. Increased incidence of type II diabetes mellitus in Mexican Americans. *Diabetes Care* 1991; 14: 102–8.

10 Kissebah AH, Vydelingum N, Murray R *et al.* Relation of body fat distribution to metabolic complications of obesity. *J Clin Endocrinol Metab* 1982; 54: 254–60.

11 Kissebah AH, Evans DJ, Peiris A, Wilson CR. Endocrine characteristics in regional obesities: role of sex steroids. In: Vague J, Björntorp P, Guy-Grand B, Rebuffé-Scrive M, Vague P, eds. *Metabolic complications of human obesities*. Elsevier Science, Amsterdam, 1985; 115–30.

12 Björntorp P. Visceral fat accumulation: the missing link between psychosocial factors and cardiovascular disease? *J Intern Med* 1991; 230: 195–201.

13 Rodnick KJ, Haskell WL, Solomon R, Widstrom A, Reaven GM. Improved insulin action in muscle, liver, and adipose tissue in physically trained human subjects. *Am J Physiol* 1987; 253: E489–95.

14 Adamo M, LeRoith D, Simon J, Roth J. Effect of altered nutritional states on insulin receptors. *Annu Rev Nutr* 1988; 8: 149–66.

15 Facchini F, Hollenbeck CB, Jeppesen J, Chen Y-D1, Reaven GM. Insulin resistance and cigarette smoking. *Lancet* 1992; 339: 1128–30.

16 Schumacher MC, Hasstedt SJ, Hunt SC, Williams RR, Elbein SC. Major gene effect for insulin levels in familial NIDDM pedigrees. *Diabetes* 1992; 41: 416–23.

17 Clark PM, Levy JC, Cox L, Burnett M, Turner RC, Hales CN. Immunoradiometric assay of insulin, intact pro-insulin and 32–33 split pro-insulin and radioimmunoassay of insulin in diet-treated type II (non-insulin-dependent) diabetic subjects. *Diabetologia* 1992; 35: 469–74.
18 Nagi DK, Hendra TJ, Ryle AJ *et al.* The relationships of concentrations of insulin, intact pro-insulin and 32–33 split pro-insulin with cardiovascular risk factors in Type II (non-insulin-dependent) diabetic subjects. *Diabetologia* 1990; 33: 532–7.
19 Ferrannini E, Cobelli C. The kinetics of insulin in man.I.General aspects. *Diab Metab Rev* 1987; 3: 335–65.
20 Roth J, Kahn CR, Lesniak MA *et al.* Receptors for insulin, NSILA-s and growth hormone: applications to disease states in man. *Rec Progr Horm Res* 1975; 31: 95–120.
21 Unger RH, Grundy S. Hyperglycaemia as an inducer as well as a consequence of impaired islet cell function and insulin resistance: implications for the management of diabetes. *Diabetologia* 1985; 28: 119–21.
22 Ferrannini E, Haffner SM, Stern MP. Essential hypertension: an insulin resistant state. *J Cardiovasc Pharmacol* 1990; 15 (Suppl 5): S18–25.
23 Ferrannini E, Haffner SM, Stern MP *et al.* High blood pressure and insulin resistance: influence of genetic background. *Eur J Clin Invest* 1991; 21: 280–6.
24 Ferrannini E, DeFronzo RA. The association of hypertension, diabetes and obesity: a review. *J Nephrol* 1989; 1: 3–15.
25 Zavaroni I, Bonora E, Pagliara *et al.* Risk factors for coronary heart disease in healthy persons with hyperinsulinemia and normal glucose tolerance. *N Engl J Med* 1989; 320: 702–6.
26 Ferrannini E. The haemodynamics of obesity: a theoretical analysis *J Hypertens* 1992; 10: 1417–23.
27 Del Prato S, Ferrannini E, DeFronzo RA. Evaluation of insulin sensitivity in man. In: Clarke WL, Larner J, Pohl SL, eds. *Methods in diabetes research. II. clinical methods*, John Wiley & Sons, New York; 1986: 35–76.
28 Kahn CR, Smith RJ, Chin WW. Mechanism of action of hormones that act at the cell surface. In: Wilson JD, Foster DW eds. *Williams textbook of endocrinology* (8th ed), WB Saunders Company, Philadelphia, 1992; 91–134.
29 Bogardus C, Lillioja S, Nyomba BL *et al.* Distribution of *in vivo* insulin action in Pima Indians as mixture of three normal distributions. *Diabetes* 1989; 38: 1423–32.
30 Lillioja S, Mott DM, Zawadski JK *et al. In vivo* insulin action is familial characteristic in Pima Indians. *Diabetes* 1987; 36: 1329–35.
31 Martin BC, Warram JH, Rosner B, Rich SS, Soeldner JS, Krolewski AS. Familial clustering of insulin sensitivity. *Diabetes* 1992; 41: 850–4.
32 Haffner SM, Stern MP, Hazuda HP, Pugh JA, Patterson JK. Hyperinsulinemia in a population at high risk for non-insulin-dependent diabetes mellitus. *N Engl J Med* 1986; 315: 220–4.
33 Haffner SM, Stern MP, Hazuda HP, Mitchell BD, Patterson JK. Increased insulin concentrations in nondiabetic offspring of diabetic parents. *N Engl J Med* 1988; 319: 1297–301.
34 Eriksson J, Franssila-Kallunki A, Ekstrand A *et al.* Early metabolic defects in persons at increased risk for non-insulin-dependent diabetes mellitus. *N Engl J Med* 1989; 321: 337–43.
35 Gulli G, Ferrannini E, Stern MP, Haffner SM, DeFronzo RA. The metabolic profile of non-insulin-dependent diabetes mellitus is fully established in glucose tolerant offspring of two non-insulin dependent diabetic parents. *Diabetes* 1992; 41:1575–86.
36 Sicree RA, Zimmet PZ, King HOM, Coventry JS. Plasma insulin response among Nauruans prediction of deterioration in glucose tolerance over 6 yr. *Diabetes* 1987; 36:179–86.
37 Lillioja S, Mott DM, Howard BV *et al* Impaired glucose tolerance as a disorder of insulin action: longitudinal and cross-sectional studies in Pima Indians. *N Engl J Med* 1988; 318:1217–25.
38 Haffner SM, Stern MP, Mitchell BD, Hazuda HP, Patterson JK. Incidence of type II diabetes in Mexican Americans predicted by fasting insulin and glucose levels, obesity, and body-fat distribution. *Diabetes* 1990; 39:283–8.
39 Warram JH, Martin BC, Krolewski AS, Soeldner JS, Kahn CR. Slow glucose removal rate and hyperinsulinemlia precede the development of type II diabetes in the offspring of diabetic parents. *Ann Intern Med* 1990; 113:909–15.
40 Groop LC, Bonadonna RC, DelPrato S *et al.* Glucose and free fatty acid metabolism in non-insulin dependent diabetes mellitus. Evidence for multiple sites of insulin resistance. *J Clin Invest* 1988; 84:205–13.
41 DeFronzo RA. The triumvirate: beta cell, muscle, liver: a collusion responsible for NIDDM. *Diabetes* 1988; 37:667–87.
42 Ferrannini E, Buzzigoli G, Bonadonna R *et al.* Insulin resistance in essential hypertension. *N Engl J Med* 1987; 317:350–7.
43 Pollare T, Lithell H, Berne C. Insulin resistance is a characteristic feature of primary hypertension indepedent of obesity. *Metabolism* 1990; 39:167–74.
44 Natali A, Santoro D, Palombo C, Cerri M, Ghione S, Ferrannini E. Impaired insulin action on skeletal muscle metabolism in essential hypertension. *Hypertension* 1991; 17:170–8.
45 Capaldo B, Lembo G, Napoli *et al.* Skeletal muscle is a primary site of insulin resistance in essential hypertension. *Metabolism* 1991; 40:1320–2.
46 Rooney DP, Neely RD, Ennis CN *et al.* Insulin action and hepatic glucose cycling in essential hypertension. *Metabolism* 1992; 41:317–24.
47 Saad MF, Lillioja S, Nyomba BL *et al.* Racial differences in the relation between blood pressure and insulin resistance. *N Engl J Med* 1991; 324:733–9.
48 Falkner B, Hulman S, Tannenbaum J, Kushner H. Insulin resistance and blood pressure in young black men. *Hypertension* 1990; 16:708–11.
49 Ferrari P, Weidmann P, Shaw *et al.* Altered insulin sensitivity, hyperinsulinemia, and dyslipidemia in individuals with a hypertensive parent. *Am J Med* 1991; 91:589–96.
50 Haffner SM, Ferrannini E, Hazuda HP, Stern MP. Clustering of cardiovascular risk factors in confirmed prehypertensive individuals. *Hypertension* 1992; 20:38–45.
51 Skarfors ET, Lithell HO, Selinus I. Risk factors for the development of hypertension: a 10-year longitudinal study in middle-aged men. *J Hypertens* 1991; 9:217–23.
52 Niskanen LK, Uusitupa MI, Pyöräla K. The relationship

of hyperinsulinemia to the development of hypertension in type 2 diabetic patients and in non-diabetic subjects. *J Hum Hypertens* 1991; 5:155–9.
53 Reaven GM, Lerner RL, Stern MP, Farquhar JW. Role of insulin in endogenous hypertriglyceridemia. *J Clin Invest* 1967; 46:1756–67.
54 Quiñones-Galvan A, Santoro D, Natali A *et al.* Insulin sensitivity in familial hypercholesterolemia. *Metabolism* 1993; 42: 1359–64.
55 Haffner SM, Valdez RA, Hazuda HP, Mitchell BD, Morales PA, Stern MP. Prospective analysis of the insulin resistance syndrome (Syndrome X). *Diabetes* 1992; 41:715–22.
56 Laakso M, Sarlund H, Mykkänen I. Essential hypertension and insulin resistance in non-insulin-dependent diabetes. *Eur J Clin Invest* 1989; 19:518–26.
57 Widen E, Ekstrand A, Saloranta C *et al.* Localization of insulin resistance in type 2 (non-insulin-dependent) diabetic patients with hypertriglyceridemia. *Diabetologia* 1992; 35:1140–5.
58 Hunt SC, Wu LL, Hopkins PN *et al.* Apolipoprotein, low density lipoprotein subfraction and insulin associations with familial combined hyperlipidemia: study of Utah patients with familial dyslipidemic hypertension. *Arteriosclerosis* 1989; 9: 335–4.
59 Selby JV, Newman B, Quiroga J, Christian JC, Austin MA, Fabsitz RR. Concordance for dyslipidemic hypertension in male twins. *JAMA* 1991; 265: 2079–84.
60 Haffner SM, Stern MP, Hazuda HP, Mitchell BD, Patterson JK, Ferrannini E. Parental history of diabetes is associated with increased cardiovascular risk factors. *Arteriosclerosis* 1989; 9: 928–33.
61 Florey C du V, Uppal S, Lowy C. Relation between blood pressure, weight, and plasma sugar and serum insulin levels in schoolchildren aged 9–12 years in Westland, Holland. *Br Med J* 1976; i: 1368–71.
62 Medalie JH, Papier CM, Goldbourt H, Herman JB. Major factors in the development of NIDDM in 10,000 men. *Arch Intern Med* 1975; 135: 811–17.
63 Salomaa VV, Strandberg TE, Vanhanen H, Naukkarinen V, Sarna S, Miettinen TA. Glucose tolerance and blood pressure: long term follow up in middle aged men. *Br Med J* 1991; 302: 493–6.
64 Swinburn BA, Nyomba BL, Saad MF *et al.* Insulin resistance associated with lower rates of weight gain in Pima Indians. *J Clin Invest* 1991; 88: 168–73.
65 Valdez R, Mitchell BD, Haffner SM *et al.* Predictors of weight change in a biethnic population. The San Antonio Heart Study. *Int J Obes* 1993; (in press).
66 Bouchard C. Genetic aspects of human obesity. In Björntorp P, Brodoff BN, eds. *Obesity*. JB Lippincott Company, Philadelphia, 1992; 343–51.
67 Williams RR, Hasstedt SJ, Hunt SC *et al.* Genetic traits related to hypertension and electrolyte metabolism. *Hypertension* 1991; 17 (Suppl 1): 169–73.
68 Doria A, Fioretto P, Avogaro A *et al.* Insulin resistance is associated with high sodium-lithium countertransport in essential hypertension. *Am J Physiol* 1991; 261: E68–91.
69 Mangili R, Bending JJ, Scott G, Li LK, Gupta A, Viberti GC. Increased sodium-lithium countertransport activity in red cell of patients with insulin-dependent diabetes and nephropathy. *N Engl J Med* 1988; 318: 146–50.
70 Groop L, Ekstrand A, Forsblom C, Widén E, Groop P-H, Teppo A-M, Eriksson J. Insulin resistance, hypertension and microalbuminuria in patients with Type 2 (non-insulin-dependent) diabetes mellitus. *Diabetologia* 1993; 36: 642–7.
71 Canessa M, Zerbini P. Insulin modulation of $Na^+/Li^+$ countertransport: impact on hypertension and diabetes. *Acta Diabetol* 1992; 29: 186–90.
72 Mahnensmith RL, Aronson PL. The plasma membrane sodium-hydrogen exchanger and its role in physiological and pathophysiological process. *Circ Res* 1985; 56: 443–67.
73 Draznin B, Sussman KE, Eckel RH, Kao M, Yost T, Sherman NA. Possible role of cytosolic free calcium concentrations in mediating insulin resistance of obesity and hyperinsulinemia. *J Clin Invest* 1988; 82: 1848–52.
74 Paolisso G, Scheen A, D'Onofrio F, Lefebvre PJ. Magnesium and glucose homeostasis. *Diabetologia* 1990; 33: 511–14.
75 Ram JL, Stanley PR, Sowers JR. Hypertension, insulin function, and calcium. In: Draznin B, Eckel RH ed, *Diabetes and atherosclerosis. molecular basis and clinical aspects.* Elsevier, Amsterdam, 1993: 291–306.
76 Mogensen CE. Prediction of clinical diabetic nephropathy in IDDM patients: alternative to microalbuminuria? *Diabetes* 1990; 39: 761–7.
77 Krolewski AS, Canessa M, Warram J *et al.* Predisposition to hypertension and susceptibility to renal disease in insulin-dependent diabetes mellitus. *N Engl J Med* 1988; 318: 140–5.
78 Mangili R, Bending JJ, Scott G, Li LK, Gupta A, Viberti GC. Increased sodium–lithium countertransport activity in red cells of patients with insulin-dependent diabetes and nephropathy. *N Engl J Med* 1988; 318: 146–50.
79 Parving HH, Mogensen CE, Jensen HAE, Evrin PE. Increased urinary albumin excretion rate in benign essential hypertension. *Lancet* 1974; 1190–1192.
80 Krolewski AS, Czyzyk A, Kopczynski J, Rywik S. Prevalence of diabetes mellitus, coronary heart disease and hypertension in the families of insulin dependent and insulin independent diabetics. *Diabetologia* 1981; 21: 520–4.
81 Krolewski AS, Warram JH, Cupples A, Gorman CK, Szabo AJ, Christlieb AR. Hypertension, orthostatic hypotension and the microvascular complications of diabetes. *J Chron Dis* 1985; 38: 319–26.
82 Haffner SM, Stern MP, Koslowski Gruber MK, Hazuda HP, Mitchell BD, Patterson JK. Microalbuminuria. Potential marker for increased cardiovascular risk factors in nondiabetic subjects? *Arteriosclerosis* 1990; 10: 727–31.
83 Juhan-Vague I, Alessi MC, Vague P. Increased plasminogen activator inhibitor 1 levels. A possible link between insulin resistance and atherothrombosis. *Diabetologia* 1991; 34: 457–62.
84 Alessi MC, Juhan-Vague I, Kooistra T, Declerck PJ, Collen D. Insulin stimulates the synthesis of plasminogen activator inhibitor 1 by the human hepatocellular line HepG2. *Thromb Haemostas* 1988; 60: 491–4.
85 Facchini F, Chen Y-DI, Hollenbeck CB, Reaven GM. Relationship between resistance to insulin-mediated glucose uptake, urinary uric acid clearance, and plasma uric acid concentration. *JAMA* 1991; 226: 3008–11.
86 Barker DJP, Bull AR, Osmond C, Simmonds SJ. Foetal

and placental size and risk of hypertension in adult life. *Br Med J* 1990; 301: 259–62.
87 Hales CN, Barker DJP, Clark PMS *et al.* Foetal and infant growth and impaired glucose tolerance at age 64. *Br Med J* 1991; 303: 1019–22.
88 Barker DJP, Hales CN, Fall CHD, Osmond C, Phipps K, Clark PMS. Type 2 (non-insulin-dependent) diabetes mellitus, hypertension and hyperlipidaemia (syndrome X): relation to reduced foetal growth. *Diabetologia* 1993; 36: 62–7.
89 Athens M, Valdez R, Stern M. Effect of birthweight on future development of 'Syndrome X' in adult life. *Diabetes* 1993; 42 (Suppl 1): 61A.
90 Breschi MC, Seghieri G, Bartolomei G, Gironi A, Baldi S, Ferrannini E. Relation of birthweight to maternal plasma glucose and insulin concentrations during normal pregnancy. *Diabetologia* 1993; 36: 1315–21.
91 Yudkin JS, Forrest RD, Jackson CA. Microalbuminuria as predictor of vascular disease in non-diabetic subjects. *Lancet* 1988; ii: 530–3.
92 Fuller JH, Head J. Blood pressure, proteinuria and their relationship with circulatory mortality: the WHO multinational study of vascular disease in diabetics. *Diabetes Metab* 1989; 15: 273–7.
93 Mattock MB, Morrish NJ, Viberti G, Keen H, Fitzgerald AP, Jackson G. Prospective study of microalbuminuria as predictor of mortality in NIDDM. *Diabetes* 1992; 41: 736–41.
94 Barker DJP, Winter PD, Osmond C, Margetts B, Simmonds SJ. Weight in infancy and death from ischaemic heart disease. *Lancet* 1989; ii: 577–80.
95 Eriksson K-F. Prevention of non-insulin-dependent diabetes mellitus. A population study with special reference to insulin secretion, skeletal muscle morphology and metabolic capacity. Doctoral Thesis, University of Lund, Sweden, 1992; 53–9.
96 Krolewski AS, Warram JH, Valsania P, Martin BC, Laffel LMB, Christlieb AR. Evolving natural history of coronary artery disease in diabetes mellitus. *Am J Med* 1991; 90 (Suppl 2A): 56S-61S.
97 Haffner SM, Stern MP, Hazuda HP, Mitchell BD, Patterson JK. Cardiovascular risk factors in confirmed prediabetic individuals: does the clock for coronary heart disease start ticking before the onset of clinical diabetes? *JAMA* 1990; 263: 2893–8.
98 Ducimetiere P, Eschwege E, Papoz L, Richard JL, Claude JR, Rosselin G. Relationship of plasma insulin levels to the incidence of myocardial infarction and coronary heart disease mortality in a middle-aged population. *Diabetologia* 1980; 19: 205–10.
99 Pyöräla K. Relationship of glucose tolerance and plasma insulin to the incidence of coronary heart disease: results from two population studies in Finland. *Diabetes Care* 1979; 2: 131–41.
100 Welborn TA, Wearne K. Coronary disease incidence and cardiovascular mortality in Busselton with reference to glucose and insulin concentrations. *Diabetes Care* 1979; 2: 154–60.

# Epidemiology of the Complications of Diabetes

## 15 Introduction

Aaron I. Vinik

In the next few chapters, we will review the current knowledge and information available on the complications of diabetes. Since the advent of insulin in 1922, people with diabetes are not in general dying of the acute complications, e.g. diabetic ketoacidosis and hyperosmolar non-ketotic coma but, are, instead, subject to the morbidity and potential mortality ascribable to the complications of the disorder. The major cause of both morbidity and mortality is no doubt macrovascular disease and therefore the information is generally more plentiful and more attention has been focused on this aspect of diabetes. None the less, significant morbidity derives from the neuropathic complications which are probably the most frequent complication causing the greatest morbidity if not contributing to the greatest mortality. Renal disease in diabetes is now the leading cause of admission to a renal transplant unit and eye disease is now the third leading cause of blindness in the world. Each will be presented and discussed from the point of view of their impact in the individual and society as a whole. The lessons that may be learned from epidemiologic studies will become apparent and possibly shed new light on the clues to understanding the pathogenesis, an important prerequisite if we are to develop new therapeutic strategies aimed at preventing or retarding the progression of the disease.

# 16 Macrovascular Disease in Diabetes

Braxton D. Mitchell

## INTRODUCTION

Large vessel disease is the leading cause of mortality in subjects with diabetes and a major cause of morbidity. The major manifestations of large vessel disease include heart disease, cerebrovascular disease, and peripheral vascular disease. This chapter will review briefly the epidemiology of these conditions as they occur in diabetes. The review will emphasise data obtained from population-based prospective studies, especially those which include non-diabetic controls.

## HEART DISEASE IN DIABETES

The close association between diabetes and heart disease has been recognised for a long time. It is estimated that diabetics have a two to fourfold excess risk of developing heart disease (see below) and, since heart disease occurs at a relatively high frequency in the general population, diabetes accounts for a large number of heart disease cases.

From a public health perspective, diabetes-related heart disease is gaining importance as a major contributor of morbidity and mortality. The introduction of insulin therapy in 1923, for example, dramatically lengthened the life-span of many patients with insulin-dependent diabetes but, in so doing, also increased the number of persons at risk for developing the macrovascular complications of diabetes. More recent studies have documented that the prevalence of type 2 diabetes is on the increase in many places in the world. For the period 1980 and 1987, the Centers for Disease Control reported a 9% increase in the prevalence of diabetes in the United States and found that there was a 34% increase among diabetics in the hospitalisation rates for major cardiovascular disease and stroke (1). Data from the Minnesota Heart Survey have indicated that the prevalence of diabetes among men hospitalised with a myocardial infarction in the Minneapolis–St Paul metropolitan area doubled between 1970 and 1985 and increased by 60% in women (2). In westernised countries, like the United States, some of the increase in diabetes prevalence can be attributed to the ageing of the population, but some of the increase probably also reflects an increase in the incidence of diabetes. The prevalence of diabetes is also increasing in many developing countries of the world. Populations which appear to be at particularly high risk are those making the transition from rural to urban environments, and in the process adopting westernised lifestyles and behaviours (3).

Table 16.1. *Summary of population-based prospective studies showing the relative risk of heart disease in persons with and without diabetes, according to sex*

| Study (Reference) | Length of follow-up | Endpoint[a] | Age-adjusted Relative risk (*diabetic vs. non-diabetic*) | |
|---|---|---|---|---|
| | | | Men | Women |
| Whitehall Study (39) | 10 yr | CHD mortality | 4.0 | – |
| Bedford Survey (25) | 10 yr | CHD mortality | 2.1 | 7.3[b] |
| Tecumseh Study (28) | 18 yr | CHD mortality | 3.0 | 3.0 |
| Framingham Study (23) | 20 yr | CVD | 2.2 | 2.8 |
| | 20 yr | CHD | 1.7 | 2.7 |
| | 20 yr | CVD mortality | 2.1 | 4.9 |
| Evans County Study (24) | 4.5 yr | CHD mortality | 1.0 | 2.8 |
| Israeli Ischaemic Heart Disease | 5 yr | MI mortality | 3.4 | – |
| Study (52) | 5 yr | CHD | 2.5 | – |
| US Whites (NHANES I | 9 yr | CVD mortality | 2.6 | 2.2 |
| survey) (10) | 9 yr | CHD mortality | 2.8 | 2.5 |
| Rancho Bernardo Study (26) | 14 yr | CHD mortality | 1.8 | 3.3 |
| Chicago Industry Study (27) | 9 yr | CHD mortality | 4.0 | 5.9 |

[a] Endpoint abbreviations: CHD, coronary heart disease; CVD, cardiovascular disease.
[b] Extrapolated from Figure.

## DIABETES AND CARDIOVASCULAR MORTALITY

Mortality from cardiovascular diseases is two to four times higher in diabetics than in non-diabetics (4, 5). The evidence for this comes from a number of population-based follow-up studies, the results of which are summarised in Table 16.1. Most of these studies have also indicated that diabetes is more strongly associated with cardiovascular mortality in women than in men. (see discussion below).

In most Western countries, heart disease is the leading cause of death in the general population so it is not surprising that it is also the leading cause of death in persons with diabetes. It has been estimated that cardiovascular disease accounts for approximately 50–60% of all deaths among diabetics (6–9). Based on a 9-year follow-up of NHANES I subjects in the United States, Kleinman and colleagues estimated that 75% of the excess mortality in diabetic men and 57% of the excess mortality in diabetic women was attributable to cardiovascular disease (10).

Due to the prominence of other diabetes-related causes of mortality associated with type 1 diabetes (especially mortality from renal disease), cardiovascular diseases account for a higher proportion of deaths in type 2 diabetes than in type 1 diabetes. In southern Wisconsin, for example, heart disease was reported to be the underlying cause of death in 49% of persons diagnosed with diabetes after the age of 30, but in only 30% of persons diagnosed with diabetes before age 30 (7). If one accounts for the younger age distribution of the type 1 subjects, however, the actual risk of cardiovascular death is probably higher in type 1 subjects than in type 2 subjects. Among previously diagnosed diabetics in southern Wisconsin, the association between diabetes and heart disease mortality was far stronger for younger onset diabetics (relative risk = 9.1) than for older onset diabetics (relative risk = 2.3) (7). In the Pittsburgh Epidemiology of Diabetic Complications Study, Dorman *et al.* estimated that patients with childhood onset IDDM experienced cardiovascular mortality at rates that were 11 times higher than those experienced by the general population (11). By 55 years of age, 35% of male and female juvenile onset IDDM subjects studied by Krolewski and colleagues from the Joslin Clinic had died of coronary artery disease compared to expected rates of 8% for non-diabetic men and 4% for non-diabetic women (12). In the London cohort of the World Health Organisation Multinational Study of Vascular Disease in Diabetes, however, age-adjusted coronary heart disease mortality rates were approximately equal between subjects with type 1 and type 2 diabetes (9).

## PREVALENCE AND INCIDENCE

It has long been recognised that heart disease occurs more frequently in diabetics than in non-diabetics. Because diabetics with heart disease tend to die earlier than diabetics without heart disease, prevalence data underestimate the excess occurrence of cardiovascular disease in diabetes. Nevertheless, most studies have reported that diabetics are $1\frac{1}{2}$ to 3 times more likely to have coronary heart disease (CHD) than non-diabetics, depending on the age range of the population of the study and the diagnostic criteria used (4,5). Diabetics have a higher frequency of ECG abnormalities compared to non-diabetics, including major Q wave abnormalities and S–T segment depressions (14–16). Diabetics are also more likely than non-diabetics to report a previous history of myocardial infarction, angina pectoris, and prior heart surgery (4).

A number of prospective studies of diabetes and heart disease have now been carried out, with most finding the incidence of new cardiovascular disease to be 2–4 times higher in diabetic than in non-diabetic individuals (4,5,17). As with cardiovascular mortality, the majority of these studies show that the relative impact of diabetes on incidence of non-fatal cardiovascular disease is stronger in women than in men (see next section).

There is considerable variation in the risk of developing heart disease for diabetic populations world-wide. This has been demonstrated by the World Health Organisation Multinational Study of Vascular Disease in Diabetics, in which a total of 6695 diabetic men and women were studied from 14 centres in Asia, Europe, and North America. This study used similar case definitions across study sites and found a relatively low prevalence of coronary heart disease in diabetics of Oriental background (e.g. the prevalence of angina pectoris and myocardial infarction was less than 10% in Tokyo and Hong Kong) and a relatively high prevalence in diabetics examined in Moscow, Warsaw, Berlin, and Havana (more than 20% affected) (18). More recent data from this study indicate that mortality from ischaemic heart disease is also considerably lower among diabetics from Hong Kong and Tokyo than in diabetics from Berlin, Warsaw, and London (19).

One explanation for these geographical differences in susceptibility to diabetes-related heart disease is that susceptibility to heart disease in general varies widely between populations. Diabetics in East Finland, for example, have approximately a twofold higher prevalence of CHD compared to diabetics in West Finland, but the prevalence of CHD in the general population is also higher in East Finland than in West Finland (20). Diabetic Pima Indians of the southwestern United States, who have one of the highest levels of diabetes in the world, have an unexpectedly low incidence of fatal CHD (19, 21), and one study, in fact, has reported CHD mortality among diabetic Pima Indians to be even lower than in the general Caucasian population in Framingham, Massachusetts (21). Among non-diabetic Pima Indians, however, it turns out that CHD is relatively uncommon (15, 21).

## SEX DIFFERENCES IN THE IMPACT OF DIABETES ON HEART DISEASE

In the general population, women have a lower risk of CHD compared to men, although the female protection against CHD becomes less pronounced after menopause. Data from a number of studies have suggested that among diabetic individuals, the sex difference in CHD is also decreased, thus implying that the relative impact of diabetes on cardiovascular disease is greater in women than in men. In the Framingham Study, for example, the incidence of cardiovascular disease in diabetic men was two times higher than in non-diabetic men, while the incidence in diabetic women was three times higher than in non-diabetic women (22, 23). Similar patterns have been reported from other population-based follow-up studies (24–27), although at least two have reported that having a history of diabetes increased the risk of CHD mortality by about the same degree in men and women (10, 28). Table 16.1 summarises the results from nine population-based prospective studies which have examined the impact of diabetes on fatal or non-fatal cardiovascular disease in men and/or women.

Data from the Multinational Study of Vascular Disease in Diabetics also suggest that women with diabetes lose their protection against cardiovascular disease relative to men. At baseline, the prevalence of ischaemic heart disease, as measured by Minnesota-coded ECGs, was found in this study to be nearly identical between diabetic men and women (29). The London cohort of this study has now been followed prospectively for 8 years, and the incidence of ischaemic ECG abnormalities and total ischaemic heart disease (ischaemic ECG abnormalities, angina pectoris, and myocardial infarction) was also roughly similar between men and women. Women with IDDM were also just as likely to develop myocardial infarction as men with IDDM, although myocardial infarction incidence was significantly higher in men with NIDDM than in women with NIDDM (13).

At least one study has reported a greater impact of diabetes in men than in women. Uusitupa *et al.* studied 133 newly diagnosed NIDDM patients and 144 non-diabetic controls from Eastern Finland and found the 5-year incidence of myocardial infarction to be 19.4% in diabetic men compared to 11.0% in diabetic women. In this population diabetes accounted for a 6-fold excess of myocardial infarction in men and a 3.7-fold excess in women (30).

Most of the population-based studies of diabetes and cardiovascular disease have included populations in which the overwhelming majority of diabetics had type 2 diabetes. This implies that the relative impact of type 2 diabetes on heart disease is stronger in women than in men. In the London cohort of the Multinational Study of Vascular Disease in Diabetics, however, women with type 2 diabetes were less likely to die of cardiovascular disease than their male counterparts as evidenced by the fact that their age-adjusted cardiovascular mortality was 2.5 times lower than that of men with type 2 diabetes. The age-adjusted cardiovascular disease mortality rates for type 1 patients, however, were virtually identical between men and women, suggesting that in this study type 1 diabetes had a particularly adverse impact on women (9).

## NON-ATHEROSCLEROTIC HEART DISEASE IN DIABETES

The vast majority of heart disease in diabetes is atherosclerosis-related. This is supported by the fact that the same risk factors associated with CHD in non-diabetic populations (e.g. obesity, high levels of total cholesterol, low levels of HDL cholesterol, hypertension, and smoking) also predict CHD in diabetic populations, and, moreover, these risk factors carry approximately the same magnitude of risk for diabetics as they do for non-diabetics (see discussion below). Numerous autopsy studies of coronary arteries have also shown that relative to non-diabetics, the arteries of diabetics show more evidence of atherosclerosis, including more fatty streaks, more raised atherogenic lesions, more fibrous plaques, and a greater extent of coronary stenosis (31–34). These findings, in part, have led to the conclusion that diabetes is associated with accelerated atherosclerosis.

There is debate as to whether diabetics also

are more likely than non-diabetics to experience heart disease that is unrelated to atherosclerosis (35, 36). Much of the epidemiological data comes from the Framingham Study, in which diabetes was associated with a 2.2 times excess risk for congestive heart failure in men and a 5.4 times excess risk in women. When the analysis was adjusted for age, systolic pressure, smoking, and left ventricular hypertrophy ECG abnormalities, the association between diabetes and congestive heart failure remained significant but was diminished slightly, to 1.8 in men and 3.8 in women (37). Subgroup analyses revealed that nearly all of the excess risk of congestive heart failure among the diabetic subjects was confined to subjects treated with insulin (38). It is not known whether the excess risk of congestive heart failure associated with diabetes can be attributed entirely to atherosclerosis or whether other pathogenic processes, such as small vessel disease, may be involved (36).

## RISK FACTORS FOR HEART DISEASE IN DIABETES

The factors associated with the development of heart disease in diabetes appear to be quite different from those responsible for the development of diabetic microvascular disease. The incidence of both retinopathy and diabetic renal disease, for example, is strongly associated with both the duration of diabetes and the level of glycaemic control, suggesting that the metabolic derangements that accompany diabetes play an important role in the aetiology of these disorders. In contrast, the incidence of heart disease in diabetes is not strongly correlated with either the duration of diabetes or the level of glycaemic control. The lack of a strong correlation between heart disease and these variables may reflect the fact that heart disease has a variety of causes, and diabetes is only one.

### Hyperglycaemia

Although the risk of heart disease is clearly higher in diabetics than in non-diabetics, it is difficult to evaluate the importance of hyperglycaemia *per se* as a risk factor for heart disease. Multivariate analyses that include both level of glucose and diabetes in the same model are difficult to interpret since diabetes, by definition, includes all individuals in the upper tail of the glucose distribution. To assess the independent effect of hyperglycaemia on heart disease risk, a number of studies have therefore examined the relationship between glucose levels and heart disease in individuals without diabetes. As discussed below, these studies have provided conflicting evidence as to whether blood glucose levels below the threshold for diabetes are a risk factor for heart disease.

Several studies have compared the incidence of cardiovascular disease between subjects with impaired glucose tolerance and subjects with normal glucose tolerance. In the Whitehall Study, cardiovascular mortality was approximately two times higher in men with impaired glucose tolerance than in men with normal glucose tolerance (39, 40). Similarly, the Paris Prospective Study reported that total cardiovascular mortality was approximately two times higher in men with impaired glucose tolerance than in men with normal glucose tolerance, although there was no evidence for a difference in CHD mortality between the two groups (41). The Honolulu Heart Program found no difference in CHD mortality rates between men with previously diagnosed diabetes and men with glucose intolerance but no prior history of diabetes. In both groups, however, CHD mortality was approximately 3 times higher than in men with normal glucose tolerance (42).

Impaired glucose tolerance was also associated with coronary heart disease mortality in the Bedford Survey, although the association was stronger in women than in men (25). In a review of 11 studies conducted in middle-aged men in eight countries, however, the International Collaborative Group concluded that evidence for an association between impaired glucose tolerance and CHD mortality was inconclusive (43, 44). In these studies, CHD mortality was compared between non-diabetic men in the top 20% of the glucose distribution with non-diabetic men in the bottom 20% of the glucose distribution. In four of the 11 studies, a relative risk of approximately 2 or more was reported, although in four other studies the relative risks were approximately 1, indicating no association between glucose level and CHD mortality. Moreover, of the four studies showing a positive association between glucose levels and CHD mortality, in only one did the relative risk remain statistically significant when other cardiovascular risk factors were accounted for in the analysis. In three of the 11 studies, however, higher glucose levels were significantly associated with total cardiovascular deaths in multivariate analysis (44).

Among those studies reporting a correlation between glucose levels and cardiovascular disease, further analyses have focused on whether the association is linear or whether there is a threshold for glucose below which glucose levels are not associated with disease. Data from some studies suggest that the relationship may be linear. In Japanese men in Hawaii, 1-hour post-load glucose levels were significantly associated with 9-year CHD and cardiovascular mortality in linear fashion, and the associations remained significant after adjustment for other cardiovascular risk factors (42). After 12 years of follow-up, the incidence of both fatal CHD and non-fatal myocardial infarction continued to increase linearly with increasing glucose concentration (45). A linear relationship between casual (non-fasting) glucose levels in the 70 to 199 mg/dl range and 10-year incidence of cardiovascular disease was reported in women in the Framingham Heart Study, although there was no association between glucose levels and CHD incidence in men (46). The Rancho Bernardo Study, on the other hand, reported a linear relationship between fasting glucose and CHD incidence in men, although, in women, a threshold effect was observed, with only those women with glucose values greater than 110 mg/dl experiencing higher risk (47, 48).

In the Puerto Rico Heart Health Study, there was no evidence for a linear effect of elevated glucose levels on the risk of CHD death in non-diabetic men, although men with glucose values greater than 140 mg/dl had a higher CHD death rate than men with lower glucose values, even after excluding subjects under treatment for diabetes (49).

A number of other studies, however, have suggested that the relationship between glucose levels and cardiovascular disease may not be linear. In the Whitehall Study, for example, non-diabetic men whose baseline glucose values were in the upper 5% of the blood glucose distribution were two times more likely to die of CHD than men whose glucose values were in the lower 95% of the glucose distribution. In men in the lower 95% of the distribution, no dose–response relationship was observed, however (14). In a 10-year follow-up of non-diabetic men enrolled in the Paris Prospective Study, men in the highest quintile (top 20%) of both the fasting and the 2-hour glucose distribution experienced significantly higher CHD mortality than men in the lower four quintiles of the glucose distribution, although there was no evidence for a dose–response relationship (50). Similarly, in the Helsinki Policeman Study, 10-year incidence of CHD was significantly higher in men in the top 20% of the 1-hour post-load glucose distribution than in men in the lower 80%, but again there was no evidence for a dose–response relationship. Neither fasting nor 2-hour post-load glucose levels, however, were associated with CHD incidence (51). Among non-diabetics in the Tecumseh Community Health Survey, hyperglycaemia was marginally associated with CHD mortality in men, although the effect was not linear. Hyperglycaemia was not associated with CHD mortality in women (28).

In some studies, hyperglycaemia has been found to be more strongly associated with cardiovascular disease in women than in men. For example, the relative risks between hyperglycaemia and CHD death reported from the Chicago Industry Study were 1.6 in men and 3.1 in women (27), and relative risks from the Bedford Survey were 1.4 in men and 5.4 in women (25). A significant correlation between glucose levels and cardiovascular disease incidence was also found in women in the Framingham Heart Study, but not in men (46). In the Rancho Bernardo Study, non-diabetic women with fasting glucose values greater than 110 mg/dl were more likely to develop CHD than women with glucose values below this level, although a linear relationship between glucose and CHD was noted in men (47, 48). In the Tecumseh Community Health Survey, however, hyperglycaemia was marginally associated with CHD mortality in men, but there was no association in women (28).

## Duration of diabetes

Among individuals with diabetes, the duration of diabetes is not strongly associated with the risk of CHD. In the Israeli Ischaemic Heart Disease Study, for example, the 5-year incidence of fatal myocardial infarction was elevated by about 3.4-fold in both newly and previously diagnosed diabetics as compared to non-diabetics. Patients with previously diagnosed diabetes did, however, have a 3.2-fold higher incidence of angina pectoris compared to non-diabetics, while angina incidence among newly diagnosed diabetics was surprisingly only 60% as high as that in non-diabetics (52). CHD mortality rates were slightly higher in previously diagnosed diabetic men in the Paris Prospective Study compared to newly diagnosed diabetic men (4.3 per 1000 vs. 3.0 per 1000), but both were considerably higher than the CHD mortality rates in men with normal glucose tolerance (1.4 per 1000) (50). Men newly diagnosed with type 2 diabetes in the Whitehall Study actually experienced higher CHD mortality rates than did previously diagnosed men, although the difference was not statistically significant (40).

The lack of a correlation between duration of diabetes and presence of heart disease has also been confirmed by autopsy studies. In their study of 229 diabetic necropsy patients, Waller *et al.* found no correlation between duration of diabetes and the prevalence of severe coronary stenosis due to atherosclerotic plaques (31). In another group of 185 diabetic patients autopsied by Vigorita *et al.*, the degree of coronary atherosclerosis as assessed by post-mortem coronary angiography correlated poorly with duration of diabetes, although diabetics had significantly more than non-diabetics (32).

## Traditional CHD risk factors

In addition to being associated with heart disease *per se*, numerous studies have documented that diabetes is also associated with an adverse level of other cardiovascular risk factors. Relative to non-diabetics, diabetics tend to have higher systolic and diastolic blood pressures, higher triglyceride levels, and lower levels of HDL-cholesterol (53), and these differences are not explained by the greater obesity of diabetics relative to non-diabetics. Elevated levels of blood pressure and depressed levels of HDL-cholesterol occur in adolescents with type 1 diabetes (54), as well as in patients with type 2 diabetes.

It seems natural to wonder if the association between diabetes and coronary heart disease is mediated by diabetes-induced changes in these other risk factors. This does not appear to be the case, since multivariate analyses which adjust for differences in cardiovascular risk factors between diabetics and non-diabetics reduce only slightly the magnitude of the association between diabetes and heart disease (17, 20, 25, 29, 71).

Among non-diabetic individuals, triglyceride levels are correlated with the prevalence of coronary heart disease, although most studies agree that the association is not independent of other known cardiovascular risk factors. Among individuals with glucose intolerance, at least two studies have reported hypertriglyceridaemia to be an independent risk factor for coronary heart disease. In the Paris Prospective Study, elevated levels of triglycerides were a stronger predictor of CHD death in subjects with abnormal glucose tolerance than were cholesterol, glucose, insulin, or body mass index (56). Serum triglycerides were also significantly associated with the prevalence of major Q-wave abnormalities among diabetics examined in the Multinational Study of Vascular Disease in Diabetics, and the association remained highly significant even after adjustment for age, adiposity, cholesterol, and systolic blood pressure (29). In neither of these studies, however, was HDL-cholesterol levels measured, and so it is unknown whether the triglyceride–heart disease association was independent of HDL-cholcsterol levels.

Individuals who have elevated levels of one cardiovascular risk factor are more likely to have elevated levels of other cardiovascular risk factors, and this clustering appears to be more common in diabetics than in non-diabetics (55). Because diabetics frequently have elevated levels of multiple cardiovascular risk factors simultaneously, it has been speculated that the excess CHD risk experienced by diabetics might be attributable to an interaction between cardiovascular risk factors. Most studies addressing this issue, however, have found no evidence for this hypothesis; that is, although risk factor levels tend to be higher in diabetics, there is no evidence that any of these risk factors has a greater effect in diabetics than in non-diabetics (22, 29, 39). One exception, however, is the Rancho Bernardo Study, which noted that cigarette smoking was a far stronger risk factor for cardiovascular death in diabetics than in non-diabetics (57). Cigarette smoking was also a powerful predictor of cardiovascular mortality for individuals with type 1 diabetes in the Pittsburgh IDDM Study, although non-diabetics were not examined as part of this study so the effect of smoking in non-diabetics could not be assessed (58). In the Whitehall Study, hypertension was more strongly associated with 10-year CHD mortality in men than either smoking, cholesterol concentration, or obesity (39), but whether hypertension is a stronger risk factor for CHD in diabetics than in non-diabetics remains to be seen.

Several studies have suggested that diabetes may be associated with a greater degree of lipoprotein abnormalities in women than in men (59–61). While diabetics of both sexes have higher levels of triglycerides and LDL-cholesterol and lower levels of HDL-cholesterol than non-diabetics, the impact of diabetes appears to be worse for women than for men. These observations are consistent with the idea that diabetes has a relatively greater impact on CHD incidence in women than in men (see earlier discussion).

### Hyperinsulinaemia

It seems unlikely that the aetiology of heart disease in diabetes (particularly type 2 diabetes) can be explained solely by an association between diabetes and accelerated atherosclerosis. Jarrett, for example, has argued that, if diabetes were causally related to atherosclerosis, then the incidence of CHD should be correlated with the duration of diabetes (40, 62). Contrary to this expectation, however, the available data suggest that CHD incidence and mortality is roughly similar between previously and newly diagnosed diabetics. In addition, subjects with impaired glucose tolerance clearly have an elevated risk of CHD compared to subjects with normal glucose tolerance, with some studies, in fact, showing the excess risk associated with impaired glucose tolerance to be as high as in subjects with overt diabetes. Numerous prospective studies have now shown that, even after adjusting for the adverse effect of diabetes on traditional cardiovascular risk factors, the association between diabetes and CHD remains very strong. These findings lend further support to the hypothesis that the effect of diabetes on heart disease is mediated only in part by an effect of diabetes on traditional cardiovascular risk factors.

Evidence that insulin resistance, marked by hyperinsulinaemia, may be involved in the aetiology of heart disease in diabetes has been reviewed recently (17, 63) and by Ferrannini (see Chapter 14). First, there is evidence that insulin may promote atherosclerosis directly (64), and it may induce adverse changes in other cardiovascular risk factors as well (e.g. triglycerides, HDL-cholesterol, and blood pressure) (17, 63, 65). At least two studies have retrospectively examined the baseline characteristics of non-diabetic subjects who were known later to have developed diabetes. In the Rancho Bernardo Study, these pre-diabetic subjects had higher triglyceride levels and systolic blood pressures at baseline examination compared to subjects who remained non-diabetic throughout the follow-up period (66). Similar results were obtained from the San Antonio Heart Study, with additional analyses of these data revealing that the differences in cardiovascular risk factors between those who eventually converted to diabetes and those who did not diminish considerably when their fasting insulin levels were taken into account (67).

Only a few prospective studies have examined the relationship between insulin levels and CHD incidence. In the Paris Prospective Study, fasting insulin was a stronger predictor of CHD death and non-fatal myocardial infarction among non-diabetic men than was fasting glucose, and the effect of fasting insulin was independent of other cardiovascular risk factors. HDL-cholesterol levels, however, were not measured (50). Plasma insulin levels were also predictive of CHD in the Helsinki Policeman Study, even after adjustment for glucose levels and other cardiovascular risk factors (68). In Busselton, Australia, one-hour serum insulin concentrations were associated with 12-year mortality from cardiovascular disease in men, but not in women. Moreover, the association appeared to be independent of other major cardiovascular risk factors (69).

The relationship between insulin treatment and CHD is unclear. In the University Group Diabetes Program, the incidence of CHD was no higher in subjects taking insulin than in subjects in the placebo group (70). Diabetic men taking insulin did not have a higher incidence of CHD compared to other previously diagnosed diabetic men in the Puerto Rican Heart Program (49). In the Framingham Heart Study, however, women treated with insulin had a significantly higher risk of cardiovascular death than diabetic women undergoing other types of treatment, although no relationship was observed between cardiovascular mortality and type of treatment in men (71).

## SURVIVAL FOLLOWING MYOCARDIAL INFARCTION IN DIABETICS

In addition to experiencing an increased susceptibility to myocardial infarction (MI), diabetics who survive an MI are also at increased risk for developing future CHD events. In the Perth Coronary Register, which followed patients beginning at 28 days post-MI, patients with a history of diabetes were 2.1 times more likely than patients without such a history to die within 9 years and the relative risk decreased only slightly after adjustment for other prognostic factors (72). Diabetics are also twice as likely to die within the first month following an MI compared to non-diabetics (73). One study reported operative mortality in patients undergoing aortocoronary bypass to be two times higher in diabetic patients compared to age- and sex-matched non-diabetic controls, even though the major coronary arteries appeared similar on angiography in both groups of patients (74).

Some studies have reported that diabetic women have a worse prognosis following an MI than diabetic men. In the Framingham Heart Study, diabetic women were 2.7 times more likely to experience a recurrent MI and 2.3 times more likely to die of CHD than non-diabetic women. In contrast, diabetic men were 1.3 times more likely to experience a recurrent MI and 1.7 times more likely to die of CHD than non-diabetic men. Furthermore, diabetic women surviving a MI were more likely to have a recurrent MI and to die of CHD than diabetic men surviving a MI (75). No sex difference in 30-day mortality was reported among the type 2 diabetics followed by Singer *et al.*, however (76).

Some of the excess risk for recurrent CHD that is associated with diabetes is accounted for by the fact that diabetics may have a more adverse cardiovascular risk factor profile and more severe pre-existing heart disease by virtue of their diabetes. Diabetic MI patients had significantly more frequent A-V and intraventricular conduction disorders than age- and sex-matched non-diabetic MI patients in a large study of hospitalised MI cases studied in Warsaw, and diabetics with arrhythmias and/or conduction disorders experienced a particularly poor prognosis (77). Singer *et al.* found that diabetes was associated with a 1.6-fold higher rate of mortality within 30 days, but further analyses revealed that diabetes had the most adverse effect on mortality in patients whose pre-MI cardiovascular status was relatively normal (76).

## CEREBROVASCULAR DISEASE

After coronary heart disease, cerebrovascular disease is the second leading cardiovascular cause of death among diabetics. In the Framingham Heart Study, it was estimated that 14.3% of atherothrombotic brain infarctions (ABI) in women and 10.1% of ABI in men were attributable to diabetes (37). Since data pertaining to cerebral haemorrhage and embolic brain infarction were not analysed, the total burden of cerebrovascular disease was actually higher. In other studies, cerebrovascular disease was reported as the underlying cause of death in 12–16% of all diabetic deaths (78, 79). In Japan, where cerebrovascular disease is very common and CHD mortality relatively low, cerebrovascular disease is the leading cause of death among diabetics (5).

There are relatively few population-based epidemiological studies which have assessed the frequency of cerebrovascular disease in diabetic populations. At baseline examination, a history of stroke was reported in 2.3% of men and 2.6% of women enrolled in the Multinational Study of Vascular Disease in Diabetics, although this study had no non-diabetic comparisons (18). Studies that have included diabetic comparisons have, in general, found the frequency of cerebrovascular disease to be 2–3 times higher in diabetics than in non-diabetics (6, 22, 37, 39, 80, 81). In the Framingham Heart Study, the incidence of fatal and non-fatal atherothrombotic brain infarction (ABI) was estimated to be 4.7/1000 per year in diabetic men and 6.2/1000 per year in diabetic women, rates that were approximately 2.5 and 3.6 times higher than in non-diabetic men and women, respectively (22). The incidence of cerebrovascular disease among diabetics in the London cohort of Multinational Study of Vascular Disease in Diabetics was 5.9/1000 per year, although as previously mentioned, non-diabetics were not studied (13). A slightly smaller effect of diabetes on stroke incidence was found in Rochester, Minnesota, where the incidence of first stroke among diabetics during 1945–69 was only 1.7 times greater than the rate expected from the general population (82). The Whitehall Study reported cerebrovascular mortality to be two times higher in diabetic men than in non-diabetic men (39), while in Finland, even greater differentials have been reported (5).

## RISK FACTORS

There is evidence from some studies that elevated blood glucose levels below the threshold for diabetes may be a risk factor for stroke. In the Whitehall Study, men with glucose intolerance were three times more likely to die of stroke than men with normal glucose tolerance. Diabetics, in contrast, were approximately four times more likely to die of stroke compared to men with normal glucose tolerance (39). In women, but not men, enrolled in the Framingham Heart Study, glucose levels were significantly associated with the incidence of total cardiovascular disease, a category that included angina pectoris, myocardial infarction, coronary death, coronary insufficiency, stroke, transient ischaemic attacks, and intermittent claudication (46). In Japanese–American men in Honolulu, the incidence of thrombo-embolic stroke was significantly higher in men with 1-hour post-load glucose levels greater than 122 mg/dl than in men with glucose levels below this value, although there was no evidence for a dose–response relationship. Glucose levels were not associated with the incidence of haemorrhagic stroke (81).

In non-diabetics, hypertension is one of the most important risk factors identified for stroke. Because hypertension is associated with diabetes, some have questioned whether the association between diabetes and stroke is mediated by hypertension. In Rochester, Minnesota, hypertensive diabetics were 1.7 times more likely to have a stroke than hypertensive non-diabetics, but non-hypertensive diabetics were only 1.1 times more likely to have a stroke than non-hypertensive non-diabetics (83), thus raising the possibility that the increased incidence of stroke could be attributable to the increased prevalence of hypertension among diabetics. Other studies, however, have found diabetes to be independently associated with stroke incidence even after adjustment for hypertension. In the Framingham Study, for example, the relative risk between diabetes and ABI decreased from 2.6 to 2.2 in men and from 3.8 to 2.2 in women once age, systolic blood pressure, plasma cholesterol, cigarette smoking, and left ventricular hypertrophy by ECG were accounted for (23). Among men enrolled in the Whitehall Study, hyperglycaemia remained significantly associated with the 10-year stroke mortality even after adjustment for systolic blood pressure and other cardiovascular risk factors (39).

While hypertension was identified as the dominant risk factor for ABI in the Framingham Study, serum cholesterol and cigarette smoking were also associated with the incidence of ABI, and, in men, these latter variables appeared to be at least as strongly associated with ABI as with CHD (84). Cigarette smoking was also significantly associated with mortality from stroke among men from the Whitehall Study (39).

In a university-based diabetes clinic, 20% of adults were found to have evidence of carotid artery occlusive disease (CAOD) by measurement of ocular changes in carotid arterial blood flow and phonoangiography. In multivariate analysis, higher systolic blood pressure, higher cholesterol, and reduced adiposity were found to correlate with CAOD prevalence, although there was no association between CAOD prevalence and gender, duration of diabetes, type of diabetes, or glycaemic control (85)

## PERIPHERAL VASCULAR DISEASE

Peripheral vascular disease (PVD) is the third most common manifestation of macrovascular disease in diabetes. Peripheral vascular disease is characterised by diminished blood flow to the legs and feet, and, although it is not a life-threatening condition, this disease is associated with considerable morbidity. The most serious complications of PVD include ulcers and gangrene, the latter which can lead to amputations. Diabetics are approximately 15 times more likely than non-diabetics to have a lower extremity amputation, and it has recently been estimated that 45% of all lower extremity amputations in the United States are in persons with diabetes (86).

As with the other manifestations of macrovascular disease, the diagnosis of PVD is difficult. Patients with advanced disease may experience pain in the legs during exercise, or intermittent claudication. The disease may also be detected subclinically on physical examination by the absence of peripheral arterial pulses, or by use of more sensitive measures, including radiography for arterial calcification.

### PREVALENCE AND INCIDENCE

There are relatively few prospective studies of peripheral vascular disease in diabetic individuals. While PVD does occur in non-diabetic individuals, available data suggest that it occurs 2–5 times more frequently in diabetics than in non-diabetics (30, 87, 88). About 8% of diabetics residing in Rochester, Minnesota, between 1945 and 1969 already had evidence of peripheral pulse defects at the time of diagnosis of their diabetes (89). In the WHO Multinational Study of Vascular Disease in Diabetics, approximately 3% of diabetics reported a history of either intermittent claudication or amputation (18). After 14 years or more of diabetes, 5.7% of subjects enrolled in the University Group Diabetes Program (UGDP) trial experienced intermittent claudication (90).

Some (18, 89, 91), but not all (37, 90), studies have reported PVD to be more common in diabetic men than in diabetic women, although these gender differences may represent artefacts of patient selection. In the Framingham Heart Study, diabetic men were 4.0 times more likely to develop intermittent claudication than non-diabetic men, but diabetic women were 6.4 times more likely to develop intermittent claudication than non-diabetic women. After adjustment for systolic blood pressure, smoking, cholesterol, and left ventricular hypertrophy on ECG, the impact of diabetes of intermittent claudication was approximately similar between men and women (37). In another study in which a male excess of PVD was found among diabetics, the excess was completely accounted for by the higher prevalence of smoking in men (91).

The incidence of peripheral vascular disease has been reported from several studies. The incidence of peripheral pulse defects among diabetics in Rochester, Minnesota, was estimated to be about 2% per year (89). In the Framingham Heart Study, the incidence of intermittent claudication among diabetics without symptoms at baseline was about 1% per year (37). In the UGDP trial, however, the incidence of intermittent claudication was estimated to be 2% per year in diabetic men and 3% per year in diabetic women (90). Other clinic-based studies have reported higher rates of PVD (30, 91).

## RISK FACTORS

Diabetic patients with PVD have a higher prevalence of other cardiovascular risk factors compared to diabetic patients without PVD. Peripheral vascular disease has been associated with cigarette smoking and hypertension in several cross-sectional studies (90, 91), and these associations have also been observed in prospective studies (87, 92). In the Framingham Heart Study, the incidence of intermittent claudication was highest in diabetics on oral agents and in women taking insulin (87). In neither the Framingham Heart Study (87) nor the WHO Multinational Study (18) was the prevalence of PVD associated with the duration of diabetes. In Rochester, Minnesota, however, the incidence of peripheral pulse defects was correlated with both age and duration of diabetes (89).

## REFERENCES


1 Wetterhall SF, Olson DR, DeStefano F *et al.* Trends in diabetes and diabetic complications, 1980–1987. *Diabetes Care* 1992; 15; 960–7.

2 Sprafka JM, Burke GL, Folsom AR *et al.* Trends in prevalence of diabetes mellitus in patients with myocardial infarction and effect of diabetes on survival: the Minnesota heart survey. *Diabetes Care* 1991; 14; 537–43.

3 Stern MP. Kelly West Lecture. Primary prevention of type II diabetes mellitus. *Diabetes Care* 1991; 14: 399–410.

4 Barrett-Connor E, Orchard T. Diabetes and heart disease. In *Diabetes in America*. Diabetes Data Compiled 1984. National Diabetes Data Group, 1985; NIH Publ No. 85–1486.

5 Pyörälä K, Laakso M. Macrovascular disease in diabetes mellitus. In: Mann YI, Pyörälä K, Teuscher A. (eds.), *Diabetes in Epidemiologic Perspective*. Churchill Livingstone; 1983: 183–247.

6 Panzram G. Mortality and survival in Type 2 (non-insulin-dependent) diabetes mellitus. *Diabetologia* 1987; 30: 123–31.

7 Moss SE, Klein R, Klein BE. Cause-specific mortality in a population-based study of diabetes. *Am J Public Health* 1991; 81: 1158–62.

8 Ochi JW, Melton LJ, Palumbo PJ, Chu CP. A population-based study of diabetes mortality. *Diabetes Care* 1985; 8: 224–9.

9 Morrish NJ, Stevens L, Head JA, Fuller JH *et al.* A prospective study of mortality among middle-aged diabetics (the London cohort of the WHO multinational study of vascular disease in diabetics) I: causes and death rates. *Diabetologia* 1990; 33: 538–41.

10 Kleinman JC, Donahue RP, Harris MI *et al.* Mortality among diabetics in a national sample. *Am J Epidemiol* 1988; 128: 389–401.

11 Dorman JS, LaPorte, RE, Kuller LH *et al.* The Pittsburgh insulin-dependent diabetes mellitus (IDDM) morbidity and mortality study: mortality results. *Diabetes* 1984; 33: 271–6.

12 Krolewski AS, Kosinski EJ, Warram JH *et al.* Magnitude and determinants of coronary artery disease in juvenile onset, insulin-dependent diabetes mellitus. *Am J Cardiol* 1987; 59: 750–5.
13 Morrish NJ, Stevens LK, Fuller JH, Keen H *et al.* Incidence of macrovascular disease in diabetes mellitus: the London cohort of the WHO multinational study of vascular disease in diabetics. *Diabetologia* 1991; 34: 584–9.
14 Fuller JH, Shipley MJ, Rose G, Jarrett RJ, Keen H. Coronary heart disease and impaired glucose tolerance: the Whitehall study. *Lancet* 1980; i: 1373–6.
15 Ingelfinger JA, Bennett, PH, Liebow IM, Miller M. Coronary heart disease in the Pima Indians. Electrocardiographic findings and postmortem evidence of myocardial infarction in a population with a high prevalence of diabetes mellitus. *Diabetes* 1976; 25: 561–5.
16 Ducimetiere P, Eschwege E, Richard J *et al.* Relationship of glucose tolerance to prevalence of ECG abnormalities and to annual mortality from cardiovascular disease: results of the Paris Prospective Study. *J Chron Dis.* 1979; 32: 759–66.
17 Donahue RP, Orchard TJ. Diabetes mellitus and macrovascular complications: an epidemiological perspective. *Diabetes Care* 1992; 15: 1141–55.
18 World Health Organization Multinational Study of Vascular Disease in Diabetics. Prevalence of small vessel and large vessel disease in diabetic patients from 14 centres. *Diabetologia* 1985; 28(suppl 1): 615–40.
19 Head J, Fuller JH. International variations in mortality among diabetic patients; the WHO Multinational Study of Vascular Disease in Diabetics. *Diabetologia* 1990; 33: 477–82.
20 Laaksko M, Ronnemaa, R, Pyörälä K *et al.* Atherosclerotic vascular disease and its risk factors in non-insulin-dependent diabetic and non-diabetic subjects in Finland. *Diabetes Care* 1988; 11: 449–63.
21 Nelson RG, Sievers ML, Knowler WC *et al.* Low incidence of fatal coronary heart disease in Pima Indians despite high prevalence of non-insulin-dependent diabetes. *Circulation* 1990; 81: 987–95.
22 Kannel WB, McGee DL. Diabetes and cardiovascular risk factors: The Framingham Study. *Circulation* 1979; 59: 8–13.
23 Kannel WB, McGee DL. Diabetes and glucose tolerance as risk factors for cardiovascular disease: The Framingham Study. *Diabetes Care* 1979; 2: 120–6.
24 Heyden S, Heiss G, Bartel AG *et al.* Sex differential in coronary mortality among diabetics in Evans County, Georgia. *J Chron Dis* 1980; 33: 265–73.
25 Jarrett RJ, McCartney P, Keen H. The Bedford Survey: ten-year mortality rates in newly diagnosed diabetics, borderline diabetics and normoglycaemic controls and risk indices for coronary heart disease in borderline diabetics. *Diabetologia* 1982; 22: 79–84.
26 Barrett-Connor EL, Cohn BA, Wingard DL, Edelstein SL. Why is diabetes mellitus a stronger risk factor for fatal ischemic heart disease in women than in men? The Rancho Bernardo study. *J Am Med Assoc* 1991; 265: 627–31.
27 Pan W-H, Cedres LB, Liu K *et al.* Relationship of clinical diabetes and asymptomatic hyperglycemia to risk of coronary heart disease mortality in men and women. *Am J Epidemiol* 1986; 123: 504–16.
28 Butler WJ, Ostrander LD, Carman WJ, Lamphiear DE. Mortality from coronary heart disease in the Tecumseh study: long-term effect of diabetes mellitus, glucose tolerance and other risk factors. *Am J Epidemiol* 1985; 121: 541–7.
29 West KM, Ahuja MMS, Bennett PH *et al.* The role of circulating glucose and triglyceride concentrations and their interactions with other 'risk factors' as determinants of arterial disease in nine diabetic population samples from the WHO multinational study. *Diabetes Care* 1983; 6, 361–9.
30 Uusitupa MIJ, Niskanen LK, Siitonen O *et al.* 5-year incidence of atherosclerotic vascular disease in relation to general risk factors, insulin level, and abnormalities in lipoprotein composition in non-insulin-dependent diabetic and non-diabetic subjects. *Circulation* 1990; 82: 27–36.
31 Waller BF, Palumbo PJ, Lie JT, Roberts WC. Status of the coronary arteries at necropsy in diabetes mellitus with onset after age 30 years: analysis of 229 diabetic patients with and without clinical evidence of coronary heart disease and comparison to 183 control subjects. *Am J Med* 1980; 69: 498–506.
32 Vigorita VJ, Moore GW, Hutchins GM. Absence of correlation between coronary arterial atherosclerosis and severity or duration of diabetes mellitus of adult onset. *Am J Cardiol* 1980; 46: 535–42.
33 Robertson WB, Strong JB. Atherosclerosis in persons with hypertension and diabetes. *Laborat Invest* 1968; 18: 538–51.
34 Zdanov VS, Vihert AM. Atherosclerosis and diabetes mellitus. *Bull World Health Org* 1976; 53: 547–53.
35 Regan TJ. Congestive heart failure in the diabetic. *Am Rev Med* 1983; 34: 161–8.
36 Crepaldi G, Nosadini R. Diabetic cardiopathy: is it a real entity? *Diabetes/Metab Rev* 1988; 4: 273–88.
37 Kannel WB, McGee DL. Diabetes and cardiovascular disease: The Framingham Study. *J Am Med Assoc* 1979c; 241: 2035–8.
38 Kannel WB, Hjortland M, Castelli WP. Role of diabetes in congestive heart failure: The Framingham Study. *Am J Cardiol* 1974; 34: 29–34.
39 Fuller JH, Shipley MJ, Rose G *et al.* Mortality from coronary heart disease and stroke in relation to degree of glycaemia: the Whitehall Study. *Br Med J* 1983; 287: 867–70.
40 Jarrett JR, Shipley MJ. Type 2 (non-insulin-dependent) diabetes mellitus and cardiovascular disease – putative association via common antecedents. Further evidence from the Whitehall study. *Diabetologia* 1988; 31: 737–40.
41 Eschwege E, Ducimetiere P, Papoz L, *et al.* Blood glucose and coronary heart disease. *Lancet* 1980; ii, 472–3.
42 Yano K, Kagan A, McGee D, Rhoads GG. Glucose intolerance and nine-year mortality in Japanese men in Hawaii. *Am J Med* 1982; 72: 71–80.
43 Stamler R, Stamler J, Dyer A *et al.* Asymptomatic hyperglycemia and cardiovascular diseases in three Chicago epidemiologic studies. *Diabetes Care* 1979; 2: 142–3.
44 International Collaborative Group. Joint discussion. *J Chron Dis* 1979; 32: 829–37.
45 Donahue RP, Abbott RD, Reed DM, Yano K. Postchallenge glucose concentration and coronary heart disease in men of Japanese ancestry: Honolulu Heart Program. *Diabetes* 1987; 36: 689–92.
46 Wilson PWF, Cupples A, Kannel WB. Is hyperglycemia associated with cardiovascular disease? The Framingham Study. *Am Heart J* 1991; 121: 586–90.

47 Scheidt-Nave C, Barrett-Connor E, Wingard DL, Cohn BA *et al.* Sex differences in fasting glycemia as a risk factor for ischemic heart disease death. *Am J Epidemiol* 1991; 133: 565–76.
48 Barrett-Connor E, Wingard DL, Criqui MH, Suarez L. Is borderline fasting hyperglycemia a risk factor for cardiovascular death? *J Chronic Dis* 1984; 37: 773–9.
49 Cruz-Vidal M, Garcia-Palmieri M, Costas R. Abnormal blood glucose and coronary heart disease: The Puerto Rico Heart Health Program. *Diabetes Care* 1983; 6: 556–61.
50 Eschwege E, Richard JL, Thibult N *et al.* Coronary heart disease mortality in relation with diabetes, blood glucose and plasma insulin levels: The Paris Prospective Study, ten years later. *Hormone Metab Res Suppl* 1985; 15: 41–6.
51 Pyörälä K. Relationship of glucose tolerance and plasma insulin to the incidence of coronary heart disease: results from two population studies in Finland. *Diabetes Care* 1979; 2: 131–41.
52 Herman JB, Medalie JH, Goldbourt U. Differences in cardiovascular morbidity and mortality between previously known and newly diagnosed adult diabetics. *Diabetologia* 1977; 13, 229–34.
53 Steiner G. Diabetes and atherosclerosis: an overview. *Diabetes*: 1981; 30 (suppl 2): 1–7.
54 Cruikshanks KJ, Orchard TJ, Becker DJ. The cardiovascular risk profile of adolescents with insulin-dependent diabetes mellitus. *Diabetes Care* 1985; 8: 118–24.
55 Wingard DL, Barrett-Connor E, Criqui MH, Suarez L. Clustering of heart disease risk factors in diabetic compared to non-diabetic adults. *Am J Epidemiol* 1983; 117: 19–26.
56 Fontbonne A, Eschwege E, Cambien F *et al.* Hypertriglyceridaemia as a risk factor of coronary heart disease mortality in subjects with impaired glucose tolerance or diabetes: results from the 11-year follow-up of the Paris Prospective Study. *Diabetologia* 1989; 32, 300–4.
57 Suarez L, Barrett-Connor E. Interaction between cigarette smoking and diabetes mellitus in the prediction of death attributed to cardiovascular disease. *Am J Epidemiol* 1984; 120: 670–5.
58 Moy CS, LaPorte RE, Dorman JS, Songer TJ *et al.* Insulin-dependent diabetes mellitus mortality; the risk of cigarette smoking. *Circulation* 1990; 82: 37–43.
59 Walden CE, Knopp RH, Wahl PW, Beach KW *et al.* Sex differences in the effect of diabetes mellitus on lipoprotein triglyceride and cholesterol concentrations. *N Eng J Med* 1984; 311: 953–9.
60 Gordon T, Castelli WP, Hjortland MC *et al.* Diabetes, blood lipids, and role of obesity in coronary heart disease risk for women. The Framingham Study. *Ann Int Med* 1977; 87: 393–7.
61 Barrett-Connor E, Witzum JL, Holdbrook M. A community study of high density lipoproteins in adult non-insulin-dependent diabetics. *Am J Epidemiol* 1983; 117: 186–92.
62 Jarrett RJ. Type 2 (non-insulin-dependent) diabetes mellitus and coronary heart disease – chicken, egg, or neither? *Diabetologia* 1984; 26: 99–102.
63 Donahue RP, Orchard TJ, Becker DJ *et al.* Sex differences in the Cardiovascular risk profile: a possible role for insulin. The Beaver County study. *Am J Epidemiol* 1987; 125: 600–7.
64 Stout RW. Insulin and atheroma: 20-yr perspective. *Diabetes Care* 1990; 13: 631–54.
65 Mitchell BD, Haffner SM, Hazuda HP, Valdez R *et al.* The relation between serum lipid levels and 8-year changes in lipid, lipoprotein, and blood pressure levels. *Am J Epidemiol* 1992; 136: 12–22.
66 McPhillips JB, Barrett-Connor E, Wingard DL. Cardiovascular risk factors prior to the diagnosis of impaired glucose tolerance and non-insulin-dependent diabetes mellitus in a community of older individuals. *Am J Epidemiol* 1990; 131: 443–53.
67 Haffner SM, Stern MP, Hazuda HP, Mitchell BD, Patterson JK. Cardiovascular risk factors in confirmed prediabetic individuals. Does the clock for coronary heart disease start ticking before the onset of clinical diabetes? *J Am Med Assoc* 1990; 263: 2893–8.
68 Pyörälä K, Savolainen E, Kaukola S, Haapakoski J. Plasma insulin as coronary heart disease risk factor: relationship to other risk factors and predictive value during 9 ½ year follow-up of the Helsinki Policeman Study population. *Acta Med Scand* (suppl) 1985; 701: 38–52.
69 Welborn TA, Wearne K. Coronary heart disease incidence and cardiovascular mortality in Busselton with reference to glucose and insulin concentrations. *Diabetes Care* 1979; 2: 154–60.
70 Klimt CR, Knatterud GL, Meinert CL, Prout TE. A study of the effects of hypoglycemic agents on vascular complications in patients with adult-onset diabetes. *Diabetes* 1979; 19: 747–830.
71 Garcia MJ, McNamara PM, Gordon T *et al.* Morbidity and mortality in diabetics in the Framingham population: sixteen year follow-up study. *Diabetes* 1974; 23: 105–11.
72 Martin CA, Thompson PL, Armstrong BK *et al.* Long-term prognosis after recovery from myocardial infarction: a nine year follow-up of the Perth coronary register. *Circulation* 1983; 68: 961–9.
73 Rytter L, Troelsen S, Beck-Nielsen H. Prevalence and mortality of acute myocardial infarction in patients with diabetes. *Diabetes Care* 1985; 8: 230–4.
74 Verska JJ, Walker WJ. Aortocoronary bypass in the diabetic patient. *Am J Cardiol* 1975; 35: 774–7.
75 Abbott RD, Donahue RP, Kannel WB, Wilson PWF. The impact of diabetes on survival following myocardial infarction in men vs. women: The Framingham Study. *J Am Med Assoc* 1988; 260: 3456–60
76 Singer DE, Moulton AW, Nathan DM. Diabetic myocardial infarction: interaction of diabetes with other preinfarction risk factors. *Diabetes Care* 1989; 38: 350–7.
77 Czyzk A, Krowlewski AS, Szablowska S, Alot A *et al.* Clinical course of myocardial infarction among diabetic patients. *Diabetes Care* 1980; 3: 526–9.
78 Manson JE, Colditz GA, Stampfer MJ *et al.* A prospective study of maturity-onset diabetes mellitus and risk of coronary heart disease and stroke in women. *Arch Intern Med* 1991; 151: 1141–7.
79 Wong JS, Pearson DW, Murchison LE, Williams MJ *et al.* Mortality in diabetes mellitus: experience of a geographically defined population. *Diabetic Med* 1991; 8: 135–9.
80 Kuller LH, Dorman JS, Wolf PA. Cerebrovascular disease and heart disease. In *Diabetes in America*, Diabetes Data Compiled 1984, National Diabetes Data Group (NIH publ. no. 85–1486).
81 Kagan A, Popper JS, Rhoads GG. Factors related to

stroke incidence in Hawaii Japanese men. *Stroke* 1980; 11: 14–21.
82 Palumbo PJ, Elveback LR, Whisnant JP. Neurologic complications of diabetes mellitus: transient ischemic attack, stroke, and peripheral neuropathy. *Adv Neurol* 1978; 19: 593–9.
83 Roehmholdt ME, Palumbo PJ, Whisnant JP, Elveback LR. Transient ischemic attack and stroke in a community-based diabetic cohort. *Mayo Clin Proc* 1983; 58: 56–8.
84 Gordon T, Kannel WB. Predisposition to atherosclerosis in the head, heart, and legs: The Framingham Study. *J Am Med Assoc* 1972; 221: 661–6.
85 Kuebler TW, Bendick PJ, Fineberg SE *et al.* Diabetes mellitus and cerebrovascular disease: prevalence of carotid artery occlusive disease and associated risk factors in 482 adult diabetic patients. *Diabetes Care* 1983; 6: 274–8.
86 Most RS, Sinnock P. The epidemiology of lower extremity amputations in diabetic individuals. *Diabetes Care* 1983; 6: 87–91.
87 Brand FN, Abbott RD, Kannel WB. Diabetes, intermittent claudification and risk of cardiovascular events. *Diabetes* 1989; 38: 504–9.
88 Palumbo PJ, Melton LJ. Peripheral vascular disease and diabetes. In *Diabetes in America*. Diabetes Data Compiled 1984, National Diabetes Data Group, 1985 (NIH publ no 85–1486).
89 Melton LJ III, Macken KM, Palumbo PJ, Elveback LR. Incidence and prevalence of clinical peripheral vascular disease in a population based cohort of diabetic patients. *Diabetes Care* 1980; 3: 650–4.
90 Kreines K, Johnson E, Albrink M *et al.* The course of peripheral vascular disease in non-insulin-dependent diabetes. *Diabetes Care* 1985; 8: 235–43.
91 Beach KW, Strandness DE Jr. Arteriosclerosis obliterans and associated risk factors in insulin-dependent and non-insulin-dependent diabetes. *Diabetes* 1980; 29: 882–8.
92 Palumbo PJ, O'Fallon WM, Osmundson PJ, Zimmerman BR. Progression of peripheral occlusive arterial disease in diabetes mellitus. What factors are predictive? *Arch Int Med* 1991; 151: 717–21.

# 17 Diabetic Neuropathy

Aaron I. Vinik

## INTRODUCTION

Diabetic neuropathy encompasses a wide range of abnormalities affecting both peripheral and autonomic nerve function. The disorder may be manifested either clinically, through a number of different symptoms, or subclinically, with abnormalities detectable only by careful testing. Frequently, the diagnosis of diabetic neuropathy is difficult to make because the manifestations are non-specific and may occur in a number of other conditions. Neuropathy is not confined to a single type of diabetes, but can occur in IDDM, NIDDM, and in various forms of acquired diabetes (1–3). Although there is considerable uncertainty as to the prevalence of neuropathy among diabetic persons, it is generally accepted that neuropathy is the most common, and often the most troublesome, of the major complications afflicting individuals with diabetes.

## PREVALENCE AND INCIDENCE OF NEUROPATHY

Estimates of the prevalence of neuropathy vary widely in the literature (1–12). These apparently disparate results can be explained by small groups studied, the diversity of patients entered and the inconsistencies in the definition of neuropathy. Some authors have used pain as their total definition (1), others have required signs of nerve dysfunction (2), whereas some have required at least two of the following to be present: signs, abnormalities in quantitative sensory testing or electrophysiology (11). A variety of tools for testing have been introduced into the arena of diabetes investigation for the measurement of symptoms (3, 13–15) and signs (5, 16). As a result of these advances, the American Diabetes Association established guidelines for the diagnosis of diabetic neuropathy which, in essence, requires that there are symptoms, signs, abnormalities in quantitative sensory tests and abnormal electrophysiology. Modified nerve disability scoring systems (NDS) have evolved which ascribe numerical values to the ankle jerk, vibration, pin prick and temperature sensation. Neuropathy symptom scores have been developed which evaluate burning, numbness and tingling and fatigue, cramping or aching in the limbs. Scores are given based upon the presence of the symptom and the site, lower or upper limb or elsewhere (1–3, 13–16). These more objective measures are moving in the direction of standardisation of the means whereby a reasonable approximation of the true prevalence of neuropathy can be obtained.

None the less useful prevalence data for diabetic neuropathy are relatively sparse, and it is difficult to obtain reliable estimates of the prevalence of neuropathy among the different diabetic populations. Few population-based studies have been undertaken, and since the prevalence of undiagnosed diabetes in the general population is estimated to be at least as great as the prevalence of diagnosed diabetes (12), most published studies entail substantial selection biases, since they are limited to that portion of the diabetic population with access to clinic care. In addition, lack of consensus as to the appropriate diagnostic criteria for diabetic neuropathy has resulted in a wide range of prevalence estimates reported in the literature, ranging from 0% to 93% (17).

Probably the best data regarding prevalence of neuropathy come from the extensive study of nearly 4400 clinic patients undertaken by Pirart, who reported a prevalence rate ranging from 7% for individuals within one year of diagnosis of diabetes to 50% for those with diabetes for more than 25 years. (13–15). Neuropathy was defined in this study as loss of Achilles reflexes with symptoms or objective signs of polyneuropathy. Comparable prevalence rates were reported by Franklin *et al.*, who also used a combination of symptoms and objective information to diagnose neuropathy in their study of NIDDM patients in the San Luis Valley Diabetes Study (16). While Brown and Asbury have estimated that at least one-half of all patients receiving insulin have symptomatic neuropathy (9), and Goodman *et al.* reported pain and paresthesias to be present in 62% of all cases in their series (18), Boulton *et al.* have suggested that most prevalence studies have overestimated the true prevalence of symptomatic neuropathy by using diagnostic criteria that are non-specific. Thus, these researchers defined symptomatic neuropathy as the presence of symptoms and signs of nerve dysfunction in the absence of peripheral vascular disease and found that 10.4% of insulin-treated patients less than age 60 in their clinic population had symptomatic neuropathy. An additional 8.9% had absent knee and ankle reflexes in the absence of significant symptoms, and an additional 6.3% had absent foot pulses (19). This estimate is similar to that obtained by Fry *et al.* who observed symptoms in association with 'significant signs' present in 13% of their patients (20). A cross-sectional study of randomly selected diabetic patients was performed using a standardised questionnaire and physical examination in 118 hospitals in the UK. A total of 6487 diabetic patients were studied, with equal distribution between the sexes, median age of 59 years and duration of diabetes of 8 years. One-third of the patients were IDDM and the remainder NIDDM. The overall prevalence of clinical neuropathy was 28.5% (IDDM 22.7% and NIDDM 32%). The prevalence increased with age from 5% in the 20–39 year group to 44.2% in the 70–79 year age group. Duration of diabetes had a very significant effect, 20.8% < 5 years and 36.8 after 10 years. What is of greater interest is the very narrow range of prevalence figures from a low of 21.7% in East Anglia to a high of 34.6% in northern England while Scotland, Wales and Ireland had figures within these extremes. Franklin *et al.* (16) stated that neurological techniques and prevalence are specific to the population tested. This may be true if equivalent methods are not used for the evaluation. In the San Luis valley study (3) a prevalence of 25.8% of 279 NIDDM was found not unlike that in the British studies, comparable with 44% of 400 patients in the Pittsburgh epidemiology study (7). If, however, only severe symptoms are recorded, then the prevalence falls to around 10.7% (8), especially if rigorous electrophysiological criteria are applied, and 14% if only pinprick sensation is used as the index (9). These differences in prevalence are based upon endpoints measured. In a study from Finland in 142 newly diagnosed NIDDM aged 45–64 years, symptomatic neuropathy was found in only 1.5% of patients and in 2.3% if signs were used as the endpoint. No subjects had both symptoms and signs. If electrophysiological studies were used, then 15.2% of newly diagnosed diabetics had neuropathy. These figures appear to be surprisingly low in light of other observations on other population groups (Table 17.1). In a series of 1175 unselected patients from a diabetes out-

Table 17.1. *Epidemiology of diabetic populations*

| | Incidence | Established | | Duration | | Age | Control | | Comment |
|---|---|---|---|---|---|---|---|---|---|
| | | IDDM | NIDDM | <5 y | >20 y | y | Good | Poor | |
| Rochester Diabetes Project (21) | 133/100 000 pop/y | | 10% | 4% | 15% | | 10% | 24% | Retrospective study NIDDM 1945–90 |
| Rochester Diabetes Management Study (11, 22, 23) | | 39%<br>asymptomatic<br>15 | 32%<br><br>13 | | | | | | Population-based cross-sectional survey. Quantitated endpoints. All pts with diabetes in 1986. 380 subjects, 27% IDDM, 73% NIDDM |
| San Luis Valley (24–26) | | — | 26 | 17 | 53 | 20–44 10%<br>65–74 32% | | | Case control, modern criteria validated measures. VPT >HbA1c (11.2 vs 10.2) >males/females 34/20% |
| 1989 Health Interview Survey (27, 28) | | 30 | 37 | 30 | 45 | | | | 84 572 >18 yr 2405 diabetes questionnaire vs. 20 035 non-diabetes. Gender= Hisp>Black>White |
| NHANES II (29) | | | | | | 35–74<br>12.5% | | | ORO BP, duration, control, SE status, ankle reflexes/knee |
| National Hospital Discharge Survey (30) | | | | | | | | | ICD-9 code neuropathy in 265 693 hospital patients |
| DCCT (31) | | 37 | — | | | | | | 278 correlates IDDM signs 37%, symptoms 6% older males, taller, >duration, lower C-peptide |
| Pittsburgh Epidemiology Study (32–34) | | | | | 50 | | | | Cohort 628 IDDM correlates glycaemia, trig, O BP, phys. activity |

patient clinic, Pirart found that 12% already had signs of diabetic neuropathy at the time of diagnosis of diabetes (13–15). Ankle reflexes were absent in 19.6% of a diabetic population studied by Boulton (19), and Nilsson *et al.* found that Achilles reflex was absent in 10.5% of short duration diabetics and 15.2% of long duration diabetics. Interestingly, though, Nilsson also observed absence of Achilles reflexes in 8.5% of non-diabetic controls and in 25% of non-diabetic controls over the age of 60 (35). Loss of ankle vibration and/or Achilles tendon reflexes were found among 40.8% of 503 Mexican subjects with NIDDM, although in this group 32.2% of subjects had symptoms attributable to peripheral neuropathy (36). Using a broader set of criteria, Haimanot found that 54.0% of diabetics had objective sensory deficits in the extremities, reduction or loss of deep tendon reflexes, and autonomic disturbances or mononeuropathy without an obvious alternative cause (37). Prevalence ranged from 42.0% for individuals with duration of diabetes less than five years to 80.0% for individuals with duration of 15 years or more. Moreover, these findings were present in only 8% of a non-diabetic control population.

Clinically, detectable diabetic neuropathy is more common than generally thought, if its presence is sought by careful examination. In a cohort of 278 healthy insulin-dependent diabetic subjects enrolled in the feasibility phase of the Diabetes Control and Complication Trial (DCCT), clinical peripheral polyneuropathy was detectable in 39% of the subjects on careful examination despite the fact that patients with known neuropathy of sufficient severity to require medical attention were excluded (38). Thus, the prevalence of detectable but subtle (and often asymptomatic) peripheral somatic neuropathy in a generally healthy cohort of subjects with IDDM of less than 15 years' duration is quite high.

Although uncommon, neuropathy may occasionally occur in diabetic children. Reductions in motor nerve conduction velocities have even been documented among diabetic children (39, 40) as have reductions in vibratory sensation (41). Symptomatic neuropathy is found only rarely among young diabetics.

## SEX DIFFERENCES

In the study by Pirart who longitudinally followed 4400 diabetic patients for over 26 years (2) the sex incidence favoured males. Pirart did not, however, use symptoms in the diagnosis and included patients with mononeuropathies and amyotrophies in the analysis which might favour a male predominance. In the San Luis Valley cross-sectional study a male predominance was also found (3) which differs from the equal sex incidence found in the British studies. Thus, there may, indeed, be sex differences in different populations, but this may also depend on the nature of testing for the presence of neuropathy.

## DURATION AND AGE

An increasing prevalence of neuropathy has been found fairly uniformly to accompany increasing duration of diabetes (2, 3, 7, 9) which has recently been confirmed using newer methodologies by Young and colleagues (4). The correlation with duration of diabetes is independent of age which incidentally also correlates with prevalence of neuropathy.

## TYPE OF DIABETES

Many studies have failed to make the distinction between type of diabetes and the prevalence of neuropathy (1, 2, 7, 9), or have only examined IDDM (5) or NIDDM (3, 6). The study from Britain was sufficiently large with enough patients in the two groups to allow a comparison to be made. The overall prevalence of neuropathy in the NIDDM was significantly greater in the NIDDM (32.1%) compared with 22.7% in IDDM. These differences remained, if age was corrected for, and the trend was maintained throughout the range of known duration of diabetes. Although these differences may be explained by the long prodromal period for diabetes in NIDDM, or a genuine difference in the pathogenesis in the two groups, it must not be forgotten that many NIDDM are masquerading as slowly evolving IDDM and are often found to have antibodies to islet proteins and GAD and may indeed be IDDM. Recent evidence that neuropathy may have an autoimmune cause would support the notion that there may be differences in the pathogenesis of the disorder in the two groups and will require that future prevalence studies focus upon a clearer distinction between the different types of diabetes.

## WHY EVALUATE?

Neuropathy is the most frequent of the diabetic complications and leads to the greatest morbidity and ultimately mortality. It had been established that the loss of an ankle reflex predicts the development of a neuropathic foot ulcer (38) and subsequent loss of limbs. When all the variables are entered into the equation such as age, duration of diabetes, tobacco, alcohol and the genetic predisposition, the neuropathy is=*n* subjects over the age of 50 is 50% dictating a need for regular examinations of the feet, proper footcare and appropriate education.

## AUTONOMIC NEUROPATHY AND OTHER NEUROPATHIC SYNDROMES

There are few published estimates of the prevalence of other syndromes of somatic neuropathy, mainly because these conditions occur so infrequently. In two African populations, the prevalence of mononeuropathy (including mononeuropathy multiplex) among patients with diabetes was reported to be 3.7% (37) and 1.1% (42). Prevalence rates for radiculopathy and amyotrophy in these populations ranged from 0% to less than 2%. In a sample of 351 patients admitted to an inpatient diabetes clinic, we observed prevalence rates for mononeuropathy, radiculopathy, and amyotrophy to be 3.0%, 3.5%, and 2.1%, respectively.

No adequate studies are available on the prevalence of symptomatic autonomic neuropathy. A wide range has been reported in the prevalence rates for different autonomic symptoms, but these rates are difficult to interpret because of the high frequency with which many of these symptoms can occur in the non-diabetic population. Impotence, for example, may be present in as many as 50% of diabetic men, although this condition is not infrequent in the non-diabetic population. In one study, Jeyarajah *et al.* found that 38.5% of their patients experienced one or more of the autonomic symptoms (intermittent diarrhoea, sweating abnormality, giddiness on standing, gastric fullness, or hypoglycaemic unawareness), but only one-half had abnormal autonomic function tests (43).

Estimates of the prevalence of autonomic neuropathy based on the presence of abnormalities of cardiovascular autonomic reflexes have ranged in the literature from 14% to nearly 50% (43–47). Burke *et al.*, who observed that 14% of their clinic patients experienced both an abnormal heart rate variation during deep breathing and an abnormal heart rate response to standing, then observed that 61.9% of these patients also experienced one or more of the following symptoms: postural dizziness, chronic diarrhoea, impotence, postprandial sweating, dysphagia, or urinary symptoms (47). At the other extreme, Jeyarajah *et al.* observed autonomic function test abnormalities in 46.2% of their diabetic patients, but also in 15% of their healthy controls (43). The prevalence of autonomic function test abnormalities has been found to be associated both with duration of diabetes (46) and with age (43), although these correlations may not hold for all indices of autonomic function.

It was formerly thought that diabetic autonomic neuropathy was a disease only of insulin-dependent diabetes but, as has been recently reported by Veglio and colleagues, the prevalence is equal in NIDDM or even greater than that of IDDM (48). It has also been noted that the age of the individual is more important a predictor of the appearance of autonomic neuropathy than duration of neuropaths to sudden demise for which no apparent reason has been found. Epidemiological data suggest that autonomic neuropathy may co-segregate with factors predisposing to macrovascular events. A striking association has been found between autonomic neuropathy and hypertension, elevation of LDL-cholesterol, and a reduction of HDL cholesterol (49), as well as, somewhat surprisingly, an increased prevalence amongst females and those individuals with a raised body mass index (50). It is therefore not surprising that these individuals are those most susceptible to an attenuated life span because of co-segregation of all the risk; factors for cardiovascular mortality with autonomic neuropathy.

## Risk factors

Despite very poor control of their diabetes, up to 50% of all diabetic subjects never develop symptoms of neuropathy, even after 20 or more years of diabetes (13–15). Conversely, some unfortunate subjects develop neuropathy soon after the onset of diabetes, even when glycaemic control is relatively good. These well-known observations implicate the involvement of factors other than glycaemia in the etiology of diabetic neuropathy.

A genetic predisposition for the development of diabetic neuropathy has been sought (13–15, 35, 51–53) but, as yet, not identified. At least two studies have failed to find an association between signs of peripheral neuropathy and family history of NIDDM (13–15, 35), thus suggesting that there is not a single gene responsible for both NIDDM and peripheral neuropathy. Chochinov *et al.* speculated that other genetic factors may be involved, and measured vibration sensation in diabetic subjects, in their immediate family members, and in normal controls. They found that, although vibration sensation was reduced in the diabetic subjects, sensation in family members was, however, not reduced and was no different than in normal controls (53). The question that has not been adequately investigated, though, is whether there are genes that segregate independently of diabetes that affect susceptibility to neuropathy but are expressed only in the presence of diabetes. There may be heritable defects (i.e. genes), for example, that predispose neural (and vascular) tissue to further injury in the metabolic milieu of diabetes. An example would be a genetic predisposition to autoimmune destruction of nerves. Seventy-nine patients with IDDM whose disease started before the age of 21 years and were followed for 15–21 years who had complete evaluation of cardiovascular autonomic function evaluated and were classified as having intact, mildly impaired and significantly impaired autonomic function. The HLA-DR3/4 phenotype was present in more than 50% of the patients with significant autonomic neuropathy and conferred relative odds of 6.2 for the development of autonomic neuropathy when compared with other HLA-DR phenotypes. The association was independent of other risk factors including sex, ideal body weight and smoking, nor did it relate to glycaemic control although the patients with significant autonomic neuropathy had the worst HbA1 levels. These findings raise the possibility that autoimmune mechanisms contribute to the pathogenesis of cardiovascular autonomic neuropathy. There are several indications that autoimmunity may participate in the disorder. Activated DR-positive lymphocytes were found in patients with cardiac autonomic neuropathy and organ-specific, complement fixing antiganglioside antibodies have been found in the sera of patients with IDDM with autonomic neuropathy as well as anti-GAD antibodies in a small group of patients. More detailed understanding of the specific antigens and the immune mechanisms involved in neuropathy and an extensive population survey is required before these issues can be further elaborated.

The relationship between neuropathy and various constitutional factors has been investigated by several researchers. Gadia *et al.* recently reported an inverse correlation between vibratory sensation and height and between peroneal motor nerve conduction velocities and height in a group of subjects with NIDDM and suggested that body stature may be a proxy for neurone length, with larger neurones being more susceptible to metabolic injury than shorter neurons (54). Moreover, a causal relationship between height and peripheral neuropathy could explain the association between male gender and peripheral neuropathy among subjects with IDDM recently reported in the Diabetes Control and Complications Trial (55). Grenfell, on the other hand, observed an association between presence of nephropathy and short stature among individuals with onset of diabetes during childhood and hypothesised that poor diabetic control may retard growth in childhood, thus making short stature a marker for the early development of complications (56). At least two studies have investigated a possible relationship between obesity (per cent ideal body weight) and presence of peripheral polyneuropathy and both failed to find an association (13–15, 57) notwithstanding the association of an increased BMI and autonomic neuropathy (50).

The relationship between pubertal changes and development of neuropathy was investigated by Sosenko *et al.*, who found that vibration sensation was significantly reduced in postpubertal children as compared to prepubertal children (41). This observation needs to be confirmed; possibly the increased physiological stress on the body that occurs during puberty increases susceptibility to neuropathy.

Nutritional factors, including vitamin deficiencies, have long been recognised as possible contributing factors to the development of neuropathy, including diabetic neuropathy (58). Deranged Vitamin $B_{12}$ metabolism is one possible pathway that has been implicated theoretically (59), but there are no data available supporting this hypothesis. Some researchers have suggested that the interaction of malnutrition with diabetes might account for the high prevalence of neuropathy seen in the diabetic population in underdeveloped countries (60).

## NATURAL HISTORY

Slowing of nerve conduction velocities (NCV) are among the earliest neuropathic abnormalities that occur in diabetes and are often present even at the diagnosis of diabetes (61–64). After diagnosis, slowing of NCV generally progresses and is correlated with duration of diabetes (65). Sensory fibres are usually affected first, followed by motor fibres (66).

Although slowing of NCV is common in diabetes, and often occurs early in the course of the disease, there is considerable uncertainty as to the relevance of these abnormalities to the future development of either subclinical manifestations or clinically apparent diabetic neuropathy. While most studies have documented that symptomatic patients are more likely to have slower nerve conduction velocities than patients without symptoms (19, 37, 43, 66–68), NCV does not appear to be related to the severity of symptoms (69).

The relationship between the objective signs of neuropathy and neuropathic symptoms is also not well defined. The observed manifestations of neuropathy are thought to depend on the type of nerve fibre affected. Small nerve fibre damage, which usually, although not always, precedes large nerve fibre damage, is manifested first in the lower limbs, with a loss of thermal sensitivity, and reduced light touch and pin prick sensation occurring early (70). When pain occurs, NCV is often normal or only minimally reduced (71), suggesting that pain is an early (small fibre) manifestation of diabetic polyneuropathy. When pain is present, it typically resolves on its own, but whether this is reflective of the reversibility of early nerve damage or progression to nerve death is not clear. Large fibre neuropathies are manifested by reduced vibratory sensation and depressed tendon reflexes. In two follow-up studies, progressive reduction of vibratory sensation and loss of tendon reflexes have been observed in patients who at the same time, reported an improvement in pain symptoms (72, 73). The situation is further complicated by the fact that most diabetic peripheral neuropathy is of the 'mixed' variety with both large and small nerve fibre involvement. In our own clinic population only 15.0% of diabetic subjects with clinically confirmed symptoms of neuropathy had no objective signs of neuropathy, although 63.7% of patients with signs had no symptoms. Twenty-eight other investigators have reported even smaller proportions of 'pure' small nerve fibre and 'pure' large nerve fibre neuropathies (70).

Autonomic neuropathy may be a prerequisite in the development of foot ulceration in diabetes that is conventionally classified as a manifestation of distal symmetric polyneuropathy (74, 75). Animal studies have suggested that autonomic neuropathy alone may precipitate plantar ulceration (76). Callus formation, which predates plantar foot ulceration, may arise in part from excess blood flow as it disappears if peripheral vascular disease develops (77). Chariot arthropathy (neuroarthropathy) is an underdiagnosed complication of the diabetic neuropathic foot in which bone fractures occurs, and are followed by bone disorganisation and increased risk of secondary ulceration. This is traditionally ascribed solely to distal symmetric polyneuropathy in diabetes. High peripheral blood flow causing weakening of bones in the foot may predispose to fractures in the insensitive foot (78, 79).

Much remains to be learned of the natural history of diabetic autonomic neuropathy. Testing of cardiovascular reflexes has revealed that signs of autonomic neuropathy may occur relatively early in the course of diabetes. (43, 46, 80–82). Both sympathetic and parasympathetic nerve fibres may be affected, with parasympathetic dysfunction preceding sympathetic dysfunction (46, 79–82). Improvements in the methods to measure sympathetic function have now shown, though, that sympathetic damage may occur earlier than previously thought (83). Using infrared pupillometry, Ziegler *et al.*, for example, have demonstrated that the speed of pupillary dilation may be slowed even at the diagnosis of IDDM (64).

Approximately 75% of all parasympathetic nerve fibres are in the vagus nerves (10th cranial nerve), where they pass to the entire thoracic and abdominal regions of the body. Early autonomic nerve dysfunction has been attributed to vagal damage, with manifestations appearing in a number of organ systems. A battery of diagnostic tests to assess cardiovascular autonomic function has been devised which measure heart rate responses under various conditions. Among the defects indicative of cardiac autonomic damage demonstrable by these tests are: an increase in resting heart rate (tachycardia), abnormal heart rate response to the Valsalva manoeuvre, loss of beat to beat variability in heart rate, and loss of the immediate heart rate response to standing (46, 80–82, 84, 85). These tests were initially thought to reflect cardiac parasympathetic integrity, but it is now appreciated that the autonomic pathways involved in these reflexes are complex, and these tests may reflect both parasympathetic and sympathetic innervation (86). Once these tests become abnormal, they usually remain abnormal (87, 88).

Autonomic neuropathy (AN) is a well-recognised and serious complication of diabetes. Its prevalence in insulin-dependent diabetes mellitus (IDDM) ranges from as low as 16% (89) in newly diagnosed IDDM patients to as much as 75% (90) in established diabetes. A number of studies have indicated prevalences somewhere between these two extremes (46, 86, 91, 92, 93–95), dependent primarily on the methods used for sampling and measurement. The presence of autonomic neuropathy is typically confirmed and measured using a battery of cardiovascular reflexes developed primarily by Ewing and colleagues (80–82, 91, 96, 97). The San Antonio

Conference on Diabetic Neuropathy (98) suggested the use of heart-rate response to Valsalva manoeuvre, deep breathing, and standing; as well as blood pressure response to standing or tilting and sustained hand grip in order to fully assess cardiovascular autonomic status. That conference also indicated that a scoring system should be used to permit a hierarchical staging of the levels of sensitivity of these tests. However, specific scoring systems have not yet been adopted universally (99, 100). The sensitivity of symptoms and even clinical signs for the detection of AN has been shown to be substantially less than that of cardiovascular and other tests, as these standardisable tests often identify clinically unrecognised autonomic impairment (81, 86, 91, 94, 95).

In light of the increased mortality associated with autonomic neuropathy (81, 89, 90, 96, 101–109) and its possible involvement in other complications of diabetes, it is crucially important to define the long-term course of autonomic neuropathy measurements and symptoms, as well as its relationship to other complications. There have been few previous reports comprehensively describing the natural history and progression of autonomic neuropathy over time in terms of both symptoms and autonomic function tests (101, 102, 110).

Sampson and colleagues studied the progress of autonomic neuropathy in three groups of IDDM followed for 10–15 years. They found that heart rate variability declined at a rate of 1.02 ± 0.47 per annum in diabetics with an initially normal heart rate variability. Symptoms were not found to remit, even over a decade, but they did not commonly progress. Forty-nine had symptomatic autonomic neuropathy and an abnormal heart rate variability, 24 were asymptomatic with an abnormal heart rate variability (<12) and 38 had normal heart rate variability. The 10-year survival rates were 74%, 91.7% and 89.5%, respectively. The 18 deaths were renal failure ($n$=40), myocardial infarction ($n$=3) and sudden unexpected death. The chief autonomic symptoms in this series were diarrhoea, postural hypotension, and gustatory sweating which, although persistent, apparently did not deteriorate or become disabling. The development of symptoms in patients with abnormal reflexes was an unusual event (101). O'Brien *et al.* screened 506 randomly selected patients with IDDM for autonomic neuropathy. Of these, 484 were traced five years later and 44 (9%) had died (89). Renal failure was significantly associated with autonomic failure and the cumulative 5-year mortality was 27% compared with 5% in those with normal autonomic function. Discriminant analysis showed that autonomic neuropathy was the most important independent predictor of death.

These relationships were investigated in a cohort of randomly selected insulin-dependent diabetics who were initially studied in 1981 and who were assessed again nine years later (111).

Sympathetic failure usually follows vagal denervation and may involve the following processes: cardiac denervation (in combination with parasympathetic denervation), loss of peripheral and splanchnic (visceral) vasoconstriction, and loss of vasomotor control and increase of peripheral blood flow (83). Among the symptoms which may be manifested by these defects are postural hypotension, sweating disturbances, and hypoglycaemic unawareness. Direct injury to small myelinated and unmyelinated sympathetic nerve fibres signalling pain and temperature may also occur, leading possibly to painful peripheral neuropathy.

Although symptomatic peripheral neuropathy usually precedes the development of symptomatic autonomic neuropathy (7, 112), signs of parasympathetic neuropathy may sometimes appear before signs of peripheral neuropathy (112). In contrast, sympathetic nerve abnormalities are rarely found in the absence of signs of peripheral neuropathy (112). Isolated abnormalities on autonomic function tests are occasionally found, however, in non-diabetic individuals (43).

The mortality for diabetic autonomic neuropathy has been estimated to be of the order of

Table 17.2. *Influences of autonomic neuropathy on mortality in insulin-dependent diabetes*

| Reference | Subject | Selection criteria | Length of follow-up | Overall mortality (%) |
|---|---|---|---|---|
| (113) | 40 | Autonomic symptoms and abnormal AFT* | 19 months–5 years | 53 |
| (87) | 64 | Autonomic symptoms and abnormal AFT | 3–5 years | 27 |
| (114) | 16 | Abnormal beat-to-beat | 5 years | 19 |
| (101) | 41 | Abnormal AFT | 5 years | 24 |
| (106) | 30 | Abnormal AFT | 5 years | 46 |
| (11) | 84 | Abnormal AFT | 5 years | 27 |

* AFT=Autonomic function test.

44% within $2\frac{1}{2}$ years of diagnosis of symptomatic autonomic neuropathy (80–82). The early studies by Ewing and colleagues in Scotland caused much concern because most people died of conditions other than autonomic neuropathy including renal failure and the only patients followed were those who were symptomatic. Table 2 is a summary of currently available data on the influence of autonomic neuropathy on mortality and insulin-dependent diabetes. It can be seen that, although Ewing's observations were thought to be an overestimate, it is apparent that, based upon asymptomatic subjects with only abnormalities, in autonomic function tests the overall mortality rate may be as high as 25–40% (115).

## REFERENCES


1 Deckert T. Late diabetic manifestations in 'pancreatogenic' diabetes mellitus. *Acta Med Scand* 1960; 168: 439–46.
2 Galton DJ. Diabetic retinopathy and haemochromatosis. *Br Med J* 1965; 1: 1169.
3 Bank S, Marks IN, Vinik AI. Clinical and hormonal aspects of pancreatic diabetes. *Am J Gastroenterol* 1975; 64: 13–22.
4 Young RJ, Zhou YQ, Rodriguez E, Prescott RJ *et al.* Variable relationship between peripheral somatic and autonomic neuropathy in patients with different syndromes of diabetic polyneuropathy. *Diabetes* 1986; 35: 192–7.
5 Thomas PK, Eliasson SG. Diabetic neuropathy. In: Dyck PJ, Thomas PK, Lambert EH, Bunge R, ed. *Peripheral neuropathy,* Philadelphia: WB Saunders, 1984; 1773–810.
6 Sullivan JF. The neuropathies of diabetes. *Neurology* 1958; 8: 243–9.
7 Ellenberg M. Diabetic neuropathy. In Ellenberg M, Rifkin H, ed. *Diabetes Mellitus: theory and practice,* New York: McGraw-Hill; 1982: 777–801.
8 Greene DA, Pfeifer MA. Diabetic neuropathy. In: Olefsky JM, Sherwin RS, ed. *Diabetes mellitus: management and complications,* New York: Churchill Livingstone, 1985; 223–54.
9 Brown MJ, Asbury AK. Diabetic neuropathy. *Ann Neurol* 1984; 15: 2–12.
10 American Diabetes Association, American Academy of Neurology. Consensus statement: Report and recommendations of the San Antonio conference on diabetic neuropathy. *Diabetes Care* 1988; 11: 592–7.
11 Dyck PJ, Kratz KM, Lehman KA, Karnes JL *et al.* The Rochester diabetic neuropathy study: design, criteria for types of neuropathy, selection bias, and reproducibility of neuropathic tests. *Neurology* 1991; 41: 799–807.
12 Orchard TJ, Dorman JS, LaPorte RE, Ferrell RE *et al.* Host and environmental interactions in diabetes mellitus. *J Chronic Dis* 1986; 39: 979–99.
13 Pirart J. [Diabetes mellitus and its degenerative complications: a prospective study of 4,400 patients observed between 1947 and 1973 (author's transl)]. *Diabet Metab* 1977; 3: 97–107.
14 Pirart J. [Diabetes mellitus and its degenerative complications: a prospective study of 4,400 patients observed between 1947 and 1973 (2nd part) (author's transl)]. *Diabet Metab* 1977; 3: 173–82.
15 Pirart J. [Diabetes mellitus and its degenerative complications: a prospective study of 4,400 patients observed between 1947 and 1973 (3rd and last part) (author's transl)]. *Diabet Metab* 1977; 3: 245–56.
16 Franklin G, Kahn L, Baxter J. *An epidemiologic study of neuropathy in the San Luis Valley.* Amherst, MA: SER Meetings; 1987.
17 Bruyn GW, Garland H. Neuropathies of endocrine origin. In: Vinkin PJ, Bruyn GW, eds *Handbook of clinical neurology,* Amsterdam: North-Holland Publishing Company. 1970; 29–71.
18 Goodman JI, Baumoel S, Frankel L *et al. The diabetic neuropathies.* Springfield, IL: Charles C. Thomas; 1953

19 Boulton AJ, Knight G, Drurym J, Ward JD. The prevalence of symptomatic, diabetic neuropathy in an insulin-treated population. *Diabetes Care* 1985; 8: 125–9.
20 Fry IK, Hardwick C, Scot GW. Diabetic neuropathy: a survey and follow-up of 66 cases. *Guy's Hosp Rep* 1962; 111: 113–29.
21 Palumbo PJ, Elveback LR, Whisnant JP. Neurologic complications of diabetes mellitus: transient ischemic attack, stroke, and peripheral neuropathy. *Adv Neurol* 1978; 19: 593–601.
22 Melton LJ, Ochi JW, Palumbo PJ, Chu CP. Sources of disparity in the spectrum of diabetes mellitus at incidence and prevalence. *Diabetes* 1983; 6:427–31.
23 Dyck PJ, Kratz KM, Karnes JL *et al.* The prevalence by staged severity of various types of diabetic neuropathy, retinopathy, and nephropathy in a population-based cohort: The Rochester diabetic neuropathy study. *Neurology* 1993; 43: 817–24.
24 Hamman RF, Marshall JA, Baxter J *et al.* Methods and prevalence of non-insulin-dependent diabetes mellitus in a biethnic Colorado population. *Am J Epidemiol* 1989; 129;295–311.
25 Franklin GM, Kahn LB, Baxter J, Marshall JA, Hamman RF. Sensory neuropathy in non-insulin-dependent diabetes mellitus. The San Luis Valley Diabetes Study. *Am J Epidemiol* 1990; 131: 633–43.
26 Hamman RF, Franklin GA, Mayer EJ *et al.* Microvascular complications of NIDDM in Hispanics and non-Hispanic whites. San Luis Valley Diabetes Study. *Diabetes Care* 1991; 14: 655–64.
27 National Center for Health Statistics Current estimates from the National Health Interview Survey, 1989. Vital and Health Statistics Ser. 10 1990; No. 176.
28 Harris MH, Eastman R, Cowie C. Symptoms of neuropathy in adults with NIDDM in the US population. *Diabetes Care,* 1993; 16: In Press.
29 National Center for Health Statistics Plan and operation of the Second National Health and Nutrition Examination Survey. Vital and Health Statistics. Ser. 1, No. 15. Washington, DC, USGPO, DHHS publication no. (PHS) 81–1981; 1317.
30 NHDS, National Hospital Discharge Survey Govt. Printing Office 1991.
31 The Diabetes Control and Complications Trial Research Group. The effect of intensive diabetes treatment on the development and progression of long-term complications in insulin-dependent diabetes mellitus: The Diabetes Control and Complications Trial. *N Engl J Med* 1993; 329:In press,
32 Maser RE, Steenkiste AR, Dorman JS *et al.* Epidemiological correlates of diabetic neuropathy. *Diabetes* 1989; 38: 1456–61.
33 Maser RE, Nielsen VK, Dorman JS, Drash AL, Becker DJ, Orchard TJ. Measuring subclinical neuropathy: does it relate to clinical neuropathy? Pittsburgh Epidemiology of Diabetes Complications Study-V (published erratum appears in *J Diabet Complications* 1991; 5:205) *J Diabetic Complications* 1991; 5: 6–12.
34 Maser RE, Becker DJ, Drash AL *et al.* Pittsburgh Epidemiology of Diabetes Complications Study. Measuring diabetic neuropathy follow-up study results. *Diabetes Care* 1992; 15: 525–7.
35 Nilsson SV, Nilsson JE, Frostberg N, Emilsson T. The Kristianstad survey. II. Studies in a representative adult diabetic population with special reference to comparison with an adequate control group. *Acta Med Scand* Suppl 1967; 469: 1–42.
36 Paisey RB, Arrendondo G, Villalobos A, Lozano O *et al.* Association of differing dietary, metabolic, and clinical risk factors with microvascular complications of diabetes: a prevalence study of 503 Mexican type II diabetic subjects. II. *Diabetes Care* 1984; 7: 428–33.
37 Haimanot RT, Abdulkadir J. Neuropathy in Ethiopian diabetics: a correlation of clinical and nerve conduction studies. *Trop Geog Med* 1985; 37: 62–8.
38 DCCT Research Group. Diabetic control and complications trial: research of feasibility study. *Diabetes Care* 1987; 10: 1–119.
39 Marcus J, Ehrlich R, Kelly M, Murphy EG. Nerve conduction in childhood diabetes. *Can Med Assoc J* 1973; 108: 1116–19.
40 Kruger M, Brunko E, Dorchy H, Noel P. Fermoral versus peroneal neuropathy in diabetic children and adolescents – relationships to clinical status, metabolic control and retinopathy. *Diabete Metab* 1987; 13: 110–15.
41 Sosenko JM, Boulton AJ, Kubrusly DB, Weintraub JK *et al.* The vibratory perception threshold in young diabetic patients: associations with glycemia and puberty. *Diabetes Care* 1985, 8: 605–7.
42 Osuntokun BO, Akinkugbe FM, Francis TI, Reddy S *et al.* Diabetes mellitus in Nigerians: a study of 832 patients. *West Afr Med J Niger Pract* 1971; 20: 295–312.
43 Jeyarajah R, Samarawickrama, P, Jameel, MM. Autonomic function tests in non-insulin dependent diabetic patients and apparently healthy volunteers. *J Chronic Dis,* 1986; 39: 479–84.
44 Sharpey-Schafer EP, Taylor PJ. Absent circulatory reflexes in diabetic neuritis. *Lancet* 1960; i: 559–62.
45 Ewing DJ, Irving JB, Kerr F, Wildsmith JA, Clark BF, *et al.* Cardiovascular responses to sustained handgrip in normal subjects and in patients with diabetes mellitus: a test of autonomic function. *Clin Sci Mol Med* 1974; 46; 295–306.
46 Drybert T, Benn J, Christiansen JS, Hilsted J *et al.* Prevalence of diabetic autonomic neuropathy measured by simple bedside tests. *Diabetologia* 1981; 20: 190–4
47 Burke CM, O'Doherty A, Flanagan A, O'Connel BM *et al.* Autonomic neuropathy in a diabetic clinic. *Irish Med J* 1984; 77: 202–5.
48 Veglio MP, Carpano-Maglioli P, Tonda L, Quadri R *et al.* Autonomic neuropathy in non-insulin-dependent diabetic patients: correlation with age, sex, duration and metabolic control of diabetes. *Diabete Metab* 1990; 16: 200–6.
49 Maser RE, Pfeider MA, Dorman JS *et al.* Diabetic autonomic neuropathy and cardiovascular risk. Pittsburgh Epidemiology of Diabetes Complications Study III. *Arch Internal Med* 1990; 150: 1218–22.
50 Bergstrom B, Lilja B, Osterlin S, Sundkvist G. Autonomic neuropathy in non-insulin-dependent (type II) diabetes mellitus. Possible influence of obesity. *Int Med* 1990; 227: 57–63.
51 Boulton AJ, Worthm RC, Drury J, Hardisty CA *et al.* Genetic and metabolic studies in diabetic neuropathy. *Diabetologia* 1984; 26: 15–19.
52 Shenfield GM, McCann VJ, Tjokresetio R. Acetylator status and diabetic neuropathy. *Diabetologia* 1982; 22: 441–4.

53 Chochinov RH, Ullycot GL, Moorhouse JA. Sensory perception thresholds in patients with juvenile diabetes and their close relatives. *New Eng J Med* 1972; 286: 1233–37.

54 Gadia MT, Ayyar DR, Ramos LB, Natori N *et al.* The association between neurologic dysfunction and body stature. *Diabetes* 1986; 35 (suppl 1): 103A (Abstract).

55 Greene DA, Brown M, Gilbert P, Nielsen VK *et al.* Age and gender are factors in the development of diabetic neuropathy: baseline neurologic assessment in the Diabetes Control and Complications Trial (DCCT). *Diabetes* 1986; 35 (suppl 1): 12A (Abstract).

56 Grenfell A, Migdalis I, Leslie DG. Short stature and diabetic complications. *Transpl Proc* 1986; 18(6): 1500.

57 Weinberg CR, Pfeifer MA. Development of a predictive model for symptomatic neuropathy in diabetes. *Diabetes* 1986; 35: 873–80.

58 Rudy A, Epstein SH. Review of 100 cases of 'diabetic neuropathy' followed from 1–10 years. *J Clin Endocrinol Metab* 1945; 5: 92–109.

59 Bhatt HR, Linnell JC, Matthews DM. Can faulty vitamin B-12 (cobalamin) metabolism produce diabetic neuropathy? [letter]. *Lancet* 1983; ii: 572.

60 Chuttani PN, Chawla LS. Diabetic neuropathy in India. *Ind J Med Res* 1974; 62: 99–109.

61 Fraser DM, Campbell IW, Ewing DJ, Murray A *et al.* Peripheral and autonomic nerve function in newly diagnosed diabetes mellitus. *Diabetes* 1977; 26: 546–50.

62 Ward JD, Barnes CG, Fisher DJ, Jessop JD *et al.* Improvement in nerve conduction following treatment in newly diagnosed diabetics. *Lancet* 1971; 428–30.

63 Christensen NJ. Diabetic macroangiopathy blood flow and radiological studies. In Camerini-Davalos RA, Cole HS, eds. *Vascular and neurological changes in early diabetes*, New York: Academic Press: 1973; 129–34.

64 Ziegler D, Cicmir I, Wiefels K, Mayer P. Peripheral and autonomic nerve dysfunction in newly diagnosed insulin-dependent diabetics (IDDM). *Diabetes* 1986; 35 (suppl 1): 102A (Abstract).

65 Gregersen G. Diabetic neuropathy: influence of age, sex, metabolic contol, and duration of diabetes on motor conduction velocity. *Neurology* 1967; 17: 972–80.

66 Lamontagne A, Buchthal F. Electrophysiological studies in diabetic neuropathy. *J Neurol Neurosurg Psychiat* 1970; 33: 442–52.

67 Mulder DW, Lambert EH, Bastron JA, Sprague RG. The neuropathies associated with diabetes mellitus: a clinical and electromyographic study of 103 unselected diabetic patients. *Neurology* 1961; 11(4): 275–84.

68 Skillman TG, Johnson EW, Hamwi GJ, Driskill HJ. Motor nerve conduction velocity in diabetes mellitus. *Diabetes* 1961; 10(1): 46–51.

69 Greene DA, Brown MJ, Braunstein SN, Schwartz SS *et al.* Comparison of clinical course and sequential electrophysiological tests in diabetics with symptomatic polyneuropathy and its implications for clinical trials. *Diabetes* 1981; 30: 139–47.

70 Jaspan J. *Personal communication.*

71 Archer AG, Watkins PJ, Thomas PK, Sharma AK *et al.* The natural history of acute painful neuropathy in diabetes mellitus. *J Neurol Neurosurg Psychiat* 1983; 46: 491–9.

72 Bischoff A. The natural course of diabetic neuropathy: a follow-up. *Hormone Metab Res* 1980; 9 (suppl 1): 98–100.

73 Mayne N. The short-term prognosis in diabetic neuropathy. *Diabetes* 1968; 17: 270–3.

74 Edmonds ME, Nicolaides K, Watkins PJ. The importance of autonomic neuropathy in the etiology of diabetic neuropathic foot ulceration. *Diabetologia* 1981; 21: 506–7 (Abstract).

75 Deanfield JE, Daggett PR, Harrison MJ. The role of autonomic neuropathy in diabetic foot ulceration. *J Neurol Sci* 1980; 47: 203–10.

76 Barkowshi M. An experimental study on the role of arteriovenous anastomoses in the pathogenesis of the trophic ulcer. *Arch Immunol Ther Exp (Warsz)* 1973; 21: 363–75.

77 Edmonds ME. The diabetic foot: pathophysiology and treatment. *Clin Endocrinol Metab* 1986; 15: 889–916.

78 Stevens MJ, Roberts VC, Watkins PJ. Selective neuropathy and preserved vascular responses in the diabetic Charcot foot. *Diabetologia* 1992 (in press).

79 Edmonds ME, Roberts VC, Watkins PJ. Blood flow in the diabetic neuropathic foot. *Diabetologia* 1982; 22: 9–15.

80 Ewing DJ, Clarke BF. Diagnosis and management of diabetic autonomic neuropathy. *Br Med J* 1982; 285: 916–18.

81 Ewing DJ Clarke BF. Diagnosis and management of diabetic autonomic neuropathy. *Br Med J* 1982; 285: 916–18.

82 Ewing DJ, Clarke BF. Cardiovascular reflex tests: In the natural history of diabetic autonomic neuropathy. *New York State J Med* 1982; 82: 903–8.

83 Watkins PJ, Edmonds ME. Sympathetic nerve failure in diabetes. *Diabetologia* 1983; 25: 73–7.

84 Hilsted J. Testing for autonomic neuropathy. *Ann Clin Res* 1984; 16: 128–35.

85 Hilsted J. Testing for autonomic neuropathy. *Ann Clin Res* 1984; 16: 128–35.

86 Ewing DJ, Martyn CN, Young RJ, Clarke BF. The value of cardiovascular autonomic function tests: 10 years experience in diabetes. *Diabetes Care* 1985; 8: 491–8.

87 MacKay JD, Page MM, Cambridge J, Watkins PJ. Diabetic autonomic neuropathy. The diagnostic value of heart rate monitoring. *Diabetologia* 1980; 18: 471–8.

88 Ewing DJ, Campbell IW, Clarke BF. Mortality in diabetic autonomic neuropathy. *Lancet* 1976; 1: 601–3.

89 O'Brien IAR, McFadden JP, Corrall RJM. The influence of autonomic neuropathy on mortality in insulin-dependent diabetes. *Quart J Med* 1991; 79: 495–502.

90 Navarro X, Kennedy WR, Sutherland DER. Autonomic neuropathy and survival in diabetes mellitus: effects of pancreas transplantation. *Diabetologia* 1991; 34(Suppl 1): S108–12.

91 Ewing DJ, Clarke BF. Diabetic autonomic neuropathy: present insights and future prospects. *Diabetes Care* 1986; 9: 648–65.

92 Hilsted J, Jensen SB. A simple test for autonomic neuropathy in juvenile diabetics. *Acta Med Scand* 1979; 205: 385–7.

93 Zola B, Kahn JK, Juni JE, Vinik AI. Abnormal cardiac function in diabetic patients with autonomic neuropathy in the absence of ischemic heart disease. *J Endocrinol Metab* 1986; 63: 208–14.

94 Kennedy, WR, Navarro X, Sakuta M, Mandell H, Knox CK, Sutherland DER. Physiological and clinical correlates of cardiorespiratory reflexes in diabetes mellitus. *Diabetes Care* 1989; 12: 399–408.
95 Fisher BM, Frier BM. Usefulness of cardiovascular tests of autonomic function in asymptomatic diabetic patients. *Diabetes Res Clin Pract* 1989; 6: 157–60.
96 Ewing DJ, Campbell IW, Clarke BF. Assessment of cardiovascular effects in diabetic autonomic neuropathy and prognostic implications. *Ann Int Med* 1980; 92: 308–11.
97 Ewing DJ, Borsey DQ, Bellavere F, Clarke BF. Cardiac autonomic neuropathy in diabetes: comparison of measures of R-R variation. *Diabetologia* 1981; 21: 18–24.
98 Factors in development of diabetic neuropathy. Baseline analysis of neuropathy in feasibility phase of Diabetes Control and Complications Trial (DCCT). The DCCT Research Group. *Diabetes* 1988; 37: 476–81.
99 Kempler P, Varadi A, Tamas G. Which battery of cardiovascular autonomic function tests? Suggestion for a rational diagnostic model. *Diabetologia* 1990; 33: 640.
100 Ewing DJ. Which battery of cardiovascular autonomic function tests? *Diabetologia* 1990; 33: 180–1.
101 Sampson MJ, Wilson S, Karagiannis P, Edmonds M, Watkins PJ. Progression of diabetic autonomic neuropathy over a decade in insulin-dependent diabetics. *Quart J Med* 1990; 75: 635–46.
102 Ewing DJ, Campbell IW, Clarke BF. The natural history of diabetic autonomic neuropathy. *Quart J Med* 1980; 193: 95–108.
103 Watkins PJ, MacKay JD. Cardiac denervation in diabetic neuropathy. *Ann Int Med* 1980; 92: 304–7.
104 Kahn JK, Zola B, Juni JE, Vinik AI. Radionuclide assessment of left ventricular diastolic filling in diabetes mellitus with and without cardiac autonomic neuropathy. *J Am Coll Cardiol* 1986; 7: 1303–9.
105 Zola BE, Vinik AI. Effects of autonomic neuropathy associated with diabetes mellitus on cardiovascular function. *Curr Sci* 1992; 3: 33–41.
106 Kahn JK, Sisson JC, Vinik AI. QT interval prolongation and sudden cardiac death in diabetic autonomic neuropathy. *J Clin Endocrinol Metab* 1987; 64: 751–4.
107 Kahn JK, Sisson JC, Vinik AI. Prediction of sudden cardiac death in diabetic autonomic neuropathy. *J Nucl Med* 1988; 29: 1605–6.
108 Bellavere F, Ferri M, Guarini L, Bax G, Piccoli A, Cardone C, Fedele C. Prolonged QT period in diabetic autonomic neuropathy: a possible role in sudden cardiac death? *Br Heart J* 1988; 59: 379–83.
109 Ewing DJ, Boland O, Neilson JMM, Cho CG, Clarke, BF. Autonomic neuropathy, QT interval lengthening, and unexpected deaths in male diabetic patients. *Diabetologia* 1991; 34: 182–5.
110 Sundqvist G, Lilja B. Autonomic neuropathy in diabetes mellitus: a follow-up study. *Diabetes Care* 1985; 8: 129–33.
111 Levitt NS, Stansberry KB, Wynchanck S, Vinik AI. The Natural History of Autonomic Neuropathy in a Cohort of IDDM. *Diabetes* 1993; 42 (Suppl 1), 100A.
112 Sundkvist G. Autonomic nervous function in asymptomatic diabetic patients with signs of peripheral neuropathy. *Diabetes Care* 1981; 4: 529–34.
113 O'Brien IAR, Lewin IG, O'Hare JP, Arendt J *et al.* Abnormal circadian rhythm of melatonin in diabetic autonomic neuropathy. *Clin Endocrinol (Oxf)* 1986; 24: 359–64.
114 Clark BF, Campbell IW, Ewing DJ. Prognosis in diabetic autonomic neuropathy. *Horm Metab Res Suppl* 1980; 9: 101–4.
115 Hasslacher C, Bassler G. Prognosis of cardiac autonomic neuropathy in diabetes. *MMW Munch Med Wochenschr* 1983; 125: 375–7.

# 18 Diabetic Foot Infections

Steven B. Leichter

## INTRODUCTION

Few complications of diabetes cause as much morbidity, mortality, and disability as pedal infections. It is estimated that diabetic patients who develop pedal infection have hospital stays that are twice as long and twice as costly as the average hospital stay attributable to diabetes (1). Amputations due to pedal disease in diabetic patients constitute up to 45% of all lower extremity amputations in the United States (2). Diabetic patients are twice as likely to require special aids for mobility as non-diabetic persons (3). And diabetic patients who suffer a unilateral amputation have up to a 25% death rate within 5–7 years after the amputation (4).

These observations underscore the importance of a much richer fabric of information to emerge about diabetic foot infections within the last few years. Investigations on patient characteristics, predisposing metabolic factors, vascular insufficiency, pedal biomechanics, and the characteristics of infection have all together yielded a more sophisticated picture of this feared complication. As these data are assimilated, they will no doubt lead to more standard and more effective therapies.

## RISK FACTORS FOR THE DEVELOPMENT OF PEDAL INFECTION

### Age and duration of diabetes

Pedal infection seems to be a relatively late complication of diabetes. In two studies in which the duration of diabetes prior to amputation was noted, the pedal infection occurred at a mean of 13–18 years after the known onset of diabetes (5, 6). Studies of Pima Indians show that the longer the duration of diabetes, the higher the risk of occurrence of infection and amputation (7). Foot infection also occurs in a late middle age to maturely aged population (8). There may be a direct temporal relationship between the occurrence of peripheral neuropathy and the occurrence of pedal infection. A similar association has been suggested for peripheral vascular disease and pedal infection (9, 10). Both of these complications increase in prevalence among diabetic patients with ageing.

### Microvascular disease and hypertension

The prevalence of other microvascular complications of diabetes is high among patients with pedal infection. Peripheral neuropathy is present in more than 80% of affected patients (5, 7, 11). At least two studies have demonstrated that renal insufficiency and retinopathy are found in the majority of patients (5). Hypertension, a predisposing risk factor for microvascular complications, is also common.

### Gender differences

There may, or may not, be a sex bias in the occurrence of pedal infection. The most definitive data reflect rates of amputation from all causes among diabetic individuals, not occurrence of pedal infection (3). The data assume that these amputations are primarily due to peripheral vascular disease and pedal infection, although this is not documented. These data suggest that diabetic men are more likely to suffer amputation than women (3). Diabetic men less than 44 years of age were more than twice as likely to undergo amputation than diabetic women of the same age. These differences narrow, but are not abolished, with increasing age. A similar study of 477 diabetic amputees among 253 000 Eastern Finns reported an opposite sex bias (6). The group of 477 amputees consisted of almost twice as many diabetic women as diabetic men. Smaller studies on diabetic patients with pedal infection do not reflect a significant sex bias (5). These studies are not population based. Interestingly, many studies do not report the sex distribution of the subjects (12–14). Many others have been carried out at Veterans' Administration Medical Centers, which would have a preponderance of male subjects.

## METABOLIC CHARACTERISTICS OF PATIENTS WITH PEDAL INFECTION

Since diabetic foot infection tends to occur in patients in middle age or older, it is not surprising that the majority of patients have type II diabetes, and that they have the metabolic characteristics often seen in such patients (5, 12). They tend to have reduced serum HDL-cholesterol levels, elevated serum triglyceride concentrations, and little or no abnormality of LDL-cholesterol concentrations. However, on an age-adjusted basis, patients with type I diabetes are somewhat more likely to suffer pedal infection than those with type II diabetes (12). Studies on patients in the United States suggest that the majority of diabetic individuals with pedal infection are taking insulin at the time they present with the infection (5, 12). This is not true in similar evaluations carried out in Finland, although the majority of patients with pedal infection in that country appears to have type II diabetes (6).

Whether patients who suffer pedal infection tend to have poor control of hyperglycaemia is unclear. Patients in two studies had no significant difference in haemoglobin A1c levels in patients with foot infection versus uninfected diabetic patients (12, 15). However, Pima Indians undergoing amputation for pedal infection did have higher levels of serum glucose than controls (7). In both controlled and uncontrolled series, the mean levels of haemoglobin A1c were relatively high (5, 12, 15).

Subnormal serum zinc concentrations have now been observed in patients with pedal infection in two large series. Leichter *et al.* (5) first reported over a 60% prevalence of zinc deficiency in these patients. Reiber *et al.* (12) observed that infected patients who undergo amputation are more likely to have zinc deficiency and reduced zinc protoporphyrin/haem rations than patients who do not undergo amputation.

There is potential significance to these data regarding zinc deficiency. Zinc deficiency has been associated with dysfunctions in wound healing (15) and immune response to infection (16). Zinc deficiency may have been suspected in these patients because of the high prevalence of diabetic nephropathy in these subjects, and the possible association between proteinuria and zincuria in diabetic patients (17).

There is also concern in recent studies about the nutritional competence of these patients.

Reiber *et al.* (12) noted an increased risk of hypoproteinaemia and reduced serum carotene levels in patients undergoing amputation. Reduced nutritional competence may afflict a large minority of older patients undergoing orthopaedic surgery or amputation for pedal problems associated with diabetes (18). Whether there are problems conferred by the diabetic condition is unclear.

## PEDAL BIOMECHANICS AND THE LOCATION OF PEDAL INFECTIONS

There has long been the assumption that diabetic neuropathy confers alterations in the physiomechanical characteristics of the foot and thereby leads to soft tissue breakdown and pedal infection (19, 20). Although pedal disease has been reported in patients without neuropathy (15) the majority of patients are neuropathic at the time the infection is diagnosed (5, 12, 21). Many of these patients also have vascular insufficiency. Injury to the foot due to the anaesthesia or proprioceptive loss from neuropathy has been cited as one aspect of this problem (19–21). Bony deformities due to pedal osteopaenia and Charcot remodelling of the foot are another (20). These changes may substantially alter weight bearing and pressures on skin and soft tissues on the plantar surface of the foot and disrupt intact tissue (22–24). The ability of skin and subcutaneous tissues to cushion the foot against these pressures may be compromised by reduced thickness of soft tissues in the foot of patients with diabetic neuropathy (25).

These factors have been suggested as influences of the location of pedal lesions. Most lesions appear to occur in the distal part of the foot (26). The risk of amputation may be significantly higher with lesions in the proximal part of the foot (25).

## VASCULAR INSUFFICIENCY VS. NEUROPATHY

In most, but not all, studies, the majority of patients with pedal infection have demonstrable vascular insufficiency. Estimates of prevalence among different studies vary widely, from 15% to almost 70% (5, 21, 26, 27). Attitudes about the relative importance of vascular disease to the development of pedal infection also vary. Since neuropathy is usually observed to be more prevalent among infected patients, some groups argue that neuropathy is relatively more important in the occurrence of pedal disease than vascular insufficiency (28, 29). Other investigators suggest that vascular insufficiency may be an important determinant both of the occurrence of pedal infection, and the risk of major amputation (4, 30, 31).

## CHARACTERISTICS OF INFECTION

There has been a vigorous interest in the epidemiology of the pedal lesions themselves, particularly the bacteriology of these lesions. One obvious source of such interest is the influence such data have on the use of treatments in this clinical situation, such as antibiotic therapy. It is important to keep this in mind when assessing studies on this aspect of pedal infection.

Patients with diabetic foot infection may have surprisingly indolent infections, considering the potential gravity of this complication. In three studies, the mean intervals between the onset of infection and presentation for definitive treatment were noted to be 3.2 (12), 5.5 (5), and 9.0 (32) months. In another study of 60 patients, the interval was as long as 6 months (33). These long intervals may reflect the possibility that the clinical presentation may not appear as serious as the underlying infection really is (15, 33). In many cases, less aggressive attempts at treatment may have been used, before definitive therapy was applied (5).

There is no standard classification of pedal

infection, although it is generally recognised that there are certain important variables that group these lesions (33, 34). These include the presence or absence of ulceration, ischaemic disease or gangrene, and bacteraemia or sepsis (33). Another set of criteria which has attracted much support is that of Wagner, which evaluates the physical appearance and depth of lesions (37). The relative rates of occurrence of these problems is presently unknown. Whether these different types of problems are associated with different clinical courses, bacterial pathogens, or outcomes is unclear. However, certain features have been suggested as indicative of specific characteristics. Bacteraemia or soft tissue gas is a worrisome complication with regard to outcome (15, 35, 36). An uncomplicated cellulitis without ulceration may be associated with a gram positive aerobic organism (37, 38).

Despite these variations among patient groups in different studies, there are few disparities among studies on the bacteriology of these lesions (34). Aerobic gram positive organisms and aerobic gram negative organisms are the most common organisms recovered from these wounds. Fifty per cent or more of these lesions have aerobic gram positive organisms in them, and up to 50% have various aerobic gram negative organisms. Up to 20% of these wounds yield no organisms on routine culture (5). Two or more organisms are recovered from most of these lesions (5, 34–36). (Staphylococcus and streptococcus species are often the most common organisms recovered. The importance of enterococcus as a pathogen in these lesions has been recognised within recent years (5, 35, 36).

The one area of substantial variation among studies is the prevalence and, by implication, relative importance of anaerobes in these infections. Seven studies have reported a relatively high prevalence of anaerobic organisms, particularly bacteroides, in pedal infection (13, 32, 35, 36, 39–42).

However, anaerobic organisms were recovered from only a minority of patients in nine other studies (34). Bacteroides species were recovered in less than 20% of these patients in seven of these nine studies. These disparate results have led to an active debate about the importance of antibiotic coverage for anaerobic organisms in the design of treatment, especially at the beginning of therapy, before the results of cultures are known.

### Osteomyelitis

Another unsettled area is the relative importance of osteomyelitis. Estimates of the prevalence of osteomyelitis among pedal infections has ranged between 13 and 68% (5, 35, 36, 42–44). Uncertainty about the best methods for firmly establishing the diagnosis may partly explain this variation (29, 43). Whether therapy should be altered if osteomyelitis is present is controversial. Some investigators have reported that the presence of osteomyelitis is not necessarily an absolute indication for amputation, provided treatment is sufficiently aggressive and has a sufficiently long duration (45).

## PATTERNS OF CARE

The issues outlined above illustrate some of the reasons for the lack of standard therapeutic approaches in cases of pedal infection. Pedal infection in diabetic patients is a common, costly, and potentially debilitating complication. However, its severity may be underestimated, the presence of underlying osteomyelitis may not always be appreciated, and the indolent nature of these lesions may inappropriately delay referral for definitive treatment.

These worrisome trends may be emphasised by the patterns of care for pedal infection. Diabetes is known to be more prevalent in poorer Americans (45) and in black Americans (46). In statewide studies, black diabetic patients were significantly more likely to suffer amputation than white patients (3). Patients who have poor knowledge about their own diabetes care or foot care are significantly more likely to suffer pedal infection than those who are knowledgeable (33). Thus, this problem may be more likely to occur in poorer, less educated patients, who would be less capable of making good judgements about whether their lesion requires more aggressive intervention or not. In the current medical practice climate, the characteristics of these infections and the demography of patients most likely to have them raise concerns about advocacy of outpatient, less aggressive treatment for pedal infection. Although up to 75% of patients may have successful resolution of the infection with outpatient, oral antibiotic therapy (38), these other factors should encourage care programmes to structure careful defences for the welfare of the remaining 25% of patients, who may be least likely to defend themselves.

## REFERENCES


1 Leichter SB, Hernandez C, Fisher A *et al.* Diabetes in Kentucky. *Diabetes Care* 1982; 5: 126–34.
2 Drury TF. Disability among adult diabetics, in National Diabetes Data Group, *Diabetes in America* (Bethesda, US Public Health Service, NIH Publication No. 85–1468, 1985), p. XXVIII–1–22.
3 Most RS, Sinnock P. The epidemiology of lower extremity amputations in diabetic individuals. *Diabetes Care* 1983; 6: 87–91.
4 Whitehouse FW, Jurgensen C, Block MA. The later life of a diabetic amputee. Another look at the fate of the second leg. *Diabetes* 1968; 17: 520–21.
5 Leichter SB, Allweiss P, Harley J *et al.* Clinical characteristics of diabetic patients with serious pedal infection. *Metabolism* 1988; 37 (Suppl 1): 22–4.
6 Sitonen OI, Niskanen LK, Laakso M *et al.* Lower-extremity amputation in eastern Finland: a population-based study in eastern Finland. *Diabetes Care* 1993; 16: 16–20.
7 Nelson RG, Gohdes DM, Everhart JE, Hartner JA *et al.* Lower extremity amputation in NIDDM: 12 year follow-up study in Pima Indians. *Diabetes Care* 1988; 11: 8–16.
8 Bild DE, Selby JV, Sinnock P *et al.* Lower-extremity amputation in people with diabetes: epidemiology and prevention. *Diabetes Care* 1989; 12: 24–31.
9 Pirart J. Diabetes mellitus and its degenerative complications: a prospective study of 4400 patients observed between 1947 and 1973. *Diabetes Care* 1978; 1: 168–88.
10 Melton LJ, III, Macken KM, Palumbo PJ, Elveback LR. Incidence and prevalence of clinical peripheral vascular disease in a population-based cohort of diabetic patients. *Diabetes Care* 1980; 3: 650–4.
11 Beach KW, Strandness DE, Jr. Arteriosclerosis obliterans and associated risk factors in insulin-dependent and non-insulin-dependent diabetes. *Diabetes* 1980; 29: 882–8.
12 Reiber GE, Peccoraro RE, Koepsell TD. Risk factors for amputation in patients with diabetes mellitus: a case-control study. *Ann Int Med* 1992; 117: 97–105.
13 Kahn O, Wagner W, Bessman AN. Mortality of diabetic patients treated surgically for lower limb infection and/or gangrene. *Diabetes* 1974; 23: 287–92.
14 Sapico FL, Bessman AN, Canawati HN. Bacteremia in diabetic patients with infected lower extremities. *Diabetes Care* 1982; 5: 101–4.
15 Delbridge L, Appleberg M, Reeve TS. Factors associated with development of foot lesions in the diabetic. *Surgery* 1983; 78: 82.
16 Engel ED, Erlick NE, Davis RH. Diabetes mellitus: Impaired wound healing from zinc deficiency. *J Podiat Med Assoc* 1981; 10: 536–43.
17 Allen JI, Bell E, Boosalia MG *et al.* Association between zinc excretion and lymphocyte dysfunction in patients with lung cancer. *Am J Med* 1985; 79: 209–15.
18 Jensen JE, Jensen TG, Smith TK *et al.* Nutrition in orthopedic surgery. *J Bone Joint Surg* 1982; 64-A: 1263–72.
19 Dickhaut SC, DeLee JC, Page CP. Nutritional status: importance in predicting wound-healing after amputation. *J Bone Joint Surg* 1982; 64-A: 71–5.
20 Levin ME. Medical evaluation and treatment, In: Levin ME, O'Neal LW, eds. *The diabetic foot.* St. Louis: CV Mosby; 1988: 1–50.
21 Brand, P. The diabetic foot. In Rivkin, H Porte D Jr D, ed. *Diabetes Mellitus in theory and practice,* New York: Elsevier, 1990; 792–823.
22 Guy RJC, Clark CA. Malcolm PN, Watkins PJ. Evaluation of thermal and vibration sensation in diabetic neuropathy. *Diabetologia* 1985; 28: 131–7.
23 Stokes IAF, Faris IB, Hutton WC. The neuropathic ulcer and loads on the foot in diabetic patients. *Acta Orthop Scand* 1975; 46: 839–47.
24 Ctercteko GC, Dhanendran M, Hutton WC *et al.* Vertical forces acting on the feet of diabetic patients with neuropathic ulceration. *Br J Surg* 1981; 68: 608–14.
25 Boulton AJM, Hardisty CA, Betts RP *et al.* Dynamic foot pressures and other studies as diagnostic and management aids in diabetic neuropathy. *Diabetes Care* 1983; 6: 25–33.
26 Gooding GAW, Stess RM, Graf PM *et al.* Sonography of the sole of the foot: evidence for loss of foot pad thickness in diabetes and its relationship to ulceration of the foot. *Investig Radiol* 1986; 21: 45–8.
27 Kaufman J, Breeding L, Rosenberg N. Anatomic location of acute diabetic foot infection. *Am Surg* 1987; 53: 109–12.
28 Holewski JJ, Moss KM, Stess RM *et al.* Prevalence of foot pathology and lower extremity complications in a diabetic outpatient clinic. *J Rehabil Res Dev* 1989; 26: 35–44.
29 LoGero FW, Coffman JD. Vascular and microvascular disease of the foot in diabetes. *New Engl J Med* 1984; 311: 1615–8.
30 Gruenfeld C. Diabetic foot ulcers: etiology, treatment, and prevention. *Adv Internal Med* 1991; 37: 103–31.
31 Apelqvist J, Castenfors J, Larsson J. *et al.* Prognostic value of systolic ankle and toe blood pressure levels in the outcome of diabetic foot ulcer. *Diabetes Care* 1989; 12: 373–8.

32 Wheat LJ, Allen SD Henry M *et al.* Diabetic foot infections: bacterial analysis. *Arch Int Med* 1986; 146: 1935–40.

33 Griffiths GD, Wieman T-J. Metatarsal head resection for diabetic foot ulcers. *Arch Surg* 1990; 125: 832–5.

34 Karanfilian R, Lynch TG, Zirul VT *et al.* The value of laser Doppler velocimetry and transcutaneous oxygen tension determination in predicting healing of ischemic forefoot ulcerations and amputations in diabetic and non-diabetic patients. *J Vasc Surg* 1986; 4: 511–16.

35 Lipsky BA, Pecoraro RE, Wheat JL. The diabetic foot: soft tissue and bone infection. *Infect Dis Clin N Am* 1990; 4: 409–32.

36 Lipsky BA, Pecoraro RE, Larson SA *et al.* Outpatient management of uncomplicated lower extremity infections in diabetic patients. *Arch Int Med* 1990; 150: 790–7.

37 Wagner FW. The diabetic foot and amputation of the foot. In: Mann RA, ed. *Surgery of the foot*, St. Louis: CV Mosby, 1986; 421–55.

38 Jones EW, Edwardsm R, Finch R *et al.* A microbiological study of diabetic foot lesions. *Diabetes Med* 1984; 2: 213–15.

39 Fierer J, Dale D, Davis C. The fetid foot: lower-extremity infections in patients with diabetes mellitus. *Rev Infect Dis* 1979; 1: 210–17.

40 LeFrock JL, Blais F, Schell RF *et al.* Cefoxitin in the treatment of diabetic patients with lower extremity infections. *J Clin Microbiol* 1983; 22: 80–3.

41 Louie TJ, Bartlett JG, Tally FP *et al.* Aerobic and anaerobic bacteria in diabetic foot ulcers. *Ann Int Med* 1976; 85: 461–3.

42 Scer KS, Steele FJ. The septic foot in patients with diabetes. *Surgery* 19; 104: 661–6.

43 Leichter SB, Schaefer JC, O'Brian JT. New concepts in managing diabetic foot infections. *Geriatrics* 1991; 46: 24–30.

44 Gibbons GW, Eliopoulos GM. Infection of the diabetic foot. In Hoar CS, Kozak GP, eds. *Management of diabetic foot problems*. Philadelphia: WB Saunders Co, 1984: 97–102.

45 Wheat LJ. Diagnostic strategies in osteomyelitis. *Am J Med* 1985; 78 (Suppl 6B): 218–24.

46 Newman LG, Waller J, Palestro C *et al.* Unsuspected osteomyelitis in diabetic foot ulcers. *J Am Med Assoc* 1991; 266: 1246–51.

# 19 Ocular Complications of Diabetes

Alan L. Wagner

## INTRODUCTION

Blindness existed well before the origin of the written word. Susruta noted the disease of the 'honey urine' in the earliest of Hindu medical texts. Classical texts credit Aretaeus of Cappadocia (AD 81–138) with the observation that diabetes was 'a melting down of the flesh and limbs to urine'. With these, and many other references to what has now become known as diabetes mellitus, it was not until Jaëger's 1856 (1) paper that specific changes in the fundi of those who suffered from diabetes mellitus were first noted. In 1890, Hirschberg wrote the first comprehensive treatise on the multiple manifestations of diabetes mellitus and the eye (2). The primary changes reflected in the eye from the presence of diabetes mellitus have been subject to intense scrutiny and several methods of standardisation. This process has been one of constant evolution.

A reference text published in 1967 (3) stated that 'diabetes . . . a chronic and incurable disease . . . (with) the result is that diabetes is one of the common causes of blindness as the years go by owing to improvements in insulin therapy and longer expectation of life.' This reflected the increased incidence of blindness from diabetes in New York state from a rate of 4.5% in 1941 to 16.6% in 1957 (4). By the mid-1960s it was the leading cause of new blindness between the ages of 25 and 64 in the US (5). The apparent epidemic growth in the complications of diabetes initiated multiple retrospective and recent prospective studies to detect the causes and associated factors that modulate the impact of diabetes on the eye.

The reported prevalence of vision loss due to diabetes, i.e. the total number of any population having the disease, must be viewed sceptically. Even if diabetes or its complications were reportable by law, the medical and support personnel as well as the patients' lack of co-operation would not allow for reporting many of the cases. Under-reporting will occur more frequently where blindness has an attendant negative social impact. In the United States, many localities have made blindness reportable but not mandatory to do so; hence there remains a significant degree of underreporting. Furthermore, reportable loss of vision depends upon the locally set thresholds, skill of the examiners, cross-sectional age profile of the group studied, screening technique utilised, size of the sample, and representativeness of the sample relative to the larger population.

The United States first used a population census to determine blindness. The accuracy of the data relied upon the honesty of the respondent, and an assumed understanding of the definition of blindness. Social pressures and lack of a standardised examination lead to a significant under-reporting of the incidence and prevalence of blindness. Institutionalised patients were not reflected in the tally. It is reasonable to expect that the institutionalised population would have a much higher rate of infirmities, including blindness.

A captured population (case series, registers, and schools for the blind) provides valuable information as to the spectrum of a disease's impact upon the cohort; however, it may not reflect accurately upon the assumed supporting population. Patients in these groups may travel long distances and represent other populations. A hospital or clinic may only study or treat one particular type of disease while excluding others (6–9).

Comparison of blindness across country borders is perilous due to the aforementioned variables. The incidence and prevalence of the reported loss of vision in non-industrialised countries from diabetes is minimal. Anterior segment disease (corneal scarring, cataracts) is the most frequent cause of loss of vision from birth to the mid-20s and, thereafter, glaucoma takes an ever-enlarging role. As the age of the population progresses, females are more frequently afflicted owing to their increased longevity as the population mix changes.

In answer to the above concerns, two separate approaches have been used to estimate the epidemiology of ocular complications in diabetes. Multicentre prospective randomised control treatment trials (10–16) and population based sampling (17–19). This information, in turn, has been used comparatively, and in a summary fashion, to not only provide recommendations for improved patient care and reduced morbidity from diabetes, but also to argue in favour of support of the improved delivery of ophthalmic care to patients with diabetes to afford substantial financial and visual savings to the patient as well as to the government (20, 21).

## PREVALENCE AND INCIDENCE

Disability due to the impact of diabetes upon the eye arises primarily from retinal disease, proliferative diabetic retinopathy and/or macular oedema, and secondarily from cataracts. Figs. 19.1–19.5. reflect the prevalence of vision loss and its relation to both duration of diabetes, and the age at the time of the patient's first eye examination for both younger and older onset diabetics (19).

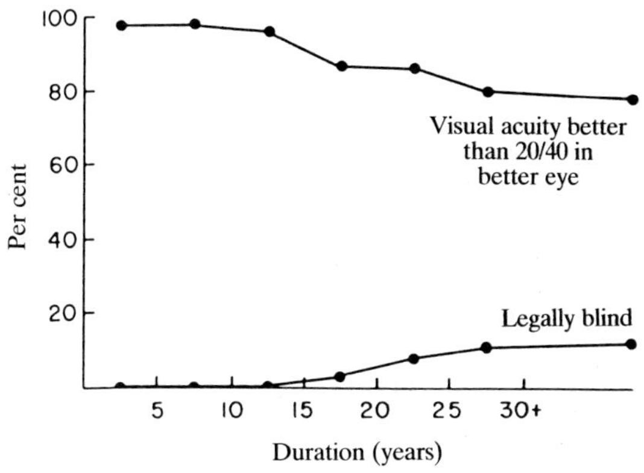


Fig. 19.1. Per cent of younger onset diabetic persons with visual acuity of 20/40 or better, and of those with legal blindness by duration of diabetes.

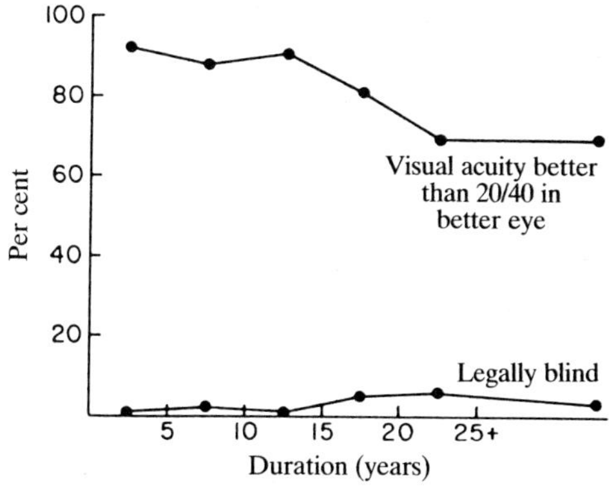


Fig. 19.2. Per cent of older onset diabetic persons with visual acuity of 20/40 or better, and of those with legal blindness by duration of diabetes.

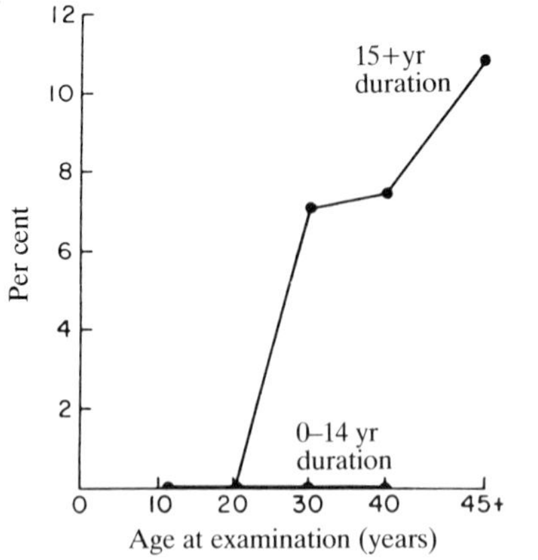


Fig. 19.3. Per cent of younger onset diabetic persons with legal blindness by duration of diabetes and age at examination.

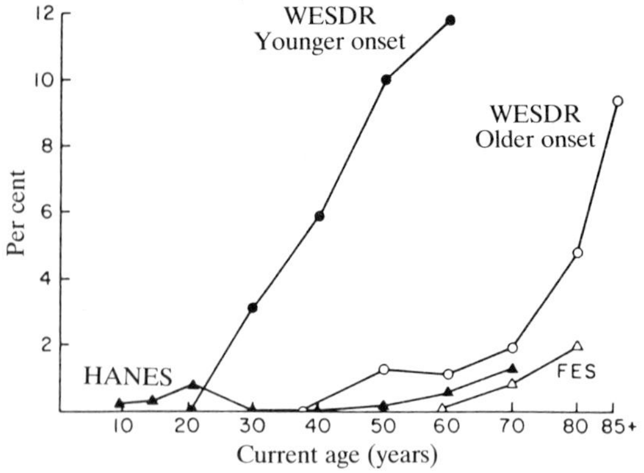


Fig. 19.5. Per cent of persons with visual acuity of 20/200 or worse in better eye in Wisconsin Epidemiologic Study of Diabetic Retinopathy (WESDR) in the Health and Nutrition Examination Survey (HANES)[19] and in the Framingham Eye Study (FES)[5] by current age.

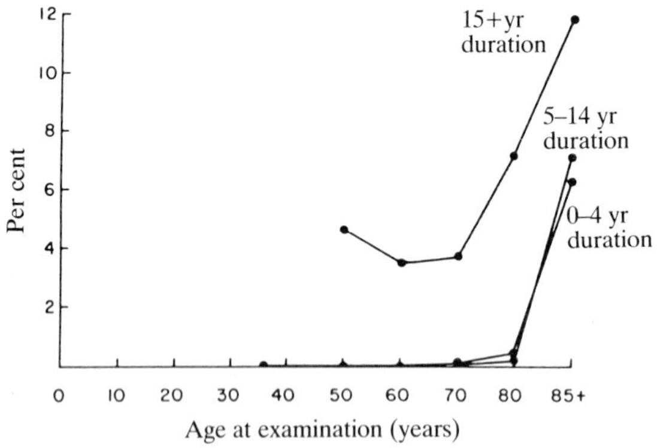


Fig. 19.4. Per cent of older onset diabetic persons with legal blindness by duration of diabetes and age at examination.

The best data on epidemiology of visual dysfunction arises from the longitudinal studies done by Ronald and Barbara Klein at the University of Wisconsin. In early onset diabetics, the visual function ranged from 20/40 best corrected visual acuity in 96.4% of the males aged 0–17 years of age to 76.9% in males 45–54 years of age. Legal blindness (less than or equal to 20/200 visual acuity) was first seen in males 25–34 years of age. In the 25–34 year age group, 3.3% were disabled compared to 12.8% in those aged 45–54 years. Females had a similar presentation except for higher rates of moderate to severe visual impairment at 55 years and older. Those diagnosed as being a diabetic after the age of 30 had a 0.4% reported frequency of legal blindness and 6.2% in those aged 75 and older. Again, females showed similar relationships except for a higher rate of moderate to severe visual impairment in those 85 years and older.

None the less, Rand (22) argues persuasively that the cross-sectional nature of Klein's above study still presents a major underestimation of the true frequency of visual disability in diabetes. Patients with diabetes at death are much more likely to be blind or visually disabled than those of equal age who do survive. Utilising the Klein data set and adjusting for mortality related to duration of diabetes, the prevalence data fall 150% to 240% short of 'true' loss of vision, 20/200 or worse. A crucial assumption is that 25% of those who died were blind. This treatment of the epidemiological information presented in similar studies targeting those populations with increased genetic/environmental susceptibility such as children in Finland, American and Asian Indians, Mexican Americans, Australian Aborigines, and those living in the Western Pacific would imply that there is a greater frequency of blindness than when only the prevalence data are evaluated. Populations studied utilising incidence data (23–26) are felt to more accurately reflect their population.

The above studies rely on appropriate examination and follow-up. When known diabetics are without appropriate ophthalmologic follow-up (greater than 2 years since the last examination), 61% had clinical characteristics consistent with diabetic retinopathy, glaucoma, cataract or other eye abnormalities. Of the subjects, 17% were found to have eye disease that required immediate treatment, referral, or accelerated follow-up. Of the Beaver Dam Eye Study, 48% diabetics had this problem (27) (see Figs. 19.6, 19.7).

## DIFFERENCES BETWEEN IDDM AND NIDDM

The development of diabetic retinopathy is disease duration specific. Figs. 19.6 and 19.7 illustrate this finding for type I and type II diabetics. The enormity of this problem is clear when the incidence of diabetes is 13 per 100 thousand in the United States population under the age of 20 (14–16) (Table 19.1).

In type I diabetes, the annual incidence of the progression of the patient's eyes to background diabetic retinopathy in the first four years is 5%

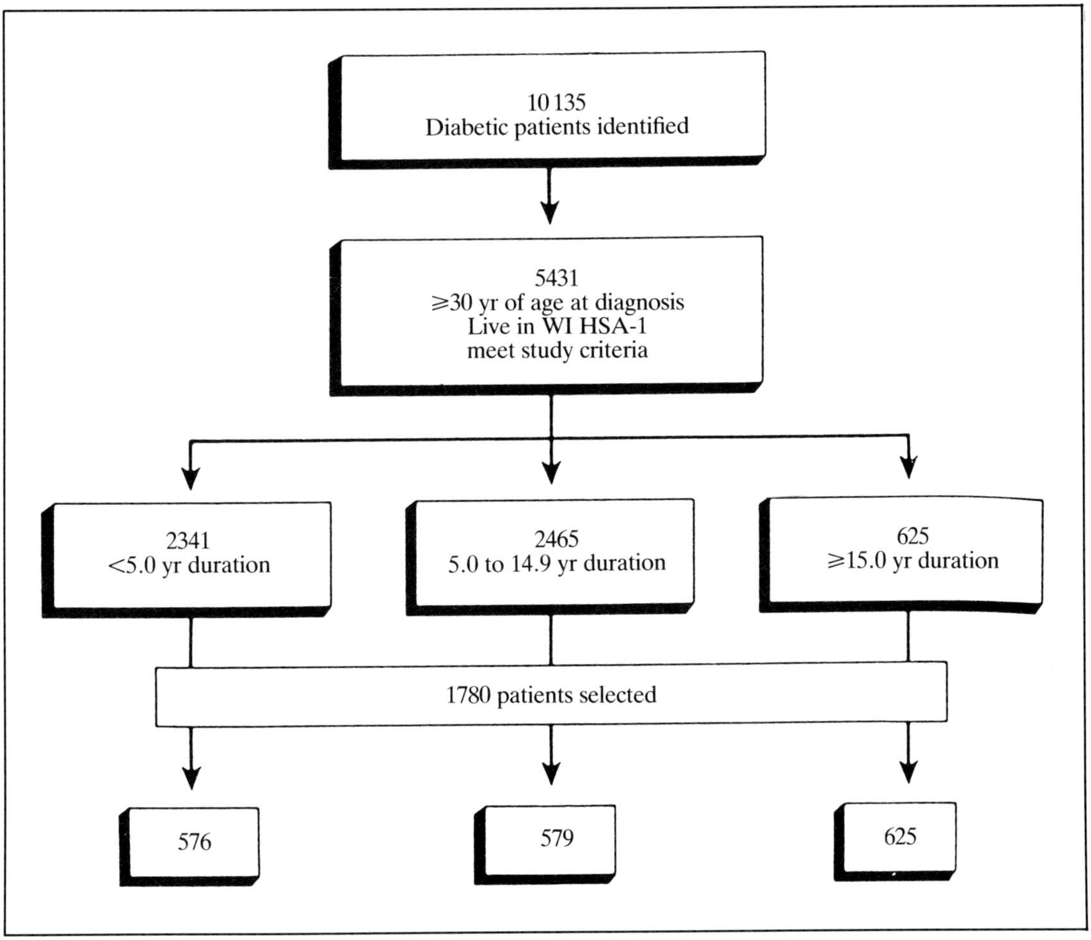


Fig. 19.6. Schematic diagram showing patient selection for examination phase of study. WI HSA-1 indicates Wisconsin Health Service Area 1.

Table 19.1. *Age-specific incident cases of Type I diabetes in the United States* (20)

| | | | | | |
|---|---|---|---|---|---|
| Age at onset | <20 | 20–29 | 30–49 | 50–69 | 70+ |
| Annual incidence per 100 000[a] | 13.00 | 6.50 | 3.80 | 4.40 | 3.70 |
| 1988 US population (millions)[b] | 71.33 | 41.06 | 70.01 | 42.96 | 20.37 |
| Annual incident cases | 9272 | 2669 | 2660 | 1890 | 754 |

[a] Derived from Refs. 14–16.
[b] Obtained from Vital Statistics of the US.

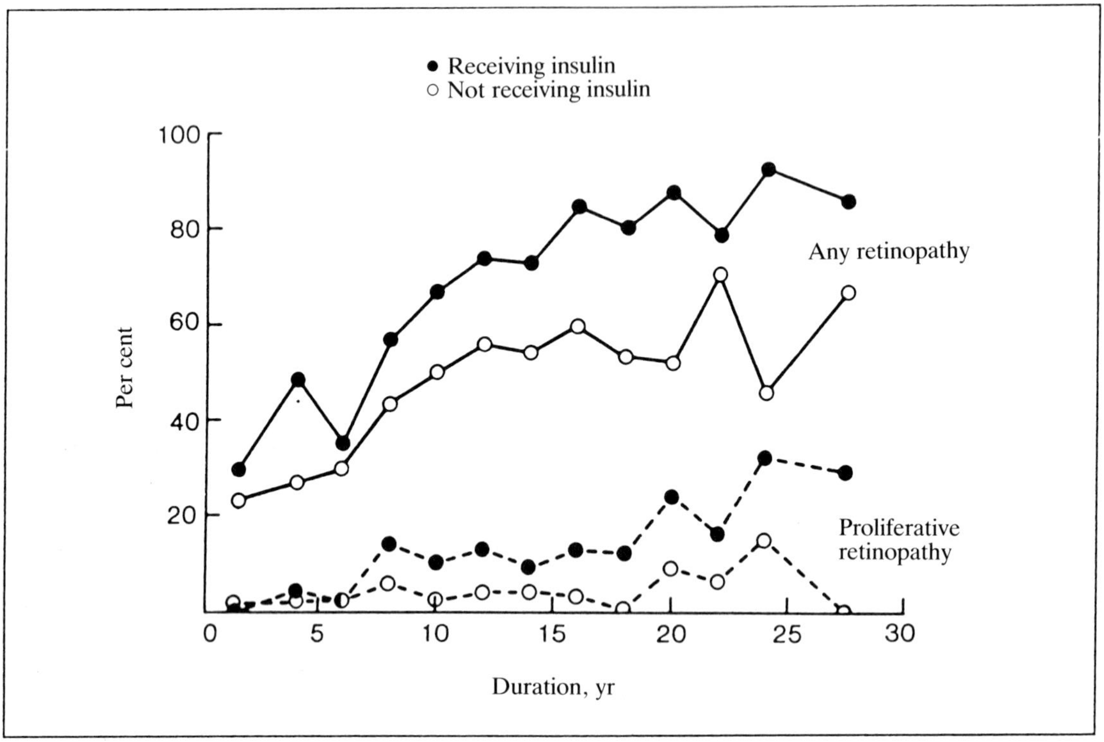


Fig. 19.7. Frequency of retinopathy or proliferative retinopathy by duration for insulin-taking and non-insulin-taking persons.

per year. After 5 years it increases to 20%. The progression to proliferative diabetic retinopathy is first noted 6 years after the diagnosis. Between year 6 and 10 of having diabetes the annual incidence of progression is 0.8%. After 10 years the annual incidence of progression increases to 6.2%. Macular oedema first appears between year 6 and 7 with an annual incidence of 0.5% and at 8 or more years, 2.5%.

The development of the various subtypes of diabetic retinopathy related to duration of diabetes mellitus clearly illustrates the usual step wise progression of the disease process.

Age of onset of diabetes was found to play an independent role in the development of severe retinopathy. Those patients who developed diabetes mellitus before age 15, when compared to

Table 19.2 *Patients with different levels of retinopathy and duration of diabetes (<10y or >10y)* (28)

| | Degree of retinopathy[a] | | | | | |
|---|---|---|---|---|---|---|
| | N | S | M | PP | P | UK |
| Total | | | | | | |
| % | 31.8 | 28.1 | 3.4 | 5.4 | 23.6 | 7.8 |
| *n* | 159 | 141 | 17 | 27 | 118 | 39 |
| Duration <10 y | | | | | | |
| % | 74.8 | 13.4 | 0 | 2.4 | 0 | 9.4 |
| *n* | 95 | 17 | 0 | 3 | 0 | 12 |
| Duration >10 y | | | | | | |
| % | 17.2 | 33.3 | 4.6 | 6.5 | 31.5 | 7.2 |
| *n* | 64 | 124 | 17 | 24 | 118 | 27 |

[a] N=Normal, S=simplex, M=maculopathy, PP=preproliferative, UK=unknown.

a duration matched cohort of type I diabetics, were found to have a higher incidence of proliferative diabetic retinopathy (28). This study specifically answers the suggestions of multiple authors (19, 29–33).

## RISK FACTORS

### Hyperglycaemia

Chronic hyperglycaemia is felt to be the primary cause of diabetic retinopathy and this has been supported by multiple studies. (19, 29–31). The question of severity of retinopathy relative to levels of haemoglobin Alc has been raised by several authors (19, 34–36). Poor metabolic control (high haemoglobin Alc values) was correlated with an increased risk of the development and the severity of the retinopathy (7). These findings are supported by a five-year study showing an increase in capillary loss and leakage of fluorescein evaluated by fluorescein angiography in a conventional treatment group compared to an intensified treatment group where the difference in the average haemoglobin Alc concentration was significant to a level of $P$ <0.001. The effect of plasma glucose on the haemodynamics of the macular capillary bed is still an unresolved issue (37, 38).

### Hypertension

The correlation between systemic hypertension and severity of retinopathy is strong (19, 35, 36). One study found hypertension only to be a significant factor after diabetes of 10 or more years' duration. The benefits of antihypertensive medication, measured as the relationship between systolic blood pressure and retinopathy, has been observed (39). Although the linkage is strong between retinopathy and hypertension, a causal relationship has yet to be identified. Hypertension can occur either before or after the development of retinopathy. A possible clue is the linkage of hypertension to nephropathy. An inconsistent correlation of systolic blood pressure and retinopathy with severe loss of vision was noted with increased albuminuria (40). Other authors have found a positive correlation between alterations in serum creatinine and creatinine clearance in patients with proliferative retinopathy compared to those with mild background retinopathy. There was no correlation of proteinuria with the presence of retinopathy unless the patient had been diabetic for greater than 10 years. The relationship of nephropathy to retinopathy, its timing and development, is still unclear, and cannot be used to accurately prognosticate the development of proliferative diabetic retinopathy (41–43).

## Pregnancy

Pregnancy frequently accelerates diabetic retinopathy. The amount of change is usually due to the severity of the pre-existing diabetic retinopathy (44). If no retinopathy is present at the onset of pregnancy, on average, 12% are found to develop mild to significant background diabetic retinopathy changes (45–48). Gestational diabetics do not appear to develop retinopathy acutely.

Diabetic women who possess background diabetic retinopathy at the time of pregnancy frequently have progression of their condition (47%) (45). Of this population, 5% develop proliferative diabetic retinopathy changes. Of these patients, 85% required panretinal photocoagulation to control the proliferans. In all cases, the degree and severity of the retinopathy regressed post-partum. The use of panretinal photocoagulation to control proliferative diabetic retinopathy during pregnancy has significantly reduced the likelihood of catastrophic loss of vision. Some suggest that, with appropriate intervention, the likelihood of complications during pregnancy may be no greater than that in the non-pregnant age-matched group (48). The data from the 1950s (49) that supported the concept of therapeutic abortion for women with proliferative diabetic retinopathy at the onset of gestation are no longer routinely supported, since retinopathy during pregnancy responds to laser photocoagulation.

The mechanism of the worsening of diabetic retinopathy during pregnancy is still unknown. Frequently, these high risk pregnancies are treated with an intensive blood glucose control regimen. Many authors have reported rapid progression of diabetic retinopathy in diabetic populations that are not pregnant when blood sugar is rapidly brought to a much lower and tighter range (50–52). With childbearing individuals, a previous pregnancy does not increase the risk of the development of proliferative diabetic retinopathy. Duration of the diabetes is the primary factor (53). Response to operative intervention, panretinal photocoagulation, vitrectomy, is the same as with non-pregnant patients (54). Should a vitreous haemorrhage occur at the time of delivery, and spontaneous clearing not occur, the use of a vitrectomy would be indicated. With newer operative procedures (vitrectomy) available, this would not be considered a catastrophic event as it was when similar data was collected in the 1960s.

## REFERENCES


1 Jaëger. *Beitr z Path d Auges, Wien* 1856; 33.
2 Hirschberg. *Dtsh Med Wschr* 1890; 16, 1181, 1236.
3 Duke-Elder, Sys. *Ophthalmic. diseases of the retina*, CV Mosby Co.: St. Louis 1967; 445.
4 Dube. *New York State J Med* 1963; 63: 2783.
5 Klein HA, Moorehead HB. Statistics on blindness in the model reporting area, 1969–70 (Bethesda, MD): US Department of Health, Education & Welfare, 1973 (DHW Publ No (NIH) 73–427), 1970.
6 Parving HH, Hommel E, Skott P, Edberg B *et al.* Prevalence of microalbuminuria, arterial hypertension, retinopathy in patients with insulin-dependent diabetes. *Br Med J* 1988; 296: 156–60.
7 Knowles HC. Long-term juvenile diabetes treated with unmeasured diet. *Trans Assoc Am Phys* 1971; 84: 95–101.
8 Borch-Johnsen KB, Deckert T. Complications of diabetes; the changing scene. In: Kggmm Albertic *et al.* eds. *International textbook of diabetes mellitus*, 1992; 1213–22.
9 Lestradet H, Papoz L, Hellouin DE, Menibus CL *et al.* Long term study of mortality in vascular complications in juvenile-onset (Type I) diabetes. *Diabetes* 1981; 30: 175–9.
10 The Diabetic Retinopathy Study Research Group. Photocoagulation treatment of proliferative diabetic retinopathy. Clinical application of diabetic retinopathy study (DRS) findings, DRS Report Number 8. *Ophthalmology* 1981; 88: 583–600.
11 The Diabetic Retinopathy Study Research Group. Four risk factors for severe visual loss in diabetic retinopathy. The third report from the diabetic retinopathy study. *Arch Ophthalmol* 1979; 97: 654–5.
12 Diabetic keto-acidosis, hyperosmolar, non-ketotic coma, lactic acidosis, and hypoglycemia. Fishbein, HA. Diabetes in America. PHS publication No. 85–1468.
13 Aiello LM, Ferris FL III. Photocoagulation for diabetic macular edema [letter]. *Arch Ophthalmol* 1981; 105: 163.
14 LaPorte RE, Cruickshanks KJ. Incidence and risk factors for insulin-dependent diabetes. In *National diabetes data group*. Diabetes in America: Diabetes Data Compiled 1984 [Bethesda, MD]: US Department of Health and Human Services 1985 chap. 8, 1–2 [NIH Publ. No. 85–1468].
15 Lorenzi M, Cagliero E, Schmidt NJ. Racial differences in incidence of juvenile-onset type I diabetes: epidemiologic studies in southern California. *Diabetologia* 1985; 28: 734–8.

16 Melton LJ III, Plaumbo PJ, Chu CP. Incidence of diabetes mellitus by clinical type. *Diabetes Care* 1983; 6: 75–86.
17 Klein R, Klein BEK, Moss SE *et al.* Retinopathy in young-onset diabetic patients. *Diabetes Care* 1985*a*; 8: 311–15.
18 Klein R, Klein BEK, Moss SE. A population-based study of diabetic retinopathy in insulin-using patients diagnosed before 30 years age. *Diabetes Care* 1985*b*; 8(suppl 1): 71–6.
19 Klein R, Klein BEK, Moss SE *et al.* The Wisconsin Epidemiology Study of Diabetic Retinopathy, II. Prevalence and risk of diabetic retinopathy when age at diagnosis is less than 30 years. *Arch of Ophthalmol* 1984; 102: 520–6.
20 Javitt JC, Aiello LP, Bassi LJ, Chiang YP *et al.* (1991). Detecting and treating retinopathy in patients with type I diabetes mellitus. *Ophthalmology*, 98, 1565–74.
21 Olivera EM, Duhalde EP, Gagliardino JJ. Costs of permanent and temporary disability induced by diabetes. *Diabetes Care* 1991; 14: 593–6.
22 Rand II Visual Impairment in diabetes (Discussion). *Ophthalmology* 91: 8–9.
23 Zimmet PZ. Kelly West Lecture 1991. Challenges in diabetes epidemiology from West to the rest. *Diabetes Care* 1992; 15: 232–51.
24 Diabetes Epidemiology Research International Group. Secular trends in incidents of childhood IDDM in 10 countries. *Diabetes* 1990; 39: 858–64.
25 Diabetes Epidemiology Research International Study Group. The epidemiology and immunogenetics of IDDM in Italian Heritage population. *Diabetes/Metab Rev* 1990; 6: 63–9.
26 Tuomilehto J, Lounamaa R, Tuomilehto-Wolf E *et al.* Epidemiology of childhood diabetes mellitus in Finland-background of a nationwide study of Type I (insulin-dependent) diabetes mellitus. Childhood diabetes in Finland study group, *Diabetologia* 1992; 35: 70–6.
27 The Beaver Dam Eye Study Retinopathy in adults with newly discovered and previously diagnosed diabetes mellitus. *Ophthalmology* 1992; 99: 58–62.
28 Agardh E, Torffvit O, Agardh C-D. The prevalence of retinopathy and associated medical risk factors in type I (insulin-dependent) diabetes mellitus. *J Int Med* 1989; 226: 47–52.
29 Frank RN, Hoffman WH, Podgor MJ, Joondeph HC *et al.* Retinopathy in juvenile-onset diabetes of short duration. *Ophthalmology* 1980; 87: 1–9.
30 Frank RN, Hoffman WH, Podgor MJ, Joondephm HC *et al.* Retinopathy in juvenile-onset type I diabetes of short duration. *Diabetes* 1982; 31: 874–82.
31 Palmberg P, Smith M, Waltman S, Krupin T *et al.* The natural history of retinopathy in insulin-dependent juvenile-onset diabetes. *Ophthalmology* 1981; 88: 613–8.
32 Knowles HC Jr, Guest GM, Lampe J, Kessler M *et al.* The course of juvenile diabetes treated with unmeasured diet. *Diabetes* 1965; 14: 239–73.
33 Nanda N, Murphy RP, Plotnick L, Auer C *et al.* The effects of puberty on the prevalence of diabetic retinopathy. *Investig Ophthalmol Vis Sci* 1986; 27 (Suppl): 5.
34 Constable IJ, Knuiman MW, Welborn TA *et al.* Assessing the risk of diabetic retinopathy. *Am J Ophthalmol* 1984; 97: 53–61.
35 Bodansky HJ, Cudworth AG, Drury PL, Kohner EM. Risk factors associated with severe proliferative retinopathy in insulin-dependent diabetes mellitus. *Diabetes Care* 1982; 5: 97–100.
36 Hanna AM, Roy M, Zinman B *et al.* An evaluation of factors associated with proliferative diabetic retinopathy. *Clin Investig Med* 1985; 8: 109–19.
37 Davies EG, Hyer SL, Kohner EM. Macular blood flow response to acute reduction of plasma glucose in diabetic patients measured by the blue light entoptic technique. *Ophthalmology* 1990; 97: 160–4.
38 Sinclair SH. Macular retinal capillary hemodynamics in diabetic patients. *Ophthalmology* 1991; 98: 1580–6.
39 Teuscher A, Schnell H, Wilson PWF. Incidence of diabetic retinopathy and relationship to baseline plasma glucose and blood pressure. *Diabetes Care* 1988; 11: 246–51.
40 Parving H, Hommel E, Mathiesen E, Skott P *et al.* Prevalence of microalbuminuria arterial hypertension retinopathy and neuropathy in patients with insulin-dependent diabetes. *Br Med J* 1988; 296: 156–60.
41 Vigstrup J, Morgensen CE. Proliferative diabetic retinopathy: at risk patients identified by early detection of microalbuminuria. *Acta Ophth* 1985; 63: 530–4.
42 Agardh E, Tallroth G, Bauer B, Cavallin-Sjoberg U *et al.* Retinopathy and nephropathy in insulin-dependent diabetics: an inconsistent relationship? *Diabetic Med* 1987; 4: 248–50.
43 Feldman JN, Hirsch SR, Beyer BS, James WA *et al.* Prevalence of diabetic nephropathy at time of treatment for diabetic retinopathy. In: Friedman EH, L'Esperance FA, ed. *Diabetic renal — retinal syndrome*, Grune & Stratton, Ltd, London, 1982; 9–12.
44 Aiello LM, Rand LI, Briones JC, Weiss JN *et al.* Nonocular clinical risk factors in the progression of diabetic retinopathy. In: Little HL, Jack RL, Patz A, Forsham PH, eds. *Diabetic retinopathy*, New York: Thieme-Stratton, Inc. 1983; 31–32.
45 Sunness JS. The pregnancy woman's eye. *Survey Ophthalmol* 1988; 32: 219–38.
46 Moloney JBM, Drury MI. The effect of pregnancy on the natural course of diabetic retinopathy. *Am J Ophthalmol* 1982; 93: 745–56.
47 Soubrane G, Canivet J, Coscas G. Influence of pregnancy on the evolution of background retinopathy: preliminary results of a prospective fluorescein angiography study. In: Ryan SJ, Dawson AR, Little HL, eds. *Retinal disease*, Grune & Stratton, Orlando, FL, 1985.
48 Bresnick GH. Background diabetic retinopathy. In: Ryan SJ ed *Retina*, 1989; vol. 2, Chap. 71: 327–66.
49 Beetham WP. Diabetic retinopathy in pregnancy. *Trans Am Ophthalmol Soc* 1950; 48: 205–19.
50 Laatikainen L, Larinkari J, Teramo K, Raivio KO. Occurrence and prognostic significance of retinopathy in diabetic pregnancy. *Metab Pediat Syst Ophthalmol* 1980; 4: 191–5.
51 Lawrence RD. Acute retinopathy without hyperpiesis in diabetic pregnancy. *Br J Ophthalmol* 1948; 32: 461–5.
52 White P. Pregnancy and diabetes: medical aspects. *Med Clin N Am* 1965; 49: 1015–24.
53 Klein BEK, Klein R. Gravidity and diabetic retinopathy. *Am J Epidemiol* 1984; 119: 564–9.
54 Singerman LJ. Diabetic retinopathy in juvenile-onset diabetics. I. Laser therapy in high risk proliferatives. II. Effects of pregnancy, In: Fine SL, Owens SL, eds. *Management of the retinal vascular and macular disorders*, The Williams & Wilkins Co., Baltimore, 1983; 43–6.

# 20 Diabetic Nephropathy

John T. O'Brian

## PREVALENCE

Diabetic nephropathy is now the most common cause of new onset end stage renal disease (ESRD). Direct health care costs in this country alone exceeded 2 billion dollars in 1990 (1). Without treatment, GFR falls at an average of 1 ml per minute per month, leading to ESRD in a mean period of 5–7 years, although a large variation among individuals is seen. Incidence data indicate that diabetic nephropathy will develop in approximately 35% of patients with IDDM (2). The figures for NIDDM are less certain, but lie between 15 and 60% of NIDDM patients depending on their ethnic origin with an unusually high incidence in American blacks. Caucasian patients tend to have lower frequencies (3–5), but prevalence figures of 50–60% after 20 years of diabetes occur among Japanese and the Pima Indians (6, 7). The majority of patients with proteinuria eventually will progress to ESRD or die prematurely from cardiovascular complications (8–10). In addition, proteinuric patients display up to a 40-fold increased risk of cardiovascular mortality compared with matched diabetic patients without proteinuria (11). Cardiovascular disease (CVD) is the most common cause of mortality in Western NIDDM patients with proteinuria (12), whereas in the Japanese, with a low incidence of CVD, ESRD is foremost (13).

## IMPORTANCE OF MICROALBUMINURIA

One of the most intriguing recent observations in diabetology relates to the seminal importance of microalbuminuria in the pathogenesis of diabetic nephropathy. Viberti and co-workers first described microalbuminuria as a risk factor for renal disease, in that patients with microalbuminuria were 20 times more likely to develop clinical proteinuria than patients with normoalbuminuria (14), an observation that was upheld by subsequent investigations (15–18). Meta-analysis showed that microalbuminuria had a predictive power of >80% for the development of renal disease. Messent, in a reanalysis of an original patient cohort after a 23-years follow-up, noted that microalbuminuria was a significant predictor of premature cardiovascular mortality, with a 3-fold relative risk (19). In NIDDM, studies have shown that microalbuminuria is a predictor for proteinuria, and also a prognostic indicator of early mortality from CVD (20–22). Microalbuminuria is also predictive of cardiovascular mortality in mature non-diabetic subjects (23–26), and has been suggested by Haffner (27) and Ferranini (26) as important in essential hypertension as well.

In addition to the foregoing, microalbuminuria is associated with other risk factors for cardiovascular disease. Microalbuminuric patients display average, blood pressure values that are 10 mmHg above that of matched IDDM patients without microalbuminuria, and the relation to arterial pressure is independent of blood glucose control (28). However, changes in arterial pressure have been shown to be correlated with changes in albumin excretory rate (AER) (29). Poor blood glucose control is another independent association of microalbuminuria (28). Microalbuminuria is exceedingly rare in the first 5 years after onset of IDDM (30) tending to support the view that it is an early warning sign of glomerular disease, not a marker of susceptibility.

Renal biopsy studies in microalbuminuric IDDM patients have revealed that significant glomerular abnormalities may be discernible at this stage of the disease, although most patients have normal, or even supernormal GFR (31). Chavers and associates point out that thickening of glomerular basement membrane, expansion of the mesangium and increased mesangial matrix volume fraction all occur at this early stage (9, 10). The more marked the microalbuminuria and elevated BP the more marked they found the associated anatomic changes. The recently held NIH/ADA consensus conference suggested that microalbuminuria was indeed not a surrogate marker for renal disease but direct evidence thereof. This view has recently been challenged, and not all microalbuminuria is associated with histological change in the kidney. The reasons for this discrepancy are not yet apparent.

Diabetic dyslipidaemia, is seen in both IDDM and NIDDM patients with microalbuminuria. Elevated levels of total and VLDL triglycerides, total and LDL cholesterol, apoB, and reduced levels of HDL have all been observed (32). Lipoprotein (a), which is believed to be an independent risk factor for atherosclerosis in the general population, may also be elevated in IDDM patients with microalbuminuria (33). Fibrinogen, another independent risk factor for macrovascular disease, has also been documented to be elevated in this group of patients. Atherogenic profiles such as these may be causal to the excess cardiovascular mortality described in patients with microalbuminuria. There is a body of evidence which supports the contention that dyslipidaemia *per se* is a contributory factor to the renal disease, and fatty infiltration of the kidney has been observed.

Just as it has been established that microalbuminuria is a potent predictor of subsequent nephropathy and cardiovascular complications, so also has it been shown that addressing the above risk factors may favourably influence the progression at least to overt nephropathy. Blood glucose control is a definite determinant of diabetic renal disease, but once overt nephropathy has developed, Viberti and co-workers showed that restoration of near-normoglycaemia did not appear to retard progression to renal failure (34, 35). However, in two well-done studies in IDDM patients with microalbuminuria (36, 37), tight glucose control using CSII therapy was effective in reducing AER compared with patients on CIT. Of microalbuminuric patients treated with CIT 28% in the first study progressed to overt clinical proteinuria over 2 years. By contrast, overt nephropathy did not develop in any of the patients receiving CSII. The beneficial effect of strict glucose control has been confirmed by longer term studies (29), which show no progression of microalbuminuria in patients receiving intensified insulin therapy.

Reduction of elevated blood pressure in IDDM patients with established nephropathy has been demonstrated in several studies to slow the rate of fall in GFR and to arrest increasing albuminuria (38–40). ACE inhibitors, one class of drugs used in these studies, had a specific renoprotective effect (41–43). Microalbuminuric IDDM patients show significantly lower BP and a lower rate of progression of AER while receiving enalapril (44). Captopril has been shown to reduce AER and retard the development of proteinuria in normotensive microalbuminuric IDDM patients, independently of a reduction in systemic BP (45), in support of evidence from animal models of diabetic renal disease (41) in which ACE inhibition lowers intraglomerular pressure, independent of systemic pressure changes. However, there is some evidence to suggest that only patients with hypertension are likely to show a reduction in AER, and that this effect may not be specific to the ACE inhibitors alone (46). In addition to lowering intraglomerular pressure, ACE inhibitors may improve glomerular performance characteristics. Treatment of proteinuric diabetic patients with ACE inhibitors reduces clearance of large neutral dextrans without any measurable change in either renal haemodynamics or systemic BP (42, 47). ACE inhibitors also have been suggested to improve insulin sensitivity (48) in some but not all studies (49). Angiotensin II induces hypertrophy in cultured aortic smooth muscle cells *in vitro* (50, 51) and ACE inhibition has been shown to prevent such effects in both hypertensive and normotensive animals (52, 53). In IDDM patients with microalbuminuria, treatment with ACE inhibitors reportedly has reduced left ventricular hypertrophy (54), and in the spontaneously hypertensive rat, low doses of lisinopril reverse the myocardial fibrosis seen in this model (55). Renal effects of administration of ACE inhibitors include a marked attenuation of maturational growth of glomerular structure and function (56), and, in subtotally nephrectomised animals, ameliorates not only the development of glomerulosclerosis, but also the marked hypertrophy that precedes it (57). Early studies had suggested that ACE inhibitors decrease proteinuria in non-hypertensive diabetics, but the number of subjects studied is relatively small.

Reduction of animal protein in the diet to approximately 0.6 g/kg/day in IDDM patients with clinical proteinuria significantly slows the rate of GFR decline over at least the ensuing 3 to 5 years (58, 59). The mechanism of action of low protein diets in amelioration of renal function is not fully understood, but appears to implicate the intrarenal synthesis of prostaglandin E and kinins (60–62), possibly via insulin sensitivity (63). The effects of low protein diets are independent of BP, but the response is heterogeneous, with some patients showing no improvement in the rate of disease progression. Restriction of dietary protein by the same amount in microalbuminuric IDDM patients, has lowered AER as well (64), but whether it actually delays the onset of clinical proteinuria remains to be investigated. Dietary protein restriction of this degree seems to have no long-term detrimental effects on nutritional status. Because compliance with a low protein diet is difficult, some investigators have substituted vegetable for animal protein to contrast any differential effects on renal function. A vegetable protein diet with a 'normal' protein content (1g/kg/day) induced renal haemodynamic changes similar to those obtained by a low protein diet in a group of non-diabetic volunteers (65). Thus, it might be possible in the future to design diets that achieve a normal total protein content without adverse renal effects. The NIH has instituted a multicentre study to examine the effects of two levels of protein restriction, 0.6 and 0.4 g/kg body weight, controlling for the differences in phosphate restriction. This is an important study, which may help to define the need for such severe diets in a population whose average protein consumption is 1.6 gm/kg/day.

No evidence currently available assesses which interventions are successful in reducing microalbuminuria, thus leading to an amelioration of abnormalities in glomerular morphology which are already detectable in these patients, thereby preventing the progression to ESRD. Knowledge of the factors involved in the pathophysiological transition from normoalbuminuria to microalbuminuria is essential to the formulation of effective preventive efforts.

One factor suggested as a prognostic indicator of diabetic renal disease preceding the development of microalbuminuria is glomerular hyperfiltration (66). Studies in animals suggest that haemodynamic factors may significantly contribute to glomerulopathy in diabetes (67,68). Hyperfiltration appears early in the course of both IDDM (2–4), and NIDDM (2–6), although of lesser degree in the latter than the former. The role of glomerular hyperfiltration in the pathogenesis of human diabetic nephropathy remains controversial. In one long-term follow-up study, no association between increased AER and initial glomerular hyperfiltration was demonstrated (69). In another, the effect of long-standing glomerular hyperfiltration was investigated (70), and it was concluded that long-standing hyperfiltration had no detectable harmful effects on kidney function, a fact underscored by more recent observations (71). However, other studies have reached different conclusions (66), and initial glomerular hyperfiltration was significantly associated with the development of micro- or macroalbuminuria. It has been shown that hyperfiltration is related to the degree of blood glucose control, and intensified insulin treatment reduces GFR toward normal levels (72–74). Improvement in metabolic control has also been reported by some, but not all, investigators to decrease renal size (74–76). Excess renal production of prostaglandins and kinins has been postulated to mediate glomerular hyperfiltration (61, 77).

Inhibitors of PGE have been shown to reduce GFR in hyperfiltering IDDM patients, although controversy exists in this regard (76, 77). In the animal model, treatment with a kallikrein inhibitor lowers GFR. A similar effect on glomerular hyperfiltration is obtained by short-term low protein diets in the diabetic (78). Based on the foregoing, the predictive value of glomerular hyperfiltration is thus unclear.

Whether dyslipidaemia, often seen early in diabetic nephropathy, actually plays a role in its pathogenesis, is unclear. Hypertriglyceridaemia precedes the development of proteinuria and glomerular injury in the obese Zucker rat, and lipid levels increase *pari passu* with the rise in urinary albumin excretion in this model (79). Lowering lipid levels protects these animals against glomerulosclerosis, without affecting haemodynamic parameters (79). In both the spontaneously hypertensive and Wistar–Kyoto rat, cholesterol feeding results in an increase in both serum cholesterol and urinary albumin excretion (80). Hyperlipidaemia *per se* is not associated with glomerulopathy in the general population, and thus its role in the pathogenesis of diabetic kidney disease remains unknown (81).

It is important to realise that an aggregation of risk factors for the development of diabetic renal disease and CVD may even predate the onset of microalbuminuria. Patients with microalbuminuria have a more severe degree of morphologic renal abnormalities than that in their normoalbuminaemic counterparts. While preliminary intervention studies are encouraging, we must improve our ability to predict the subset of patients at risk for diabetic renal disease and CVD at onset of diabetes mellitus. The following are some important antecedents.

Clustering of diabetic nephropathy in families was first reported by Seaquist *et al.* who noted that 82% of diabetic siblings of probands with diabetic nephropathy have evidence of nephropathy, compared with only 17% of diabetic siblings of probands without nephropathy (82). This was later confirmed by Borch-Johnsen *et al.* (83). In NIDDM, a familial influence on the development of nephropathy has also been described in the Pima Indian (84). Inherited factors thus seem to play an important role in determining susceptibility to diabetic nephropathy, but the true nature of these factors is unknown. Higher levels of arterial pressure are seen in parents of type I patients with elevated AER (85, 86). Patients with established nephropathy not only have a more strongly positive history of hypertension in their parents, but also higher mean arterial pressure during adolescence, with a relative risk of developing overt nephropathy of 3.8, if one or both parents were hypertensive (87). Thus, a family history of hypertension confers an increased susceptibility to the development of proteinuria at least in some groups of diabetic patients.

Whether or not familial aggregation of CVD occurs in diabetic patients with nephropathy was explored in a study of parental cardiovascular morbidity and mortality of IDDM patients with and without proteinuria. The prevalence of CVD was significantly greater in parents of proteinuric patients, and CVD as a direct cause of death was significantly higher in parents of patients with nephropathy (90). Among diabetic patients with nephropathy, a positive family history of CVD was significantly more prevalent among those who had already suffered a cardiovascular event. A familial predisposition to CVD thus increases the risk of nephropathy in diabetes, and the risk of CVD increases in diabetics with nephropathy, arguing for a commonality of causation, at least in part.

Studies of the Na–Li transport system (Na–Li CT), the activity of which is genetically determined, have enhanced our understanding of the potentially inherited susceptibility to diabetic renal disease and CVD. Elevated activity of this system is a recognised marker of essential hypertension and its associated cardiovascular complications (91). Increased activity has been described in IDDM patients with microalbuminuria and clinical proteinuria (88, 92–94). The hereditary nature of this phenomenon has been confirmed by family studies demonstrating a higher Na–Li CT activity in parents of diabetic patients with proteinuria compared with parents of diabetic patients without proteinuria (92, 95, 96). Further, a close correlation has been found in Li–CT activity of identical twins discordant for IDDM (95, 96). Rates of Na–Li CT activity in IDDM were also found to be correlated with AER and arterial BP (95, 96). The activity of this membrane transport system emerged as the strongest determinant of proteinuria, followed by arterial pressure, duration of diabetes, and blood glucose control (95, 96). A significant interaction between rates of Na–Li CT and blood glucose control as determinants of proteinuria was also found in this study, with the highest frequency of proteinuria occurring in those patients with glycohaemoglobin values above the median and with a Na–Li CT activity above the normal range. A previous retrospective study had shown an eight fold increase in the risk of nephropathy when increased Na–Li CT was linked with evidence of a history of poor blood glucose control (88). One possible explanation for this interaction can be derived from observations using a euglycaemic hyperinsulinaemic clamp, in which non-proteinuric normotensive IDDM patients with raised Na–Li CT activity were less insulin sensitive than a matched control group with normal Na–Li CT (95, 96).

A similarly reduced sensitivity has been described in patients with essential hypertension and high Na–Li CT compared with matched hypertensive patients with normal transport rates (97). Thus, insulin resistance might, to some extent, explain the relationship between Na–Li CT and worse glucose tolerance both in diabetes and essential hypertension. The activity of the Na–Li CT shares many similarities with a membrane transport system that is crucial in the regulation of cell growth, intracellular pH and cell volume, and sodium reabsorption in the proximal renal tubules; the Na–H antiport (98). An overactivity of the Na–H antiport has been demonstrated in RBCs of patients with essential hypertension and in leukocytes of IDDM patients with macroalbuminuria (98). The activity of this cation transport was recently measured, in cultured skin fibroblasts of IDDM patients with and without nephropathy, and in healthy, non-diabetic control subjects. It was found that Na–H antiport activity and serum-stimulated DNA synthesis were both elevated significantly in IDDM patients with nephropathy compared with the other two groups. These findings suggest that abnormalities of cell function are intrinsic to diabetic patients who develop nephropathy. An abnormal cellular host response to the hyperglycaemia of diabetes may trigger hypertrophic and vasoconstrictive mechanisms which lead to the lesions of hypertension, renal disease, and CVD. The explanation of the molecular and genetic determinants of altered cell function in diabetic patients susceptible to renal and vascular damage has yet to be fully elucidated.

## REFERENCES

1 United States Renal Data Service: Annual data report. *Am J Kidney Dis* 1990; 16 (Suppl. 2): 22–7.
United States Renal Data Service: Annual data report 1990. *Am J Kidney Dis* 1990; 16 (Suppl. 2): 16–21.
2 Andersen AR, Christiansen JS, Andersen JK, Kreiner S *et al.* Diabetic nephropathy in type 1 (insulin-dependent) diabetes: an epidemiological study. *Diabetologia* 1983; 25: 496–501.
3 Fabre J, Balant LP, Dayer PG, Fox HM *et al.* The kidney in maturity onset diabetes mellitus: a clinical study of 510 patients. *Kidney Int* 1982; 21: 730–8.
4 Klein R, Kleine BEK, Moss S, DeMets DL. Proteinuria in diabetes. *Arch Internal Med* 1988; 148: 181–6.
5 Hasslacher C, Ritz E, Wahl P, Michael C. Similar risks of nephropathy in patients with type 1 or type 2 diabetes mellitus. *Nephrol/Dialysis/Transpl* 1989; 4: 859–63.
6 Nelson RG, Kunzelman CL, Pettitt DJ, Saad, MF *et al.* Albuminuria in type 2 (non-insulin-dependent) diabetes mellitus and impaired glucose tolerance in Pima Indians. *Diabetologia* 1989; 32: 870–6.
7 World Health Organization multinational study of vascular disease in diabetics: prevalence of small vessel and large vessel disease in diabetic patients from 14 centers. *Diabetologia* 1985; 28: 615–40.
8 Mogensen CE. Progression of nephropathy in long term diabetics with proteinuria and effect of initial anti hypertensive treatment. *Scand J Clin Laborat Invest* 1976; 36: 383–8.
9 Viberti GC, Bilous RW, Mackintosh D, Keen H. Monitoring glomerular function in diabetic nephropathy. *Am J Med* 1983*a*; 74: 256–64.
10 Viberti GC, Bilous RW, Mackintosh D, Bending JJ *et al.* Long-term correction of hyperglycaemia and progression of renal failure in insulin-dependent diabetes. *Br Med J* 1983*b*; 286: 598–602.
11 Borch-Johnsen K, Anderson PK Deckert T. The effect of proteinuria on relative mortality in type 1 (insulin-dependent diabetes mellitus). *Diabetologia* 1985; 28: 590–6.
12 Nelson RG, Pettitt DJ, Carraher MJ, Baird HR *et al.* Effect of proteinuria on mortality in NIDDM. *Diabetes* 1988; 37: 1499–504.
13 Saski A, Horiuchi N, Hasegawa K, Uehara M. Risk factors related to the development of persistent albuminuria among diabetic patients observed in long-term follow-up. *J Jap Diabetes Soc* 1986; 29: 1017–23.
14 Viberti GC, Hill RD, Jarrett, RD *et al.* Microalbuminuria as a predictor of clinical nephropathy in insulin-dependent diabetes mellitus. *Lancet* 1982; 1430–2.
15 Mathiesen ER, Oxenboll B, Johansen K, Svendsen PA *et al.* Incipient nephropathy in type I (insulin-dependent) diabetes mellitus. *Diabetologia* 1986; 29: 640–3.
16 Parving HH, Oxenboll B, Svendensen PA, Christiansen JS *et al.* Early detection of patients at risk of developing diabetic nephropathy. A longitudinal study of urinary albumin excretion. *Acta Endocrinol* 1982; 100: 550–5.
17 Mogensen CE. Microalbuminuria predicts clinical proteinuria and early mortality in maturity onset diabetes. *New Engl J Med* 1984*a*; 310: 356–60.
18 Mogensen CE. Microalbuminuria predictors clinical proteinuria and early mortality in maturity onset diabetes. *N Eng J Med* 1984*b*; 310: 356–60.
19 Messent J, Elliot JG, Jarrett RJ, Hill RD *et al.* The prognostic significance of microalbuminuria in type 1 (insulin-dependent) diabetes mellitus: a 23 year follow-up study. *Kidney Inter* 1992; 41: 936–9.
20 Mogensen CE, Christiansen CK. Predicting diabetic nephropathy in insulin-dependent diabetic patients. *N Eng J Med* 1984; 311: 89–93.
21 Jarrett JW, Viberti, GC, Argyropoulos A, Hill RD *et al.* Microalbuminuria predicts mortality in non-insulin-dependent diabetes. *Diabetic Med* 1984; 1: 17–9.
22 Schmitz A, Vaeth M. Microalbuminuria: a major risk factor in non-insulin-dependent diabetes. A 10 year follow-up study of 503 patients. *Diabetic Med* 1988; 5: 126–34.
23 Mattock MB, Morrish NJ, Viberti GC, Keen H *et al.* Microalbuminuria as a predictor of morality in NIDDM: a prospective study. *Diabetes* 1992*a*; 41: 731–5.
24 Mattock MB. Morrish NJ, Viberti G, Keen H *et al.* Prospective study of microalbuminuria as a predictor of mortality in NIDDM. *Diabetes* 1992*b*; 41(6): 736–4.
25 Damsgaard EM, Froland A, Jorgensen OD, Mogensen CE. Eight to nine year mortality in known non-insulin-dependent diabetics and controls. *Kidney Int* 1992; 41: 731–5.
26 Ferranini E, Haffner SM, Mitchell BP. Hyperinsulinaemia: the key feature of a cardiovascular and metabolic syndrome. *Diabetologia* 1991; 34: 416–22.
27 Haffner SM, Stern MP, Hazuda HP, Mitchell BD *et al.* Cardiovascular risk factors in confirmed prediabetic individuals. Does the clock for coronary heart disease start ticking before the onset of clinical diabetes? *J Am Med Assoc* 1990; 263: 2893–8.
28 Wiseman MJ, Viberti GC, Mackintosh D, Jarrett RJ *et al.* Glycaemia, arterial pressure and micro albuminuria in type 1 (insulin-dependent) diabetes mellitus. *Diabetologia* 1984; 2: 401–5.
29 Feldt-Rasmussen B, Mathiesen ER, Deckert T. Effect of 2 years of strict metabolic control on progression of incipient nephropathy. *Lancet* 1986; i: 1300–4.
30 Viberti GC, Pickup JC, Jarrett RJ, Keen H. Effect of control of blood glucose on urinary albumin and beta-2 microglobulin in insulin-dependent diabetes. *N Eng J Med* 1979; 300: 638–341.
31 Walker JD, Close CF, Jones SL, Rafftery M *et al.* Glomerular structure in type 1 (insulin-dependent) diabetic patients with normo and microalbuminuria. *Kidney Int* 1992; 41: 741–8.
32 Jones SL, Close CJ, Mattock MB, Jarrett RJ *et al.* Plasma lipids and coagulation factor concentrations in insulin-dependent diabetics with microalbuminuria. *Br Med J* 1989; 289: 487–90.
33 Winocour PH, Bhatnager D, Ishola M, Arrol S *et al.* Lipoprotein (a) and microvascular disease in type 1 (insulin-dependent) diabetes. *Diabetic Med* 1991; 8: 922–7.

34 Kroc Collaborative Study Group. Blood glucose control and the evolution of diabetic retinopathy and albuminuria. A preliminary multicenter trial. *N Eng J Med* 1984a; 211: 365–72.
35 Kroc Collaborative Study Group. Blood glucose control and the evolution of diabetic retinopathy and albuminuria. *N Eng J Med* 1984*b*; 6: 365.
36 Feldt-Rasmussen B, Mathiesen ER, Jensen T, Lauritzen R *et al.* Effect of improved metabolic control on loss kidney function in type 1 (insulin-dependent) diabetic patients: an update of the Steno studies. *Diabetologia* 1991; 34: 164–70.
37 Parving HH, Andersen AR, Smidt UM, Hommel E *et al.* Effect of antihypertensive treatment on kidney function in diabetic nephropathy. *Br Med J* 1987; 294: 137–44.
38 Bjorck S, Mulec H, Johnsen SA, Norden G *et al.* Renal protective effect of enalapril in diabetic nephropathy. *Br Med J* 1992; 304: 339–43.
39 Anderson S, Rennke HG, Brenner BM. Therapeutic advantage of converting enzyme inhibitors in arresting progressive renal disease associated with systemic hypertension in the rat. *J Clin Investig* 1986; 77: 1993–2000.
40 Morrelli E, Loon N, Meyer T, Peters W, Myers *et al.* Effects of converting enzyme inhibition on barrier function in diabetic glomerulopathy. *Diabetes* 1990; 39: 76–82.
41 Remuzzi A, Puntorieri S, Battaglia C, Bertani T *et al.* Angiotensen converting enzyme inhibition ameliorates glomerular filtration of macromolecules and water and lessens glomerular injury in the rat. *J Clin Investig* 1990; 85: 541–9.
42 Marre M, Chatillier G, Leblanc, H, Guyene TT, Menard J *et al.* Prevention of diabetic nephropathy with enalapril in normotensive diabetics with microalbuminuria. *Br Med J* 1988; 297: 1092–5.
43 Mathiesen ER, Hommel E, Giese J, Parving HH. Efficacy of captopril in postponing nephropathy in normotensive insulin-dependent diabetic patients with microalbuminuria. *Br Med J* 1991; 303: 81–7.
44 Melbourne Diabetic Nephropathy Study Group. Comparison between perindopril and nifedipine in hypertensive and normotensive diabetic patients with microalbuminuria. *Br Med J* 1991; 302: 210–16.
45 Pinto, J, Walker JD, Turner CD, Beesley M *et al.* Renal response to lowering of arterial pressure by angiotensen converting enzyme inhibitor or diuretic therapy in insulin-dependent diabetic patients with nephropathy (abstract). *Kidney Int* 1990; 37: 516 (Abstract).
46 McMurrary, J, Fraser D. Captopril, enalapril and blood glucose (abstract). *Lancet* 1986; i: 1035 (Abstract).
47 Berne C, Pollare T, Lithell H. Effects of antihypertensive treatment on insulin sensitivity with a special reference to ACE inhibitors. *Diabetes Care* 1991; 14 (Suppl 4): 39–47.
48 Geisterfer AAT, Peach MJ, Owens GK. Angiotensen II induces hypertrophy, not hyperplasia, of cultured rat aortic smooth muscle cells. *Cir Res* 1988; 62: 749–56.
49 Campbell-Boewell M, Robertson AL. Effects of angiotensin II and vasopressin on human smooth muscle cells *in vitro*. *Exp Mol Path* 1981; 35: 265–76.
50 Owens GK. Influence of blood pressure on development of aortic medial smooth muscle hypertrophy in spontaneously hypertensive rats. *Hypertension* 1987; 91: 178–87.
51 Wang DH, Prewitt RL. Captopril reduces aortic and microvascular growth in hypertensive and normotensive rats. *Hypertension* 1990; 15: 68–77.
52 Tan LB, Weber KT. Prevention of structural changes in the heart in hypertension by angiotensin converting enzyme inhibition. *J Hypertension* 1993; (in press).
53 Sampson M, Chambers J, Springings D, Drury PL. Regression of left ventricular hypertrophy with 1 year of antihypertensive treatment in type 1 diabetic patients with early nephropathy. *Diabetic Med* 1991; 8: 106–10.
54 Anderson S, Rennke HG, Garcia DC, Brenner RM. Short- and long-term effects of antihypertensive therapy in the diabetic rat. *Kidney Int* 1989; 36: 526–36.
55 Fogo A, Yoshida Y, Yared A, Ishikawa I. Importance of angiogenic angiotensin II in the glomerular growth of maturing kidneys. *Kidney Int* 1990; 38: 1068–74.
56 Zeller K, Whittaker E, Sullivan I, Raskin P *et al.* Effect of restricting dietary protein on the progression of renal failure in patients with insulin-dependent diabetes mellitus. *N Eng J Med* 1991; 324: 78–84.
57 Walker JD, Bending JJ, Dodds RA, Mattock MB *et al.* Restriction of dietary protein and progression of renal failure in diabetic nephropathy. *Lancet* 1989; ii: 1411–14.
58 Cohen D, Dodds R, Viberti GC. Effect of protein restriction in insulin-dependent diabetics at risk of nephropathy. *Br Med J* 1987; 294: 795–8.
59 Kontessis P, Jones SL, Dodds R, Trevisan R *et al.* Renal, metabolic and hormonal responses to ingestion of animal and vegetable proteins. *Kidney Int* 1990; 38: 136–44.
60 Jaffa AA, Harvey JN, Sutherland SE, Margolius HS *et al.* Renal kalikrein responses to dietary protein: a possible mediator of hyperfiltration. *Kidney Int* 1989; 36: 1003–10.
61 Axelrod L. Insulin, prostaglandins, and the pathogenesis of hypertension. *Diabetes* 1991; 40: 1223–7.
62 Messent J on behalf of MCS Group. Arterial blood pressure and glycaemia in the progression from normoalbuminuria to microalbuminuria in type 1 diabetes – the 4 year findings. *Diabetic Med* 1992; 9 (Suppl): A20.
63 Chase HP, Garg SK, Marshall G, Berg CL *et al.* Cigarette smoking increases the risk of albuminuria among subjects with type 1 diabetes. *J Am Med Assoc* 1991; 265: 514–17.
64 Hostetter T. Human renal response to a meat meal. *Am J Physiol* 1986; 250: F13–18.
65 Hischberg RR, Zipser RD, Sklomowitz LA, Kopple JD. Glucagon and prostaglandins are mediators of amino acid induced rise in renal haemodynamics. *Kidney Int* 1988; 33: 1147–55.
66 Brenner BM. Hemodynamically medicated glomerular injury and the progressive nature of kidney disease. *Kidney Int* 1983; 23: 647–55.
67 Lervang HH, Jensen S, Borchner-Mortensen J, Ditzel J. Early glomerular hyperfiltration and the development of late nephropathy in type 1 (insulin-dependent) diabetes mellitus. *Diabetologia* 1988; 31: 723–9.
68 Schmitz A, Christensen CK, Solling K. No microalbuminuria or other adverse effects of long standing hyperfiltration in humans with one kidney. *Am J Kidney Dis* 1989; 13: 131–6.
69 Messent J, Jones SL, Wiseman M, Viberti GC. Glomeru-

lar hyperfiltration and albuminuria: a 8 year prospective study. *Diabetologia* 1991; 34 (Suppl 2): A3.
70 Rudberg S, Persson B, Dahlquist G. Increased glomerular hyperfiltration rate as a predictor of diabetic nephropathy – an 8 year prospective study. *Kidney Int* 1992; 41: 822–8.
71 Christiansen JS, Gammelgaard J, Tronier B, Svendsen PA *et al.* Kidney function and size in diabetics before and during initial insulin treatment. *Kidney Int* 1982; 21: 683–8.
72 Wiseman MJ, Saunders AJ, Keen H, Viberti GC. Effect of blood glucose on increased glomerular filtration rate and kidney size in insulin-dependent diabetics. *N Eng J Med* 1985; 312: 617–21.
73 Tuttle KR, Bruton L, Perusek MC, Lancaster JL *et al.* Effect of strict glycaemic control on renal hemodynamic response to amino acids and renal enlargement in insulin-dependent diabetes mellitus. *N Eng J Med* 1991; 324: 1626–32.
74 Feldt-Rasmussen B, Hegedus L, Mathiesen ER, Deckert T. Kidney volume in type 1 (insulin-dependent) diabetic patients with normal or increased urinary albumin excretion: effect of long-term improved metabolic control. *Scand J Clin Laborat Invest* 1992; 51: 31–6.
75 Harvey JN, Edmundson AW, Mayfield RAK. Renal kallikrein in IDDM patients with glomerular hyperfiltration *Diabetes* 1990; 39 (Suppl 1): 72A (Abstract).
76 Christiansen JS, Feldt-Rasmussen B, Parving HH. Short-term inhibition of prostaglandin synthesis has no effect on the elevated glomerular filtration rate of early insulin-dependent diabetes. *Diabetic Med* 1985; 2: 17–20.
77 Estmatjes E, Fernandez MR, Halperin I *et al.* Renal hemodynamic abnormalities in patients with short-term insulin-dependent diabetes mellitus: role of renal prostaglandins. *J Clin Endocrinol Metab* 1985; 60: 1231–6.
78 Wiseman MJ, Bognetti E, Dodds R, Keen H *et al.* Changes in renal function response to protein restricted diet in type 1 (insulin-dependent) diabetes patients. *Diabetologia* 1987; 30: 154–9.
79 Kasiske BL, O'Donnell MP, Keane WF. The Zucker rat model of obesity, insulin resistance, hyperlipidaemia, and renal injury. *Hypertension* 1992; 19: 110–5.
80 Cooper ME, Vranes DA, Panagiotopoulos S, Allen TJ *et al. Clin Exp Pharmaco Physiol* 1990; 17: 225–8.
81 Keane WF, Kasiske BC O'Donnell MP, Kim Y. The role of altered lipid metabolism in the prognosis of renal disease: experimental evidence. *Am J Kidney Dis* 1991; 17: 38–42.
82 Seaquist ER, Goetz FC, Rich S, Barbosa J. Familial clustering of diabetic kidney disease. Evidence for genetic susceptibility to diabetic nephropathy. *N Eng J Med* 1989; 32: 1161–5.
83 Borch-Johnsen K, Norgaard K, Hommel E, Mathiesen EM *et al.* Is diabetic nephropathy an inherited complication? *Kidney Int* 1992; 41: 719–22.
84 Pettitt DJ, Saad MF, Bennett PM, Nelson RG *et al.* Familial predisposition to renal disease in two genertations of Pima Indians with type 2 (non-insulin-dependent) diabetes meilitus. *Diabetologia* 1990; 33: 438–43.
85 Viberti GC, Keen H, Wiseman MJ. Raised arterial pressure in parents of proteinurtic insulin-dependent diabetics. *Br Med J* 1987; 295: 515–17.
86 Krolewski AS, Canessa M, Warram JH, Laffel LMB *et al.* Predisposition to hypertension and susceptibility to renal disease in insulin-dependent diabetes mellitus. *N Eng J Med* 1988; 318: 140–5.
87 Barzily J, Warram JH, Bak M, Laffel LMB *et al.* Predisposition to hypertension: risk factor for nephropathy and hypertension in IDDM. *Kidney Int* 1992; 41: 723–30.
88 Jensen JS, Mathiesen ER, Norgaard K, Hommel E *et al. Diabetologia* 1990; 33: 619–24.
89 Viberti GC, Earle K. Predisposition to essential hypertension and the development of diabetic nephropathy. *Am J Nephrol* 1993; (in press).
90 Mangili R, Bending JJ, Scott G, Li LK *et al.* Increased sodium–lithium countertransport in red cells of patients with insulin-dependent diabetes and nephropathy. *N Eng J Med* 1988; 318: 146–50.
91 Jones SL, Trevisan R, Tariq T, Semplcini A *et al.* Sodium–lithium countertransport in microalbuminuric insulin-dependent diabetic patients. *Hypertension* 1990; 15: 570–5.
92 Earle K, Walker J, Hill C, Viberti GC. Familial clustering of cardiovascular disease in patients with insulin-dependent diabetes and nephropathy. *N Eng J Med* 1992; 326: 673–7.
93 Walker JD, Tariq T, Viberti GC. Sodium–lithium countertransport activity in red cells of patients with insulin-dependent diabetes and nephropathy and their parents. *Br Med J* 1990; 301: 635–8.
94 Leslie RDG, Hardman T, Dubrey S, Lant AF. Increased lithium–sodium countertransport activity in identical twins discordant for type 1 diabetes (Abstract). *Diabetologia* 1991; 34 (Suppl 2): A67 (Abstract).
95 Lopes de Faria JB, Friedman R, Tariq T, Viberti GC. Prevalence of raised sodium–lithium countertransport activity in type 1 (insulin-dependent) diabetic patients. *Kidney Int* 1992*a*; 41: 877–82.
96 Lopes de Faria JB, Jones SL, MacDonald F, Chambers J *et al.* Sodium–lithium countertransport activity and insulin resistance in normotensive IDDM patients. *Diabetes* 1992*b*; 41: 610–15.
97 Trevisan R, Nosadini R, Fioretto P, Semplicini A *et al.* Clustering of risk factors in hypertensive insulin-dependent diabetics with high sodium lithium countertransport. *Kidney Int* 1992; 41: 855–61.
98 Trevisan RT, Li LK, Messent J, Tariq T *et al.* Na+ – H+ antiport activity and cell growth in cultured skin fibroblasts of insulin-dependent diabetic patients with nephropathy. *Diabetes* 1993; (in press).

# 21 The Personal, Social and Economic Burden of Diabetic Complications

Leon-Paul Georges

The complications of diabetes mellitus are associated with enormous burdens for the individual and for society in general. They impact on the individual's social, psychological, and economic fabric. They create disability, foreshortened life-span, and result in high utilisation of health resources, all of which impact adversely on the nation's economy. These burdens are poorly understood by society in general and often underestimated by otherwise well-informed health-care providers.

## PSYCHOSOCIAL IMPACT

Diabetic individuals make up an extremely diverse group. They range in age from infants to the elderly. They come from all walks of life, represent all races, religions and cultural heritages. This diversity is reflected in the wide range of personal and psychosocial issues encountered.

From the time that the diagnosis of diabetes mellitus is first established, the diabetic individual faces the realisation that life-spoiling complications, and even reduced life-span, may occur even with the utmost efforts committed to good care. Worry for the future is nearly always a major concern (1).

The adult diabetic person often does not share knowledge of the illness with acquaintances, friends, or associated workers. In this regard, it has been referred to as an 'invisible' disease. Thus, behavioural and functional impairments may not be recognised as being related to the diabetic state. The diabetic person with complications may be denied the usual benefits of compassion, sympathy for the sick and concessions to the problems encountered with their illness that others might receive.

The complex and demanding treatment regimens that all diabetics must deal with become even more complex with the onset of chronic complications. Patients are expected to make daily decisions and perform varied tasks which affect their health in both the short and long term. Once complications arise, they may feel betrayed or angry because they believed that their good self-care would be rewarded. They become vulnerable to falling self-esteem and unresolved conflicts (2).

The evolution of complications to levels of severity which interfere with personal function are likely to be accompanied by an increased perception of stress, more actual negative life events and more psychological symptoms (3). These individuals continuously face the psychological burden of recognising that they may be unable, through no fault of their own, to carry out social or work-related goals at any time.

Even the slightest miscalculation may lead to significant embarrassment at the least, or even severe incapacity. Hypoglycaemic unawareness may result in acute, transient behavioural changes which may cause embarrassment, social rejection, or even loss of employment. With diabetic enteropathy, for instance, there may be the constant fear that an episode of uncontrollable diarrhoea may result in public embarrassment. Neuropathic consequences such as instability of gait and inability to perform fine hand movements may be considered evidence of public drunkenness, drug use or worse.

For some families, the development of complications is associated with a disruption of a delicate balance and results in family dysfunction or disorganisation. A fragile interfamilial balance may not be able to withstand the assault of one more major stress (2). When such difficulties are not dealt with frankly by the diabetic person and the health-care team, and when there is an inadequate support cast, severe emotional destabilisation may occur. Individuals without appropriate supportive care may withdraw, not only from the day-to-day concerns with their health management, but from society in general and lead a reclusive existence.

## EMPLOYMENT

In the United States, federal and state laws prohibit discriminatory hiring practices based solely on medical conditions or handicaps. The American Diabetes Association's often stated position is that a diabetic person should be eligible for employment in any position for which he or she is individually qualified. None the less, discrimination in the workplace against the person with diabetes remains a major concern. The prospect of being unable to earn a livelihood is one of the most threatening aspects of any chronic disease. When one cannot qualify for proper employment, or when one is suboptimally employed, drastic changes in life-style as well as psychological state, occur.

As is true of the general population, participation in the work-world differs with age, sex, race, education, health status and many other factors. Men with diabetes are almost twice as likely as women with diabetes to participate in the work force. Black diabetic individuals have lower employment rates than do white diabetic individuals. Those with little education have much lower rates than those with more years of training. Diabetic persons with limitations due to their diabetes or its complications are less likely to work than those without such limitations.

Employment practices vary widely. Often employers fear that diabetic employees may be injured, or may injure others during the course of their work. There is also the concern that diabetics may miss excessive periods of work because of illness. While some studies have shown diabetic workers to lose more time at work due to illness than non-diabetics (4, 5), other studies have shown the reverse (5–7).

A recent study in the United States (8) compared more than 150 insulin-dependent diabetic individuals with a similar number of non-diabetic siblings to evaluate the effect of diabetes on employability. The IDDM patients reported more job refusals, and were less likely to be employed, indicating that hiring practices may still be discriminatory. On the other hand, once hired, the employment experiences of both groups appear to be similar, provided that no diabetic complications develop. Diabetic individuals are at greater risk of losing their jobs, once diabetic complications occur.

That diabetics experience difficulties in obtaining employment because of their disease when compared to non-diabetic individuals, is not a problem limited to the United States alone. Robinson *et al.* (4) surveyed employment experiences by diabetic persons in the United Kingdom. A random sample of diabetics aged 17–65 years was compared to a non-diabetic controlled group. Although absence from the workplace due to illness over a 12-month period was not significantly different, diabetic workers had four times the difficulty obtaining an appropriate job and three times the chance of losing it because of their disease.

Driving licence regulations vary widely within many other countries. Today, the right to drive an automobile is no longer simply an issue of personal privilege, but increasingly a necessity in modern life. In the United States, more individuals use automobiles to travel back and forth to work than any other form of transportation. Many states deny diabetic individuals the right to drive motorised vehicles when they experience specific complications (9, 10). Aside from visual impairment, the most common causes are histories of severe hypoglycaemic events and seizures. Krosnick (11) listed hypoglycaemia, poor judgement, poor or blurred vision, defective reflexes or impaired sensation to the feet as the main reasons why one state limits licencure, and requires a physician's exhaustive report once a motor violation or accident has occurred.

Traffic accidents are one of the leading causes of death in much of the world. Past reports had indicated that drivers with chronic conditions including diabetes had more than twice as many accidents per millions of miles of driving than did drivers with no known conditions (12).

There are but few well-controlled studies measuring the effects of diabetes on accident rates. For the most part, they have failed to demonstrate higher incidents of major motor vehicle accidents among persons with diabetes. A recent study (13) concluded that, while diabetic drivers have more accidents than non-diabetic drivers, the risk was small enough not to warrant restrictions on driving privileges. None the less, while some individual US states allow trucks to be driven within the state, interstate truck driving is prohibited by rulings of the Federal Highway Administration of the US Department of Transportation.

These concerns are not unique to the United States. There are great differences in licensing regulations among European countries (12–14). In one country, everyone, not only diabetics, must have examinations that may include blood and urine testing, while in another there are no firm regulations, the decision resting with a physician's judgement. One nation refused licensing to insulin-using diabetic persons to drive a taxi or bus but permitted truck driving.

Thus, people with diabetes and its complications are more likely to experience problems in obtaining employment and staying employed, than people without diabetes. Additionally, choice of profession may be restricted by statutes which affect licensing opportunities and other limitations owing to the nature of the disease, the functional limitations it imposes and, at least in part, by preconceived prejudices.

## IMPAIRMENT AND DISABILITY

The chronic complications of diabetes mellitus result in significant degrees and scope of functional impairment. The overall impact depends on the number of systems affected and the degrees of severity of each. No matter which facet of functional impairment/disability is examined, adult diabetics are more likely to be disabled than are adults in the general population.

Absence of major extremities and severe visual impairments are relatively more frequent among diabetics than they are among non-diabetics.

Diabetics are more likely than non-diabetics to be limited in their usual activities, whether those are working, housekeeping, going to school, leisure activities, or whatever else is measured. Diabetics are more likely to have limited mobility both inside and outside their neighbourhood and to need the assistance of other persons in carrying out essential activities of daily living particularly bathing and dressing (14).

The most common complication of diabetes mellitus, for instance, peripheral sensory–motor diabetic neuropathy may result in wide-ranging functional impact on an individual. The diabetic individual with even moderate degrees of neuropathy may need assistance in everyday household work, may be unable to climb stairs without assistance, may be unable to sit or stand for long periods and may be unable to drive to work or school. Diminished muscular strength, easy fatigability and altered sensation may each separately or in combination, diminish ability to perform usual activities either socially or in the workplace.

Over half of adult diabetics are estimated to be limited in their activities because of one or more chronic conditions or impairments. Diabetics with limitation of activity are much more likely to perceive their health as only fair or poor and to have higher rates of restricted activity days, bed disability days, and work-lost days than diabetics who are not limited (15). About 30% of diabetics with limitation of activity due to diabetes account for 70% of all restricted-activity days due to diabetes.

The degree of functional impairment demonstrably affects work performance. A 1978 Social Security Administration Survey of Disability and Work showed that one-half of all adult diabetics were limited in their activities to the degree that it impacted on their work. In studying the percentage of persons age 20 to 64 years, who were work disabled in the United States in 1978, it was shown that 'severe work disability' (meaning the individual was unable to work at all) in diabetics was four times that of the general population. The rate of those considered occupationally disabled (able to work regularly but not full-time or not at the same kind of job they were trained to do) was twice that of the general population for diabetics. The study also showed that diabetics were twice as likely as the general population to be limited in the type or kind of work that was offered even though they were able to work full-time (14).

## ECONOMIC BURDEN

Diabetes mellitus is a leading cause of morbidity and premature mortality in the general population. Diabetes itself is a major factor in the economic cost of living for the person afflicted with it (16, 17).

During the past few decades, medical cost expenditures have risen extensively throughout the world (16). The rise in health costs have exceeded cost increases reported in other segments of the economy. In the United States, the design and financing of the health-care system is geared toward the treatment of acute illness. However, today most morbidity and mortality is caused by chronic diseases such as diabetes (18). While there have been calls from many quarters in recent years for reform of the US health-care system, most of the recommended changes address health-care access and financing, and are not designed to implement models of chronic care.

The economic issues related to diabetes complications are substantial. The most common complications associated with diabetes are impaired vision, coronary artery disease, stroke, renal disease, peripheral vascular disease, hypertension, lower limb ulceration, gangrene and amputation. Diagnosis, assessing the severity of and treating these complications requires the use of a diversity of health-care resources. The long-term consequences of diabetes therefore, impact on the overall welfare of society by drawing upon scarce medical resources, and contributing to lost production, as well as adversely effecting individuals' health status.

The total health-care resources spent on treating and caring for diabetic patients will be related to the prevalence and incidence of the disease itself. In the United States, the incidence of new cases of insulin-dependent diabetes mellitus is relatively stable at 12–14 new cases per year, per 100 000 in the group of children from birth to 16 years of age. Throughout the world, however, there are pockets with much higher incidences (18). Recent studies in Scotland have shown that the incidence of type I diabetes has more than doubled over the last 15 years (19,20) and in Sardinia (21) and Finland (23) the incidence of new cases may be as high as 40 per 100 000 population. A large increase in the incidence of non-insulin-dependent diabetes mellitus has been demonstrated in the United States where 500 000 or more new cases of diabetes occur per year (24). These data suggest that the economic impact of diabetes as a percentage of total health-care expenditures will continue to rise, irrespective of the health-care financing modality utilised.

The economic costs of health-care are usually divided into two categories: the direct and indirect costs of disease (25, 26). The direct costs include expenditures for diagnosis and medical care and treatment of the illness (physician services, home-health services, nursing home care, hospital care, devices, drugs and other medical needs). These costs are relatively easy to estimate for any given disease by surveys and studies. Indirect costs of a specific illness are considered those due to the societal costs of morbidity, disability, and premature mortality. These are non-medical costs and must be estimated through lost earnings from premature mortality, and the cost of absenteeism from work. These require economic assumptions including life expectancy, years of productivity lost, estimations of earning capacity and the present and future value of currency. A third category 'welfare effects' or 'psychological costs' includes considerations such as disability and distress which result in deterioration in quality-of-life associated with the illness. This latter category has been inadequately studied to date and is generally not included in estimates of the overall cost of a disease (25, 26).

Because diabetes is related to other acute and chronic conditions that are often considered the reason for medical expenses incurred by diabetic persons, it is difficult to estimate the full economic impact of the complications of this disease. Recent reviews in the United States, New Zealand and France all agree that the economic impact of the complications of diabetes is considerably underestimated (27–29).

In part, this has been due to the costing methodology utilised in which all attributed costs are based upon primary diagnosis data only. Studies utilising this methodology demonstrated that the total economic impact of diabetes rose in the United States from $2.6 billion in 1969 to 13.8 billion dollars in 1984 (32). Several reasons have been cited for the apparent increase in the economic cost of diabetes over the years, and in the increase seen in the percentage of total cost related to health-care. These include the inflation of medical care prices, the increased prevalence of diabetes, the increased utilisation of medical services among diabetic patients and the development of new treatment technologies for diabetes. From 1969 to 1980 the estimated health-care costs of diabetes rose 380% while the medical care component of the consumer price index rose 134% (31, 32).

A recent United States study has estimated the overall cost of non-insulin-dependent diabetes mellitus alone to be $19.8 billion per year. Direct health-care expenditures were estimated at $11.6 billion and lost productivity at $8.2 billion (33).

Fox and colleagues (29, 35), estimated the cost of diabetes in 1987 to be 20.4 billion dollars, equalling 4% of the measured total USA health expenditures. Direct costs were estimated at 54% and indirect at 46% (14% due to premature death and 32% due to disability). Their follow-up study utilising patient records identified for the 1987 National Hospital Discharge Summary evaluated the economic impact of the complications of diabetes. They reported 7 million hospital days attributed to diabetic complications during the study year. Hospitalisation for diabetic nephropathy reached a peak of 6.74/1000 between the ages of 45 and 54 years, compared to 0.14 to 1.80/1000 in controls. Diabetic patients up to 45 years of age were 46 times more likely to be hospitalised due to neuropathy. The risk of cardiovascular complications was also high. Diabetic patients were 22 times more likely to be admitted for skin ulcers/gangrene, 15 times more likely due to peripheral vascular disease, and 10 times due to atherosclerosis. The risk of cerebrovascular accident and heart disease was 6 to 10 times greater in diabetic patients. Ophthalmic complications increased with age. Diabetic complications accounted for 2% of the total hospital admissions in the United States in 1987. The total cost of the treatment of late diabetic complications was estimated at +5091 million (cardiovascular 74%; renal diseases 10%; nephropathy 3.6%; ophthalmic disorders 1.5%; other unspecified diseases 10%).

The report indicated that the rate of hospitalisation for diabetics were $2\frac{1}{2}$ times that of other adults and 5 times that of other children. Utilisation of direct services other than hospitalisation were also high with a reported 15–20% of nursing home population being diabetic.

There are limited data on the cost of diabetes from countries other than the United States of America. Jonsson (34) estimated the total cost of diabetes care in Sweden to be 1317 billion Swedish Kronor in 1978. Forty-three per cent were direct costs. Laing and Williams (35) estimated direct costs of diabetes in 1986–87 for England and Wales to be 484 million pounds. Triomphe (29) estimated the average cost of diabetes in France was 7711 French francs for each IDDM patient, and 5892 French francs for each NIDDM patient in 1984. In Australia, the cost of diabetes was estimated at 1.2 billion Australian dollars for 1986 (36). In Canada, the cost estimation was 1.8 billion Canadian dollars for 1985 (37).

Because each country uses its own methodology, the cost comparative data is much less valuable than if there was a standardized methodology for measuring costs across the world. Were comparative values available, it would be of great interest to evaluate the distribution of costs in different countries. The advantages or disadvantages of different health-care practices and reimbursement mechanisms between countries might be discernible from such comparisons. Truly comparable data are not available for such analysis at this time.

In conclusion, diabetes health related costs have risen significantly over the past two decades. The economic impact of the complications of diabetes is substantial in every country in which it has been measured, by whatever methodology. As the world's population ages, and as the number of diabetic persons increases, health-care costs due to diabetic complications will continue to increase unless changes in health-care delivery are undertaken. The mismatch between the nature of chronic diseases such as diabetes and the structure of health-care systems designed to deal with acute illness, will continue to give rise to significant barriers to the translation of scientific knowledge into improved health-care and health for people with diabetes (39). Access to adequate health-care, education and preventative screening have all been shown to be effective in decreasing the burden of diabetic complications (37, 38, 40). They must be actively incorporated in diabetic care and related health models.

## REFERENCES

1 Hauser ST, Jacobson AM, Powers S, Noam G. Ego development and self image complexity in early adolescence: longitudinal studies of psychiatric and diabetic patients. *Arch Gen Psychia* 1983; 40: 325.
2 Jacobsen AM, Leibovich J. Diabetes mellitus: psychological issues in patient management. *Contemp Issues Endocrinol Metabol* 1985; 1: 353–76.
3 Jacobsen AM, Rand L, Hauser ST. Psychological stress and glycemic control in patients with and without proliferative diabetic retinopathy. *Psychosomatic Med* 1985; 47(4): 372–81.
4 Robinson N, Yateman NA, Protopapa LE, Bush L. Employment problems in diabetes. *Diabetic Med* 1990; 7: 16–22.
5 Welsh RA. Employment of diabetics in a post office region. *J Soc Occupat Med* 1986; 36: 80–5.
6 Waclawski ER. A case control study of sickness absence among insulin-treated diabetic employees. *Diabetic Med* 1990; 7(1): 41–4.
7 Beardwood JT Jr. The Committee on Employment, ADA. Analysis of a survey concerning employment of diabetics in some major industries. *Diabetes* 1957; 6: 550–4.
8 Weaver NK, Peret JT. The diabetic industry. *Med Bull* (standard oil, NJ) 1958; 18: 304–16.
9 Dublin LI, Marks HH. The diabetic in industry and his employer. *Indust Med Surg* 1950; 19: 279–82.
10 Songer TJ, LaPorte RE, Dorman JS, Ochard TJ *et al.* (1989). Employment spectrum of IDDM. *Diabetes Care* 1989; 12: 615–22.
11 Krosnick A. Yes, you can get a driver's licence. *Diabetes Forecast* 1982; 35: 16.
12 Hansotia P, Brostesk. The effect of epilepsy or diabetes mellitus on the risk of automobile accidents. *N Engl J Med* 1991; 324: 22.

13 Alvsjo. Social rights of diabetic patients in Europe. *Swedish Diabetic Assoc* 1986; 4–30.
14 Diabetes and Driving, Diabetes conquest 1984 (Winter): S11–13.
15 The Carter Center of Emory University. Closing the gap: the problem of diabetes mellitus in the United States. *Diabetes Care* 1985; 8: 391–406.
16 Simanis JG. Health-care expenditure: international comparisons, 1970–80. *Social Security Bull* 1987; 50: 19–24.
17 Diabetes Epidemiology Research International Mortality Study Group. International evaluation of cause-specific mortality and IDDM. *Diabetes Care* 1991; 14: 55–60.
18 LaPorte RE, Tajima N, Akerblom HR *et al.* Geographic difference in the risk of insulin-dependent diabetes mellitus: the importance of registries. *Diabetes Care* 1985; 8: 101–7.
19 Patterson CC, Thorogood M, Smith PG *et al.* Epidemiology of type 1 diabetes in Scotland 1968–76. Evidence of an increasing incidence. *Diabetologia* 1983; 124: 238–43.
20 Waugh NR. Insulin-dependent diabetes in a Scottish region: Incidence and urban/rural differences. *J Epidemiol Community Health* 1986; 40: 240–3.
21 Diabetes Epidemiology Research International Study Group. The epidemiology and immunogenetics of IDDM in Italian Heritage population. *Diabetes/Metab Rev* 1990; 6: 63–9.
22 Rice DP. Estimating the cost of illness. Health Economic Series No 6, PHS Publ. No. 947–6. Washington, DC: US Government Printing Office, 1966.
23 Rice DP, Hodgson TA, Kopstein AN. The economic cost of illness: a replication and update. *Health Care Fin Rev* 1985; 7: 61–80.
24 Hodgson TA, Meiners MR. Cost-of-illness methodology: a guide to current practices and procedures. *Milbank Mem Fund Quart* 1982; 60: 429–62.
25 Gerard K, Donaldson C, Maynard AK. The cost of diabetes. *Diabetic Med* 1989; 6: 164–70.
26 Shiell A, Gerard K, Donaldson C. Disease costing: an aid to decision making? *Health Policy* 1987; 8: 317–23.
27 Jacobs J, Sena M, Fox N. The cost of hospitalization for the late complications of diabetes in the United States. *Diabetic Med* 1991; 8: 523–9.
28 Phillips DE, Mann JI. Diabetes – inpatient utilization, cost and data validity. Dunedin 1985–9. *N Z Med J*, Aug 12: (939) 1992; 105: 313–15.
29 Triomphe A. The socio-economic cost of diabetic complications in France. *Diabetic Med* 1991; 8: 530–2.
30 Songer TJ. The economics of diabetes care. In: *International textbook of Diabetes mellitus*. John Wiley & Sons, 1992; 1643–54.
31 Medical Care Component of the Consumer Price Index, 1940–77. *Soc Secur Bull* 1978; 41: 67.
32 Medical Care Component of the Consumer Price Index 1977–84. *Soc Secur Bull* 1984; 47: 62.
33 Huse DM, Oster G, Killen AR, Lacey JM *et al.* The economic costs of non-insulin-dependent diabetes mellitus. *J Am Med Assoc* 1989; 262: 2708–13.
34 Jonsson B. Diabetes – the cost of illness and the cost of control. An estimate for Sweden 1978. *Acta Med Scand* 1983; 671 (suppl): 19–27.
35 Laing W, Williams R. Diabetes, a model for health-care management. *Office Health Econ* 1989; paper No 92. London.
36 Diabetes in Australia Canberra: Australian Diabetes Foundation, 1986.
37 Bain M, Ross SA. Socio-economic impact of diabetes. Status of diabetes in Canada. Report of a symposium held at Le Chateau, Montibello, Quebec, 21–23 May, 1985.
38 Pugh JA, Tuley MR, Hazuda HP, Stern MP. The influence of outpatient insurance coverage on the microvascular complications of non-insulin-dependent diabetes in Mexican Americans. *J Diabetes Complications* 1992; 6: 236–24.
39 LaPorte RE, Tajima N, Akerblom HR *et al.* Geographic difference in the risk of insulin-dependent diabetes mellitus: the importance of registries. *Diabetes Care* 1985; 8: 101–7.
40 Miller LV, Goldstein J. More efficient care of diabetic patients in a county-hospital setting. *N Engl J Med* 1972; 286: (26) 1388–91.

# 22 Mortality among Persons with Diabetes

Leon-Paul Georges

The diagnosis of diabetes mellitus confers with it a lifetime of consequences which affect nearly all aspects of an individual's being. Life-style changes which impact heavily on the diabetic individual's daily routine and activities are required from the onset. Careful attention to the details of therapy as currently applied, undoubtedly improves long-term outcomes. None the less, susceptibility to life-spoiling and life-shortening complications remains a very real threat for the individual, as well as for society as a whole. Diabetes continues to be, not only a major source of individual disability and national health costs, but a leading cause of death as well (1, 2).

## MORTALITY RATES

Mortality has traditionally been under-reported in diabetes. Accurate data collection has been impaired by a variety of circumstances, the major one being the lack of reliability in listing the cause(s) of demise on the official death certificate.

The death certificate is the most commonly utilised instrument in calculating leading causes of death. In the United States, deaths are recorded on death certificates that contain space for the condition or disease that is considered to be the primary or originating cause of death. This is the cause that is utilised in calculating national death rates and for ranking the leading causes of death. Contributing causes are also listed. These are other diseases and conditions that were also present at death. The full impact of diabetes on mortality is understated when it is either not listed, or listed only as a contributing cause, for instance, in an individual whose primary cause of death is listed as coronary artery disease or acute myocardial infarction. Fully three-quarters of recorded diabetic deaths are not attributed to diabetes even though the direct cause of death may have been due to a condition caused or worsened by the diabetic state (3, 4).

Utilising data from the 1986 National Mortality Followback Survey, Bild and Stevenson (5) showed that diabetes was recorded on only 30% of the death certificates of 2766 decedents who had a proven history of diabetes mellitus. It was listed as the underlying cause in only 9.6%. When other listed causes of death included conditions that may have been related to diabetes such as cardiovascular disease, diabetes was listed between 45 and 70% of the time. They concluded that diabetes is often not recorded on death certificates and that the likelihood of it being recorded is related to age, duration of diabetes, and co-morbidity.

International studies suggest that a similar problem exists outside of the US as well. A study in nine European countries documented wide variability in death certificate coding practices from country to country (6). In France (7), a recent study demonstrates that diabetes is completely omitted on the death certificate of many diabetic subjects, and that, using mortality statistics derived from death certificates, underestimates the prevalence of diabetes and its effects on French public health. In Australia (8), the diagnosis of diabetes was stated on only 65% of the death certificates of known diabetics. Although cardiovascular disease was assigned as the direct cause of death in 63%, in only 24% was diabetes listed as a direct or antecedent cause. A Kuwait study (9) demonstrated that diabetes mellitus was under-estimated in that country as the cause of death by 60% compared to death certification through hospital records.

Additionally, reporting variations by age, sex or race have been well described in determining when diabetes is listed as the leading cause of death (3). The likelihood of selecting diabetes decreases with the increasing age of the deceased. This may reflect the prominent role that cardiovascular disease assumes with increasing age of death. The proportion of diabetic deaths that involve virtually all the other causes of death decline with increasing age of death.

The relative ranking of mortality from diabetes does vary by sex. Diabetes is selected as the leading cause of death more often for females than for males. Diabetes was the ninth leading underlying cause of death among white and non-white males in 1978, whereas for females, the comparable ranking was sixth and fifth, respectively. Diabetes is selected more often for non-whites than for whites.

Mortality from diabetes also displays a seasonal pattern in that diabetic deaths are more frequently reported in the winter months and are less prevalent in the summer months. Seasonal variations in diabetes mortality may be a result of diabetic deaths being linked to cardiovascular–renal disease deaths which also exhibit a similar seasonal pattern.

When assessing death rates or other measures of mortality related to a disease process such as diabetes mellitus, one must compare it to the death rate in the general population. In the general population the mortality rate is age related with a relatively high mortality rate during the first years of life. Thereafter, survival rates remain constant until age 35–40, following which mortality rates gradually rise. Survival declines progressively with each decade of life thereafter so that only half the men remain alive at age 72 and half of the women at age 80 (10). When one compares mortality among diabetics to that of the general population by computing the ratio of the number of deaths among diabetics to the expected number of deaths in the general population, a clear picture of excess mortality in the diabetic population emerges. Survival of diabetic individuals is appreciably below that of the general population at all ages.

## INSULIN-DEPENDENT DIABETES MELLITUS

Before the discovery and availability of insulin, the diagnosis of IDDM was a death sentence, and one which was relatively quickly imposed. Death, mainly due to keto-acidosis, occurred within a year or two of diagnosis (11). Once insulin became available, life expectancy increased dramatically. As a result of insulin therapy, there was an immediate reduction in mortality. A remarkable 350-fold reduction in mortality of young children with diabetes was accomplished over a period of the next 40 years (12). Unfortunately, with time it became clear that insulin treatment alone did not normalise survival rates. Although markedly reduced in number, deaths due to acute complications continued to occur. Survival beyond the first few years allowed previously unrecognised long-term complications to become evident. Today, IDDM continues to be disproportionately associated with premature mortality. Death rates for persons with IDDM are nearly eight times that for the general population with greater than 20% of affected individuals dying each year (12–14).

The primary sources of data on IDDM mortality in the US are from the cohort studies of the Childrens Hospital of Pittsburgh (14) and the Joslin Clinic (15, 16). The mortality results from these two centres are remarkably consistent and appear to reflect the general mortality of persons with IDDM. The overall mortality rate for white male and female IDDMs in the Pittsburgh study was similar for males (6.4/1000) and females (5.8/1000) but was much higher than for the general population. There was a higher relative mortality in the black diabetic population compared to white diabetics. By comparing mortality rates for persons with IDDM with those for the general population, it was shown that males were 5.4 times more likely to die than the general United States population of males, and females were 11.5 times more likely to die. The risk markedly accelerated after age 25 and was 20 times that seen in the general population.

The major source of IDDM mortality data outside the US is the Steno Memorial Hospital, Denmark. Their recent reports have demonstrated an improved prognosis for IDDM persons with a consistently decreasing trend in relative mortality with calendar year of diagnosis (17–19). These observations are supported by others and the improvement in mortality appears primarily related to the decreasing incidence of proteinuria (20–22).

Recently, attention has been drawn to striking differences in all-cause IDDM mortality among nations. The Diabetes Epidemiology Research International study examined mortality patterns of four population-based cohorts of IDDM cases from Allegheny County, Pennsylvania, Finland, Israel and Japan (23). Life-table analysis revealed that at 20-year duration of diabetes, 5.5% of the cohorts had died in Allegheny County in contrast to only 3.1% in Finland and 4.6% in Israel. The Japanese cohort exhibited markedly higher age-adjusted mortality rates that the other three (Japan 681, US 230, Finland 171 and Israel 131). A standardised protocol developed to evaluate cause-specific mortality demonstrated a surprisingly high percentage of deaths (>25% in each country) due to acute diabetes related complications (23) suggesting that much of the premature mortality associated with IDDM may be potentially preventable. Songer and colleagues (24) suggest that, in the United States, health system barriers, such as access to care and the financial burden of diabetes care, may be contributing to adverse outcomes, and that perhaps one-half of the IDDM deaths at ages 25–37 years may be preventable.

## NON-INSULIN-DEPENDENT DIABETES MELLITUS

While persons with NIDDM are less likely to experience the acute metabolic complications of diabetes than persons with IDDM, their vulnerability to the long-term complications impacts unfavourably on their survival. At 25 years past diagnosis, survival is only 70–80% of that expected in the general adult population. The Diabetes National History Study conducted at the Joslin Clinic (25) demonstrated that survival decreased as age at diagnosis increased. A new analysis grouping patients according to age at diagnosis in 20-year intervals has been performed (10) beginning with age 30 instead of age 20 as in the earlier publication. Diabetes which is clinically manifest after the age of thirty is predominantly non-insulin dependent. The newer analysis shows progressively poorer prognosis as age at diagnosis increases and a lack of sex difference in prognosis which is strikingly different from the larger sex difference seen in the general population. For males, there was no excess mortality until after age 50, but for females there was a noticeable excess mortality before age 45. After age 50, survival for both sexes declined rapidly so that median survival was reached 12 years earlier than the general population for women and 5 years earlier for men. Since women in the general population survive longer than males, these data reflect a greater impact of NIDDM on women than men. Additionally, while recent trends show a decline in coronary related NIDDM deaths (similar to that in the general population) the decline was found to be mainly among men, with little decline in women deaths.

Recent reports have addressed mortality rates in American Indians and Mexican Americans. NIDDM is associated with an overall age-sex-adjusted death rate in PIMA Indians 1.7 times that in non-diabetic persons (26). Compared with a general state population, Oklahoma Indians with NIDDM experienced an observed/expected ratio for number of deaths of 2.92 for men and 4.09 for women (27). Mexican Americans with NIDDM studied in Texas (28) also experienced premature (one-third of deaths were in individuals less than 65 years of age) and excessive mortality compared to the general population.

It is difficult to contrast mortality experience of persons with IDDM and with NIDDM. The older literature grouped all diabetic deaths rather than separate insulin dependent and non-insulin dependent. One can, however, estimate the type of diabetes by age of onset criteria, assuming that the vast majority of individuals in whom diabetes occurs prior to age 30–35 will be insulin dependent. Data collected prior to 1970 demonstrated that, among insurance applicants, there was more than 11-fold excess mortality for individuals when diabetes developed before the age of 15 compared to mortality in the general population. Whereas diabetes diagnosed after age 40 was associated with approximately a two–three-fold excess mortality. Thus, an individual with diabetes diagnosed at age 14 was expected to live only to age 47 (33 years' expectation). An individual diagnosed at age 49 had a 20-year expectancy of life and was expected to live to age 69 (28a). The indication being that youth-onset diabetes has substantially greater impact on mortality than does older-onset diabetes.

## CAUSE OF DEATH

### Acute complications

#### Diabetic keto-acidosis and hyperosmolar coma

Diabetic keto-acidosis (DKA) and hyperosmolar coma are among the most serious complications of diabetes mellitus. If misdiagnosed and either untreated or undertreated, they carry a high mortality (29, 30). At least half of the patients for instance, who present in hyperosmolar coma have not been previously known to be diabetic. The diagnosis therefore, may be seriously delayed and the length of delay may be related to an adverse outcome. A number of complications which worsen the prognosis can accompany DKA-hyperosmolar syndromes. The extent of these complications relate directly to the duration of symptoms and invariably to the rate at which hyperosmolarity is relieved. They include urinary tract and pulmonary infections, venous and arterial embolisation, cerebral oedema, disseminated intravascular coagulopathy and cardiac arrhythmias secondary to hypokalaemia (30a).

The incidence of the acute complications of diabetes mellitus remains high. Faisch and colleagues (31) showed that DKA accounted for 1.6% of all diabetic admissions in Rhode Island. The annual incidence rate was 46/10 000 diabetic persons. Fishbein and the National Diabetes Data Group (USA) described the annual DKA rate as 3–8 episodes per 1000 diabetic persons. The rate in females is 1.5 times higher than in males, and is highest in young, individuals (0–9 years) (32, 33). The same group estimated mortality due to DKA to be 9–10% of all diabetic deaths, 50% higher in females than in males, three times higher for non-whites than whites and to occur in 57/100 000 diabetics per year.

Numerous studies (14, 18, 32) have reported a decline in recent years from death due to the acute complications of diabetes mellitus. The Diabetes Epidemiology Research International Mortality Study Group, however, noted a similarly high percentage of death (>25% in each country) from acute diabetes-related complications. In a four-nation (US, Japan, Israel and Finland) cohort study, mortality associated with acute complications of diabetes was either the first or second leading cause of diabetic death in all countries. Because deaths from acute diabetic complications occur at such a young age, they are probably the leading cause of premature life lost for persons with IDDM (23).

### Hypoglycaemia

Severe hypoglycaemia is a common occurrence in insulin-treated diabetic persons (32, 34). It is the most common complication of insulin treatment and the aspect of the disease that IDDM patients fear the most from day to day. It has been estimated that one-fourth to one-third of all patients on conventional insulin therapy will have at least one episode of hypoglycaemia severe enough to require assistance from another person, each year. While there is a wide variation in the reported frequency of severe hypoglycaemia, it is clear that the frequency increases with more intensive insulin regimens attempting to normalise plasma glucose (35, 36). There is also a pattern of individual susceptibility with greater risk in those patients with a prior history of severe hypoglycaemia. The overall incidence of severe hypoglycaemia, especially severe nocturnal hypoglycaemia may be under-reported (37, 38).

Death due to hypoglycaemia in diabetic persons has been thought to be uncommon. The Joslin Clinic mortality experience from 1922–1979 (38) attributed death due to hypoglycaemia in only 85 of 33 330 deaths. Other studies in Denmark and the United Kingdom also described hypoglycaemia as only a rare cause of death (39–41). However, severe brain damage with characteristic anatomic changes occur with hypoglycaemia. The extent of the brain damage and risk of death appears to correlate best with the length of hypoglycaemic coma (42, 43). Tattersall and Gill's (44) report on a series of unexplained deaths in young insulin-dependent diabetic individuals brings a new perspective. Twenty-two individuals were found 'dead in bed' presumably from severe hypoglycaemic episodes. All were on human insulin therapy, lived alone and only four had severe chronic complications of diabetes, making it unlikely that autonomic neuropathy was responsible. Fourteen had histories of at least one prior severe nocturnal hypoglycaemic episode. The authors conclude that physicians should be cautious when recommending normoglycaemia or a normal glycated haemoglobin as the target in patients who sleep alone.

### Autonomic neuropathy

Persons with diabetic autonomic neuropathy are at risk of dying suddenly with no apparent cause found on autopsy examination (45, 46). While diabetic autonomic neuropathy may involve any of the body's systems, it is often undetected clinically. The prevalence of this disorder, when established by utilising varying cardiovascular reflex tests is 17–40% (47) while it may be variably related to the presence of sensory–motor neuropathy, the disturbance in neurological function usually coexists. Approximately 50% of patients with peripheral neuropathy will have asymptomatic autonomic neuropathy.

Once symptoms of autonomic neuropathy are present, the anticipated mortality is 15–40% within 5 years. There is some disagreement as to the actual cause of death. Most favour cardiac causes, some implicate respiratory causes (48–50). When symptoms of gastroparesis are present, 35% die within 3 years' time, presumably from aspiration and pneumonia.

Little is known as to the distribution of this disorder among various populations or of possible differences in expression of its lethalness.

## Chronic complications

### Vascular disease

The majority of the devastating complications of diabetes mellitus, those causing premature mortality, are due to pathologic changes which occur in both small and large blood vessels.

### Macrovascular disease

#### Cardiovascular

The risk of cardiovascular disease in diabetes is increased two–three-fold over age- and sex-matched non-diabetics. Both IDDM and non-IDDM diabetics are at increased risk of heart disease that is indistinguishable epidemiologically, pathologically or clinically from atherosclerotic heart disease seen in non-diabetics (51).

In the Framingham Study (52), the relative risk for cardiovascular death in diabetics versus non-diabetic subjects was 2.1 for men and 4.9 for women. This strikingly increased cardiovascular risk, especially in women, has now been well documented (53, 54).

The increased coronary heart disease mortality in diabetics may be attributable to both the higher incidence rate and to the reported increased probability of death in the acute state of infarction (55, 56). The latter is apparently not related to the size of the infarction (57, 58) but may be related to poor metabolic control (59, 60).

The majority of epidemiological studies concerning diabetic cardiovascular mortality included mainly patients with NIDDM. Panzram (61) reviewed studies from the USA, Europe and Japan. The ratio of observed to expected deaths from all causes was elevated from 1.15 to 3.01, including both age-adjusted and age-specific data. The ratios for coronary heart disease mortality were higher than those for all-cause mortality. In Japan, excess mortality due to CHD is of recent origin and the proportion of cardiovascular death remains lower than that in Europe and North America. When Japanese migrated to Hawaii, however, the proportion of deaths attributed to CHD became nearly equal to that in the Hawaiian, European diabetic patients (62). Comparatively decreased CHD mortality in other populations has also been noted. Prevalence rates of macrovascular complications in the WHO multinational study on vascular diseases in diabetes varied widely (63). These data raise the suspicion that increased CHD risk associated with NIDDMs may not be related to diabetes itself.

For IDDM, long-term follow-up studies from the Joslin Clinic (10, 16) demonstrated that the excessive mortality in early onset IDDM increased rapidly in the third decade of life. By age 55, CHD mortality was 35% for diabetic men and women compared to 8% for aged-matched non-diabetic men and 4% for non-diabetic women in the Framingham Heart Study. The Steno Study (18, 19) has demonstrated a linkage between all cause mortality as well as coronary heart disease in IDDM patients with proteinuria. In IDDM patients who remain free of proteinuria there is a substantially reduced relative mortality risk. The onset of proteinuria was followed by a significantly increased incidence of fatal and non-fatal CHD. It may be that much of the excess CHD of IDDM can be attributed to diabetic renal disease.

#### Cerebrovascular

While diabetic persons are known to have a higher incidence of atherosclerotic diseases affecting the coronary and peripheral arteries, it has been less certain that this is true for the cerebrovascular system. Diabetes does seem to be more prevalent in the population of patients who present with stroke (64). In the Framingham Study, the incidence of stroke was doubled in diabetes (65).

In IDDM there are few pertinent studies. Fuller (66) reviewed death certificates in England and Wales for 1975 and 1976. Only 3.7% mentioned diabetes. For those individuals in the 15–45 years of age range, and therefore thought likely to be insulin-dependent diabetics, there was a significant increase in cerebrovascular disease in females. In a recently published German study (67) in which 229 IDDM patients and 157 NIDDM patients were followed after laser photocoagulation therapy for diabetic retinopathy, stroke was the most frequent macrovascular complication, present in 8.4% of IDDM patients and 16.5% of NIDDM patients.

Other studies, however, have not shown significant increases in diabetic stroke deaths. A Polish study (68) compared diabetic patients age 30–68 years at diagnosis with those in the general population. Excess mortality from cerebrovascular disease was similar in men and women treated with insulin but the difference was not statistically different. In the United Kingdom (69) a population-based cohort study identified 915 deaths in 4186 patients with diabetes mellitus over a 5-year period. Cerebrovascular disease which accounted for 16% of deaths was not statistically different in the diabetic population compared to 14% in the non-diabetic population. While the data are quite variable, there is a general consensus that cerebrovascular disease is more common, at least in NIDDM than in the general population. Prospective studies such as those by K.L. Chan (70) (unpublished observations) have demonstrated a significantly higher incidence of ultrasound evidence of high-grade carotid artery stenosis in NIDDM patients (8.2%) compared to controls (0.7%). Although age alone could not account for the observed difference, the prevalence rose sharply after age 60. There was a higher correlation between carotid stenosis and focal neurological symptoms. Variability in the reported incidence of cerebrovascular disease may well reflect methodological problems.

## MICROVASCULAR DISEASE

The two predominant forms of microvascular disease associated with diabetes mellitus are retinopathy and nephropathy. Along with cardiovascular disease (macrovascular), diabetic nephropathy is a major determinant of the excess mortality seen in diabetic persons. Together, they account for 50–80% of all diabetic deaths (10, 71).

Diabetic nephropathy is clinically defined by the presence of persistent proteinuria (more than 0.5 grams in 24 hours) in a diabetic person without other urinary tract/renal disease or heart failure. It is accepted today that microalbuminuria is an indicator of early diabetic renal disease and that its measurement may be utilised to screen for the disorder before routine tests can demonstrate proteinuria (72).

While diabetic nephropathy is a relatively common complication in both IDDM and NIDDM, epidemiological studies suggest that only a subset of diabetic individuals is at risk to develop clinically important diabetic nephropathy (19, 20). The incidence is greater in IDDM and low age at onset and male sex are associated with higher risk for nephropathy (19).

Deckert (17) was the first to show that clinical nephropathy, as manifest by persistent proteinuria, was associated with increased diabetic mortality. More recent studies have described the excess mortality as being attributable not only to renal failure but also to cardiovascular disease and have shown that the high mortality of IDDM patients is confined almost entirely to patients developing diabetic renal disease (18, 74). Jensen and colleagues (75), showed, in a case control study, that within 6 years of onset of proteinuria, the cumulative incidence of coronary heart disease was 8 times greater for the proteinuric than non-proteinuric diabetics.

## REFERENCES


1 Covar MG, Harris MI, Hadden WC. The scope of diabetes in the United States population. *Am J Public Health* 77(12), 1549–50.
2 The Carter Center of Emory University. Closing the gap: the problem of diabetes mellitus in the United States. *Diabetes Care* 1985; 8: 391–406.
3 Harris MI, Entmacher PS. Mortality from diabetes. *Diabetes in America*. NIH Publication No 85–1468, 1985.
4 Palumbo PJ, Elveback LR, Chu CP, Connoll DC *et al.* Diabetes mellitus incidence, prevalence, survivorship and causes of death. *Diabetes* 1976; 25: 566–73.

5 Bild DE, Stevenson JM. Frequency of recording of diabetes on U.S. death certificates: analysis of 1986 national mortality followback survey. *J Clin Epidemiol* 1992; 45(3): 275–81.
6 Jougla E, Papoz L, Balkau B, Maquin P *et al.* Death certificate coding practices related to diabetes in European Countries – The 'EURODIAB Subarea C Study'. *In J Epidemiol* 1992; 21(2): 343–51.
7 Balkau B, Papoz L. Certification of cause of death in French diabetic patients. *J Epidemiol Community Health* 1992; 46(1): 63–5.
8 Whittal DE, Glatthaar C, Knuiman MW, Welborn TA. Deaths from diabetes are under-reported in national mortality statistics. *Med J Aust* 1990; 152(11): 598–600.
9 Moussa MA, Shafie MZ, Khogali MM, el-Sayed AM *et al.* Reliability of death certificate diagnosis. *J Clin Epidemiol* 1990; 43(12): 1285–95.
10 Krolewski AS, Warram JH, Christlieb AR. Onset, course, complications and prognosis of diabetes mellitus. In *Joslin's diabetes mellitus*, 12th edn, Marble A., Krall LP, Bradley RF, Christlieb AR, Soeldner JS eds. Philadelphia: Lea & Febiger, 1985; 251–77.
11 Joslin EP. *The treatment of diabetes mellitus*, 4th edn. Lea & Feibiger, N. Philadelphia; 1928.
12 Dorman JS, LaPorte RE. Mortality in insulin-dependent diabetes. In *Diabetes in America*. NIH Pub No. 85–1468, 1985.
13 Connel FA, Louden JM. Diabetes mortality in persons under 45 years of age. *Am J Public Health* 1983; 73: 1174–77.
14 Dorman JS, LaPorte RE, Juller LH, Cruickshank K *et al.* The Pittsburgh insulin-dependent diabetes mellitus morbidity and mortality study: Mortality results. *Diabetes* 1984; 33: 271–6.
15 Entmacher PS, Root HF, Marks HH. Longevity of diabetic patients in recent years. *Diabetes* 1964; 13: 373–7.
16 Krolewski AS, Kosinski EJ, Warram JH *et al.* Magnitude and determinants of coronary artery disease in juvenile onset, insulin-dependent diabetes mellitus. *Am J Cardiol* 1987; 59: 750–5.
17 Deckert T. The influence of supervision in exogenous insulin secretion on the course of insulin-dependent diabetes mellitus. *Acta Endocrinol* 1980; 94 (suppl 238): 31–8.
18 Green A, Borch-Johnsen K, Anderson PK, Hougaard P *et al.* Relative mortality of Type I (insulin-dependent) diabetes in Denmark, 1933–81. *Diabetology* 1985; 28: 339–42.
19 Kofoed-Enevoldsen A, Borch-Johnsen K, Kreiners, Nerupj J *et al.* Declining incidence of persistence proteinuria in Type-I (insulin-dependent) diabetic patients in Denmark. *Diabetes* 1987; 36: 205–9.
20 Krolewski AS, Warram JH, Christlied AR, Busick EJ *et al.* The changing natural history of nephropathy in Type-I diabetes. *Am J Med* 1985; 78: 785–94.
21 Noss SE, Klein R, Klein BE. Cause-specific mortality in a population-based study of diabetes. *Am J Public Health* 1991; 81(9): 1158–62.
22 Hasslacher C, Borgholte G, Panradl U, Wahl P. Improved prognosis of type I and type II diabetics with nephropathy. *Med Klin* 1990; 85: 643–6.
23 Diabetes Epidemiology Research International Mortality Study Group. International evaluation of cause-specific mortality and IDDM. *Diabetes Care* 1991; 14: 55–60.
24 Songer TJ, DeBerry K, LaPorte RE, Tuomilehto J. International comparisons of IDDM mortality – clues to prevention and the role of diabetes care. *Diabetes Care* 1992; 15(1): 15–21.
25 Hirohata, T, MacMahon, B & Root, HF (1967). The natural history of diabetes I mortality. *Diabetes* 16, 875.
26 Sievers ML, Nelson RG, Knowles WC, Bennett PH. Impact of NIDDM on mortality and cause of death in PIMA Indians. *Diabetes Care* 1992; 15(11): 1541–9.
27 Lee ET, Russell D, Jorge N, Kenny S *et al.* A follow up study of diabetic Oklahoma Indians mortality and cause of death. *Diabetes Care* 1993; 16(1): 300–5.
28 Hanis CL, Ehu HH, Lawson K, Hewett-Emmett D *et al.* Mortality of Mexican Americans with NIDDM. Retinopathy and other predictors in Starr County, Texas. *Diabetes Care* 1993; 16(1): 82–9.
28a Goodkin G. Mortality factors in diabetes. *J Occup Med* 1975; 17: 716–21.
29 Schade D, Eaton RP, Alberti KGM *et al. Diabetic coma – keto acidotic and hypersomolar.* Albuquerque: New Mexico. University of New Mexico Press, 1981.
30 Fulop M. The treatment of severely uncontrolled diabetes mellitus. *Adv Internal Med* 1984; 29: 327.
30a Siperstein MD. Diabetic keto-acidosis and hyperosmolar coma. Diabetes mellitus: perspectives on therapy. *Endocrinol Metab Clin North Am* 1993; 21: 415–32.
31 Faisch, GA, Fishbein HA, Ellis SE. The epidemiology of diabetic acidosis: a population-based study. *Am J Epidemiol* 1983; 117: 551–8.
32 Fishbein HA. Diabetic Keto-acidosis, hyperosmolar, nonketotic coma, lactic acidosis, and hypoglycemia. In: *Diabetes in America*. Harris MI, Hamman RF, eds. PHS publication No. 85–1468, 1985
33 Potter J, Clarke P, Gale, EAM, Dave SH *et al.* Insulin-induced hypoglycemia in an accident and emergency department: The tip of an iceberg. *Br Med J* 1982; 285: 1180–2.
34 Casparie AF, Elving LD. Severe hypoglycemia in diabetic patients: Frequency, causes, prevention. *Diabetes Care* 1985; 8: 141–45.
35 Teusch SM, Herman WH, Dweyers DM, Lane JM. Mortality among young diabetic patients using continuous subcutaneous insulin infused pumps. *N Eng J Med* 1984; 310: 361–8.
36 DCCT Research Group. Diabetic control and complications trial: Research of feasibility study. *Diabetes Care* 1987; 10: 1–119.
37 Gale, EAM, Tattersall RB. Unrecognized nocturnal hypoglycemia in insulin treated diabetes. *Lancet* 1979; i: 1049–52.
38 Marble A, Kroll LP, Bradly RF, Christlieb AR, Soeldner JS, eds. In: *Joslin's diabetes mellitus*, 12th edn, Philadelphia: Lea & Feibiger, 1985; 402–3.
39 Malins JM. *Clinical diabetes mellitus*. London: Eyre and Spottiswood, 1968; 439.
40 Deckert T, Poulsen JC, Larsen M. Prognosis of diabetics with onset before the age of thirty-one. *Diabetologia* 1978; 14: 363–70.
41 Shenfield GM, Bhalla IP, Elton RA, Duncan LJP. Fatal coma in diabetes. *Diabete Metab (Paris)* 1980; 6: 151–5.
42 Patrick AW, Campbell, IW, Fatal hypoglycemia in insulin-treated diabetes mellitus. Clinical features and neuropathological changes. *Diabetes Med* 1990; 7: 349–54.

43 Auer RN. Hypoglycemic brain damage stroke. *Prog rev* 1986; 17: 699–708.

44 Tattersall RB, Gill GV. Unexplained deaths of type-I diabetic patients. *Diabetes Med* 1991; 8: 49–58.

45 Ewing DJ, Campbell IW, Clarke BF. Mortality in diabetic autonomic neuropathy. *Lancet* 1976; i: 601–3.

46 Page MM, Watkins PJ. Cardiorespiratory arrest in diabetic autonomic neuropathy. *Lancet* 1978; i: 14–6.

47 Vinik AI, Holland MT, LeBeau JM, Liuzzi FJ *et al. Diabetes Care* 1992; 15: 1926–75.

48 Soler NG, Eagleton LE. Autonomic neuropathy and the ventilatory responses of diabetics to progressive hypoxemia and hypercarbia. *Diabetes* 1982; 31: 609–14.

49 Chopra JS, Fannin T. Pathology of diabetic neuropathy. *J Pathol* 1971; 104: 175–84.

50 Catterall JR, Calverly PMA, Ewing DJ, Shapiro CM *et al.* Breathing sleep and diabetic autonomic neuropathy. *Diabetes* 1984; 33: 1025–7.

51 Barrett-Connor E, Orchard T. Diabetes and heart disease. In: *Diabetes in America*, NIH Publication No. 85–1468, Harris MI, Hamman RF eds. Bethesda, Maryland, USA: Department of Health and Human Services, 1985; XVI-1–14.

52 Kannel WB, McGee DL. Diabetes and cardiovascular disease: The Framingham Study. *J Am Med Assoc* 1979; 241: 2035–8.

53 Gordon, T, Castelli WP, Hjortland MC, Kannel WB *et al.* Diabetes, blood lipids, and the role of obesity in coronary heart disease risk for women. *Ann Internal Med* 1977; 87: 393–7.

54 Barrett-Connor E, Wingard DL. Sex differential in ischemic heart disease mortality in diabetics: a prospective population based study. *Am J Epidemiol* 1983; 118: 489.

55 Honcey GE, Truelove SC. Prognostic factors in myocardial infarction. *Lancet* 1957; i: 1155–61.

56 Singer DE, Moulton AW, Nathan DM. Diabetic myocardial infarction. Interaction of diabetes with other preinfarction risk factors. *Diabetes* 1989; 38: 350–7.

57 Gwilt DJ, Petri M, Lewis PW *et al.* Myocardial infarction size and mortality in diabetic patients. *Br Heart J* 1985; 54: 466–72.

58 Oswald GA, Corcoran S, Yudkin JS. Prevalence and risks of hyperglycemia and undiagnosed diabetes in patients with acute myocardial infarction. *Lancet* 1984; i: 1264–7.

59 Sykes CA, Wright AD, Malins JM *et al.* Changes in systolic time intervals during treatment of diabetes mellitus. *Br Heart J* 1977; 39: 255–9.

60 Rytter L, Troelsen S, Beck-Nielsen H. Prevalence and mortality of acute myocardial infarction in patients with diabetes. *Diabetes Care* 1985; 8: 230–4.

61 Panzram G. Mortality and survival in type 2 (non-insulin-dependent) diabetes mellitus. *Diabetologia* 1987; 30: 123–31.

62 Kawate R, Miyanushi, M, Yamakido M *et al.* Preliminary studies of the prevalence and mortality of diabetes mellitus in Japanese in Japan and on the Island of Hawaii. *Adv Metab Bis* 1978; 9: 202–24.

63 WHO multinational study of vascular disease in diabetics: prevalence of small vessel and large vessel disease in diabetic patients from 14 centres 1985.

64 Peacock PB, Riley CP, Lampton TD, Raffel SS *et al.* The Birmingham Stroke, epidemiology and rehabilitation study. In: Steward GT ed. *Trends in epidemiology: application to health research and training*, Springfield, 1972; 281–6.

65 Garcia, MJ, McNamara PM, Gordon T *et al.* Morbidity and mortality in diabetics in the Framingham population: sixteen year follow-up study. *Diabetes* 1974; 23:105–11.

66 Fuller JH, Elferd J, Goldblatt P, Adelstein AM. Diabetes mortality; new light on an underestimated public health problem. *Diabetologia* 1983; 24: 336–44.

67 Diglas J, Willinger C, Nell U, Irsigler K. Morbidity and mortality in type I and type II diabetes mellitus after the diagnosis of diabetic retinopathy. *Dtsch Med Wochenschr* 1992; 6, 117(45): 1703–8.

68 Krolewski AS, Czyzyk A, Jancczko D, Kopezynski J. Mortality from cardiovascular disease among diabetics. *Diabetologia* 1977; 13: 345–50.

69 Wong JS Pearson DW, Murchison LE, Williams MJ *et al.* Mortality in diabetes mellitus: experience of a geographically defined population. *Diabetic Med* 1991; 8: 135–9.

70 Chan KL. 657 unpublished observations.

71 Marbel A. Insulin-clinical aspects: the first fifty years. *Diabetes* 1972; 21(2): 632–6.

72 Viberti GC, Hill RD, Jarett RJ, Argyropoulos A *et al.* Microalbuminuria as a predictor of clinical proteinuria in insulin-dependent diabetes mellitus. *Lancet* 1982; i:1430–2.

73 Medical care component of the Consumer Price Index, 1940–77. *Social Security Bull* 1978; 41:67.

74 Borch-Johnsen KB. Proteinuria: value as predictor of cardiovascular mortality in insulin-dependent diabetes mellitus. *Br Med J* 1987; 294:1651–4.

75 Jensen JS, Mathiesen ER, Norgaard K, Hommel E *et al. Diabetologia* 1990; 33: 619–24.

# 23 Glycation and Diabetic Complications

Timothy J. Lyons

## INTRODUCTION

Glycation comprises the spontaneous, non-enzymatic, reaction of glucose with proteins. In diabetes, elevated levels of glucose are present not only in plasma, but also in interstitial fluid and within cells where glucose entry is not insulin dependent. As a result, glycation of a wide variety of proteins is enhanced, and this has led to a hypothesis to explain the pathogenesis of diabetic complications. This 'glycation hypothesis' states that enhanced protein modification leads to abnormalities, e.g. in turnover rate, receptor recognition, enzyme activity, and in physico-chemical properties, and that, over time, these are sufficient to cause disease. The hypothesis is attractive because it provides a rationale for the widely held clinical belief that poor glycaemic control tends to increase the risk of diabetic complications. Strong evidence is accumulating to support this belief (1–9) (at the time of writing, the results of the Diabetes Control and Complication Trial are imminent). Clearly, however, there are exceptions to the rule, and neither increased glycation, nor indeed the degree of long-term hyperglycaemia, can be the only factor determining the development of diabetic complications. Every diabetologist is familiar with patients who, despite reasonable glycaemic control, develop severe complications at an unusually early stage. Conversely, other patients seem resistant to the development of complications despite poor long-term glycaemic control. In this chapter, the biochemistry of glycation and the evidence implicating the process in the development of complications will be reviewed. Following this, an extension of the glycation hypothesis, which may partially explain the absence of a clear relationship between glycaemic control and complications, will be proposed. Briefly, recent data suggest that the processes of glycation and free radical oxidation are closely linked. It appears that the products of combined glycation and oxidation ('glycoxidation products'), or perhaps the *rate* of their formation, may be important determinants for the development of diabetic complications. These possibilities are supported by evidence from studies, outlined below, on proteins as different as low density lipoprotein (LDL) and insoluble skin collagen. Thus in individual patients, the consequences of hyperglycaemia may be modulated by the capacity to resist oxidative stress. If this hypothesis is correct, there may be practical implications for the management of diabetic patients. For example, it may be possible to identify, at a very early stage, those patients who, for a given level of glycaemic control, are particularly vulnerable to complications, i.e. those with relatively poor antioxidant defences. Also, in addition to optimising glycaemic control, efforts to reduce 'oxidative stress', either by diet or pharmacological means, may be effective in reducing the risk of complications.

## CHEMISTRY OF GLYCATION

A brief description of the chemistry of glycation follows: for a more detailed review, the reader is referred to another recent publication (10).

### Early glycation

Glycation of proteins may be regarded as a two-stage process, and the chemical reactions involved are illustrated in Fig. 23.1. In the initial stage, covalent bonds are formed between aldehyde groups of glucose molecules and reactive amino-groups of proteins. The latter are usually located on lysine side chains and N-terminal amino acid residues. As illustrated, this reaction can only take place with glucose molecules in their 'open chain' configuration (as opposed to their 'ring' configuration). It has been suggested that, in evolutionary terms, glucose is the metabolic fuel of choice precisely because it exists predominantly in the ring form, and is therefore less reactive with proteins than most other monosaccharides. As shown in Fig. 23.1, an unstable intermediate known as a 'Schiff base' is

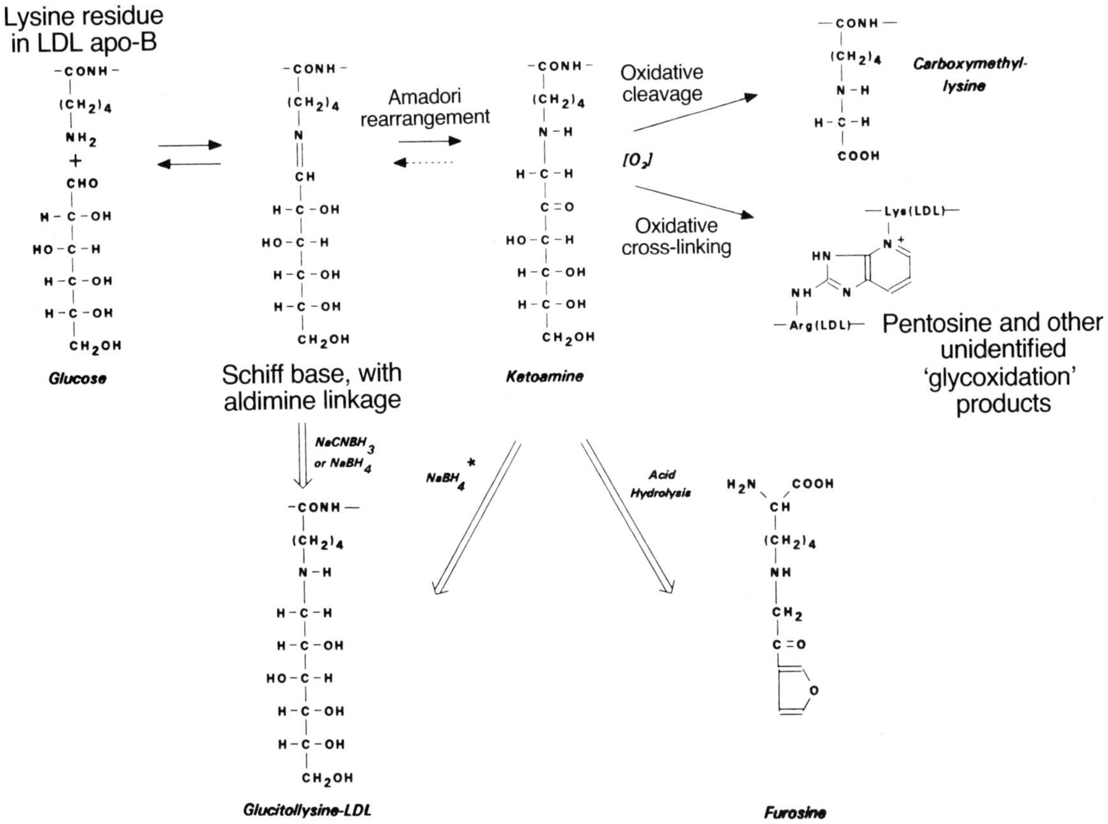


Fig. 23.1. Reactions of early and late glycation, shown affecting low density lipoprotein (LDL). Solid arrows indicate processes occurring *in vivo*, open arrows, processes occurring *in vitro*. *The reduction of the ketoamine product by sodium borohydride yields a mixture of glucitollysine and its stereo-isomer, mannitollysine. (Reprinted by permission of the American Diabetes Association, from Ref. 34.)

generated first: this part of the reaction is readily reversible. Following an Amadori rearrangement, a more stable product, fructose–lysine (FL) is formed. This adduct is *not* called glucose–lysine because of the shift in the position of the carbonyl group during the Amadori rearrangement. Although FL is relatively stable, it has recently been shown that it too may decay, releasing the carbohydrate moiety either as glucose or as more reactive hexoses such as 1- or 3-deoxyglucosone (10). Alternatively, FL may partake in further reactions in the 'browning process' as discussed below. This instability of FL explains the observation that in humans, whether diabetic or not, FL does *not* accumulate with age, even in long-lived proteins such as insoluble collagen (11, 12). Rather it exists in a steady-state relationship with ambient glucose concentration (Fig. 23.2). Thus in diabetes, skin collagen FL levels are increased significantly, but do not correlate either with age or duration of disease (Fig. 23.2). They do, however, correlate with haemoglobin $A_{1c}$ ($HbA_{1c}$), and to a greater extent with the mean of $HbA_{1c}$ values obtained at intervals over several years prior to skin biopsy (12). In diabetes, metabolic alterations directly attributable to increased FL (as opposed to the later products of browning) are perhaps most likely to predominate in short-lived proteins, since these do not exist long enough to accumulate high levels of browning products. In this chapter, the consequences of FL formation both in short-lived plasma proteins (especially lipoproteins), and in long-lived structural proteins, will be discussed.

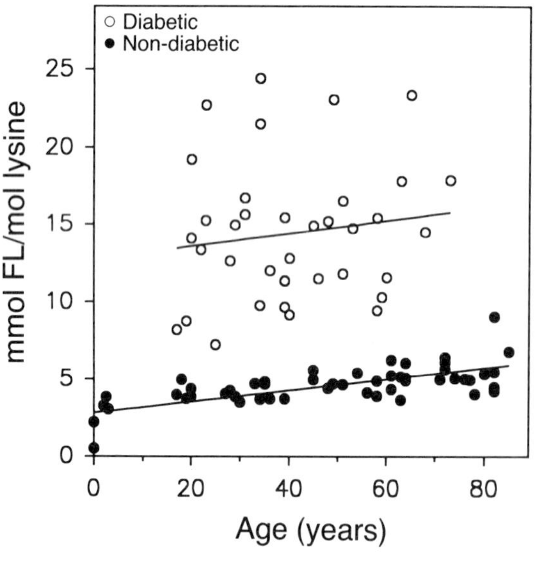


Fig. 23.2. Effects of age and diabetes on glycation of human skin collagen. The equation of the line for control subjects aged >20 years (not shown) is: mmol FL/mol Lys = [0.029 × age (years)] + 3.27 ($r$ = 0.54, $P$ <0.001). There was no significant relationship between age and skin collagen glycation in the diabetic patients. (Reprinted by permission of the American Society for Clinical Investigation, Inc., from Ref. 12.)

## Late glycation

The second stage of glycation is vastly more complex: a series of reactions involving FL or its dissociation products leads to the formation of a profusion of stable end-products. These reactions are collectively termed 'the browning reaction' or 'the Maillard reaction', and the final products are termed 'browning products', 'Maillard reaction products', or 'advanced glycosylation end-products' (AGE). Several recent review articles have addressed the browning process, which is still only partially understood (13–16). Browning products may be derived directly from FL, or may be formed from reactions between proteins and reactive sugars such as 1- and 3-deoxyglucosone released when the FL adduct dissociates, as mentioned above. The numerous final products include species which are coloured, fluorescent, and which constitute cross-links. However, only two of these final products have been identified conclusively (Fig. 23.1): $N^{E}$-carboxymethyllysine (CML) (17) (and the closely related species $N^{E}$-carboxymethylhydroxylysine and 3-($N^{E}$-lysino)-lactic acid (18)), and pentosidine (19). It is now established that both CML and pentosidine, and indeed most, if not all, glucose-derived cross-links are the products of free radical oxidation reactions affecting glycated proteins (20, 21).

CML was first identified by Ahmed *et al.* in 1986 (17), and is a product of free radical-mediated oxidative cleavage of FL (Fig. 23.1). Unlike FL, it accumulates linearly with age in skin collagen in normal individuals, and at an accelerated rate in diabetes (Fig. 23.3) (12). Also, in contrast to FL, its accumulation in skin collagen cannot be reversed by improved glycaemic control, at least in the short-term (22). CML is stable and unreactive, but unlike many 'browning' products, it is not fluorescent and cannot participate in cross-link formation *in vivo*. CML can be formed *in vitro* in reactions between proteins and carbohydrate species other than glucose, including other sugars (pentoses) and ascorbate (23). However, recent unpublished studies by the author's group have shown that plasma pentose levels are not increased in plasma from Type 1 diabetic patients, and that skin collagen CML levels are not increased in non-diabetic guinea pigs whose diets have been supplemented with ascorbate. These findings suggest that the increased levels of CML found in diabetic patients (12) are derived predominantly from glucose. Whatever the origin of the carbohydrate portion of CML, its formation always involves a free-radical oxidation reaction: *in vitro* studies have shown that no CML is formed when collagen is incubated with glucose under anti-oxidant conditions (20). For these reasons, CML may be regarded as the product of combined glycation and free radical oxidation and, at least in skin collagen, may represent a long-term index of combined glycaemic (or 'glycative') and oxidative stresses. The situation with another group of long-lived proteins, the lens crystallins, appears to be different, and is discussed below.

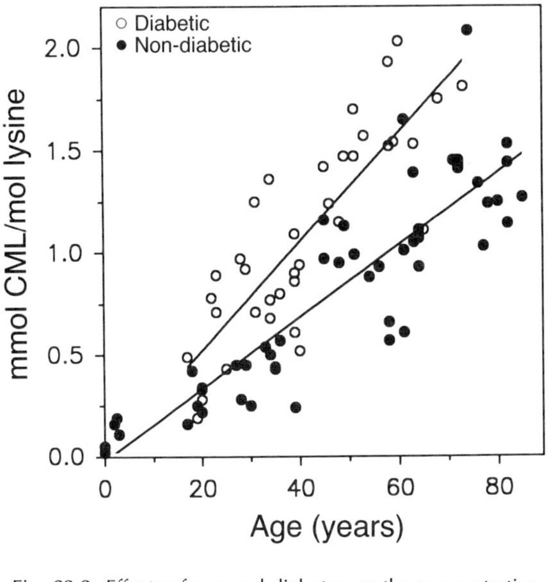


Fig. 23.3. Effects of age and diabetes on the concentration of CML in human skin collagen. The equation of the line for control subjects is: mmol CML/mol Lys = [0.018 × age] − 0.022 ($r$ = 0.89, $P$ <0.001); and for the diabetic patients: mmol CML/mol Lys = [0.027 × age] − 0.015 ($r$ = 0.84, $P$ <0.001). (Reprinted by permission of the American Society for Clinical Investigation, Inc., from Ref. 12.)

The structure of pentosidine, first determined by Sell and Monnier in 1989 (19), is also illustrated in Fig. 23.1. It is a lysine–arginine cross-link which may form between or within protein molecules. Although the structure of pentosidine is entirely different from that of CML, there are many similarities between the two compounds. Like CML, pentosidine accumulates in long-lived proteins in a linear fashion throughout life, and at an accelerated rate in the presence of diabetes (24) (Fig. 23.4). Also in skin collagen, pentosidine levels do not respond to short-term improvements in glycaemic control (22). Pentosidine, as its name suggests, was originally thought to be derived from pentoses, but it is now established that it can also be formed during interactions between proteins and other species, including glucose (25, 26). For reasons similar to those outlined above for CML, the increased levels of pentosidine in diabetes are probably the direct result of elevated glucose levels. Also like CML, the formation of pentosidine is dependent on the presence of an oxidative environment (20, 21), and thus it, too may provide an index of combined glycative and oxidative stresses. Unlike CML, pentosidine is intensely fluorescent (19, 25, 26) and, although it constitutes only a small fraction of total fluorescence in long-lived proteins such as collagen, it may

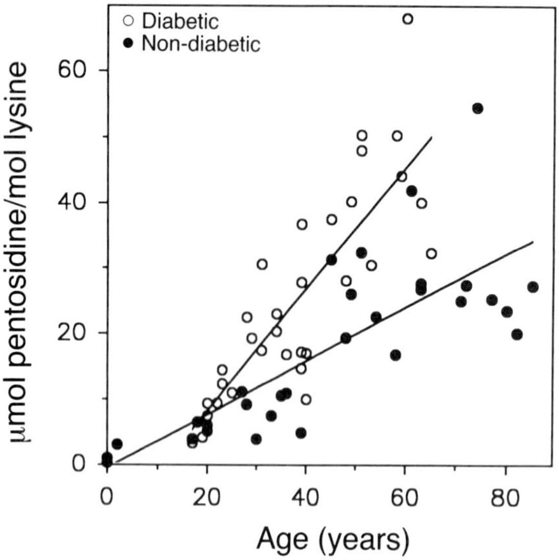


Fig. 23.4. Effects of age and diabetes on the concentration of pentosidine in human skin collagen. The equation of the line for control subjects is: μmol pentosidine/mol Lys = [0.41 × age] − 0.48 ($r$ = 0.78, $P$ <0.001); and for the diabetic patients: μmol pentosidine/mol Lys = [0.93 × age] − 10.27 ($r$ = 0.83, $P$ <0.001). (Reprinted by permission of the American Society for Clinical Investigation, Inc., from Ref. 12.)

be considered a 'biomarker' for total collagen browning (21, 26). As shown in Fig. 23.5 (upper panel), pentosidine levels correlate well with total collagen fluorescence irrespective of age or the presence of diabetes (24). The common origin of CML and pentosidine from combined glycation and oxidation reactions is emphasised by their concerted increases with advancing age and in diabetes (Fig. 23.5, lower panel).

The studies outlined above support the existence of a close inter-relation between glycation and oxidation in the browning of proteins. Indeed, recent evidence suggests that glycation of a protein may actually enhance its susceptibility to oxidative damage (27). To emphasise this inter-relation, the final products of such reactions, including CML and pentosidine, have collectively been termed 'glycoxidation products' (21). Since structural proteins tend to be the longest-lived in the body, they are likely to undergo the greatest degree of glycoxidative modification. Two of the current theories to explain the ageing process are the 'glucose theory of ageing' (28–30) and the 'free-radical

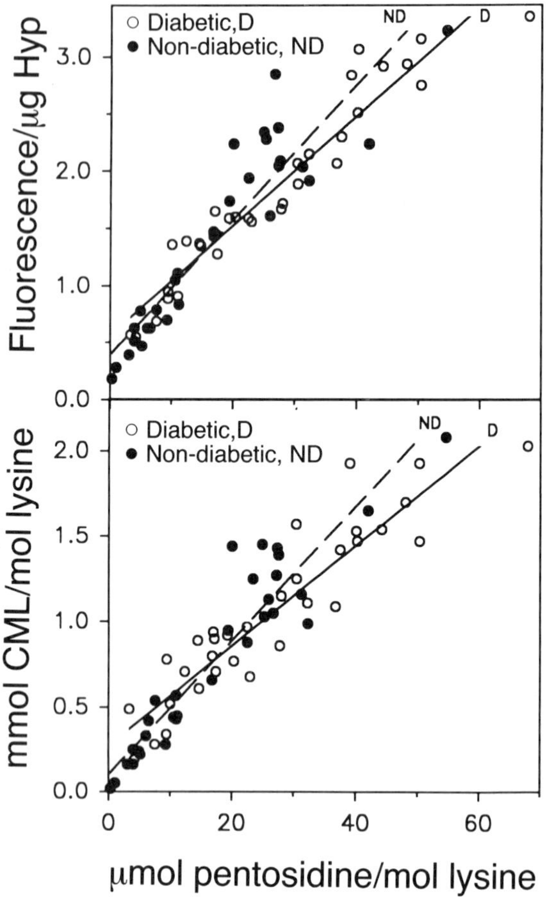


Fig. 23.5. Correlations of fluorescence (upper panel) and CML (lower panel) with pentosidine in skin collagen from the control (non-diabetic) and diabetic groups. Correlation coefficients and $P$-values are as follows: top panel, for the control subjects, fluorescence units/μg Hyp = [0.059 × (μmol pentosidine/mol Lys)] + 0.39 ($r$ = 0.92, $P$ <0.001), and for the diabetic patients, fluorescence units/μg Hyp = [0.048 × (μmol pentosidine/mol Lys)] + 0.57 ($r$ = 0.96, $P$ <0.001); bottom panel, for the control subjects, mmol CML/mol Lys = [0.039 × (μmol pentosidine/mol Lys)] + 0.10 ($r$ = 0.94, $P$ <0.001), and for the diabetic patients, mmol CML/mol Lys = [0.029 × (μmol pentosidine/mol Lys)] + 0.27 ($r$ = 0.92, $P$ <0.001). (Reprinted by permission of the American Society for Clinical Investigation, Inc., from Ref. 12.)

(oxidative) theory of ageing' (31). Clearly, both of these theories are relevant to the formation of glycoxidation products and in a biochemical sense, diabetes may be described as a disease of accelerated ageing (Figs. 23.3 and 23.4). Recent evidence, discussed below, is beginning to allow some tentative conclusions as to whether this accelerated ageing in diabetes is due to enhanced glucose-mediated changes alone, or whether enhanced oxidative stress is also involved.

While glycoxidation may have its greatest pathogenic potential in long-lived proteins, it may be equally important in some proteins which, at least in normal circumstances, are short lived. This may apply especially to lipoprotein particles, whose core lipids are susceptible to oxidative damage. Such damage, particularly affecting unsaturated fatty acids, may be enhanced by free radicals released during increased glycation of apolipoproteins on the surfaces of particles. Resulting free radical-mediated release in the core may, in turn, damage the apolipoprotein itself. Evidence is accumulating that glycated, oxidised and glycoxidised lipoproteins may contribute to the development of both macro- and microvascular diabetic complications.

In this chapter, the consequences of lipoprotein glycoxidation, and glycoxidation of long-lived proteins (lens crystallins and skin collagen), will be discussed, and will be related to the macro- and micro-vascular complications of diabetes.

## GLYCATION OF PLASMA PROTEINS

Plasma proteins are exposed to elevated ambient glucose levels in diabetes, and so it is not surprising that increased glycation has been found in all which have been studied. The evidence that the increased glycation may contribute to the development of macro- and micro-vascular complications is summarised below. Although most plasma proteins are short-lived under normal circumstances, abnormal capillary leakage in diabetes may lead to increased permeation into the extravascular space. There, the plasma proteins may become trapped by the formation of glucose-mediated cross-links, greatly prolonging their existence and leading to much greater glycoxidative modification. This process may be particularly important in the case of lipoproteins, which are unusually susceptible to oxidative damage, and which, as a result, become cytotoxic.

### Consequences of lipoprotein glycation

Abnormalities of plasma lipoprotein levels are recognised as important contributing factors to atherosclerotic disease in the non-diabetic population. In diabetes, unfavourable levels of plasma lipoproteins are frequently present, but these, combined with other recognised cardiovascular risk factors, are insufficient to explain the increased severity of atherosclerotic disease. Thus, diabetes itself has been described as an independent risk factor for the development of atherosclerosis (32). In recent years, the possibility that qualitative, as opposed to quantitative, abnormalities of lipoproteins in diabetes may contribute to the acceleration of macrovascular disease has been the subject of much investigation. More recently still, studies have begun to investigate the hypothesis that glycated, oxidised and glycoxidised lipoproteins may also mediate small vessel damage, and thereby contribute to the microvascular complications of diabetes.

Studies of lipoproteins are hampered by the complex structure of the particles. For example, individual apoproteins on the same particle may differ in age, and therefore may also differ in extent of glycation. This makes *in vitro* simulation of modifications occurring *in vivo* difficult. Also modifications separately affecting the different components of the particles may interact: as mentioned above, the process of protein glycation may generate free radicals which may damage susceptible lipids in the cores of particles, and conversely, oxidation of lipids may lead to apoprotein damage. This problem must be borne in mind when interpreting data: certainly in the earlier work, some of the effects attributed to glycation may have been the result of inadvertent oxidative damage to lipids (e.g. during isolation or *in vitro* glycation). Finally, qualitative alterations of lipoproteins in diabetes may include subtle alterations in their composition. It may be difficult to separate the effects of compositional differences from those due to glycation and oxidation. Of the major classes of lipoproteins, LDL has been the most studied (for review see 33–35): in its case, investigation is facilitated by the fact that each LDL particle has only one apo-protein, apo B-100.

The first measurement of apolipoprotein glycation following exposure to glucose, both *in vitro* and *in vivo*, was in 1981, by Schleicher *et al.* (36). These workers used the 'furosine method', in which furosine, a product of weak acid hydrolysis of FL (Fig. 23.1), is assayed. They incubated normal human lipoproteins (both LDL and HDL) with radio-labelled glucose, and found that the extent of incorporation of glucose into the apolipoprotein components of the particles (apo-$A_1$, $A_2$, B, C and E) was proportional to the period of incubation and to the ambient concentration of glucose. *In vivo*, a two-fold increase in apo-B glycation was found in LDL isolated from diabetic compared with non-diabetic human subjects. Schleicher *et al.* were the first to suggest that increased glycation of lipoproteins occurring *in vivo* might have significant pathophysiological consequences.

## Glycated LDL: interactions with human fibroblasts and murine macrophages

Shortly after the paper by Schleicher *et al.*, Gonen *et al.* (37), Witztum *et al.* (38) and Sasaki & Cottam (39) published studies investigating the metabolism of *in vitro*-glycated LDL by cultured human fibroblasts and mouse peritoneal macrophages. LDL was modified by exposing it to glucose (5–100 mM) for either one or two weeks. In some cases, sodium cyanoborohydride, a reducing agent, was added to enhance the glycation of LDL. Cyanoborohydride reduces and stabilises the Schiff base intermediate of the initial glycation reaction (Fig. 23.1). As mentioned above, Schiff base formation is readily reversible, and so its stabilisation by chemical reduction accelerates and amplifies the modification of proteins by glucose *in vitro*. However, this manoeuvre has significant disadvantages. Firstly, the resulting adduct (glucitol–lysine) differs slightly from FL and, in that sense, is non-physiological. Secondly, the degree of modification attained may be much greater than that which occurs naturally *in vivo*. With these caveats, the studies showed that recognition of 'reductively glycated' LDL by both cell types is indeed altered. Normal human fibroblasts possess the classical LDL receptor, and were unable to bind and degrade glycated LDL as effectively as control LDL. The degree of this impairment was proportional to the extent of glycation of the lipoprotein. The effect was detectable when only 6–8% of lysine residues were modified, and more extensive modification completely abolished recognition of the lipoprotein particles. Examining LDL taken from diabetic patients, a three-fold increase in glycation was found, and in later studies in which LDL was glycated *in vitro* to simulate the extent of glycation occurring in diabetes, Steinbrecher and Witztum (40) found that modification of as few as 2–5% of lysine residues, in the absence of cyanoborohydride, decreased LDL catabolism by human fibroblasts by 5–25%. Once again, the effect was proportional to the degree of glycation. In keeping with these observations, the fractional catabolic rate of radio-labelled glycated LDL injected into guinea pigs and rabbits was significantly lower than that of control LDL. These findings suggest that impaired recognition of glycated LDL could contribute to elevations of plasma LDL-cholesterol levels in diabetic patients in poor glycaemic control.

Interactions between LDL and murine peritoneal macrophages were also studied. These macrophages were chosen as model scavenger cells, but failed to distinguish between control and glycated LDL (37, 38). Contrasting results, however, were obtained with human macrophages, as detailed below.

## *In vivo* glycated LDL: interactions with human fibroblasts and macrophages

Studies performed by the author's group built upon those discussed above. A correlation between the extent of glycation of LDL and other short- and medium-term indicators of glycaemic control (mean plasma glucose, plasma protein glycation and $HbA_{1c}$) was demonstrated, as were detectable increases in LDL glycation even in normolipidaemic Type 1 diabetic patients in satisfactory glycaemic control (41). Compared with control subjects, glycation of apo-B in the diabetic patients was increased 1.6 fold, an increase similar to that of haemoglobin (1.5-fold) and total plasma proteins (2.2-fold) (41).

Cell-lipoprotein interactions using LDL isolated from diabetic patients and control subjects were investigated. Recognition of LDL from Type 1 diabetic patients by human fibroblasts was impaired (42), a result which is in agreement with those described above. In relation to the development of atherosclerosis, interactions of LDL isolated from diabetic patients with cultured human plasma-derived monocyte–macrophages were studied (43). Human monocyte–macrophages are of interest because they are the main precursors of the foam cells characteristic of early atherosclerotic plaques. Like their murine peritoneal counterparts, they are scavenger cells. However, they differed from the murine cells in their response to glycated LDL. When LDL from typical Type I diabetic patients ($HbA_{1c}$ range: 6.4–10.5%) was incubated with human macrophages, it stimulated more cholesteryl ester (CE) synthesis than did LDL from non-diabetic control subjects. Compositional differences were not detectable, and LDL from the diabetic patients appeared to differ only in the extent of apoprotein glycation, which in this study was increased, on average, 1.4-fold. Further supporting a role for glycation in the altered metabolism of LDL from diabetic patients, CE synthesis in the macrophages correlated with the extent of LDL glycation. In concert with the increased CE synthesis, intracellular CE accumulation was also increased. In a later study (44), interactions of human monocyte-macrophages with LDL isolated from patients with Type 2 diabetes and matched non-diabetic control subjects were studied. In this case, however, no increase was found in the rate of CE synthesis by macrophages exposed to LDL from the diabetic patients. This may have been because the Type 2 diabetic patients were in excellent glycaemic control and their mean LDL glycation was increased to a lesser extent (1.2-fold over control values).

These studies suggest, first, that LDL from diabetic patients, compared with that from non-diabetic control subjects, is poorly recognised by the classical LDL receptor, perhaps contributing to hyperlipidaemia in poorly controlled diabetes. Second, in human monocyte–macrophages, glycated LDL may stimulate more CE synthesis, enhancing foam cell formation, and thereby accelerating the atherosclerotic process. Since no other alteration in the particles was detected, in particular no compositional changes, it appears that these effects were dependent upon the increased *in vivo* glycation of apo-B100. While efforts were made to prevent inadvertent oxidative modification of LDL in these studies, lipid peroxidation was not actually measured.

## 'Glycated' and 'non-glycated' subfractions of LDL from donors with and without diabetes

Other recent studies by the author's group, using a different approach, and as yet unpublished, also support the enhanced atherogenicity of glycated LDL. Two fractions of intact LDL can be isolated using boronate affinity chromatography, as described by Jack *et al.* (45). Boronate affinity columns bind FL adducts on proteins, and therefore can trap intact glycated LDL particles. The method can be used to isolate 'bound' and 'non-bound' (i.e. more and less glycated)

LDL fractions from individual patients, and these can be used in lipoprotein–cell interaction studies. The two LDL fractions were isolated from a group of Type 1 diabetic patients and from a group of non-diabetic control subjects. The diabetic group had a mean $HbA_{1c}$ of 9.1%, and mild increases in mean plasma triglycerides and cholesterol. In both groups, glycation of the non-bound fractions was low, and indeed almost identical between the groups. Again in both groups, glycation of the bound fractions was increased: 2-fold in the control subjects and 3-fold in the diabetic patients. The greater increase in glycation per bound LDL particle in diabetic patients suggests that a higher proportion of lysine residues per particle were glycated. This implies that lysine residues other than those which primarily determine binding to the affinity column are glycated in the hyperglycaemic conditions present in diabetes.

The metabolic behaviour of the bound and unbound fractions was studied using human fibroblasts and human monocyte-derived macrophages. With fibroblasts, the findings were similar whether the fractions were obtained from diabetic patients or from non-diabetic subjects. Classical LDL-receptor-mediated degradation of the bound fraction was impaired compared with the non-bound LDL fraction. Non-LDL-receptor-mediated degradation was low in both fractions, and did not differ significantly between them. These results confirmed previous studies in which impaired recognition of glycated LDL by classical LDL-receptors on fibroblasts was observed, and once again the impairment correlated with the degree of glycation of the particle.

With human monocyte–macrophages, contrasting results were obtained, particularly in relation to non-LDL-receptor-mediated degradation. For bound-fraction (highly glycated) LDL, non-LDL-receptor-mediated degradation was increased two-fold if obtained from non-diabetic subjects, and to a greater extent if obtained from diabetic patients. Also with LDL isolated from diabetic patients, classical LDL-receptor-mediated degradation of the bound fraction was mildly impaired. Thus the high levels of glycation in the bound LDL particles from diabetic patients both stimulated their recognition by non-LDL-receptor-mediated mechanisms in macrophages, and impaired their recognition by the classical LDL receptor. In conclusion, these observations confirm again that in humans, glycated LDL is poorly recognised by the classical LDL receptor on fibroblasts, tending to increase plasma LDL levels, and is recognised by another high-capacity, low-affinity pathway on monocyte–macrophages, enhancing uptake by these cells and thereby enhancing foam cell formation.

## *In vitro* glycated LDL: interactions with human macrophages

Further studies were performed by the author's group to investigate and clarify the interaction of human macrophages with glycated LDL, using particles modified *in vitro* under anti-oxidant conditions (46). The *in vitro* modification produced higher levels of glycation (4-fold increases over control) than those found *in vivo* (43), and a proportionately greater effect on macrophage metabolism was observed. Thus, compared with normal LDL, the highly glycated LDL stimulated more CE synthesis, accumulation, and receptor-mediated intracellular degradation in human macrophages.

Investigations were performed to determine the pathway by which these effects were mediated. Recognition of highly glycated LDL by the classical LDL receptor in macrophages, as in fibroblasts, was diminished (46), implying that the increased uptake and degradation of the particle must be mediated through a different pathway. The scavenger receptor was an obvious contender, since another type of *in vitro*-modified LDL, acetyl-LDL, is efficiently taken up by this pathway in macrophages. However, competition studies using acetyl-LDL clearly showed that glycated LDL does not compete for the scavenger receptor pathway. To exclude the possibility that the altered recognition of glycated LDL might be a non-specific effect of glycation, the interaction of control and glycated albumin (native albumin is non-specifically taken up by macrophages) and thyroglobulin (whose molecular weight is similar to that of apolipoprotein B) with macrophages was investigated: degradation of the glycated forms of the proteins was, if anything, decreased rather than increased. To exclude the possibility that the macrophage glycoprotein receptor might be implicated, experiments were performed in the presence of increasing concentrations of yeast mannan, which is known to block this receptor. The mannan had no effect on the degradation of either control or glycated LDL. From the results of these experiments, the existence of a separate, low affinity, high capacity receptor pathway for glycated LDL was proposed.

## Lipoprotein glycation and oxidation

The possible role of enhanced oxidation of lipoproteins in the accelerated development of atherosclerosis in diabetes has been reviewed recently (33). Lipoproteins contain varying amounts of unsaturated fatty acids in their cores, and these are vulnerable to oxidative damage. Oxidised LDL is a potent stimulator of foam cell formation by macrophages (47–49) and, in the vascular wall, is cytotoxic to nearby cells (50–54) and chemotactic to monocytes (55, 56), the cells from which macrophages are derived. The processes of oxidation and glycation are closely linked (21). Both FL and simple monosaccharides may 'auto-oxidise' under physiological conditions, in the presence of traces of metal ions, generating superoxide radicals (27, 57). Thus, glycation of apolipoproteins may enhance the likelihood of oxidative damage to core lipids. Despite this, there is little evidence that oxidation of plasma lipoproteins is increased in uncomplicated diabetes, whereas glycation clearly is. Also no studies exist to demonstrate a correlation between oxidation of plasma lipoproteins and glycaemic control in diabetic patients. Nevertheless, the situation may well be different for extravasated lipoproteins sequestered in vessel walls. In these, glycation, oxidation and glycoxidation may combine to generate vicious cycles of vascular injury (33). Concomitant glycation and glycoxidation of vascular connective tissue proteins may encourage further covalent, glucose-mediated, binding of lipoproteins (58), trapping them in the media, and permitting greater degrees of modification and, hence, greater generation of free radicals, than could otherwise occur.

## LDL glycation/glycoxidation and coagulation/fibrinolysis

Increased glycation of LDL may influence platelet aggregation. Watanabe *et al.* (59) isolated LDL from young, Type 1 diabetic patients (in good-to-fair glycaemic control) and from age- and sex-matched non-diabetic control subjects. Once again, glycation of LDL from the diabetic patients was increased, while LDL composition was similar in the two groups. LDL from the diabetic patients was found to be the more potent stimulator of thromboxane B2 release and thrombin-induced platelet aggregation. LDL glycated *in vitro* also caused a marked enhancement in thrombin-, collagen-, and ADP-induced platelet aggregation, but this enhancement occurred irrespective of the concentration of glucose used in the incubation, the lowest concentration of glucose (10 mmol/l) being almost as effective as the highest (150 mmol/l). Clearly then, the effect was not linearly related to the extent of LDL glycation, and subtle alterations in the composition of platelet membranes, induced by interaction with glycated LDL, were suggested to explain the effects on platelet behaviour. Finally, when boronate affinity chromatography was used to isolate bound and non-bound fractions of LDL from Type 1 diabetic patients as described above, platelet aggregation was enhanced to a significantly greater extent by the bound (highly glycated) than the non-bound fraction (60).

The effects of modified LDL on the fibrinolytic system have also been studied. In the author's group, Jokl *et al.* (61) recently showed that LDL isolated from diabetic patients, and also normal LDL oxidized *in vitro,* failed to stimulate the expected release of the pro-fibrinolytic protein tissue plasminogen activator (tPA) by cultured human umbilical vein endothelial cells. Furthermore, they found that glycoxidised LDL increased the release of an inhibitor of fibrinolysis, plasminogen activator inhibitor 1 (PAI-1) by retinal capillary endothelial cells (62).

All of the above observations suggest that modifications of LDL occurring in diabetes may contribute to an increased tendency towards thrombosis.

## LDL glycation/glycoxidation and diabetic retinopathy

On-going studies by the author's group are investigating the hypothesis that modifications of LDL in diabetes may contribute to micro- as well as macro-vascular complications. The possibility that glycoxidised LDL may mediate an increased tendency to thrombosis in retinal vessels has already been mentioned. Other studies have shown that mild *in vitro* glycation or oxidation renders normal LDL toxic to cultured retinal capillary endothelial cells and pericytes (63). The toxicity is further enhanced by glycoxidation of LDL. These data suggest that modified LDL may contribute to the initiation of retinopathy by injuring endothelial cells, thereby causing capillary leakage, i.e. breakdown of the blood–retinal barrier. Later, when extravasated and more severely modified, LDL may also contribute to the propagation of retinopathy, causing further damage to both endothelial cells and pericytes, and perhaps to the lipid-rich retinal neural tissue as well.

## Glycation of VLDL and HDL

Increased glycation of VLDL and HDL apoproteins were demonstrated by Curtiss and Witztum (64), and as with LDL, are believed to have effects on the cellular interactions, function and metabolism of these particles. VLDL isolated from normolipeamic patients with both Type 1 and Type 2 diabetes stimulated increased CE synthesis and accumulation in cultured human monocyte-macrophages (44, 65). This effect, however, is less marked than with LDL. Subtle alterations in apoprotein composition are also present in VLDL from diabetic patients (66), so the observed metabolic differences cannot be attributed to increased glycation with confidence. Investigation of the consequences of VLDL glycation is further hampered by the difficulty of measuring the degree of modification of the several apoproteins on the VLDL particle, known to differ because of differing plasma residence times. Resorting to *in vitro*-glycated VLDL is unsatisfactory because the differential glycation of its apoproteins, occurring *in vivo,* cannot be reproduced. At present, therefore, it appears that increased glycation of VLDL apoproteins may have important consequences, but this has not yet been convincingly proven.

Similar problems must be borne in mind when interpreting studies investigating the effects of glycation of HDL. Ten years ago, Witztum *et al.* (67) showed that when HDL was glycated *in vitro,* its clearance from the circulation in guinea pigs was accelerated, an effect opposite to that observed with glycated LDL. This enhanced clearance occurred even after mild degrees of glycation, and might partially explain the low plasma levels of HDL in diabetic patients. More recently, Duell *et al.* (68) demonstrated impaired high-affinity binding of glycated HDL to fibroblasts, and a diminished capacity to remove cholesterol from peripheral cells (69). Glycation of HDL may therefore contribute to the increased risk for atherosclerotic disease in diabetic patients.

## LDL modification and the immune system

Glycation, and particularly glycoxidation, of LDL may alter its structure sufficiently to provoke an immune response (70, 71). Initial studies of this possibility (71) used LDL glycated *in vitro* in the presence and absence of cyanoborohydride (Fig. 23.1), producing heavily (60% of lysine residues glycated) and mildly (6% of lysine residues glycated) modified particles, respectively. The heavily modified particles were strongly immunogenic but, as detailed above, they contain glucitol–lysine, a product of 'reductive glycation' which does not form *in vivo*. FL, which does form *in vivo*, was not recognised by the antibody raised against reductively-glycated LDL. The FL present in mildly modified LDL proved to be a much less potent immunogen, but nevertheless, control LDL, which always contains some glycated LDL, and to a greater extent, *in vitro*-glycated LDL, both competed for the resulting antibody. The presence of antibodies against 'true' glycated LDL, i.e. that which contains FL, had no effect on its rate of clearance from plasma (72). However, the existence of even low levels of such antibodies is probably important, because LDL–immune complexes (LDL–IC) are now known to be potently atherogenic (see below). In addition, the more severely modified ('glycoxidised') lipoproteins sequestered in vessel walls are potentially more immunogenic than the less modified particles found in plasma, and are likely to stimulate *in situ* formation of immune complexes (73).

Recently it has been shown that LDL–IC are potent inducers of foam cell formation by human monocyte-derived macrophages (74–78). Transformation of these cells can be induced either by insoluble LDL–IC, presented to the macrophages as large aggregates (75), or by soluble LDL–IC presented to the macrophages adsorbed to red blood cells (RBC) (76). Both types of LDL–IC may be formed *in vivo*. Subendothelial LDL deposits are thought to stimulate LDL–IC formation *in situ*, probably resulting in insoluble aggregates. In plasma, soluble LDL–IC are likely to be formed in antigen excess: they are adsorbed to red blood cells, and then transported to organs rich in tissue macrophages (e.g. the liver) where they can be transferred to phagocytic cells and catabolised (79). *In vitro*, these red cell-bound soluble LDL–IC are 15-fold more potent than insoluble LDL–IC in inducing foam cell formation (76).

Paradoxically, while inducing foam cell formation, LDL–IC also stimulate a substantial *increase* (approximately 20-fold) in LDL receptor activity (75, 77, 78). This surprising observation has not yet been explained, but presumably represents another mechanism by which LDL–IC may accelerate foam cell formation. Additionally, LDL–IC stimulate the release of the cytokines interleukin-1 (IL-1) and tumour necrosis factor α (TNF-α) by macrophages (80), an effect which may mediate vascular injury. Acting on endothelial cells, IL-1 induces synthesis and cell surface expression of procoagulant activity (81), increases vascular permeability (82), promotes the release of platelet activating factor (83), increases neutrophil adherence (84, 85), and induces further IL-1 release by a positive feedback mechanism (86). It may indirectly stimulate fibroblast and smooth muscle cell proliferation by inducing production of platelet-derived growth factor AA (PDGF-AA) by these cells, thereby activating an autocrine growth regulating mechanism (87). Both IL-1 and TNF-α may contribute to hyperlipidaemia (88), a common feature of poorly controlled diabetes, and both can enhance the expression of vascular cell adherence molecules (VCAMs) on endothelial cells (89). However, IL-1 also induces secretion of prostaglandins by smooth muscle cells (90), and since prostaglandins have growth-inhibiting properties, the net *in vivo* effect of IL-1 release by macrophages in vascular walls remains unclear. TNF-α, which is produced not only by macrophages but also by smooth muscle cells, induces some other responses similar to those of IL-1, including cell surface expression of procoagulant activity (81) and production of IL-1 by endothelial cells (91).

In conclusion, both types of LDL-IC (soluble and insoluble) induce profound alterations in lipoprotein metabolism by monocyte-derived macrophages, and these may well promote both micro- and macro-vascular disease in diabetes.

### Consequences of glycation of other plasma constituents

#### Glycation and antithrombin III activity

Increased glycation of antithrombin III has been found to impair its thrombin-inhibiting activity (92), perhaps contributing to the enhanced tendency to thrombosis in diabetes. This inhibition of antithrombin III activity is completely reversible by an excess of sodium heparin. Consistent with this observation, an inverse correlation between antithrombin III activity and both $HbA_{1c}$ and plasma glucose, independent of plasma concentrations of antithrombin III, has been described (93). In contrast, *in vitro* glycation of fibrinogen was not found to influence its function, and therefore does not appear to promote thrombosis (94).

## GLYCATION AND GLYCOXIDATION OF STRUCTURAL PROTEINS

In this section, the effects of glycation and glycoxidation on lens crystallins will be discussed briefly. There will follow a more detailed discussion of effects on the major structural protein of the body, collagen.

### Lens crystallins

The effects of glycation and glycoxidation on lens crystallins are of interest because cataract formation, a feature of ageing, tends to occur earlier in diabetic than in non-diabetic patients (95–97). Also, lens proteins are among the longest-lived in the body, and therefore provide an interesting model for the study of the ageing process. Perhaps, in order to protect lens proteins from the effects of glucose-mediated ageing, glucose levels in the aqueous humour are normally about 50% of those in plasma (98), and in the lens itself they may only be 20% of plasma levels (99). Anti-oxidant mechanisms in the lens may also be important in the prevention of age-related changes. Consistent with this belief, dietary antioxidant therapy can prevent or delay the development of acute 'sugar' (or 'metabolic') cataracts in diabetic animals (100, 101), and lipid peroxidation products are increased in diabetic compared with non-diabetic 'senile-type' cataracts (102). On scrutiny, however, these observations do not provide very strong support for increased oxidative stress in the formation of the common senile-type cataract seen in diabetic patients. Observations concerning acute metabolic cataracts in animals are of questionable relevance not only because of species difference, but also because the acute metabolic cataract develops very differently, and is morphologically distinct from, the senile-type cataract. The observation of increased lipid peroxidation may be explained by increased permeation of lipids into the lens due to disruption of the blood–aqueous and blood–retinal barriers in diabetes. Of course, such permeation could, in itself, increase oxidative stress in the lens. Breakdown of the blood–aqueous and blood–retinal barriers in diabetes might be expected to result in disproportionate increases in glucose levels in the aqueous humour, and in the lens, in comparison with plasma. There is evidence that such large changes in glucose levels do indeed occur. DiMattio *et al.* (103) observed that permeation of glucose from the plasma to both the aqueous and vitreous compartments is abnormally high in diabetic rats. Also, damage to the ocular vasculature, with increased permeability documented by both vitreous and aqueous humour fluorophotometry (104, 105), has been identified as an early abnormality in diabetes.

Several studies investigated levels of FL and glycoxidation products in lens crystallins from non-diabetic individuals over a wide range of ages, and from diabetic and non-diabetic patients with 'senile-type' cataracts (15, 106–108). In non-diabetic patients, FL in lens crystallins changed little with advancing age (107), while CML steadily increased. These changes were similar to those observed for insoluble skin collagen (described above). Among cataract patients, those with diabetes had increases in lens crystallin FL (>4-fold) which were disproportionate to the increases in plasma glucose or $HbA_1$ (both <2-fold): this is consistent with the hypothesis that there is abnormal entry of glucose into the lens in diabetes (108). No increase in lens crystallin FL was observed in non-diabetic cataract patients, suggesting that the barriers to glucose in these patients remain intact, despite their cataracts. These findings are consistent with, but do not prove, a role for increased intra-lenticular glucose and/or FL in the acceleration of cataract formation in diabetic patients.

The results of measurements of glycoxidation products in the lens were somewhat surprising. Among cataract patients, age-corrected pentosidine levels were increased in those with diabetes, as might be expected, but CML levels were not. Indeed, age-corrected CML levels were similar in both groups of cataract patients to those in normal, non-diabetic, non-cataractous subjects. The increase in pentosidine suggests that enhanced glucose-mediated cross-linking does occur in lens crystallins in diabetic patients, and therefore could contribute to accelerated cataract formation. Such a conclusion is supported by a recent study using immunological techniques to identify AGE products in the lenses of diabetic rats (109). The absence of any increase in CML, however, suggests that, in the lens, CML may be formed primarily from species other than glucose, e.g. ascorbate (though pentosidine can also be formed from ascorbate). Consistent with an alternative origin for CML, lens crystallin CML accumulates with age in normal individuals at a much faster rate than collagen CML (23), even though proteins in the lens are exposed to much lower ambient glucose levels. Irrespective of the origin of its carbohydrate portion, the formation of CML is thought always to involve free radical oxidation. Thus the surprisingly low levels of CML in cataractous lenses from diabetic patients argue *against* the presence of increased oxidative stress in the lens in senile-type diabetic cataract.

In conclusion, senile-type cataracts, commonly seen in older diabetic patients, are morphologically similar, but biochemically distinct, from those occurring in non-diabetic patients. Increased glycation and glucose-mediated cross-linking may accelerate their formation, but it seems unlikely that increased oxidative stress is involved.

## Collagen

Of the long-lived structural proteins of the body, collagen in its various forms has been the most studied. In relation to diabetes, investigators have generally utilised skin and tendon collagen, but the nature of the glycation and browning reactions makes it reasonable to extrapolate the physico-chemical alterations observed in these collagens to those in other sites, including sites relevant to the micro- and macro-vascular complications of diabetes. Thus, glycoxidative changes occurring in Type 1 collagen in skin are considered likely to be reflected in structural collagens in vessel walls and basement membranes. Also, parallel changes probably take place in other connective tissue proteins, such as elastin, fibronectin and laminin. These proteins will not be discussed further in this chapter, but the effects of glycation on laminin have recently been well reviewed by Charonis and Tsilibary (110).

### Alterations in the physical properties of collagens with ageing and in diabetes: relationship with glycation, browning and glycoxidation

As people age, their collagen becomes increasingly insoluble, thermally stable, and resistant to enzymatic attack (111). These changes are so predictable that it is possible to determine the age of individuals with reasonable accuracy by studying their collagen (112). The altered properties of collagen with age are accompanied by, and are thought to be caused by, the formation of stable cross-links. Many of the cross-links are derived from glucose via the browning process, leading one to expect that age-related changes might be exaggerated in the presence of diabetes. Studies over the past 20 years have demonstrated that this is indeed so. In 1975, Hamlin *et al.* (113) found that prediction of the ages of patients by measurement of collagen digestibility failed in the presence of diabetes: three diabetic patients whose true ages were 33, 41 and 44 years were predicted to be aged 84, 103 and 106 years respectively. More recently, it has been shown that the browning process and the formation of cross-links in collagen are also dependent on the presence of an oxidative environment (20). The evidence that the accelerated biochemical ageing of proteins in diabetes is indeed mediated by the separate, but interrelated, processes of glycation and oxidation is presented below.

## Effects of *in vitro* modification of structural proteins on their physico-chemical properties

Initially, to determine whether increased glycation of collagen could be responsible for the changes in its physical properties, experiments were performed using collagen incubated with glucose *in vitro*. Short-term (one-week) incubations (performed under oxidative conditions) did not cause any increase in resistance to proteolytic digestion (114), although they did increase the stability of rat tail tendons (115). In longer-term incubations, spectrophotometric changes developing in lens crystallin (another very long-lived protein) were similar to those occurring with age (28), and thermal stability of basement membrane collagens was enhanced (116). Recent studies, in which rat tail collagen was incubated with glucose, have shown that, while collagen cross-linking depends on the presence of glucose, it can be inhibited by anti-oxidant conditions (20). With glucose present, the anti-oxidant conditions inhibited the formation of CML, pentosidine, and collagen fluorescence, while having no effect on the formation of FL. In summary, *in vitro* studies suggest that in collagen, the development of cross-links, increased fluorescence, and the accumulation of the specific products CML and pentosidine, are dependent not only on the presence of glucose, but also of an oxidant environment.

## Glycation, glycoxidation and browning of collagen in diabetes

In 1979, Rosenberg *et al.* (117) were the first to compare collagen glycation (FL content) in animals with and without diabetes. They demonstrated a significant increase in glycation of aortic collagen in diabetic rats, and suggested that it might be relevant to accelerated atherogenesis in diabetes. Increased glycation of collagen in diabetes was later confirmed in rat glomerular basement membranes (118), human tendon and skin (12, 119–122), and human aorta, glomerular basement membrane and tendon (123, 124).

Results of recent studies on skin collagen by the author's group have already been summarised and discussed in the section describing the chemistry of glycation (see also Figs. 23.2–23.5). Briefly, in non-diabetic subjects, collagen glycation increases only very slightly between the ages of 20 and 80 years (11, 12). In diabetes, glycation of insoluble skin collagen is increased, but is unrelated to age or duration of disease. It correlates with $HbA_1$ (121), and more closely with $HbA_1$ averaged over several years before the skin sample was taken (12). It decreases promptly after a relatively short (4-month) period of improved glycaemic control (22). All of these findings suggest that collagen glycation is in a steady-state relationship with ambient glucose concentrations.

In contrast to FL, glycoxidation products in insoluble collagen accumulate continuously from birth to death (11, 12, 19). The rate of their accumulation is accelerated in diabetic patients (12, 113, 125, 126), and thus middle-aged or even young diabetic patients may develop levels higher than those seen even in the oldest non-diabetic subject (12, 113). The extent of this excessive accumulation in individual diabetic patients may depend not only on duration of diabetes and average glycaemic control, but also on individual susceptibility to oxidative stress (12). That individuals differ in their capacity to resist oxidative stress is suggested by the degree of variation in the levels of glycoxidation products among elderly non-diabetic subjects (Figs. 23.3 and 23.4). Since these subjects have little variation in their plasma glucose levels, variations in the CML or pentosidine content of their skin collagen may be attributed to variations in oxidative stress or in anti-oxidant defences. Analysis of glycoxidation products in skin collagen and lens crystallins from diabetic patients provides no evidence that there is an inherent increase in oxidative stress caused by the presence of diabetes (12). In other words, on average, the increased accumulation of glycoxidation products in collagen from diabetic patients can be explained by the increase glycation alone (taking into account duration of diabetes) without invoking an increase in oxidative stress. Nevertheless, the accumulation of glycoxidation products, whether or not diabetes is present, is thought to be irreversible (22). This is ominous if, as suspected from the evidence discussed below, excessive accumulation of these products plays a role, directly or indirectly, in the development of diabetic complications. The ability to resist oxidative stress may therefore modulate the consequences of hyperglycaemia, and diabetic patients who have relatively poor anti-oxidant defences may be particularly vulnerable to developing complications. More optimistically, the dual origin of glycoxidation products (from both glycaemic and oxidative stresses) may lead to the ability to predict, soon after the onset of diabetes, a subgroup of patients who are particularly susceptible to complications. Also, a better understanding of the origin of these products opens up a number of possible interventions to inhibit their formation.

## Evidence relating early-stage collagen glycation products and complications

Initial studies sought a relationship between FL levels in skin collagen and complication status (121, 122). At the time it was believed that FL levels in collagen might represent a very long-term index of glycaemic control (much longer than $HbA_{1c}$). Now it is known that collagen FL responds promptly to improved glycaemic control (22), and conversely, rises rapidly after the onset of diabetes (12). Coupled with the evidence that *in vitro*, early glycation does little to alter the properties of collagen, it therefore appears unlikely that FL contributes *directly* to the development of complications. An early study by the author's group found no association between collagen FL levels and the presence or severity of limited joint mobility in Type 1 diabetic patients (121). Subsequently, Vishwanath *et al.* confirmed this, and in addition found no association between collagen FL levels and retinopathy, nephropathy or arterial stiffness (122). These results, however, do not exclude the possibility that FL in collagen may contribute *indirectly* to complications, by generating the later, more permanent, products of advanced glycation. Consistent with this, and in contrast to the findings described above, a recent study by the author's group found skin collagen FL levels to be independently associated with the presence of retinopathy and early nephropathy (microalbuminuria) (24).

## Evidence relating collagen glycoxidation products and complications

Theoretically, the accumulation of glycoxidation products, which alters the properties of collagen, is more likely than FL to cause functional abnormalities in collagen-containing tissues. Monnier and co-workers found an association between both collagen-linked fluorescence (in insoluble skin collagen) (125) and pentosidine content (127) and the severity of diabetic retinopathy, joint stiffness, and arterial stiffness. A relation-

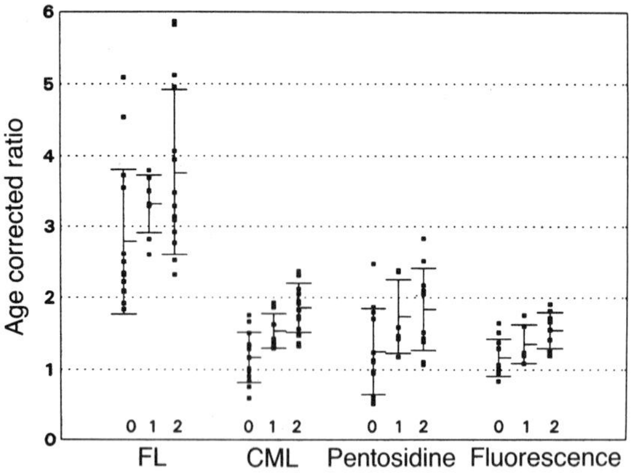


Fig. 23.6. Maillard products in skin collagen and retinopathy status. Grade 0: no retinopathy; grade 1: background retinopathy; Grade 2: proliferative retinopathy. Bars show mean ±1SD in each category. FL, CML, pentosidine and total fluorescence all increased progressively with increasing severity of retinopathy ($P < 0.05$, $P < 0.001$, $P < 0.05$, $P < 0.01$, respectively). Using logistic regression to control for duration of diabetes, FL, CML, and total fluorescence remained independently associated with retinopathy. (Reprinted by permission of the American Society for Clinical Investigation, Inc., from Ref. 24.)

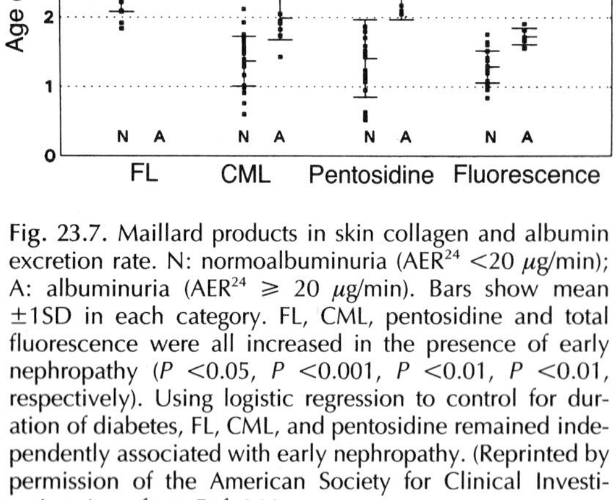


Fig. 23.7. Maillard products in skin collagen and albumin excretion rate. N: normoalbuminuria ($AER^{24}$ <20 μg/min); A: albuminuria ($AER^{24}$ ⩾ 20 μg/min). Bars show mean ±1SD in each category. FL, CML, pentosidine and total fluorescence were all increased in the presence of early nephropathy ($P < 0.05$, $P < 0.001$, $P < 0.01$, $P < 0.01$, respectively). Using logistic regression to control for duration of diabetes, FL, CML, and pentosidine remained independently associated with early nephropathy. (Reprinted by permission of the American Society for Clinical Investigation, Inc., from Ref. 24.)

ship between collagen browning and diabetic nephropathy was found in a study by Makita *et al.* (128). A recent study by the author's group has shown that levels of specific glycoxidation products and fluorescence in insoluble collagen increase with severity of retinopathy (Fig. 23.6), and with the presence of early nephropathy (Fig. 23.7) (24). Controlling for age and duration of diabetes, independent associations of CML with retinopathy and early nephropathy, and of pentosidine with early nephropathy, were demonstrated (24).

## Mechanisms by which glycoxidation of vascular wall structural proteins may contribute directly to the development of diabetic complications

Of the mechanisms summarised below, some have substantial supporting evidence, while others are more speculative.

### Abnormal vascular rigidity and tone

Monnier *et al.* showed that increased skin collagen fluorescence in Type 1 diabetic patients was associated with increased arterial stiffness (assessed *in vivo*), and with elevated systolic and diastolic blood pressures (125). The presence of increased aortic stiffness in patients with Type 1 diabetes was confirmed in autopsy studies by Oxlund *et al.* (129), but in this case the level of glycoxidation products was not determined. The loss of elasticity and compliance of arteries and arterioles in diabetes is probably due, at least in part, to increased glucose-mediated cross-linking. This may contribute directly to the development of hypertension, while arterial stiffness and hypertension together may result in abnormal endothelial shear stresses, predisposing to injury and the development of atherosclerosis. In smaller vessels, similar effects may contribute to the development of diabetic retinopathy and nephropathy.

Recent evidence suggests that both *in vitro* and *in vivo*, the presence of collagen glycoxidation products quenches the activity of nitric oxide (endothelium-derived relaxing factor, EDRF) (130). This leads to an impairment of endothelium-mediated vasodilation, which could cause abnormalities in vascular tone. Resulting abnormalities of flow, perfusion and blood pressure may contribute to arterial and arteriolar damage.

### Covalent binding of plasma constituents

Endothelial injury allows increased permeation of plasma constituents into the vessel wall, where they come into contact with elevated levels of connective tissue glycoxidation products. Brownlee *et al.*(58) found increased binding of LDL to collagen when the lipoprotein was exposed to modified collagen (containing browning products). In diabetic compared to non-diabetic animals, cross-linking of LDL to aortic collagen was increased 2.5-fold. Trapped in a high-glucose environment in the vessel wall, the LDL particles may undergo more extensive glycoxidative modification, with further increases in atherogenicity. Free radical chain reactions in the trapped LDL may damage not only the lipids within the particle, but also neighbouring structural proteins and cells. It has been shown, for instance, that products of lipid peroxidation stimulate cross-linking of collagen (131). In diabetes, these inter-related mechanisms are likely to result in various vicious cycles, leading to damage of the arterial wall and *in situ* formation of lipoprotein–immune complexes (73), further accelerating foam cell formation.

### The macrophage 'AGE-receptor'

As discussed above, monocyte/macrophages are intimately involved in the development of atherosclerotic lesions. It is now established that these cells possess a specific receptor which recognises glycoxidation products: this has been termed the 'AGE receptor', and has been shown to be distinct from other scavenger receptors (132). Macrophages expressing this receptor are capable of engulfing not just protein molecules, but also entire cells which have glycoxidation products on their surface (133). The presence of glycoxidation (or 'AGE') products in vessel walls is chemotactic to circulating monocyte/macrophages, inducing them to migrate through the vascular endothelium (134). Also, the interaction of AGE-proteins with the AGE-receptor has been shown to be accompanied by release of cytokines, TNF-$\alpha$ and IL-1 (135), which are known to mediate growth and remodelling processes, and which, as previously discussed, may accelerate the atherosclerotic process.

### Renal impairment

Accumulation of glycoxidation products may contribute to the development of renal impairment in diabetes (24, 125, 127, 128). This suggests that a generalised collagen abnormality may underlie the development of microalbuminuria, and this may partly explain the identification of microalbuminuria as a risk factor for macrovascular disease. The hypertension and lipid abnormalities associated with renal impairment may further contribute to the development of atherosclerosis.

## Glycoxidation of collagen and diabetic complications: alternative hypotheses

The results of the studies discussed above demonstrate *associations* between the levels of both FL and glycoxidation products in collagen and the presence or severity of diabetic complications. These data are compatible with, but do not prove, the hypothesis that these products may, at least in part, contribute to the development of complications. In the case of FL, the causative role may be indirect, FL being the relatively harmless precursor of damaging glycoxidation products. It is also possible that the increased levels of FL and the presence of complications may be related only in so far as both arise from a common origin: prolonged hyperglycaemia. In the case of glycoxidation products, which significantly alter the properties of collagen, a direct causative role in the development of complications is easy to envisage, and has considerable credibility. Here too, however, the case is not proven: like FL, glycoxidation products may simply reflect long-term hyperglycaemia, and complications may arise, perhaps in association with hyperglycaemia, but through other unrelated mechanisms. Evidence from recent studies by Brownlee and co-workers using aminoguanidine, a hydrazine which inhibits the browning process by binding to reactive carbonyl groups (136), has tended to refute this view. Aminoguanidine is thought to act by blocking reactive dicarbonyl browning intermediates derived from the dissociation of FL (137). It has little or no effect on the early stage of glycation, but has been successful in preventing the browning process both *in vitro* and *in vivo* (136, 137). Studies in experimental animals have shown that aminoguanidine can inhibit the cross-linking of collagen in arterial walls (136), and that it retards the development of diabetic nephropathy (138), neuropathy (139, 140) and retinopathy (141). It should be mentioned however, that the mode of action of aminoguanidine is controversial: some investigators believe that, to a significant extent, its effects are due to inhibition of nitric oxide synthase, rather than inhibition of browning (142).

### A 'glycoxidative stress' hypothesis for the development of diabetic complications

All of the above considerations may be synthesised into a new hypothesis. This states that, rather than the absolute levels of glycoxidation products in collagen, it is the *rate* of their formation (a measure of 'glycoxidative stress') which may be important in determining the risk of complications. This would explain why elderly, non-diabetic patients, despite having high levels of collagen glycoxidation products, do not develop diabetic complications. According to this hypothesis, combinations of high glycaemic and oxidative stress may mediate tissue damage. Patients experiencing these high stresses over time will accumulate a permanent 'record' in their long-lived proteins, including insoluble collagen. While the changes in collagen may be important, the real damage may result from the chronic effect of these stresses on other substrates, e.g. lipoproteins. Aminoguanidine may act by reducing glycoxidative damage not just to collagen, but also to these other substrates. For example, it has recently been shown to inhibit oxidative damage to LDL (143, 144). Patients who inherently (i.e. unrelated to their diabetes) have relatively poor anti-oxidant defences, and are unfortunate enough also to develop diabetes, may be particularly vulnerable to complications, and thus oxidative stress may be said to modulate the consequences of hyperglycaemia. This hypothesis is supported by preliminary, unpublished data from the author's group. Analysis of levels of skin collagen glycoxidation products in patients with Type 1 diabetes (24) revealed that, among patients with diabetes for over 10 years, those with retinopathy had experienced faster overall accumulation rates of CML and pentosidine (controlling for long-term glycaemia and duration of diabetes) than those without retinopathy. Indeed, patients with retinopathy appeared to have been converting FL to CML and pentosidine in skin collagen almost twice as quickly as those without retinopathy. The subset of patients whose data could be analysed in this way was very small: nevertheless, the difference in rates of accumulation almost achieved statistical significance ($p < 0.06$). Further studies are needed.

## PRACTICAL IMPLICATIONS: REDUCING GLYCOXIDATIVE STRESS

If 'glycoxidative stress' is indeed a significant risk factor in the development of macro- and microvascular complications of diabetes, then clearly it would be desirable to reduce this stress. By so doing, chronic recurring damage to short-lived species, like LDL, and cumulative damage to long-lived species, like collagen, could be minimised. Ways to inhibit the 'glycative' and 'oxidative' arms of the process may be considered separately.

## Reducing 'glycative' stress

The most obvious measure to decrease glycation is to optimise glycaemic control, minimising FL formation. Furthermore, existing FL levels may be reduced: even in long-lived proteins, improved glycaemic control has been shown to reduce FL content within a few months (22), and this should decrease the subsequent formation of glycoxidation products. In the future, pharmacological intervention using aminoguanidine, or similar agents, may inhibit browning by binding to the reactive dissociation products of FL.

## Reducing oxidative stress

At present there is little direct evidence concerning the efficacy of any treatment aimed to reduce oxidative damage to proteins and lipids in diabetes. Probucol may be effective in reducing lipid peroxidation (145), and may therefore have a protective effect in the vessel wall (146–148). Butylated hydroxytoluene may have similar effects (149, 150). Aminoguanidine, in addition to inhibiting collagen cross-linking, may also inhibit lipid peroxidation (143), but it remains an experimental agent. Another class of experimental agents, the 'leumedins' (*N*-(fluorenyl-9-methoxycarbonyl) amino acids (151)) have recently shown promise in inhibiting LDL modification (152). Relatively simple dietary interventions are perhaps the most attractive. Recently, Reaven *et al.* have shown that a diet in which mono-unsaturated fats are substituted for poly-unsaturated or saturated fats results in LDL which is less susceptible to oxidative damage (153). Dietary supplementation of free radical scavengers may be useful. Of these, ascorbate is believed to be the most important (154), and plasma levels of this, and platelet levels of Vitamin E, another free radical scavenger, tend to be abnormally low in diabetic patients (155,156). Dietary supplements of these vitamins therefore seem reasonable, providing a cheap, low-risk intervention. Unfortunately, these same advantages, by leading to widespread use, are likely to impede investigation of the efficacy of such treatments. In the future, a combination of these measures may delay the onset and slow the progression of both macro- and micro-vascular complications of diabetes, and indeed, may also be useful in certain conditions in the non-diabetic population, e.g. atherosclerosis (157). The case for long-term prospective studies to investigate the efficacy of anti-oxidant treatments is growing.

## REFERENCES

1 Pirart J. Diabetes mellitus and its degenerative complications: a prospective study of 4400 patients observed between 1947 and 1973. *Diabetes Care* 1978; 1: 168–88.
2 Klein R, Klein BEK, Moss SE, Davis MD, DeMets DL. Glycosylated haemoglobin predicts the incidence and progression of diabetic retinopathy. *J Am Med Assoc* 1989; 260: 2864–71.
3 Chase HP, Jackson WE, Hoops SL, Cockerham RS, Archer PG, O'Brien D. Glucose control and the renal and retinal complications of insulin-dependent diabetes. *J Am Med Assoc* 1989; 261: 1155–60.
4 McCance DR, Hadden DR, Atkinson AB, Archer DB, Kennedy L. Long-term glycaemic control and diabetic retinopathy. *Lancet* 1989; ii: 824–8.
5 D'Antonio JA, Ellis D, Doft BH. Diabetic complications and glycemic control. The Pittsburgh prospective insulin-dependent cohort study status report after five years of IDDM. *Diabetes Care* 1989; 12: 694–700.
6 McCance DR, Hadden DR, Atkinson AB, Johnston H, Kennedy L. The relationship between long-term glycaemic control and diabetic nephropathy. *Quart J Med* 1992; 297: 53–61.
7 Feldt-Rasmussen B, Mathiesen ER, Deckert T. Effect of two years strict metabolic control on progression of incipient diabetic nephropathy in insulin-dependent diabetes. *Lancet* 1986; ii: 1300–4.
8 Brinchmann-Hansen O, Dahl-Jorgensen K, Sandvik L, Hanssen KF. Blood glucose concentrations and progression of diabetic retinopathy: the seven year results of the Oslo study. *Br Med J* 1992; 304: 19–22.
9 Strowig S, Raskin P. Glycemic control and diabetic complications. *Diabetes Care* 1992; 15: 1126–40.
10 Lyons TJ, Thorpe SR, Baynes JW. Glycation and autoxidation of proteins in aging and diabetes. In: Ruderman N, Williamson J, Brownlee M, eds. *Hyperglycemia, diabetes, and vascular disease*. Oxford University Press, New York, 1992: 197–217.
11 Dunn JA, McCance DR, Thorpe SR, Lyons TJ, Baynes JW. Age-dependent accumulation of $N^{\varepsilon}$-(carboxymethyl)lysine and $N^{\varepsilon}$-(carboxymethyl)hydroxylysine in human skin collagen. *Biochemistry* 1991; 30: 1205–10.
12 Dyer DG, Dunn JA, Thorpe SR *et al.* Accumulation of Maillard reaction products in skin collagen in diabetes and aging. *J Clin Invest*, 1993; in press.

13 Ledl F, Schleicher E. New aspects of the Maillard reaction in foods and in the human body. *Angew Chem (Int Ed Engl)* 1990; 29: 565–94.
14 Njoroge FG, Monnier VM. The chemistry of the Maillard reaction under physiological conditions: a review. *Prog Clin Biol Res* 1989; 304: 85–107.
15 *The Maillard reaction in aging, diabetes and nutrition.* Baynes JW and Monnier VM, eds., Alan R Liss, Inc, New York, 1989.
16 Monnier VM, Sell DR, Nagaraj RH *et al.* Maillard reaction-mediated molecular damage to extracellular matrix and other tissue proteins in diabetes, aging, and uremia. *Diabetes* 1992; 41, Suppl. 2: 36–41.
17 Ahmed MU, Thorpe SR, Baynes JW. Identification of carboxymethyllysine as a degradation product of fructose–lysine in glycosylated protein. *J Biol Chem* 1986; 261: 4889–994.
18 Ahmed MU, Dunn JA, Walla MD, Thorpe SR, Baynes JW. Oxidative degradation of glucose adducts to protein. Formation of 3-(N epsilon-lysino)-lactic acid from model compounds and glycosylated proteins. *J Biol Chem* 1988; 263: 8816–21.
19 Sell DR, Monnier VM. Structure elucidation of a senescence cross-link from human extracellular matrix. Implication of pentoses in the aging process. *J Biol Chem* 1989; 264: 21597–602.
20 Fu M-X, Knecht KJ, Thorpe SR, Baynes JW. Role of oxygen in the cross-linking and chemical modification of collagen by glucose. *Diabetes* 1992; 41, Suppl. 2: 42–8.
21 Baynes JW. Role of oxidative stress in development of complications in diabetes. *Diabetes* 1991; 40: 405–12.
22 Lyons TJ, Bailie K, Dunn JA, Dyer DG, Thorpe SR, Baynes JW. Decrease in skin collagen glycosylation with improved glycemic control in patients with insulin-dependent diabetes mellitus. *J Clin Invest* 1991; 87: 1910–15.
23 Dunn JA, Ahmed MU, Murtiashaw MH, *et al.* Reaction of ascorbate with lysine and protein under autoxidizing conditions: formation of $N^{\epsilon}$-(carboxymethyl)lysine by reaction between lysine and products of autoxidation of ascorbate. *Biochemistry* 1990; 29: 10964–70.
24 McCance DR, Dyer DG, Dunn JA *et al.* Maillard reaction products and their relation to complications in insulin dependent diabetes mellitus. *J Clin Invest* 1993; In press (June '93 issue).
25 Grandhee SK, Monnier VM. Mechanism of formation of the Maillard protein cross-link pentosidine. Glucose, fructose and ascorbate as pentosidine precursors. *J Biol Chem* 1991; 266: 11649–53.
26 Dyer DG, Blackledge JA, Thorpe SR, Baynes JW. Formation of pentosidine during nonenzymatic browning of proteins by glucose. Identification of glucose and other carbohydrates as possible precursors of pentosidine *in vivo*. *J Biol Chem* 1991; 266: 11654–60.
27 Wolff SP, Dean RT. Glucose autoxidation and protein modification: the potential role of 'autoxidative glycosylation' in diabetes mellitus. *Biochem J* 1987; 245: 243–50.
28 Monnier VM, Cerami A. Non-enzymatic browning *in vivo*. Possible process for aging of long-lived proteins. *Science* 1981; 211: 491–3.
29 Cerami A, Vlassara H, Brownlee M. Glucose and aging. *Sci Am* 1987; 256: 90–6.
30 Monnier VM. Toward a Maillard reaction theory of aging. *Prog Clin Biol Res* 1989; 304: 1–22.
31 Harman D. The ageing process. *Proc Natl Acad Sci* 1981; 78: 7124–8.
32 Stamler J. Epidemiology, established major risk factors, and the primary prevention of coronary heart disease. In: Parmley W, Chatterjee K, eds. *Cardiology*. PA Lippincott, Philadelphia; 1987: 1–41.
33 Lyons TJ. Oxidized low density lipoproteins – a role in the pathogenesis of atherosclerosis in diabetes? *Diabetic Med* 1991; 8: 411–19.
34 Lyons TJ. Glycation of low density lipoprotein and its metabolic consequences. *Diabetes* 1992; 41, Suppl. 2: 67–73.
35 Lyons TJ. Glycation and oxidation: a role in the pathogenesis of atherosclerosis. *Am J Cardiol* 1993; 71: 26B-31B.
36 Schleicher E, Deufel T, Wieland OH. Non-enzymatic glycosylation of human serum lipoproteins. *FEBS Lett* 1981; 129: 1–4.
37 Gonen B, Baenziger J, Schonfeld G, Jacobsen D, Farrar P. Non-enzymatic glycosylation of low-density lipoproteins *in vitro*. *Diabetes* 1981; 30: 875–878.
38 Witztum JL, Mahoney EM, Branks MJ, Fisher M, Elam R, Steinberg D. Nonenzymatic glucosylation of low-density lipoprotein alters its biologic activity. *Diabetes* 1982; 31: 283–91.
39 Sasaki J, Cottam GL. Glycosylation of LDL decreases its ability to interact with high-affinity receptors of human fibroblasts *in vitro* and decreases its clearance from rabbit plasma *in vivo*. *Biochem Biophys Acta* 1982; 713: 199–207.
40 Steinbrecher UP, Witztum JL. Glucosylation of low density lipoproteins to an extent comparable to that seen in diabetes slows their catabolism. *Diabetes* 1984; 33: 130–4.
41 Lyons TJ, Patrick JS, Baynes JW, Colwell JA, Lopes-Virella. Glycosylation of low density lipoprotein in patients with Type 1 diabetes: correlations with other parameters of glycaemic control. *Diabetologia* 1986; 29: 685–89.
42 Lopes-Virella MF, Sherer GK, Lees AM *et al.* Surface binding, internalization and degradation by cultured human fibroblasts of low density lipoproteins isolated from type I (insulin-dependent) diabetic patients: changes with metabolic control. *Diabetologia* 1982; 22: 430–36.
43 Lyons TJ, Klein RL, Baynes JW, Stevenson HC, Lopes-Virella MF. Stimulation of cholesteryl ester synthesis in human monocyte-derived macrophages by low-density lipoproteins from type I (insulin-dependent) diabetic patients: the influence of non-enzymatic glycosylation of low-density lipoprotein. *Diabetologia* 1987; 30: 916–23.
44 Klein RL, Lyons TJ, Lopes-Virella MF. Metabolism of very low- and low density lipoproteins isolated from normolipidaemic Type 2 (non-insulin-dependent) diabetic patients by human monocyte-derived macrophages. *Diabetologia* 1990; 33: 299–305.
45 Jack CM, Sheridan B, Kennedy L, Stout RW. Non-enzymatic glycosylation of low-density lipoprotein. Results of an affinity chromatography method. *Diabetologia* 1988; 31: 126–28.
46 Lopes-Virella MF, Klein RL, Lyons TJ, Stevenson HC,

Witztum JL. Glycosylation of low-density lipoprotein enhances cholesteryl ester synthesis in human monocyte-derived macrophages. *Diabetes* 1988; 37: 550–7.
47 Henriksen T, Mahoney EM, Steinberg D. Enhanced macrophage degradation of low density lipoprotein previously incubated with cultured endothelial cells: Recognition by receptors for acetylated low density lipoproteins. *Proc Natl Acad Sci USA* 1981; 78:6499–503.
48 Steinbrecher UP, Parthasarathy S, Leake DS, Witztum JL, Steinberg D. Modification of low density lipoprotein by endothelial cells involves lipid peroxidation and degradation of low density lipoprotein phospholipids. *Proc Natl Acad Sci USA* 1984; 81: 3883–7.
49 Morel DW, DiCorleto PE, Chisolm GM. Endothelial and smooth muscle cells alter low density lipoprotein *in vitro* by free radical oxidation. *Arteriosclerosis* 1984; 4: 357–364.
50 Hessler JR, Robertson AL Jr, Chisolm GM III. LDL-induced cytotoxicity and its inhibition by HDL in human vascular smooth muscle and endothelial cells in culture. *Atherosclerosis* 1979; 32: 213–29.
51 Hessler JR, Morel DW, Lewis J, Chisolm GM. Lipoprotein oxidation and lipoprotein-induced cytotoxicity. *Arteriosclerosis* 1983; 3: 215–22.
52 Evensen SA, Galdal KS, Nilsen E. LDL-induced cytotoxicity and its inhibition by anti-oxidant treatment in cultured human endothelial cells and fibroblasts. *Atherosclerosis* 1983; 49: 23–30.
53 Morel DW, Hessler JR, Chisolm GM. Low density lipoprotein cytotoxicity induced by free radical peroxidation of lipid. *J Lipid Res* 1983; 24: 1070–6.
54 Cathcart MK, Morel DW, Chisolm GM III. Monocytes and neutrophils oxidize low density lipoprotein making it cytotoxic. *J Leukocyte Biol* 1985; 38: 341–50.
55 Quinn MT, Parthasarathy S, Fong LG, Steinberg D. Oxidatively modified low density lipoproteins: a potential role in recruitment and retention of monocyte/macrophages during atherogenesis. *Proc Natl Acad Sci USA* 1987; 84:2995–8.
56 Cushing SD, Berliner JA, Valente AJ *et al.* Minimally modified low density lipoprotein induces monocyte chemotactic protein 1 in human endothelial cells and smooth muscle cells. *Proc Natl Acad Sci USA* 1990; 87: 513–8.
57 Mullarkey CJ, Edelstein D, Brownlee M. Free radical generation by early glycation products: a mechanism for accelerated atherogenesis in diabetes. *Biochem Biophys Res Commun* 1990; 173:932–9.
58 Brownlee M, Vlassara H, Cerami A. Nonenzymatic glycosylation products on collagen covalently trap low-density lipoprotein. *Diabetes* 1985; 34:938–41.
59 Watanabe J, Wohltmann HJ, Klein RL, Colwell JA, Lopes-Virella MF. Enhancement of platelet aggregation by low density lipoproteins from IDDM patients. *Diabetes* 1988; 37:1652–57.
60 Klein RL, Lopes-Virella MF, Colwell JA. Enhancement of platelet aggregation by the glycosylated subfraction of low density lipoprotein (LDL) isolated from patients with insulin-dependent diabetes mellitus (IDDM). *Diabetes* 1990; 39 (Suppl 1):173a.
61 Jokl R, Klein RL, Colwell JA, Lopes-Virella MF. Low density lipoproteins isolated from diabetic patients alter the release of tissue plasminogen activator (tPA) by cultured human endothelial cells. *Diabetes* 1992; 41, Suppl.1:113A.
62 Jokl R, Li W, Colwell JA, Klein RL, Lopes-Virella MF, Lyons TJ. Glycoxidized LDL modifies PAI-1 release by retinal endothelial cells. *Diabetologia* 1992; 35, Suppl 1:A46.
63 Lyons TJ, Li W, Jokl R. Toxicity of low density lipoproteins to retinal capillary pericytes: an effect enhanced by lipoprotein glycation and oxidation. *Diabetes* 1992; 41, Suppl 1:111A.
64 Curtiss LK, Witztum JL. Plasma apo-lipoproteins A-I, A-II, B, C-I and E are glycosylated in hyperglycemic diabetic subjects. *Diabetes* 1985; 34: 452–61.
65 Klein RL, Lyons TJ, Lopes-Virella MF. Interaction of very-low-density lipoprotein isolated from Type 1 (insulin-dependent) diabetic subjects with human monocyte-derived macrophages. *Metabolism* 1989; 38: 1108–14.
66 Klein RL, Lopes-Virella MF. Metabolism by human endothelial cells of very low density lipoprotein subfractions isolated from Type 1 (insulindependent) diabetic patients. *Diabetologia* 1993; 36: 258–64.
67 Witztum JL, Fisher M, Pietro T, Steinbrecher UP, Elam RL. Nonenzymatic glucosylation of high-density lipoprotein accelerates its catabolism in guinea pigs. *Diabetes* 1982; 31: 1029–32.
68 Duell PB, Oram JF, Bierman EL. Nonenzymatic glycosylation of HDL resulting in inhibition of high-affinity binding to cultured human fibroblasts. *Diabetes* 1990; 39: 1257–63.
69 Duell PB, Oram JF, Bierman EL. Nonenzymatic glycosylation of HDL and impaired HDL-receptor-mediated cholesterol efflux. *Diabetes* 1991; 40: 377–84.
70 Witztum JL, Steinbrecher UP, Kesaniemi YA, Fisher M. Autoantibodies to glucosylated proteins in the plasma of patients with diabetes mellitus. *Proc Natl Acad Sci USA* 1984; 81: 3204–8.
71 Curtiss LK, Witztum JL. A novel method of generating region-specific monoclonal antibodies to modified proteins. Application to the identification of human glucosylated low density lipoproteins. *J Clin Invest* 1983; 72: 1427–38.
72 Witztum JL, Steinbrecher UP, Fisher M, Kesaniemi A. Nonenzymatic glucosylation of homologous low density lipoprotein and albumin renders them immunogenic in the guinea pig. *Proc Natl Acad Sci USA* 1983; 80: 2757–61.
73 Brownlee M, Pongor S, Cerami A. Covalent attachment of soluble proteins by non-enzymatically glycosylated collagen: role in the *in situ* formation of immune complexes. *J Exp Med* 1983; 158: 1739–44.
74 Klimov AN, Denisenko AD, Popov AV *et al.* Lipoprotein-antibody immune complexes: their catabolism and role in foam cell formation. *Atherosclerosis* 1985; 58: 1–15.
75 Griffith RL, Virella GT, Stevenson HC, Lopes-Virella MF. LDL metabolism by macrophages activated with LDL immune complexes: a possible mechanism of foam cell formation. *J Exp Med* 1988; 168: 1041–59.
76 Gisinger C, Virella GT, Lopes-Virella MF. Erythrocyte-bound low density lipoprotein (LDL) immune complexes lead to cholesteryl ester accumulation in human monocyte derived macrophages. *Clin Immunol Immunopath* 1991; 59: 37–52.

77 Lopes-Virella MF, Griffith RL, Shunk KA, Virella GT. Enhanced uptake and impaired intracellular metabolism of low density lipoprotein complexed with anti-low density lipoprotein antibodies. *Arterioscler Thromb* 1991; 11: 1356–67.
78 Gissinger C, Lopes-Virella MF. Lipoprotein–immune complexes and diabetic vascular complications. Diabetes 1992; 41, Suppl. 2: 92–96.
79 Cornacoff JB, Hebert LA, Smead WL, Vanaman ME, Birmingham DJ, Waxman FJ. Primate erythrocyte-immune complex-clearing mechanism. *J Clin Invest* 1983; 71: 236–47.
80 Munoz J, Virella G, Galbraith G, Lopes-Virella MF. LDL immune complexes activate respiratory burst and cytokine release in human monocyte-derived macrophages. *Circulation* 1992; 86: I–335.
81 Bevilacqua MP, Pober JS, Majeau GR, Cotran RS, Gimbrone MA. Interleukin-1 induces biosynthesis and cell surface expression of procoagulant activity in human vascular endothelial cells. *J Exp Med* 1984; 160: 618–22.
82 Martin S, Maruta K, Burkart V, Gillis S, Kolb H. IL-1 and INF-γ increase vascular permeability. *Immunology* 1988; 64: 301–5.
83 Breviario F, Bertocchi F, Dejana E, Bussolino F. IL-1 induced adhesion of polymorphonuclear leukocytes to cultured human endothelial cells. Role of platelet-activating factor. *J Immunol* 1988; 141: 3391–97.
84 Pohlman TH, Stanness KA, Beatty PG, Ochs HD, Harlan JM. An endothelial cell surface factor(s) induced *in vitro* by lipopolysaccharide, interleukin-1 and tumor necrosis factor α increases neutrophil adherence by a CDw18-dependent mechanism. *J Immunol* 1986; 136: 4548–53.
85 Kilpatrick JM, Hyman B, Virella G. Human endothelial cell damage induced by interactions between polymorphonuclear leukocytes and immune complex-coated erythrocytes. *Clin Immunol Immunopath* 1987; 44: 335–47.
86 Warner SJC, Auger KR, Libby P. Interleukin-1 induces interleukin-1. II. Recombinant human interleukin-1 induces interleukin-1 production by adult human vascular endothelial cells. *J Immunol* 1987; 139: 1911–17.
87 Raines EW, Dower SK, Ross R. Interleukin-1 mitogenic activity for fibroblasts and smooth muscle cells is due to PDGF-AA. *Science* 1989; 243: 393–96.
88 Feingold K, Grunfeld C. Role of cytokines in inducing hyperlipidemia. *Diabetes* 1992; 41, Suppl. 2: 97–101.
89 Luscinskas FW, Brock AF, Arnaout MA, Gimbrone MA. Endothelial-leukocyte adhesion molecule-1-dependent and leukocyte (CD11/CD18)-dependent mechanisms contribute to polymorphonuclear leukocyte adhesion to cytokine-activated human vascular endothelium. *J Immunol* 1989; 142: 2257–63.
90 Libby P, Warner SJC, Friedman GB. IL-1: a mitogen for human vascular smooth muscle cells that induces the release of growth inhibitory prostanoids. *J Clin Invest* 1988; 81: 487–98.
91 Nawroth PP, Bank I, Hadley D, Cassimeris J, Chess L, Stern D. Tumor necrosis factor/cachectin interacts with endothelial cell receptors to induce release of interleukin-1. *J Exp Med* 1986; 163: 1363–75.
92 Brownlee M, Vlassara H, Cerami A. Inhibition of heparin-catalyzed antithrombin III activity by non-enzymatic glycosylation: possible role in fibrin deposition in diabetes. *Diabetes* 1984; 33: 532–35.
93 Ceriello A, Guigliano D, Quatraro A *et al.* Daily rapid blood glucose variations may condition antithrombin biological activity but not its plasma concentration in insulin dependent diabetes: a possible role for labile non-enzymatic glycation. *Diab Metab* 1987; 13: 16–19.
94 McVerry VA, Thorpe S, Gaffney JP, Huehns ER. Non-enzymatic glycosylation of fibrinogen. *Haemostasis* 1981; 10: 261–70.
95 Van Heyningen R, Harding JJ. Risk factors for cataract: diabetes, myopia and sex. *Colloq INSERM* 1986; 147: 381–5.
96 Alberti KGMM, Hockaday TDR. In: Wetherall DJ, Ledingham JGG, Warrell DA, eds. *The Oxford textbook of medicine.* Oxford, Oxford University Press, 1987: 9.83–9.84.
97 Leske MC, Sperduto RD. The epidemiology of senile cataracts: a review. *Am J Epidemiol* 1983; 118: 152–65.
98 de Berardinis E, Tieri O, Polzella A, Iuglio N. The chemical composition of the human aqueous humour in normal and pathological conditions. *Exp Eye Res* 1965; 4: 179–86.
99 Cotlier E. The lens. In: Moses RA, ed. *Adler's physiology of the eye, clinical applications,* 7th ed. CV Mosby, St Louis, 1987: 277–303.
100 Ross WM, Creighton MO, Trevithick JR, Stewart-DeHaan PJ, Sanwal M. Modelling cortical cataractogenesis: VI. Induction by glucose *in vitro* or in diabetic rats: prevention and reversal by glutathione. *Exp Eye Res* 1983; 37: 559–73.
101 Srivastava SK, Ansari NH. Prevention of sugar-induced cataractogenesis in rats by butylated hydroxytoluene. *Diabetes* 1988; 37: 1505–8.
102 Simonelli F, Nesti A, Pensa M *et al.* Lipid peroxidation and human cataractogenensis in diabetes and severe myopia. *Exp Eye Res* 1989; 49: 181–7.
103 DiMattio J, Altszuler N, Ellis S, Zadunaisky JA. Glucose transport across ocular barriers of the streptozotocin-diabetic rat. *Diabetes* 1981; 30: 903–6.
104 Cunha-Vaz J, Faria de Abreu JR, Campos AJ, Figo GM. Early breakdown of the blood–retinal barrier in diabetes. *Br J Ophthal* 1975; 59: 649–56.
105 Waltman SR, Oestrich C, Krupin T *et al.* Quantitative vitreous fluorophotometry: A sensitive technique for measuring early breakdown of the blood–retinal barrier in young diabetic patients. *Diabetes* 1978; 27: 85–7.
106 Dunn JA, Patrick JS, Thorpe SR, Baynes JW. Oxidation of glycated proteins: age-dependent accumulation of $N^{\epsilon}$-(carboxymethyl)lysine in lens proteins. *Biochemistry* 1989; 28: 9464–8.
107 Patrick JS, Thorpe SR, Baynes JW: Non-enzymatic of protein does not increase with age in normal human lenses. *J Gerontol Biol Sci* 1990; 45: B18–B23.
108 Lyons TJ, Silvestri G, Dunn JA, Dyer DG, Baynes JW. Role of glycation in modification of lens crystallins in diabetic and non-diabetic senile cataracts. *Diabetes* 1991; 40: 1010–5.
109 Nakayama H, Mitsuhashi T, Kuwajima S, Aoki S, Kuroda Y, Itoh T, Nakagawa S. Immunochemical detection of advanced glycation end products in lens crystallins from Streptozotocin-induced diabetic rat. *Diabetes* 1993; 42: 345–50.
110 Charonis AS, Tsilibary E. Structural and functional

changes of laminin and Type IV collagen after non-enzymatic glycation. *Diabetes* 1992; 41, Suppl. 2: 49–51.

111 Hamlin CR, Kohn RR. Evidence for progressive, age-related structural changes in post-mature human collagen. *Biochim Biophys Acta* 1971; 236: 458–67.

112 Hamlin CR, Kohn RR. Determination of human chronological age by study of a collagen sample. *Exp Gerontol* 1972; 7: 377–9.

113 Hamlin CR, Kohn RR, Luschin JH. Apparent accelerated aging of human collagen in diabetes mellitus. *Diabetes* 1975; 24: 902–4.

114 Lyons TJ, Kennedy L. Effect of *in vitro* non-enzymatic glycosylation of human skin collagen on susceptibility to collagenase digestion. *Eur J Clin Invest* 1985; 15: 128–31.

115 Yue DK, McLennan S, Delbridge L, Handelsman DJ, Reeve T, Turtle JR. The thermal stability of collagen in diabetic rats: correlation with severity of diabetes and non-enzymatic glycosylation. *Diabetologia* 1983; 24: 282–5.

116 Bailey AJ, Kent MJC. Non-enzymatic glycosylation of fibrous and basement membrane collagens. In: Baynes JW and Monnier VM, eds. *The Maillard reaction in aging, diabetes and nutrition.* Alan R Liss, Inc, New York, 1989: 109–22.

117 Rosenberg H, Modrak JB, Hassing JM, Al-Turk WA, Stohs SJ. Glycosylated collagen. *Biochem Biophys Res Comm* 1979; 91: 498–501.

118 Cohen MP, Urdanivia E, Surma M, Wu V-Y. Increased glycosylation of glomerular basement membrane collagen in diabetes. *Biochem Biophys Res Comm* 1980; 95: 765–9.

119 Schneider SL, Kohn RR. Glycosylation of human collagen in aging and diabetes mellitus. *J Clin Invest* 1980; 66: 1179–81.

120 Schnider SL, Kohn RR. Effects of age and diabetes mellitus on the solubility and non-enzymatic glucosylation of human skin collagen. *J Clin Invest* 1981; 67: 1630–5.

121 Lyons TJ, Kennedy L. Non-enzymatic glycosylation of skin collagen in patients with limited joint mobility. *Diabetologia* 1985; 28: 2–5.

122 Vishwanath V, Frank KE, Elmets CA, Dauchot PJ, Monnier VM. Glycosylation of skin collagen in Type I diabetes mellitus: correlations with long-term complications. *Diabetes* 1986; 35: 916–21.

123 Vogt BW, Schleicher ED, Wieland OH. E-amino-lysine-bound glucose in human tissues obtained at autopsy. *Diabetes* 1982; 31: 1123–7.

124 Garlick RL, Bunn HF, Spiro RG. Non-enzymatic glycosylation of basement membranes from human glomeruli and bovine sources. *Diabetes* 1988; 37: 1144–50.

125 Monnier VM, Vishwanath V, Frank KE, Elmets CA, Dauchot P, Kohn RR. Relations between complications to Type I diabetes mellitus and collagen-linked fluorescence. *N Engl J Med* 1986; 314: 403–8.

126 Monnier VM, Sell DR, Abdul-Karim FW, Emancipator SN. Collagen browning and cross-linking are increased in chronic experimental hyperglycemia. Relevance to diabetes and aging. *Diabetes* 1988; 37: 867–72.

127 Sell DR, Lapolla A, Odetti P, Fogarty J, Monnier VM. Pentosidine formation in skin correlates with severity of complications in individuals with long-standing IDDM. *Diabetes* 1992; 41: 1286–92.

128 Makita Z, Radoff S, Rayfield EJ *et al.* Advanced glycosylation end products in patients with diabetic nephropathy. *N Engl J Med* 1991; 325: 836–42.

129 Oxlund H, Rasmussen LM, Andreassen TT, Heickendorff L. Increased aortic stiffness in patients with type 1 (insulin-dependent) diabetes mellitus. *Diabetologia* 1989; 32: 748–52.

130 Bucala R, Tracey KJ, Cerami A. Advanced glycosylation products quench nitric oxide and mediate defective endothelium-dependent vasodilatation in experimental diabetes. *J Clin Invest* 1991; 87: 432–8.

131 Hicks M, Delbridge L, Yue, DK, Reeve TS. Increase in crosslinking of nonenzymatically glycosylated collagen induced by products of lipid peroxidation. *Arch Biochem Biophys* 1989; 268: 249–54.

132 Vlassara H, Brownlee M, Cerami A. Novel macrophage receptor for glucose-modified proteins is distinct from previously described scavenger receptors. *J Exp Med* 1986; 164: 1301–9.

133 Vlassara H, Valinsky J, Brownlee M, Cerami C, Nishimoto S, Cerami A. Advanced glycosylation end products on erythrocyte cell surface induce receptor-mediated phagocytosis by macrophages. A model for turnover of aging cells. *J Exp Med* 1987; 166: 539–49.

134 Kirstein M, Brett J, Radoff S, Ogawa S, Stern D, Vlassara H. Advanced protein glycosylation induces transendothelial human monocyte chemotaxis and secretion of platelet-derived growth factor: role in vascular disease of diabetes and aging. *Proc Natl Acad Sci USA* 1990; 87: 9010–14.

135 Vlassara H, Brownlee M, Manogue KR, Dinarello CA, Pasagian A. Cachectin/TNF and IL-1 induced by glucose-modified proteins: role in normal tissue remodeling. *Science* 1988; 240: 1546–8.

136 Brownlee M, Vlassara H, Kooney A, Ulrich P, Cerami A. Aminoguanidine prevents diabetes-induced arterial wall protein cross-linking. *Science* 1986; 232: 1629–32.

137 Requena JR. The main mechanism of action of aminoguanidine. *Diabetologia* 1991; 34, Suppl. 2: A162.

138 Soulis-Liparota T, Cooper M, Papazoglou D, Clarke BF, Jerums G. Retardation by aminoguanidine of development of albuminuria, mesangial expansion, and tissue fluorescence in streptozotocin-induced diabetic rat. *Diabetes* 1991; 40: 1328–34.

139 Yagihashi S, Kamijo M, Baba M, Yagihashi N, Nagai K. Effect of aminoguanidine on functional and structural abnormalities in peripheral nerve of STZ-induced diabetic rats. *Diabetes* 1992; 41: 47–52.

140 Cameron NE, Cotter MA, Dines K, Love A. Effects of aminoguanidine on peripheral nerve function and polyol pathway metabolites in streptozotocin diabetic rats. *Diabetologia* 1992; 35: 946–50.

141 Hammes HP, Martin S, Federlin K, Geisen K, Brownlee M. Aminoguanidine treatment inhibits the development of experimental diabetic retinopathy. *Proc Natl Acad Sci USA* 1991; 88: 11555–8.

142 Tilton RG, Chang K, Hasan KS *et al.* Prevention of vascular dysfunction by guanidines. Inhibition of nitric oxide synthase versus advanced glycation end-product formation. *Diabetes* 1993; 42: 221–32.

143 Bucala R, Cerami, A. Phospholipids react with glucose to initiate advanced glycosylation and fatty acid oxi-

dation: inhibition of lipid advanced glycosylation and oxidation by aminoguanidine. *Diabetes* 1992; 41, Suppl. 1: 23A.
144 Bucala R, Cerami A, Makita Z *et al.* Inhibition of advanced glycosylation by aminoguanidine reduces plasma LDL levels in diabetes. *Clin Res* 1993; 41: 183A.
145 Parthasarathy S, Young SG, Witztum JL, Pittman RC, Steinberg D. Probucol inhibits oxidative modification of low density lipoprotein. *J Clin Invest* 1986; 77: 641–4.
146 Carew TE, Schwenke DC, Steinberg D. Antiatherogenic effect of probucol unrelated to its hypocholesterolemic effect: evidence that antioxidants *in vivo* can selectively inhibit low density lipoprotein degradation in macrophage-rich fatty streaks and slow the progression of atherosclerosis in the Watanabe heritable hyperlipidemic rabbit. *Proc Natl Acad Sci USA* 1987; 84: 7725–9.
147 Kita T, Nagano Y, Yokode M *et al.* Probucol prevents the progression of atherosclerosis in Watanabe heritable hyperlipidemic rabbit, an animal model for familial hypercholesterolemia. *Proc Natl Acad Sci USA* 1987; 84: 5928–31.
148 Kuzuya M, Naito M, Funaki C, Hayashi T, Asai K, Kuzuya F. Probucol prevents oxidative injury to endothelial cells. *J Lipid Res* 1991; 32: 197–204.
149 Björkhem I, Henriksson-Freyschuss A, Breuer O, Diczfalusy U, Berglund L, Henriksson P. The antioxidant butylated hydroxytoluene protects against atherosclerosis. *Arterioscler Thromb* 1991; 11: 15–22.
150 Freyschuss A, Stiko-Rahm A, Swedenborg J *et al.* Antioxidant treatment inhibits the development of intimal thickening after balloon injury of the aorta in hypercholesterolemic rabbits. *J Clin Invest* 1993; 91: 1282–8.
151 Burch RM, Weitzberg M, Blok N *et al.* *N*-(fluorenyl-9-methoxycarbonyl) amino acids, a class of antiinflammatory agents with a different mechanism of action. *Proc Natl Acad Sci USA* 1991; 355–9.
152 Navab M, Hama SY, Van Lenten BJ, Drinkwater DC, Laks H, Fogelman AM. A new antiinflammatory compound, Leumedin, inhibits modification of low density lipoprotein and the resulting monocyte transmigration into the subendothelial space of cocultures of human aortic wall cells. *J Clin Invest* 1993; 91:1225–30.
153 Reaven P, Parthasarathy S, Grasse BJ, Miller E, Steinberg D, Witztum JL. Effects of oleate-rich and linoleate-rich diets on the susceptibility of low density lipoprotein to oxidative modification in mildly hypercholesterolemic subjects. *J Clin Invest* 1993; 91: 668–76.
154 Frei B, England L, Ames BN. Ascorbate is an outstanding antioxidant in human plasma. *Proc Natl Acad Sci USA* 1989; 86:6377–81.
155 Jennings PE, Chirico S, Jones AF, Lunec J, Barnett AH. Vitamin C metabolites and microangiopathy in diabetes mellitus. *Diabetes Res* 1987; 6:151–4.
156 Karpen CW, Cataland S, O'Dorisio TM, Panganamala RV. Production of 12 HETE and vitamin E status in platelets from type 1 human diabetic subjects. *Diabetes* 1985; 34:526–31.
157 Steinberg D. Antioxidants and atherosclerosis: a current assessment. *Circulation* 1991; 84:1420–5.

# 24 The Sorbitol Pathway and Diabetic Complications

Boas Gonen & Dushan Dvornik

We now give a critical review of the evidence linking the metabolism of excess tissue glucose via the sorbitol (polyol) pathway with the initiation and progression of pathophysiological changes that usually occur over time in the nerve, kidney, and retina of patients with diabetes mellitus. Evidence supporting such link was obtained mainly by blocking the sorbitol pathway with inhibitors of aldose reductase. Whereas extensive investigations have been carried out in animals, relatively few well-designed clinical trials have been completed in man; accordingly, we present an overview of experimental data obtained in animals, and a focus on findings in patients with diabetic neuropathy.

## INTRODUCTION

It is generally accepted that an association exists between hyperglycaemia and the development of the long-term complications of diabetes (1, 2) such as neuropathy (3, 4), nephropathy (5), and retinopathy (6). Theoretically, the hyperglycaemia-derived abnormalities occurring in diabetic tissues, and the resulting clinical sequelae, could be prevented or arrested either by lowering systemic glucose to near-normal levels with intensified glycaemic control, or by pharmacotherapy aimed at interfering with the pathophysiological consequences of excess tissue glucose.

Regarding the control of hyperglycaemia *per se*, the evidence that it prevents or delays the development of long-term complications is strong (1,7) but was not compelling enough (2, 8–10) to warrant a universal recommendation that intensified insulin therapy be instituted in all diabetic patients (11, 12). However, as widely expected, the Diabetes Control and Complications Trial (DCCT) (13) has provided definitive evidence regarding the benefits of intensive insulin therapy to control the development of retinopathy, nephropathy, and neuropathy in IDDM (14).

The alternative, pharmacotherapeutic methods are aimed at preventing the chemical or biochemical reactions of the excess glucose arising in diabetic tissues susceptible to long-term complications. The question thus arises: how is the excess glucose present in a diabetic tissue transformed into tissue damage? While several mechanisms have been proposed (7,15), two of them became targets of intensive research: the sorbitol pathway, i.e. aldose reductase-catalysed metabolism of excess tissue glucose to sorbitol (16–18), and excessive protein glycation (19–21) supplemented with the glucoxidation (22, 23), and glucose autoxidation mechanisms (24, 25).

## THE SORBITOL PATHWAY THEORY

The sorbitol pathway comprises two enzymatic reactions: in tandem, glucose is reduced to sorbitol by aldose reductase with NADPH as coenzyme, and sorbitol is oxidised to fructose by sorbitol dehydrogenase with $NAD^+$ as coenzyme (Fig. 24.1).

Aldose reductase belongs to a larger family of cytosolic, monomeric oxidoreductases (26, 27) which utilise NADPH to stereoselectively reduce various aldehydes to the corresponding alcohols. Aldose reductase is noted by its presence in tissues susceptible to diabetic complications (28–32), though such tissues may also contain hexonate dehydrogenase (33). Hexonate dehydrogenase and aldose reductase differ in their affinity for glucose (34–37), reflecting structural differences in their carboxy-terminal domains (34, 38–40); like aldose reductase, however, hexonate dehydrogenase can reduce glucose to sorbitol (41).

Aldose reductase is the first example of an 'eight-stranded α/β barrel' enzyme (42) using NADPH as cofactor (43, 44). Its active site is located at the carboxy-terminal end of the β-barrel, in a deep elliptical, highly hydrophobic cavity containing at its bottom (38, 44) 1 mole (45, 46) of very tightly bound NADPH (38, 43, 44, 47–49). Since the tight binding enhances the reactivity of NADPH, and achieves essentially 'one-way' catalysis in the direction of aldehyde reduction, aldose reductase was proposed as a model of a detoxification catalyst (49) specific for a functional group (50), preferably aromatic aldehydes (48). Actually, the structural environment of the active site of aldose reductase does not favour glucose as substrate (44, 51) and, at normal glucose concentrations, sorbitol is barely detectable (17, 28), except in erythrocytes and renal medulla (52).

In 1962 the hypothesis was formulated that the development of sugar cataract is triggered by the osmotic swelling of lens fibres caused by the intracellular accumulation of polyol formed from excess sugar by the action of lens aldose reductase (53). Interest in aldose reductase was aroused when sugar cataract formation was prevented by inhibiting aldose reductase (54, 55). The recognition that, in the lens, any sugar above the catalytic capacity of hexokinase (56) flows into the sorbitol pathway was subsequently extended to other diabetic tissues which do not require insulin for glucose absorption, and which are susceptible to chronic complications (16).

The metabolism of excess glucose by aldose reductase occurring in a diabetic tissue results in a correspondingly high rate of sorbitol production and NADPH consumption (57, 58). Since sorbitol is produced faster than it is oxidised by sorbitol dehydrogenase to fructose, sorbitol accumulates (59). The accumulation is augmented by the low permeability of osmotically unstressed cell membranes to sorbitol (60), particularly in diabetic tissues (61).

The relationship between glucose and sorbitol levels is illustrated by findings in sural nerve biopsy specimens obtained from patients with diabetic neuropathy (62) (Fig. 24.2). Of note, the level of sorbitol measured in a diabetic tissue at a given time-point is not an index of aldose

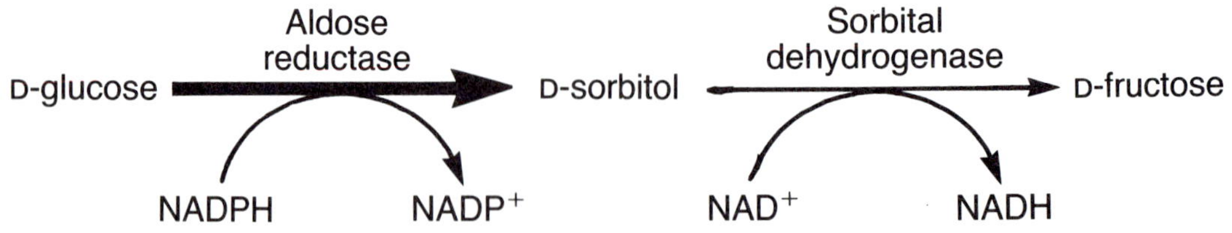


Fig. 24.1. The sorbitol (polyol) pathway.

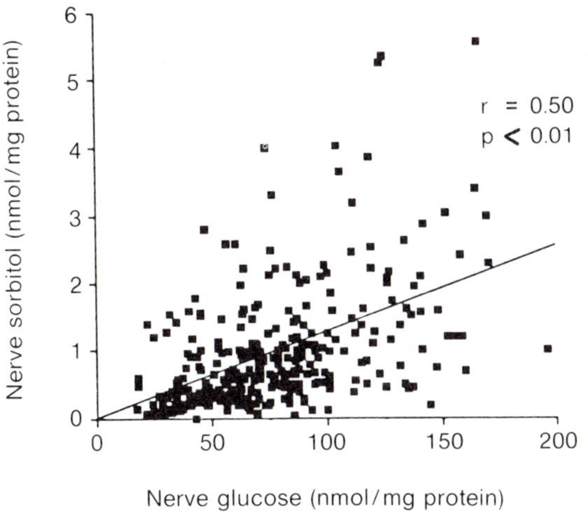


Fig. 24.2. Correlation between nerve glucose and sorbitol levels, measured in 286 human sural nerve biopsy specimens. (After Ref. 62.)

reductase activity (58, 63, 64), but reflects the dynamic equilibrium between sorbitol production (by aldose reductase) and sorbitol elimination (through effusion, and metabolism by sorbitol dehydrogenase to fructose). Sorbitol accumulation, therefore, may vary between tissues in the same species (28), and in the same tissue of different individuals, e.g. in peripheral nerve (62, 65–67), erythrocytes (68), and proximal renal tubular cells (59).

The metabolism of glucose *via* the sorbitol pathway entails excessive consumption of the pyridine nucleotides, NADPH and $NAD^+$, and their resulting deficit may contribute to the metabolic perturbations arising from the excessive sorbitol pathway activity (15, 69, 70). Variations in sorbitol pathway activity and their metabolic and functional ramifications contribute to the wide range of susceptibility to complications of long-standing diabetes (59, 63, 64, 71).

## ALDOSE REDUCTASE INHIBITION

The presence of aldose reductase in tissues susceptible to complications of chronic diabetes has led to the postulate that in such tissues, the disposal of excess glucose via the sorbitol pathway initiates a cascade of abnormalities which can progress to loss of functional and structural cell integrity (52). That increased sorbitol pathway activity acts as the trigger of such metabolic, functional, and structural changes is evidenced by the large body of experimental results showing that, in animal models of diabetic hyperglycaemia, a wide range of such abnormalities does not occur in the presence of aldose reductase (AR) inhibitors administered at the time, or soon after induction of diabetes or galactosaemia (28, 52, 72–74). The conclusion is limited by the extent of dissimilarity between human disease and animal models. However, the failure to develop human-type advanced lesions does not exclude the applicability of animal models of diabetic hyperglycaemia for the study of early pathogenetic alterations and of therapeutic responses: ‘any therapeutic manoeuvre inhibiting the initial stages of the pathological changes may offer some promise about its long term effect’(75).

Representative hyperglycaemia-induced abnormalities in the nerve, kidney, and retina of animal models of diabetic hyperglycaemia that were prevented by AR inhibitor treatment are listed in Table 24.1. So as to emphasise the link between the initial event, i.e. inhibition of aldose reductase activity and the abnormality prevented from occurring, the latter are arranged sequentially, i.e. as metabolic, functional, and structural. The sequence of metabolic abnormalities occurring in a diabetic tissue is tissue-specific (7, 91), and will be discussed accordingly.

### Nerve

Slowing of nerve conduction velocity (NCV) is observed within weeks following induction of diabetes (92). This deficit is a metabolic phenomenon, preventable by insulin (93), or by myoinositol feeding (94). In peripheral nerves of acutely diabetic rats, sorbitol accumulation is

Table 24.1. *Hyperglycaemia-induced abnormalities in the nerve, kidney, and retina of animal models of diabetic hyperglycaemia prevented by AR inhibitor treatment*

| | Abnormalities | Ref. |
|---|---|---|
| Metabolic | Polyol accumulation | 28 |
| | Myoinositol depletion (nerve, glomeruli, retina) | 28 |
| | Na, K-ATPase impairment (nerve, glomeruli) | 28 |
| | Endoneurial Na accumulation | 76 |
| | Neuropeptide depletion (nerve) | 77 |
| Functional | Decreased nerve conduction velocity | 28 |
| | Decreased axonal transport | 28 |
| | Delayed auditory brain-stem response | 78 |
| | Decreased non-cholinergic motor transmission | 79 |
| | Albuminuria | 80–85 |
| Structural | Paranodal axonal swelling | 86, 87 |
| | Axo-glial dysjunction (nerve) | 86, 87 |
| | Basement membrane thickening (retina) | 84,88 |
| | Pericyte loss, microaneurysm formation | 89, 90 |

accompanied by myoinositol depletion (95); the depletion was attributed to osmoregulatory mechanism(s) causing efflux of myoinositol (72, 95–97) and, possibly, affecting the myoinositol transporter (96).

That decreased NCV and myoinositol depletion are linked with the sorbitol pathway was demonstrated by their prevention with AR inhibitor treatment (28). The use of AR inhibitors as pathobiological probes (98) enabled the linking of individual abnormalities occurring in peripheral nerve into a plausible pathogenetic scheme (73, 99–104), e.g. by appending myoinositol depletion (105–107) and 'myoinositol uptake/Na,K-ATPase dysfunction' (108).

Based on the findings in spontaneously diabetic rats (86, 109) and in diabetic subjects (110), the scheme was expanded by linking the impaired activation of the membrane Na,K-ATPase with sodium accumulation at the nodes of Ranvier, followed by paranodal axonal swelling, axo-glial dysjunction, and paranodal demyelination (111). The structural components of the proposed scheme are supported by findings in patients with symptomatic diabetic neuropathy treated for 12 months with the AR inhibitor, sorbinil (112). Though controversial and unproven (72, 97, 113–117), the myoinositol depletion hypothesis provided a conceptual framework for a great number of investigations in animals and human subjects.

Another school of thought assigned a major pathogenetic role in diabetic neuropathy to hyperglycaemia-derived vascular insult (97), particularly in the later stages of development (118, 119). According to the 'hypoxic hypothesis' (120, 121), reduced nerve blood flow coupled with microangiopathy of *vasa nervorum* can lead to endoneurial ischaemia and hypoxic stress sufficient to impair nerve function (122, 123). The proposed linking of endoneurial vascular insufficiency with the aldose reductase-catalysed metabolism of excess nerve glucose (124) is supported by the localisation of aldose reductase in the endoneurial endothelium and pericytes (29).

Particularly intriguing is the finding that the consumption of NADPH by aldose reductase suppresses the NADPH-dependent nitric oxide biosynthesis thus causing nerve ischaemia and slowing of NCV (70). Consequently, in diabetic nerve, AR inhibitors may have a profound indirect protective effect against both metabolic and oxidative stress (125).

## Kidney

In the kidney, the relative distribution of the enzymes constituting the sorbitol pathway varies; thus, in rats, the highest aldose reductase activity was detected in the medulla and the lowest in the inner cortex, while the opposite was found for sorbitol dehydrogenase (126). Whereas in acutely diabetic rats, the activity of aldose reductase in glomeruli was unchanged, and of sorbitol dehydrogenase, increased (126), the reverse was found in glomeruli of long-term diabetic patients (127).

The coincident existence in rat inner medulla of a gradient of both aldose reductase activity and of sorbitol content (128–130) has led to the view that, in the kidney, aldose reductase may play a unique osmoregulatory role (131–135). However, since osmotically stressed renal cells can use several osmolytes to maintain proper cell volume (136–139), sorbitol is not essential for their survival. Supporting evidence is provided by the absence of any common, unusual renal side-effects across all the animal species treated chronically with structurally distinct AR inhibitors (137, 140, 141).

The lack of uniform renal effects in diabetic rats treated with AR inhibitors reflects not only the complexity of mechanisms involved in renal homeostasis, but also the structure and dose of AR inhibitor used. Nevertheless, most investigators have reported that, if administered at the time of diabetes induction (81–83, 85, 142), or soon after (84), AR inhibitors prevent (81, 83) or reduce (85, 142) the elevated urinary albumin excretion. The lack of consistent effects of AR inhibitors on the increased glomerular filtration rate (GFR) of acute diabetes (81–83, 85, 143–145) suggests that their sparing effect on albumin excretion is not mediated solely by an effect on GFR (83).

In contrast to the nerve (146), diacylglycerol production (from glucose) in glomeruli of diabetic rats is increased (147), resulting in increased activity of protein kinase C which, in turn, increases prostaglandin synthesis (148, 149). The link with the sorbitol pathway was evidenced by preventing the increase in prostaglandin synthesis with AR inhibitors (83, 143, 150); the effect was attributed to the decreased NADPH utilisation by aldose reductase (5).

So far no consistent effect of AR inhibitors on glomerular basement membrane thickening has been reported (81, 151, 152). Of note, in experimentally diabetic rats, albuminuria was reversed by islet transplantation without affecting basement membrane thickness (153).

Since the kidney cortex contains only 3% aldose reductase (30), cortical sorbitol is produced by hexonate dehydrogenase (41) which predominates in the cortex (30, 154); therefore, to prevent sorbitol production throughout the kidney, an AR inhibitor should inhibit both aldose reductase and hexonate dehydrogenase. In view of the structural similarities between aldose reductase and hexonate dehydrogenase, it is not surprising that AR inhibitors can also inhibit hexonate dehydrogenase; the extent of inhibition depends, however, on the chemical structure of the inhibitor (37, 98).

## Retina

The pathology of diabetic retinopathy and the involvement of increased sorbitol pathway activity has been recently reviewed by Tomlinson *et al.* (74). Of relevance for the present discussion is that the first histological lesion in diabetic retinopathy is a highly selective loss of intramural pericytes in retinal capillaries (155), and that this loss initiates a cascade of events that result in the development of microaneurysms, haemorrhages, and intra-retinal microvascular abnormalities. The localisation of aldose reductase in retinal pericytes (156–158) raised the possibility that sorbitol pathway action plays a role in their loss. This concept was tested by administering AR inhibitors in preventive fashion in animal models of diabetic hyperglycaemia.

Alloxan-induced diabetic dogs (159), and galactose-fed rats (89, 90) and dogs (160, 161) were shown to develop microangiopathies similar to background diabetic retinopathy in humans; when galactosaemia was maintained for up to 66 months, dogs developed advanced retinal changes, similar to those associated with pre-proliferative human diabetic retinopathy (162). Treatment of such animals with AR inhibitors produced conflicting results. In a series of studies from the National Eye Institute (NEI), complete prevention of diabetes-like histopathologies was demonstrated by light- and electron microscopy in rats fed for 28 months on a diet containing 50% galactose and 0.5% of the AR inhibitor, tolrestat (89, 90). In contrast, Kern and Engerman (163) reported no change in retinopathy development in rats fed a diet containing 50% galactose and 0.04% of the AR inhibitor, sorbinil, for up to 26 months. In dogs fed a 30% galactose diet, at the NEI, the AR inhibitors sorbinil and/or its 2-methyl derivative, administered for up to 36 months, prevented the onset and progression of retinal vascular changes (161, 164, 165). In contrast, Engerman and Kern (166) found no effect on the development of retinopathy in dogs fed the same diet and given sorbinil for up to 60 months; similarly, no effect of sorbinil treatment was detected after 60 month in alloxan-induced diabetic dogs (166). The discrepancy between the reported data remains to be resolved.

Another pathognomonic feature of diabetic retinopathy is the thickening of capillary basement membranes; that the process is linked with sorbitol pathway action was evidenced by preventing the thickening in galactose-fed rats treated with AR inhibitors (28, 84, 157).

## SORBITOL PATHWAY IN HUMAN DIABETIC TISSUES

While animal studies provide invaluable information on the role of the sorbitol pathway in the initiation and progression of lesions occurring in diabetic complications, the ultimate test of the theory (and its practical implications) has to come from human studies. The testing of the role of the sorbitol pathway in the development of complications in diabetic patients was made possible by the availability of several AR inhibitors.

To prove unequivocally the role of the metabolism of excess tissue glucose via the sorbitol pathway in the development of diabetic complications two points must be addressed: first, the magnitude of the glucose flow through the sorbitol pathway in a diabetic tissue should correlate with the degree of tissue damage; second, reduction of the flow with specific therapy should result in stabilisation or amelioration of tissue damage.

The metabolic flux rate through the sorbitol pathway, determined by [$^{13}$C] nuclear magnetic resonance spectroscopy in rabbit (57) and rat lens (58), was found to increase with glucose concentration and, at 36 mM, to account for one-third of the total glucose turnover. The activities of aldose reductase and sorbitol dehydrogenase (measured as NADPH or $NAD^+$ consumption) were determined in sural nerve specimens obtained from diabetic patients having early clinical neuropathy (167); since the power of the study was low, no correlation between nerve aldose reductase activity and myelinated fibre density was demonstrable. However, a significant correlation between nerve sorbitol levels and myelinated fibre density, and between nerve sorbitol levels and the index of pathology was found in diabetic patients with symptomatic neuropathy (113). A 42% decrease in sorbitol content, associated with active repair and regeneration was shown in sural nerve biopsy specimens from diabetic patients with clinical polyneuropathy and treated for 12 months with an AR inhibitor, sorbinil (112; see below).

Based on results obtained in diabetic rats it was believed that the erythrocyte sorbitol level would reflect the sorbitol pathway activity in other tissues (28, 168). Indeed, in man, erythrocyte sorbitol levels seem to correlate with sural nerve sorbitol levels (113). However, to extrapolate from erythrocyte sorbitol levels to AR inhibitor activity in other tissues, the following should be taken into consideration: (a) any change in erythrocyte sorbitol levels must be interpreted in relation to changes in blood glucose concentrations (168); (b) since in human erythrocytes sorbitol is produced by both aldose reductase and hexonate dehydrogenase (169), the potential hexonate dehydrogenase activity in other tissues, e.g. in the nerve, as well as the inhibitor's effect on both enzymes, must be considered; (c) in diabetes, the relative activities of aldose reductase (68, 170, 171) and sorbitol dehydrogenase in erythrocytes differ (172, 173) and may vary between tissues in the same individual; (d) above all, the tissular pharmacokinetics of an AR inhibitor (174), i.e. its uptake and elimination may vary between the erythrocytes and other tissues, e.g. peripheral nerve (28, 168, 169, 175).

Attempts are being made to correlate aldose reductase activity in erythrocytes [expressed as polyol accumulation rate (176, 177); sorbitol/glucose ratio (170, 171), or NADPH consumption (68)] with the severity of diabetic complications: the results revealed higher aldose reductase activity in Type I diabetic patients who had developed complications (71, 171, 176, 178). Based on the assumption that sorbitol pathway activity in neutrophils (179, 180) may parallel that occurring in other diabetic tissues, attempts have been made to identify it as a marker for risk of complications (181). No relationship was found, however, between aldose reductase activity in neutrophils and in sural nerve biopsy specimens collected from patients with early clinical neuropathy (167).

## STUDIES IN MAN

The promising impressions obtained in patients with slight or moderate diabetic neuropathy with alrestatin (182), the first orally effective AR inhibitor (55), prompted the formulation of a pharmacological rationale for the development of AR inhibitors as drugs to prevent, arrest, and, possibly, to reverse the sequelae of chronic diabetes initiated by the metabolism of excess tissue glucose via the sorbitol pathway (183). Indeed, over the past 27 years, thousands of compounds have been examined for their effect on aldose reductase (e.g. 184), and about a dozen have been tested in diabetic subjects (reviewed in 28, 73, 74, 117, 185–187).

Of the long-term diabetic complications, peripheral neuropathy has been the subject of the largest number of clinical trials, with results pertinent to this discussion. This may reflect the early perception that its predominant clinical manifestations (pain and paraesthesia) could be ameliorated in a matter of a few weeks, as well as the relative accessibility of peripheral nerve tissue for biochemical and morphometric analyses.

Retrospectively, it is not surprising that, in patients suffering from overt diabetic peripheral neuropathy, trials aimed primarily at clinical improvement have failed to produce unequivocal evidence of benefit. Above all, our deficient understanding of the natural history of diabetic neuropathy has made it very difficult to design proper clinical trials (188). For example, the slow (over many years) and variable (for different nerves) progression of neuropathy had to be taken into consideration; ill-defined expectations on the type and magnitude of desired clinical benefit, lack of consensus on the best ways to measure the benefit, and the inherent deficiencies of the available methods (e.g. high variability, 189, 190), all contributed to the inappropriate design of clinical trials. Thus, the most common design deficiencies included selection of patients with too advanced neuropathy, small number of patients, and short study duration.

With these important caveats in mind, results from randomised, placebo-controlled multicentre trials of systemically bioavailable AR inhibitors such as sorbinil (191, 192) and tolrestat (190, 193–195) suggested some objective and subjective improvements, but whether they can be translated into long-term clinical benefits remains to be tested.

The following general conclusions, however, can be drawn from the results of published trials of AR inhibitors. First, symptomatic improvement, e.g. reduction in neuropathic pain occurred in sporadic and inconsistent manner, and strong placebo effects, coupled with the known fluctuating nature of symptoms, were an important confounding factor.

Second, electrophysiological tests, most frequently motor NCV, were occasionally improved following AR inhibitor treatment (190, 192–197); there was no consistency between trials in which the nerves improved, nor were all tested nerves improved in a given trial. Longer studies, e.g. of 6–12 months' duration, did not show incremental improvements, and when improvements occurred, they were usually modest, e.g. 1–2 m/s in NCV. However, such changes are not uncommon in trials of improved metabolic control with insulin treatment (3, 198–200), though they seem to be smaller than those observed after a successful pancreatic transplant (e.g. 201). The improvement in NCV was most likely due to the improved metabolic milieu and better transmission across the nodes of Ranvier. It is not likely that these functional changes were the result of structural improvement, but this needs to be closely examined.

Further support for the metabolic basis of short-term changes in NCV comes from a study where treatment with an AR inhibitor, tolrestat, was discontinued, and patients (suffering mostly from advanced diabetic neuropathy) were randomised to either placebo or continued tolrestat therapy. Withdrawal of tolrestat led within weeks to worsening in NCV in three of four motor nerves tested, whereas reinstitution of tolrestat led to rapid improvement (202). That other electrophysiological tests, notably NCV and amplitude in the sensory nerves, failed to show significant worsening upon tolrestat withdrawal can be explained, at least in part, by the large number of patients who had unmeasurable baseline sural nerve amplitudes (due to advanced disease).

Third, there was a shift away from viewing pain as the predominant event in the course of diabetic peripheral neuropathy: a new definition emerged (203) based on the concept that diabetic neuropathy represents a slow, progressive loss of nerve fibres with distinct, characteristic histomorphometric features (110, 112, 113, 204). Though symptoms (most notably pain) form a common basis for diagnosis, the progression of neuropathy towards the more intractable sequelae (foot ulcers, amputation) may not be related to early symptomatic manifestations.

Three clinical trials examined the effects of AR inhibitors on the ultrastructure of the sural nerve. The trial of ponalrestat, at the dose used, failed to show any effect on sural nerve sorbitol levels (204, 205); consequently, no effects on morphometric analysis of sural nerves or on the clinical parameters tested were observed (175, 204–209).

Sorbinil, on the other hand, showed very promising results. In a small prospective study (10 patients receiving sorbinil, and six placebo), patients with diabetic neuropathy treated with sorbinil for 12 months had higher fibre density, higher percentage of normal fibres, and increased nerve regeneration/remyelination when compared to placebo-treated patients (112). In addition, several structural abnormalities (paranodal and segmental demyelination, Wallerian degeneration, myelin wrinkling, axoglial dysjunction) were significantly improved following treatment with sorbinil, compared to placebo. However, sorbinil had no effect on the endoneurial microvasculature (210), the relevance of which to the pathogenesis of peripheral neuropathy remains to be established (119, 211, 212). Two consecutive biopsies were performed on the same nerve, thus possibly confounding the interpretation of results; however, this is not likely, because the same procedure was performed on both placebo- and sorbinil-treated patients. Two conclusions can be drawn from this study: (a) the development of the structural changes was linked to the metabolic and/or functional abnormalities derived from the metabolism of excess glucose in the diabetic nerve; (b) a link between the progression of nerve lesions and the metabolic abnormalities persisted even in patients with long-standing diabetic neuropathy.

In the tolrestat-withdrawal study mentioned above, a single sural nerve biopsy was also performed after approximately five years of therapy (213). At the time of biopsy, one group of 13 patients had received tolrestat for five years and a second group of 14 patients received placebo for one year after having been treated with tolrestat for four years. Morphometric analysis showed marked nerve regeneration in both tolrestat treated groups, which was 4.7-fold higher than the regeneration observed in a group of diabetic patients used as historical control. Compared to the historical control, segmental demyelination and axo-glial dysjunction were also reduced in the treated groups; other structural parameters showed less consistent changes.

The lack of difference between the two treated groups in the results of morphometric analysis suggests that the structural changes induced by AR inhibitor treatment can persist for at least one year after drug discontinuation. The fact that a single biopsy was performed (and hence the need for a separate historic control group) weakened the positive conclusions which might be derived from this trial. In search of a definitive answer, two large, placebo-controlled, 18-month studies in diabetic patients with mild neuropathy are currently being carried out with tolrestat in the US. A contralateral sural nerve biopsy is performed at baseline and at the end of the study, with morphometric analysis constituting the primary endpoints.

What is the clinical relevance of the pathological changes observed in these 'structure-oriented' clinical trials? The data clearly suggest that nerve fibre density correlates strongly with functional measurements such as amplitude and conduction velocity, as well as with clinical assessments such as sensory perception (214–216). Whereas regeneration can accompany progressive fibre loss (113, 217), it should be considered as a favourable process because restoration of normoglycaemia with pancreatic transplant led to increased nerve regeneration and repair (218). Regeneration is likely to be clinically beneficial only if the sprouting leads to restoration of the original structural integrity, including target recognition (219, 220). Since it is likely that lost fibres cannot be fully replaced in the course of a clinical trial, a realistic outcome of interventive therapy should be in signs of regeneration coupled with prevention (or slowing) of further nerve fibre damage and loss.

Many of the clinical manifestations of diabetic neuropathy may also result from small fibre disease (221, 222), and assessment of large myelinated fibres (by electrophysiology or biopsy) may not offer a completely relevant picture of all the clinical manifestations.

While questions remain, elucidation of the relationship between morphometrically established nerve damage and measures of peripheral nerve function have considerably expanded our understanding of the natural history of diabetic neuropathy, its pathogenesis, and the probability of response to therapy.

Autonomic neuropathy was also investigated in several, relatively small clinical trials using AR inhibitors, with observation periods of up to 12 months. Improvement (of questionable clinical significance) in selected cardiovascular (223, 224) or genitourinary (225) parameters was occasionally observed, whereas other studies failed to show any effect (226–229). In a 12-month randomised, placebo-controlled study in 45 diabetic patients, tolrestat was shown to significantly improve several cardiovascular parameters, including maximum/minimum heart rate on deep inspiration, postural hypotension and lying-to-standing heart ratio (230). Since autonomic neuropathy, like peripheral neuropathy, is progressing at a very slow rate (231), well-controlled long-term studies are needed to establish the role of the sorbitol pathway in the development of this complication.

AR inhibitors have also been tested for their effect on retinopathy (73, 232–235), and incipient nephropathy (197, 236–240). With respect to diabetic retinopathy, three years of treatment with the AR inhibitor, epalrestat, reportedly produced a reduction or disappearance of microaneurysms, hemorrhages and soft exudates in patients with non-proliferative retinopathy (186). On the other hand, three years of treatment with the AR inhibitor sorbinil produced no clinically important effect on the course of retinopathy, except a slight reduction in the rate of microaneurysm increase (232). Of note, five to nine years of intensified insulin treatment was needed to retard the progression of non-proliferative retinopathy in IDDM patients (14, 241, 242). Given that the DCCT has been conducted for up to nine years, it is reasonable to assume, that for any potential benefit to be demonstrated with an AR inhibitor, trials of adequate duration need to be carried out.

In patients with incipient diabetic nephropathy, treatment with epalrestat (236), sorbinil (197), or tolrestat (240) arrested (197), or decreased (236, 240) the rate of urinary albumin excretion. Results reported for ponalrestat (on its effect on the early rise in GFR) are not consistent (237–239), perhaps reflecting ponalrestat's inability to inhibit hexonate dehydrogenase which predominates in the renal cortex (30, 37, 154). No long-term trials with AR inhibitors have been reported where the development of albuminuria and/or loss of kidney function were the endpoints.

## SUMMARY AND CONCLUSIONS

According to the sorbitol pathway theory, the metabolism of excess glucose by aldose reductase occurring in a diabetic tissue triggers a cascade of pathophysiological alterations that

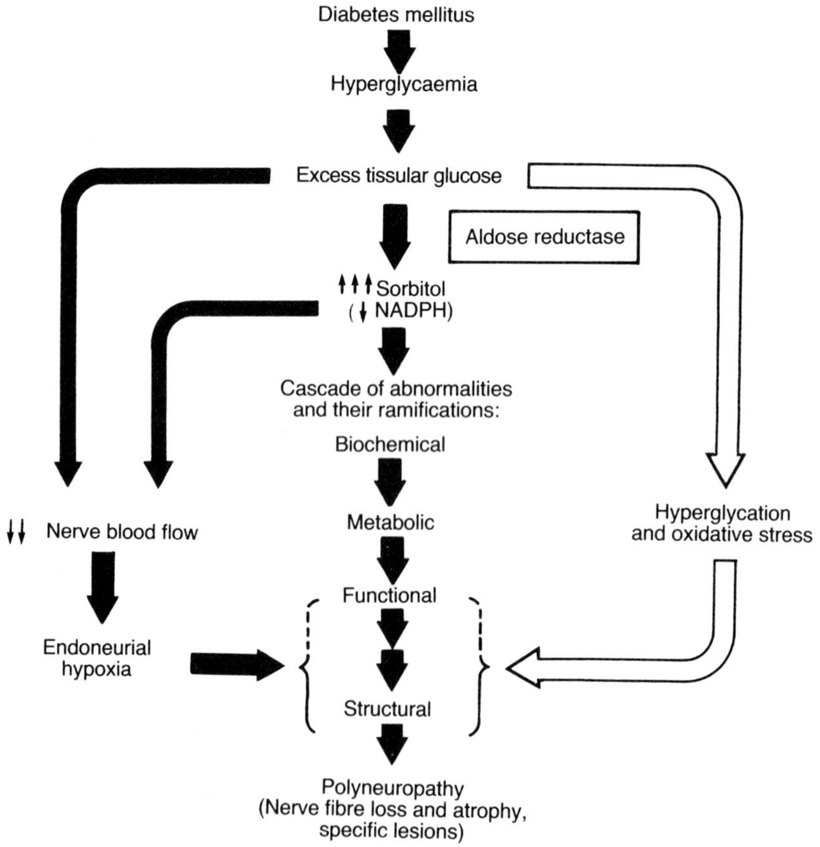


Fig. 24.3. Proposed mechanism of diabetic polyneuropathy (After Ref. 243.)

can progress to long-term complications. The theory is clearly supported by results obtained with inhibitors of aldose reductase in animal models of diabetic hyperglycaemia. Clinical trials of AR inhibitors aimed at delaying the progression of nerve damage in diabetic patients with neuropathy, on the other hand, have failed to produce unequivocal evidence of clinical benefit.

There are several differences between animal and human studies: first, whereas in animals treatment with AR inhibitors was mostly preventive, in human studies the treatment was always interventive, and at a time when the complication was clinically evident; at such time the progression of the complication may have become self-generating and independent of the operation of the sorbitol pathway. Second, animals were often administered AR inhibitors at doses relatively higher than in humans, and for longer periods of time relative to the animals' lifespan. Third, despite important similarities in hyperglycaemia-induced tissue changes between animal models and human diabetic patients, the rates of progression of abnormalities, and their functional and structural manifestations may differ.

Despite these caveats, the picture emerging from the combined human and animal experience is consistent with the view that hyperglycaemia-induced activation of the sorbitol pathway and the resulting pathophysiological alterations act as the trigger of processes which can lead to diabetic complications, whereas local hypoxia, and chronically increased glycation and oxidative stress may become pathogenetically more important at some later stage. This conclusion seems most valid for neuropathy (243) (Fig. 24.3). The paucity of human studies of sufficient duration with effective AR inhibitors coupled with uncertainties as to the relevance of certain animal models, precludes similar conclusions for retinopathy and nephropathy.

It is only through appropriately designed and conducted long-term clinical trials, using potent and effective AR inhibitors, that the precise contribution of the sorbitol pathway to the development of long-term diabetic complications will be assessed. In the meantime, AR inhibitors are expanding our understanding of the natural history of diabetic complications and the links between their metabolic, functional, and structural alterations and clinical manifestations.

## REFERENCES


1 Hanssen KF, Bangstad HJ, Brinchmann-Hansen O, Dahl-Jorgensen K. Blood glucose control and diabetic microvascular complications: long-term effects of near-normoglycaemia. *Diabetic Med* 1992; 9: 697–705.

2 Ruderman NB, Williamson JR, Brownlee M. Glucose and diabetic vascular disease. *FASEB J* 1992; 6: 2905–14.

3 Ziegler D, Mayer P, Mühlen H, Gries FA. The natural history of somatosensory and autonomic nerve dysfunction in relation to glycaemic control during the first 5 years after diagnosis of Type I (insulin-dependent) diabetes mellitus. *Diabetologia* 1991; 34: 822–9.

4 Lehtinen JM, Niskanen L, Hyvönen K, Siitonen O, Uusitupa M. Nerve function and its determinants in patients with newly diagnosed Type 2 (non-insulin-dependent diabetes mellitus) and in control subjects – a 5-year follow-up. *Diabetologia* 1993; 36: 38–62.

5 Larkins RG, Dunlop ME. The link between hyperglycaemia and diabetic nephropathy. *Diabetologia* 1992; 35: 499–504.

6 Klein R, Klein BEK, Moss SE, Davis MD, De Mets DL. Glycosylated hemoglobin predicts the incidence and progression of diabetic retinopathy. *J Am Med Assoc* 1988; 260: 2864–77.

7 Strowig S, Raskin P. Glycemic control and diabetic complications. *Diabetes Care* 1992; 15: 1126–40.

8 The DCCT Research Group. Are continuing studies of metabolic control and microvascular complications in insulin-dependent diabetes mellitus justified? *N Engl J Med* 1988; 318: 246–50.

9 Zimmerman BR. Influence of the degree of control of diabetes on the prevention, postponement and amelioration of late complications. *Drugs* 1989; 38: 941–56.

10 Santiago JV. Intensive management of insulin dependent diabetes: risks, benefits, and unanswered questions. *J Clin Endocrinol Metab* 1992; 75: 977–82.

11 Reichard P, Sule J, Rosenqvist U. Capillary loss and leakage after five years of intensified insulin treatment in patients with insulin-dependent diabetes mellitus. *Ophthalmology* 1991: 98: 1587–93.

12 Jörgens V, Grüsser M, Bott U, Mühlhauser I, Berger M. Effective and safe translation of intensified insulin therapy to general internal medicine departments. *Diabetologia* 1993; 36: 99–105.

13 The DCCT Research Group. The Diabetes Control and Complications Trial (DCCT): design and methodologic considerations for the feasibility phase. *Diabetes* 1986; 35: 530–45.

14 The DCCT Research Group: Diabetes Control and Complications Trial (DCCT): *N Engl J Med* 1993; 329: 977–86.
15 Williamson JR, Chang K, Frangos M *et al.* Hyperglycemic pseudohypoxia and diabetic complications. *Diabetes* 1993; 42: 801–13.
16 Gabbay KH. Hyperglycemia, polyol metabolism and complications of diabetes mellitus. *Ann Rev Med* 1975; 26: 521–35.
17 Dvornik D. Hyperglycemia in the pathogenesis of diabetic complications. In: Porte D, ed. *Aldose reductase inhibition: an approach to the prevention of diabetic complications.* BIC/McGraw-Hill, New York 1987: 69–151.
18 Kinoshita JH. History of aldose reductase. In: Sakamoto N, Kinoshita JH, Kador PF, Hotta N, eds. *Polyol pathway and its role in diabetic complications.* Elsevier, Amsterdam 1988: 12–19.
19 Cerami A, Stevens VJ, Monnier VM. Role of nonenzymatic glycosylation in the development of the sequelae of diabetes. *Metabolism* 1979; 28:431–7.
20 Cerami A, Vlassara H, Brownlee M. Role of advanced glycosylation products in complications of diabetes. *Diabetes Care* 1988; 11: 73–9.
21 Dominiczak MH. The significance of the products of the Maillard (browning) reaction in diabetes. *Diabetic Med* 1991; 8: 505–16.
22 Baynes JW. Role of oxidative stress in development of complications in diabetes. *Diabetes* 1991; 40: 405–12.
23 Hunt JV, Bottoms MA, Mitchinson MJ. Oxidative alterations in the experimental glycation model of diabetes mellitus are due to protein-glucose adduct oxidation. *Biochem J* 1993; 291: 529–35.
24 Wolff SP, Jiang ZY, Hunt JV. Protein glycation and oxidative stress in diabetes mellitus and aging. *Free Rad Biol Med* 1991; 10: 339–52.
25 Hunt JV, Wolff SP. Oxidative glycation and free radical production: a causal mechanism of diabetic complications. *Free Rad Res Commun* 1991; 12–13: 115–23.
26 Carper D, Nishimura C, Shinohara T *et al.* Aldose reductase and *p*-crystallin belong to the same protein superfamily as aldehyde reductase. *FEBS Lett* 1987; 22: 209–13.
27 Bohren KM, Bullock B, Wermuth B, Gabbay KH. The aldo-keto reductase superfamily. *J Biol Chem* 1989; 264: 9547–51.
28 Dvornik D. Aldose reductase inhibitors. In: Porte D, ed. *Aldose reductase inhibition: an approach to the prevention of diabetic complications.* BIC/McGraw Hill, New York 1987: 221–323.
29 Chakrabarti S, Sima AAF, Nakajima T, Yagihashi S, Greene DA. Aldose reductase in the BB rat: isolation, immunological identification and localization in the retina and peripheral nerve. *Diabetologia* 1987; 30: 244–51.
30 Terubayashi H, Sato S, Nishimura C, Kador PF, Kinoshita JH. Localization of aldose and aldehyde reductase in the kidney. *Kidney Int* 1989; 36: 843–51.
31 Powell HC, Garrett RS, Kador PF, Mizisin AP. Fine structural localization of aldose reductase and ouabain-sensitive, $K^+$-dependent *p*-nitro-phenylphosphatase in rat peripheral nerve. *Acta Neuropathol* 1991; 81: 529–39.
32 Bhatnagar A, Srivastava SA. Aldose reductase: congenial and injurious profiles of an enigmatic enzyme. *Biochem Med Metab Biol* 1992; 48: 91–121.
33 Griffin BW. Functional and structural relationships among aldose reductase L-hexonate dehydrogenase (aldehyde reductase), and recently identified homologous proteins. *Enzyme Microb Technol* 1992; 14: 690–5.
34 Morjana NA, Lyons C, Flynn TG. Aldose reductase from human *psoas* muscle. Affinity labelling of an active site lysine by pyridoxal 5′-phosphate and pyridoxal 5′-diphospho-5′-adenosine. *J Biol Chem* 1989; 264: 2906–11.
35 Kawasaki N, Tanimoto T, Tanaka A. Characterization of aldose reductase and aldehyde reductase from rat testis. *Biochem Biophys Acta* 1989; 996: 30–6.
36 Ohta M, Tanimoto T, Tanaka A. Characterization of aldose reductase and aldehyde reductase from the medulla of rat kidney. *Chem Pharm Bull* 1990; 38: 1639–43.
37 Sato S, Kador PF. Human Kidney aldose and aldehyde reductases. *J. Diab Comp* 1993; 179–87.
38 Bohren KM, Grimshaw CE, Gabbay KH. Catalytic effectiveness of human aldose reductase. Critical role of C-terminal domain. *J Biol Chem* 1992; 267: 20965–70.
39 Yamaoka T, Matshura Y, Yamashita K, Tanimoto T, Nishimura C. Site-directed mutagenesis of His-42, His-188 and Lys-263 of human aldose reductase. *Biochem Biophys Res Comm* 1992; 183: 327–33.
40 Bohren KM, Page JL, Shankar R, Henry SP, Gabbay KH: Expression of human aldose and aldehyde reductases. Site-directed mutagenesis of a critical lysine 262. *J Biol Chem* 1991; 266: 24031–7.
41 Sato S. Rat kidney aldose reductase and aldehyde reductase and polyol production in rat kidney. *Am J Physiol* 1992; 263: F799–F805.
42 Farber GK, Petsko GA. The evolution of a/β barrel enzymes. *Trends Biochem Sci* 1990; 15: 228–34.
43 Rondeau JM, Tête-Favier F, Podjarny A *et al.* Novel NADPH-binding domain revealed by the crystal structure of aldose reductase. *Nature* 1992; 355: 469–72.
44 Wilson DK, Bohren KM, Gabbay KH, Quiocho FA. An unlikely sugar substrate site in the 1.65A structure of the human aldose reductase holoenzyme implicated in diabetic complications. *Science* 1992; 257: 81–4.
45 Grimshaw CE, Shabaz M, Jahangiri G, Putney CG, McKercher SR, Mathur EJ. Kinetic and structural effects of activation of bovine kidney aldose reductase. *Biochemistry* 1989; 28: 5343–53.
46 Pavlov RA, Vartanov SS, Yaropolov AI. Regulation of aldose reductase activity. Influence of effectors on reversible isomerization of the enzymes. *Biokhimiya* 1991; 56: 1999–2015.
47 Del Corso A, Barsacchi D, Gianessi M *et al.* Bovine lens aldose reductase: tight binding of the pyridine coenzyme. *Arch Biochem Biophys* 1990; 283: 512–18.
48 Borhani DW, Harter TM, Petrash JM. The crystal structure of the aldose reductase:NADPH binary complex. *J Biol Chem* 1992; 267: 24841–7.
49 Grimshaw CE. Aldose reductase: model for a new paradigm of enzyme perfection in detoxification catalysis. *Biochemistry* 1992; 31: 10139–45.
50 Jakoby WB, Ziegler DM. The enzymes of detoxication. *J Biol Chem* 1990; 265: 20715–18.
51 Harding JJ. Aldose reductase (or is it?). *Trends Biochem Sci* 1992; 17: 494.

52 Dvornik D. Animal models of diabetic complications and their relation to aldose reductase inhibition. In: Porte D, ed. *Aldose reductase inhibition: an approach to the prevention of diabetic complications.* BIC/McGraw-Hill, New York 1987: 152–219.
53 Kinoshita JH, Merola LO, Satoh K, Dikmak E. Osmotic changes caused by the accumulation of dulcitol in the lenses of rats fed with galactose. *Nature* 1962: 194: 1084–7.
54 Kinoshita JH, Dvornik D, Kraml M, Gabbay KH. The effect of an aldose reductase inhibitor on the galactose-exposed rabbit lens. *Biochem Biophys Acta* 1968; 158: 472–5.
55 Dvornik D, Simard-Duquesne N, Kraml M *et al.* Polyol accumulation in galactosemic and diabetic rats: control by an aldose reductase inhibitor. *Science* 1973; 182: 1146–8.
56 Sochor M, Banquer NZ, Hothersall JS, McLean P. Effects of experimental diabetes on the activity of hexokinase isozymes in tissues of the rat. *Biochem Internat* 1990; 22: 467–74.
57 Gonzalez R, Barnett P, Aguayo J, Chen HM, Chylack LT Jr. Direct measurement of polyol pathway activity in the ocular lens. *Diabetes* 1984; 33: 196–9.
58 Barnett PA, Gonzalez RG, Chylack LT Jr, Cheng HM. The effect of oxidation on sorbitol pathway kinetics. *Diabetes* 1986; 35: 426–32.
59 Flath MC, Bylander JE, Sens DA. Variation in sorbitol accumulation and polyol-pathway activity in cultured human proximal tubule cells. *Diabetes* 1992; 41: 1050–5.
60 Grunewald RW, Kinne RKH. Intracellular sorbitol content in isolated rat inner medullary collecting duct cells. Regulation by extracellular osmolality. *Pflüger's Arch* 1989; 414: 178–84.
61 Grunewald RW, Kinne RKH. Sorbitol metabolism in inner medullary collecting duct cells of diabetic rats. *Pflüger's Arch* 1989; 414: 346–50.
62 Steiner K, Sima AAF, Hohman TC, Greene DA, Tolrestat Study Group. Use of morphometry in the assessment of biochemistry in sural nerve biopsies from diabetic neuropathic patients. *Diabetologia* 1992; 35 (Suppl. 1): A16.
63 Pugliese G, Tilton RG, Williamson JR. Glucose-induced metabolic imbalances in the pathogenesis of diabetic vascular disease. *Diabetes/Metab Rev* 1991; 7: 35–9.
64 Tilton RG, Baier LD, Harlow JE, Smith SR, Ostrow E, Williamson JR. Diabetes-induced glomerular dysfunction: links to a more reduced cytosolic ratio of NADH/$NAD^+$. *Kidney Int* 1992; 41: 778–88.
65 Dyck PJ, Sherman WR, Hallacher LM *et al.* Human diabetic endoneurial sorbitol, fructose, and *myo*-inositol related to sural nerve morphometry. *Ann Neurol* 1980; 8: 590–6.
66 Hale PJ, Nattrass M, Silverman SH *et al.* Peripheral nerve concentrations of glucose, fructose, sorbitol and myoinositol in diabetic and non-diabetic patients. *Diabetologia* 1987; 30: 464–7.
67 Willars GB, Newrick PG, Tomlinson DR, Ward D. Polyol metabolites and myo-inositol in sural nerve biopsies from diabetic patients. *Diabetic Med* 1987; 4: 382.
68 Hamada Y, Kitoh R, Raskin P. Crucial role of aldose reductase activity and plasma glucose level in sorbitol accumulation in erythrocytes from diabetic patients. *Diabetes* 1991; 40: 1233–40.
69 Hasan K, Santiago J, Williamson J. Acute hyperglycemia-induced increases in regional blood flow are prevented by pyruvate and by tolrestat. *Diabetes* 1993; 42 (Suppl. 1): 189A.
70 Stevens M, Dananberg J, Lattimer S, Sima A, Greene D. Sorbitol pathway mediated slowing of nerve conduction involves a nitric oxide mechanism in the streptozotocin diabetic rat. *Diabetes* 1993; 42 (Suppl. 1): 149A.
71 Hamada Y, Kitoh R, Raskin P. Association of erythrocyte aldose reductase activity with diabetic complications in Type 1 diabetes mellitus. *Diabetic Med* 1993; 10: 33–8.
72 Kinoshita JH, Nishimura C. The involvement of aldose reductase in diabetic complications. *Diabetes/Metab Rev* 1988; 4: 323–37.
73 Hotta N, Sakamoto N. Aldose reductase inhibitors. In: Alberti KGMM, Krall LP, eds. *The diabetes annual/5.* Elsevier, Amsterdam 1990: 330–61.
74 Tomlinson DR, Willars GB, Carrington AL. Aldose reductase inhibitors and diabetic complications. *Pharmac Ther* 1992; 54: 151–94.
75 Osterby R. Glomerular structural abnormalities in early and late stages of experimental diabetes: models for diabetic nephropathy. In: Shafrir E, Renold AE, eds. *Frontiers in diabetes research. Lessons from animal diabetes. II.* Libbey, London 1988; 522–7.
76 Mizisin AP, Powell HC, Myers RR. Edema and increased endoneurial sodium in galactose neuropathy. Reversal with an aldose reductase inhibitor therapy. *J Neurol Sci* 1985; 74: 35–43.
77 Diemel LT, Stevens EJ, Willars GB, Tomlinson DR. Depletion of substance P and calcitonin gene-related peptide in sciatic nerve of rats with experimental diabetes; effects of insulin and aldose reductase inhibition. *Neuroscience Lett* 1992; 137: 253–6.
78 Notvest RR, Inserra JJ. Tolrestat, an aldose reductase inhibitor, prevents nerve dysfunction in conscious diabetic rats. *Diabetes* 1987; 36: 500–4.
79 Luheshi GN, Zar MA. Inhibitory effect of streptozotocin-induced diabetes on non-cholinergic motor transmission in rat detrusor and its prevention by sorbinil. *Br J Pharmacol* 1990; 161: 411–17.
80 Bellomo G, Comstock JP, Wen D, Hazelwood RL. Prolonged fructose feeding and aldose reductase inhibition: effect on the polyol pathway in kidneys of normal rats. *Proc Soc Exp Biol Med* 1987; 186: 348–54.
81 McCaleb ML, Sredy J, Millen J, Ackerman DM, Dvornik D. Prevention of urinary albumin excretion in 6 month streptozocin diabetic rats with the aldose reductase inhibitor tolrestat. *J Diab Comp* 1988; 2: 16–18.
82 Tilton RG, Chang K, Pugliese G *et al.* Prevention of hemodynamic and vascular albumin filtration changes in diabetic rats by aldose reductase inhibitors. *Diabetes* 1989; 37: 1258–70.
83 Chang WP, Dimitriadis E, Allen T, Dunlop ME, Cooper M, Larkins RG. The effect of aldose reductase inhibitors on glomerular prostaglandin production and urinary albumin excretion in experimental diabetes. *Diabetologia* 1991; 34: 225–31.
84 McCaleb ML, McKean ML, Hohman TC, Laver N, Robison WG Jr. Intervention with the aldose reductase

inhibitor, tolrestat, in renal and retinal lesions of streptozotocin-diabetic rats. *Diabetologia* 1991; 34: 695–701.
85 Oates PJ, Ellery CA, Goldfarb S. Aldose reductase inhibitor zopolrestat reduces hyperfiltration and albuminuria in diabetic rats. *Diabetologia* 1992; 35 (Suppl. 1): A148.
86 Greene DA, Chakrabarti S, Lattimer SA, Sima AAF. Role of sorbitol accumulation and myo-inositol depletion in paranodal swelling of large myelinated nere fibers in the insulin-deficient spontaneously diabetic Bio-Breeding rat. Reversal by insulin replacement, an aldose reductase inhibitor, and myo-inositol. *J Clin Invest* 1987; 79: 1479–85.
87 Sima AAF, Prashar A, Zhang WX, Chakrabarti S. Greene DA. Preventive effect of long-term aldose reductase inhibition (ponalrestat) on nerve conduction and sural nerve structure in the spontaneously diabetic Bio-Breeding rat. *J Clin Invest* 1990; 85: 1410–20.
88 Robison WG Jr, Nagata M, Tillis TN, Laver N, Kinoshita JH. Aldose reductase and pericyte-endothelial cell contacts in retina and optic nerve. *Invest Ophthalmol Vis Sci* 1989; 30: 2293–9.
89 Robison WG Jr, Nagata M, Laver N, Hohman TC, Kinoshita JH. Diabetic-like retinopathy in rats prevented with aldose reductase inhibitors. *Invest Ophthalmol Vis Sci* 1989; 30: 2285–92.
90 Robison WG Jr, Tillis TN, Laver N, Kinoshita JH. Diabetes-related histopathologies of the rat retina prevented with an aldose reductase inhibitor. *Exp Eye Res* 1990; 50: 355–66.
91 Greene DA, Lattimer SA, Sima AAF. Tissue-specific metabolic alterations in the pathogenesis of diabetic peripheral neuropathy. In: Belfiore F, Molinatti GM, Raeven GM, eds. *Tissue-specific metabolic alterations in diabetes. 10.* Karger, Basel 1990; 83–96.
92 Elliasson SG. Nerve conduction changes in experimental diabetes. *J Clin Invest* 1964; 43: 2553–8.
93 Preston GM. Peripheral neuropathy in the alloxan-diabetic rat. *J Physiol* 1967; 189; 49P–50P.
94 Greene, DA, DeJesus PV Jr, Winegrad AI. Effects of insulin and dietary myoinositol on impaired motor nerve conduction velocity in acute streptozotocin diabetes. *J Clin Invest* 1975; 55: 1326–36.
95 Stewart MAE, Sherman WR, Kurien M, Moonsammy GI, Wisgerhof M. Polyol accumulation in nervous tissue of rats with experimental diabetes and galactosemia. *J Neurochem* 1967; 24: 1057–66.
96 Bondy C, Cowley AD, Lightman SL, Kador PF. Feedback inhibition of aldose reductase gene expression in rat renal medulla. *J Clin Invest* 1990; 86: 1103–8.
97 Greene DA, Sima AAF, Stevens MJ, Feldman EL, Lattimer SA. Complications: neuropathy, pathogenetic considerations. *Diabetes Care* 1992; 15: 1902–25.
98 Dvornik D. Aldose reductase inhibitors as pathobiochemical probes. *J Diab Comp* 1992; 6: 1–10; 154.
99 Greene DA, Lattimer S, Ulbrecht J, Carroll P. Glucose-induced alterations in nerve metabolism: current perspective on the pathogenesis of diabetic neuropathy and future direction for research and therapy. *Diabetes Care* 1985; 8: 290–9.
100 Tomlinson DR, Willars GB, Robinson JP, Lambourne JE, Calcutt NA, Compton AM. Experimental aspects of diabetic neuropathy: role of axonal transport disorders. In: Sakamoto N, Kinoshita JH, Kador PF, Hotta N, eds. *Polyol pathway and its role in diabetic complications.* Elsevier, Amsterdam 1988: 385–96.
101 Winegrad AI. Does a common mechanism induce the diverse complications of diabetes? *Diabetes* 1987; 36: 396–406.
102 Greene DA, Lattimer SA, Sima AAF. Sorbitol, phosphoinositides, and sodium-potassium ATPase in the pathogenesis of diabetic complications. *N Engl J Med* 1987; 316: 599–606.
103 Masson EA, Boulton AJM. Aldose reductase inhibitors in the treatment of diabetic neuropathy. A review of the rationale and clinical evidence. *Drugs* 1990; 39: 190–202.
104 Tomlinson DR. The pharmacology of diabetic neuropathy. *Diabetes/Metab Rev* 1992; 8: 67–84.
105 Gillon KRW, Hawthorne JN. Sorbitol, inositol and nerve conduction in diabetes. *Life Sci* 1983; 32: 1943–7.
106 Mayer JH, Tomlinson DR. The influence of aldose reductase inhibition and nerve myo-inositol on axonal transport and nerve conduction velocity in rats with experimental diabetes. *J Physiol* 1983; 340: 25P.
107 Finegold D, Lattimer SA, Nolle S, Bernstein M, Greene DA. Polyol pathway activity and myo-inositol metabolism: a suggested relationship in the pathogenesis of diabetic neuropathy. *Diabetes* 1983; 32: 988–92.
108 Greene DA, Lattimer SA. Action of sorbinil in diabetic peripheral nerve: relationship of polyol (sorbitol) pathway inhibition to a myo-inositol-mediated defect in $NA^+$, $K^+$-ATPase activity. *Diabetes* 1984; 33: 712–16.
109 Sima AAF, Lattimer SA, Yagihashi S, Greene DA. Axo-glial dysjunction. A novel structural lesion that accounts for poorly reversible slowing of nerve conduction in the spontaneously diabetic Bio-Breeding rat. *J Clin Invest* 1986; 77: 474–84.
110 Sima AAF, Nathaniel V, Bril V, McEwen TAJ, Greene DA. Histopathological heterogeneity of neuropathy in insulin-dependent and non-insulin-dependent diabetes, and demonstration of axo-glial dysjunction in human diabetic neuropathy. *J Clin Invest* 1988; 81: 349–64.
111 Greene DA, Lattimer SA, Sima AAF. Are disturbances or sorbitol, phosphoinositide, and $NA^+/K^+$-ATPase regulation involved in the pathogenesis of diabetic neuropathy? *Diabetes* 1988; 37: 688–93.
112 Sima AAF, Bril V, Nathaniel V *et al.* Regeneration and repair of myelinated fibers in sural-nerve biopsy specimens from patients with diabetic neuropathy treated with sorbinil. *N Engl J Med* 1988; 319: 548–55.
113 Dyck PJ, Zimmerman BR, Vilen TH *et al.* Nerve glucose, fructose, sorbitol, myoinositol, and fiber degeneration and regeneration in diabetic neuropathy. *N Engl J Med* 1988; 319: 542–8.
114 Greene DA, Bochenek W, Harati Y *et al.* Biochemical and morphometric response to tolrestat in human diabetic nerve. *Diabetologia* 1990; 33 (Suppl.): A92.
115 Greene DA, Sima AAF, Lattimer SA, Hachiya H, Diaz TC, Delmonte M. The elusive sorbitol-accumulation/myoinositol-depletion hypothesis of diabetic complications is alive and well but in hiding. In: Larkins R, Zimmet P, Chisholm D, eds. *Diabetes 1988.* Elsevier, Amsterdam 1989; 45–53.
116 Baxter MA. The role of myo-inositol in the pathogen-

esis of diabetic complications. *Trends Endocrinol Metab* 1991; 2: 187–90.
117 Tomlinson DR. Aldose reductase inhibitors and the complications of diabetes mellitus. *Diabetic Med* 1993; 10: 214–30.
118 Thomas PK. Diabetic neuropathy: models, mechanisms and mayhem. *Can J Neurol Sci* 1992; 19: 1–7.
119 Malik RA, Tesfaye S, Thompson SD *et al.* Endoneurial localisation of microvascular damage in human diabetic neuropathy. *Diabetologia* 1993; 36: 454–9.
120 Low PA. Recent advances in the pathogenesis of diabetic neuropathy. *Muscle & Nerve* 1987; 10: 121–8.
121 Dyck PJ. Hypoxic neuropathy: does hypoxia play a role in diabetic neuropathy? *Neurology* 1989; 39: 111–18.
122 Cameron NE, Cotter MA, Low PA. Nerve blood flow in early experimental diabetes in rats: relation to conduction deficits. *Am J Physiol* 1991; 261: E1–E8.
123 Smith WJ, Diemel LT, Leach RM, Tomlinson DR. Central hypoxaemia in rats provokes neurological defects similar to those seen in experimental diabetes mellitus: evidence for a partial role of endoneurial hypoxia in diabetic neuropathy. *Neuroscience* 1991; 2: 255–9.
124 Greene DA, Sima AAF, Pfeifer MA, Albers JW. Diabetic neuropathy. *Ann Rev Med* 1990; 41: 303–17.
125 Cameron NE, Cotter MA, Maxfield EK. Anti-oxidant treatment prevents the development or peripheral nerve dysfunction in streptozotocin-diabetic rats. *Diabetologia* 1993; 36: 299–304.
126 Corder CN, Collins JG, Brannan TS, Sharma J. Aldose reductase and sorbitol dehydrogenase distribution in rat kidney. *J Histochem Cytochem* 1977; 25: 1–8.
127 Corder CN, Braughler JM, Culp PA. Quantitative histochemistry of the sorbitol pathway in glomeruli and small arteries of human diabetic kidney. *Folia Histochem Cytochem* 1979; 17: 137–46.
128 Wirtensohn G, Lefrank S, Guder WG, Beck FX: Studies on the role of glycerophosphorylcholine and sorbitol in renal osmoregulation. In: Kovacevic Z, Guder WG, eds. *Nephrology. biochemical aspects of kidney function.* De Gruyter, Berlin 1987: 321–7.
129 Chauncey B, Leite MV, Goldstein L. Renal sorbitol accumulation and associated enzyme activities in diabetes. *Enzyme* 1988; 39: 231–4.
130 Wirtensohn G, Lefrank S, Schmolke M, Guder WG. Regulation of organic osmolyte concentrations in tubules from rat renal inner medulla. *Am J Physiol* 1989; 256: F128–35.
131 Bedford JJ, Bagnasco SM, Kador PF, Harris HW Jr, Burg MB. Characterization and purification of a mammalian osmoregulatory protein, aldose reductase, induced in renal medullary cells by high extracellular NaCl. *J Biol Chem* 1987; 262: 14255–9.
132 Burg MB, Kador PF. Sorbitol, osmoregulation, and the complications of diabetes. *J Clin Invest* 1988; 81: 635–40.
133 Yancey PH, Burg MB, Bagnasco SM. Effects of NaCl, glucose and aldose reductase inhibitors on cloning efficiency of renal medullary cells. *Am J Physiol* 1990; 258: C156–63.
134 Sands JM, Schrader DC. Coordinated response of renal medullary enzymes regulating net sorbitol production in diuresis and antidiuresis. *J Am Soc Nephrol* 1990; 1: 58–65.
135 Schmolke M, Schleicher E, Guder WG. Renal sorbitol, *myo*-inositol and glycerophosphocholine in streptozotocin diabetic rats. *Eur J Clin Chem Clin Biochem* 1992; 30: 607–14.
136 Moriyama T, Garcia-Perez A, Burg MB. Factors affecting the ratio of different organic osmolytes in renal medullary cells. *Am J Physiol* 1990; 259: F 847–58.
137 Moriyama T, Garcia-Perez A, Olson AD, Burg MB. Intracellular betaine substitutes for sorbitol in protecting renal medullary cells from hypertonicity. *Am J Physiol* 1991; 260: F 494–7.
138 Yancey PH, Haüer RG, Freudenberger TH. Effects of an aldose reductase inhibitor on organic osmotic effects in rat renal medulla. *Am J Physiol* 1990; 259: F 733–8.
139 Edmands S, Yancey PH. Effects on rat renal osmolytes of extended treatment with an aldose reductase inhibitor. *Comp Biochem Physiol* 1992; 103C: 499–502.
140 Kador PF. The role of aldose reductase in the development of diabetic complications. *Med Res Rev* 1988; 8: 325–52.
141 Harrison HE, Stribling D, Armstrong FM, Perkins CM. Aldose reductase in the etiology of diabetic complications. I. Introduction. *J Diab Comp* 1989; 3: 6–11.
142 Beyer-Mears A, Cruz E, Edelist T, Varagiannis E. Diminished proteinuria in diabetes mellitus by sorbinil, an aldose reductase inhibitor. *Pharmacology* 1986; 32: 52–60.
143 Craven PA, DeRubertis FR. Sorbinil suppresses glomerular prostaglandin production in the streptozotocin diabetic rat. *Metabolism* 1989; 38: 649–54.
144 Bank N, Mower P, Aynedjian HS, Wilkes BM, Silverman S. Sorbinil prevents glomerular hyperperfusion in diabetic rats. *Am J Physiol* 1989; 256: F1000–6.
145 Daniels BS, Hostetter TH. Aldose reductase inhibition and glomerular abnormalities in diabetic rats. *Diabetes* 1989; 38: 981–6.
146 Greene, DA, Lattimer SA. Protein kinase C agonists acutely normalize decreased ouabain-inhibitable respiration in diabetic rabbit nerve. Implications for (Na,K)-ATPase regulation and diabetic complications. *Diabetes* 1986; 35: 242–5.
147 Craven PA, DeRubertis FR. Protein kinase C is activated in glomeruli from streptozotocin diabetic rats. Possible mediation by glucose. *J Clin Invest* 1989; 83: 1667–75.
148 Kreisberg JI, Patel PY. The effects of insulin, glucose and diabetes on prostaglandin production by rat kidney glomeruli and cultured mesangial cells. *Prostaglandins Leukotrienes Med* 1983; 11: 431–42.
149 Schambelan M, Blake S, Sraer J, Bens M, Nivez MP, Wahbe F. Increased prostaglandin production by glomeruli isolated from rats with streptozotocin-induced diabetes mellitus. *J Clin Invest* 1985; 75: 404–12.
150 Frey J, Zager P, Jackson J, Eaton P, Scavini M. Aldose-reductase activity mediates renal prostaglandin production in streptozotocin diabetic rats. *Kidney Int* 1989; 35: 292.
151 Mauer SM, Steffes MW, Azar S, Brown DM. Effects of sorbinil on glomerular structure and function in long-term-diabetic rats. *Diabetes* 1989; 38: 839–46.
152 Osterby R, Gundersen HJG. Glomerular basement membrane thickening in streptozotocin diabetic rats despite treatment with an aldose reductase inhibitor. *J Diab Comp* 1989; 3: 149–53.

153 Steffes MW, Brown DM, Basgen JM, Matas AJ, Mauer SM. Glomerular basement membrane thickness following islet transplantation in the diabetic rat. *Lab Invest* 1979; 41: 116–18.
154 Sands JM, Terada L, Bernard M, Knepper MA. Aldose reductase activities in microdissected rat renal tubule segments. *Am J Physiol* 1989; 256: F563–9.
155 Kuwabara T, Cogan DG. Retinal vascular patterns. VI. Mural cells of the retinal capillaries. *Arch Ophthalmol* 1963; 69: 492–502.
156 Akagi Y, Kador PF, Kuwabara T, Kinoshita JH. Aldose reductase localization in human retinal mural cells. *Invest Ophthalmol Vis Sci* 1983; 24: 1516–19.
157 Robison WG Jr, Nagata M. Aldose reductase in mural cell loss and retinal capillary basement membrane thickening. In: Sakamoto N, Kinoshita JH, Kador PF, Hotta N, eds. *Polyol pathway and its role in diabetic commplications*. Elsevier, Amsterdam; 1988: 267–75.
158 Hohman TC, Nishimura C, Robison WG. Aldose reductase and polyol in cultured pericytes of human retinal capillaries. *Exp Eye Res* 1989; 48: 55–60.
159 Engerman R, Bloodworth J, Nelson S. Relationship of microvascular disease in diabetes to metabolic control. *Diabetes* 1977; 26: 760–9.
160 Engerman RL, Kern TS. Experimental galactosemia produces diabetic-like retinopathy. *Diabetes* 1984; 33: 97–100.
161 Kador PF, Akagi Y, Terubayashi H, Wyman M, Kinoshita JH: Prevention of pericyte ghost formation in retinal capillaries of galactose-fed dogs by aldose reductase inhibitors. *Arch Ophthalmol* 1988; 106: 1099–102.
162 Takahashi Y, Wyman M, Ferris F III, Kador PF. Diabetes-like preproliferative retinal changes in galactose-fed dogs. *Acta Ophthalmol.* 1992; 110: 1295–302; and 1993; 111: 585.
163 Kern TS, Engerman RL. Galactose-induced retinal lesions in rats and effects of aldose reductase inhibition. *Diabetes* 1992; 41 (Suppl. 1): 20A.
164 Kador PF, Akagi Y, Takahashi Y, Ikebe H, Wyman W, Kinoshita JH. Prevention of retinal vessel changes associated with diabetic retinopathy in galactose-fed dogs by aldose reductase inhibitors. *Arch Ophthalmol* 1990; 108: 1301–9.
165 Kador PF, Takahashi Y, Wyman M, Kinoshita JH. The role of aldose reductase in retinal vessel changes associated with diabetic retinopathy in galactose-fed dogs. In: *Proc. NEI-JDF Workshop on aldose reductase inhibitors, NIH Publ. 91–3114*, 1991: 75–88.
166 Engerman RL, Kern TS. Aldose reductase inhibition fails to prevent retinopathy in diabetic and galactosemic dogs. *Diabetes* 1993; 42: 820–5.
167 Dent MT, Veves A, Tebbs SE *et al.* Neutrophil aldose reductase activity as a potential marker for neuropathy and cataract in diabetes. *Diabetic Med* 1991; 8: 911–6.
168 Price DE, Grant PJ, Airey CM, Stickland MH, Kemp J, Wales JK. Red cell sorbitol levels during hyper and hypoglycaemic clamp studies in insulin-dependent diabetic patients. *Diabetic Med* 1987; 4: 229–32.
169 Nakayama T, Tanimoto T, Kador PF. Human erythrocyte aldose and aldehyde reductase. In: Weiner H, Flynn TG, eds. *Enzymology and molecular biology of carbonyl metabolism*. 2. Liss, New York 1989: 265–77.
170 Malone JI, Knox G, Harvey C. Sorbitol accumulation is altered in Type 1 (insulin-dependent) diabetes mellitus. *Diabetologia* 1984; 27: 509–13.
171 Aida K, Tawata M, Shindo H, Onaya T: Clinical significance of erythrocyte sorbitol-blood glucose ratios in Type II diabetes mellitus. *Diabetes Care* 1990; 13: 461–7.
172 Lyons PA, Wise PH, Palmer TN. The polyol pathway in the human erythrocyte and its response to diabetes. *Biochem Soc Trans* 1988; 16: P 363.
173 Nagasaka Y, Fujii S, Kaneko T. Human erythrocyte sorbitol metabolism and the role of sorbitol dehydrogenase. *Diabetologia* 1988; 31: 766–70.
174 Dvornik D. Aldose reductase inhibitors (ARI). *Proc. NEI-JDF Workshop on aldose reductase inhibitors, NIH-Publ. 91–3114*, 1991: 39–58.
175 Sundkvist G, Armstrong FM, Bradburg JE *et al.* United Kingdom/Scandinavian Ponalrestat Trial: Peripheral and autonomic nerve function in 259 diabetic patients with peripheral neuropathy treated with ponalrestat (an aldose reductase inhibitor) or placebo for 18 months. *J Diab Comp* 1992; 6: 123–30.
176 Thompson L, Pfeifer M. Association between RBC sorbitol and the presence of diabetic neuropathy. *Diabetes* 1987; 36 (Suppl. 1): 99A.
177 Airey CM, Price DE, Kemp JV, Perkins CM, Wales JK. The effect of aldose reductase inhibition on erythrocyte polyols and galactitol accumulation in diabetic patients. *Diabetic Med* 1989; 6: 804–8.
178 Airey CM, Walmsley D, Arnold PH, Wales JK. Erythrocyte polyol concentrations in diabetic retinopathy. *Diabetic Med* 1988; 5 (Suppl. 2): 29.
179 Wilson RM, Reeves WG. Neutrophil phagocytosis and killing in insulin-dependent diabetes. *Clin Exp Immunol* 1986; 63: 478–84.
180 Wilson RM, Tomlinson DR, Reeves WG. Neutrophil sorbitol production impairs oxidative killing in diabetes. *Diabetic Med* 1987; 4: 37–40.
181 Dent MT, Tebbs SE, Gonzalez KM, Ward JD, Wilson RM. Neutrophil aldose reductase activity and its association with established diabetic complications. *Diabetic Med* 1991; 8: 439–42.
182 Fagius J, Jameson S. Effect of aldose reductase inhibitor treatment in diabetic polyneuropathy – a clinical and neurophysiological study. *J Neuro Neurosurg Psychiat* 1981; 4: 991–1001.
183 Dvornik D. Chronic complications of diabetes. *Ann Rev Med Chem* 1978; 13: 159–66.
184 Humber L. The medicinal chemistry of aldose reductase inhibitors. In, Ellis GP, West GB, eds. *Progr Med Chem* 24. Elsevier, Amsterdam 1987; 299–343.
185 Stribling D. Clinical trials with aldose reductase inhibitors. *Exp Eye Res* 1990; 50: 621–4.
186 Hotta N, Kakuta H, Ando F, Sakamoto N. Current progress in clinical trials of aldose reductase inhibitors in Japan. *Exp Eye Res* 1990; 50: 625–8.
187 Krans HMJ. Recent clinical experience with aldose reductase inhibitors. *J Diab Comp* 1992; 6: 15–20.
188 Stribling D. Designing clinical trials with aldose reductase inhibitors. In: Sakamoto N, Kinoshita JH, Kador PF, Hotta N, eds. *Current concept of aldose reductase and its inhibitions*. Elsevier, Amsterdam 1990: 139–47.
189 Abraham RR, Levy DM, Abraham RM, Simpson R. Variability of neurological measurements in diabetic neuropathy. In: Sakamoto N, Kinoshita JH, Kador PF, Hotta N, eds. *Polyol pathway and its role in diabetic complications*. Elsevier, Amsterdam; 1988: 438–45.

190 Macleod A, Sonksen P. The effect of the aldose reductase inhibitor tolrestat on diabetic polyneuropathy: a meta-analysis. *Diabetologia* 1991; 40 (Suppl. 1): 555A.
191 Greene DA, Porte D, Bril V, Clements RS, Shamoon H, Zeidler A. Clinical response to sorbinil treatment in diabetic neuropathy. *Diabetologia* 1989; 32: 493A.
192 Gieron MA, Malone JI, Lowitt S, Korthals JK. Improvement in peripheral nerve function after one year of sorbinil. *Neuro Report* 1991; 2: 348–50.
193 Boulton AJM, Levin S, Comstock J. A multicentre trial of the aldose-reductase inhibitor, tolrestat, in patients with symptomatic diabetic neuropathy. *Diabetologia* 1990; 33: 431–7.
194 Gonen B. Tolrestat. summary of clinical experience. *Proc. NEI-JDF Workshop on Aldose Reductase Inhibitors. NIH Publ. 91–3114.* 1991: 129–35.
195 Macleod AF, Boulton AJM, Owens DR *et al.* A multicentre trial of the aldose-reductase inhibitor, tolrestat, in patients with symptomatic diabetic peripheral neuropathy. *Diabete Metab* 1992; 18: 14–20.
196 Judzewitsch RG, Jaspan J, Polonsky KS *et al.* Aldose reductase inhibition improves nerve conduction velocity in diabetic patients. *N Engl J Med* 1983; 308: 119–25.
197 Jennings PE, Nightingale S, Le Guen C *et al.* Prolonged aldose reductase inhibition in chronic peripheral diabetic neuropathy: effects on microangiopathy. *Diabetic Med* 1990; 7: 63–8.
198 Gregersen G. Variations in motor conduction velocity produced by acute changes of the metabolic state in diabetic patients. *Diabetologia* 1968; 4: 273–7.
199 Porte D, Graf RJ, Halter JB, Pfeifer MA, Halar E. Diabetic neuropathy and plasma glucose control. *Am J Med* 1981; 70: 195–200.
200 Young RJ, Macintyre CCA, Martyn CM *et al.* Progression of subclinical polyneuropathy in young diabetic patients with type 1 (insulin-dependent) diabetes: associations with glycaemic control and microangiopathy (microvascular complications). *Diabetologia* 1986; 29: 156–61.
201 Solders G, Tyden G, Persson A, Groth CG. Improvement in nerve conduction in diabetic neuropathy. A follow-up study 4 yr after combined pancreatic and renal transplantation. *Diabetes* 1992: 946–51
202 Santiago JV, Sonksen PH, Boulton AJM *et al.* Withdrawal of the aldose reductase inhibitor tolrestat in patients with diabetic neuropathy: effect on nerve function. *J Diab Comp* 1993; 7: 170–78.
203 Proceedings of a consensus development conference on standardized measures in diabetic neuropathy. *Muscle & Nerve* 1992; 15: 1143–70.
204 Greene DA: Effects of aldose reductase inhibitors on the progression of nerve fiber damage in diabetic neuropathy. *J Diab Comp* 1992; 6: 11–14.
205 Stribling D: Ponalrestat efficacy trials. *Proc. NEI-JDF Workshop on Aldose Reductase Inhibitors. NIH Publ. 91–3114. 1991:* 139–43.
206 Ziegler D, Mayer P, Rathmann W, Gries FA. One year treatment with the aldose-reductase inhibitor, ponalrestat, in diabetic neuropathy. *Diab Res Clin Pract* 1991; 14: 63–74.
207 Krentz AJ, Honigsberger L, Ellis SH, Hardman M, Nattrass M. A 12-month randomized controlled study of the aldose reductase inhibitor ponalrestat in chronic symptomatic diabetic neuropathy. *Diabetic Med* 1992; 9: 463–8.
208 Florkowski CM, Rowe BR, Nightingale S, Harvey TC, Barnett AH. Clinical and neurophysiological studies of aldose reductase inhibitor ponalrestat in chronic symptomatic diabetic peripheral neuropathy. *Diabete* 1991; 40: 129–33.
209 Gill SJ, Wiliams G, Ghatei MA, Hetreed AH, Mather HM, Bloom SR. Effect of the aldose reductase inhibitor, ponalrestat, on diabetic neuropathy. *Diabete Metab* 1990; 16: 296–302.
210 Sima AAF, Nathaniel V, Prashar A, Bril V, Greene DA. Endoneurial microvessels in human diabetic neuropathy: endothelial cell dysjunction and lack of treatment effect by aldose reductase inhibitor. *Diabetes* 1991; 40: 1090–9.
211 Malik RA, Newrick PG, Sharma AK *et al.* Microangiopathy in human diabetic neuropathy: relationship between capillary abnormalities and the severity of neuropathy. *Diabetologia* 1989; 32: 92–102.
212 Bradley J, Thomas PK, King RHM, Llewelyn JG, Muddle JR, Watkins PJ. Morphometry of endoneurial capillaries in diabetic sensory and autonomic neuropathy. *Diabetologia* 1990; 611–18.
213 Sima AAF, Greene DA, Brown MD *et al.* Effect of hyperglycemia and the aldose reductase inhibitor tolrestat on sural nerve biochemistry and morphometry in advanced diabetic peripheral polyneuropathy. *J Diab Comp* 1993; 7: 157–69.
214 Llewelyn JG, Gilby SG, Thomas PK, King RHM, Muddle JR, Watkins PJ: Sural nerve morphometry in diabetic autonomic and painful sensory neuropathy. *Brain* 1991; 114: 867–92.
215 Veves A, Malik RA, Lye RH *et al.* The relationship between sural nerve morphometric findings and measures of peripheral nerve function in mild diabetic neuropathy. *Diabetic Med* 1991; 8: 917–21.
216 Sima AAF. Structure–function interactions in therapeutic response of diabetic neuropathy. *J Diab Comp* 1992; 6: 40–4.
217 Said G, Goulon-Goeau C, Slama G, Tchobroutsky G. Severe early-onset polyneuropathy in insulin-dependent diabetes mellitus: a clinical and pathological study. *N Eng J Med* 1992; 326: 1257–63.
218 Beggs JL, Johnson PC, Olafsen AG *et al.* Signs of nerve regeneration and repair following pancreas transplantation in an insulin-dependent diabetic with neuropathy. *Clin Transplant* 1990; 4: 133–41.
219 Fawcett JW, Keynes RJ. Peripheral nerve regeneration. *Ann Rev Neurosci* 1990; 13: 43–60.
220 Schwartz M. Molecular and cellular aspects of nerve regeneration. *CRC Crit Rev Biochem* 1987; 22: 89–110.
221 Said G, Slama G, Selva J. Progressive centripetal degeneration of axons in small fibre type diabetic polyneuropathy. A clinical and pathological study. *Brain* 1983; 3106: 791–807.
222 Thomas PK, Brown MJ. Diabetic polyneuropathy. In: Dyck PJ, Thomas PK, Asbury AK, Winegrad AI, Porte D Jr, eds. *Diabetic neuropathy.* Saunders, Philadelphia 1987: 56–65.
223 Roy TM, Broadstone VL, Peterson HR *et al.* The effect of an aldose reductase inhibitor on cardiovascular performance in patients with diabetes mellitus. *Diab Res Clin Pract* 1990; 10: 91–7.

224 Sundkvist G, Lilja B, Rosen I, Agardh CD. Autonomic and peripheral nerve function in early diabetic neuropathy. Possible influence of a novel aldose reductase inhibitor on autonomic function. *Acta Med Scand* 1987; 221: 445–53.
225 Green A, Jaspan J, Kavin H, Chung S, Schoenberg H. Influence of long-term aldose reductase inhibitor therapy on autonomic dysfunction of urinary bladder, stomach and cardiovascular systems in diabetic patients. *Diab Res Clin Pract* 1987; 4: 67–75.
226 Martyn CH, Reid W, Young RJ, Ewing DJ, Clarke BF. Six-month treatment with sorbinil in asymptomatic diabetic neuropathy. *Diabetes* 1987; 36: 987–90.
227 Lewin IG, O'Brien IAD, Morgan MH, Corral RJM: Clinical and neurophysiological studies with the aldose reductase inhibitor sorbinil in symptomatic diabetic neuropathy. *Diabetologia* 1984; 26: 445–8.
228 O'Hare JP, Morgan MH, Alden P, Chissel S, O'Brien IA, Corral RJM. Aldose reductase inhibition in diabetic neuropathy: clinical and neurophysiological studies of one year's treatment with sorbinil. *Diabetic Med* 1988; 5: 537–42.
229 Faes TJC, Yff GA, De Weerdt O, Lanting P, Heimans JJ, Bertelsmann FW: Treatment of diabetic autonomic neuropathy with an aldose reductase inhibitor. *J Neurol* 1993; 240: 156–60.
230 Giugliano D, Marfella R, Quatraro A *et al.* Tolrestat for mild diabetic neuropathy: a 52-week, randomized, placebo-controlled trial. *Ann Int Med* 1993; 118: 7–11.
231 Sampson MJ, Wilson S, Karagiannis P, Edmonds M, Watkins PJ. Progression of diabetic autonomic neuropathy over a decade in insulin-dependent diabetics. *Quart J Med* 1990; 75: 635–46.
232 Sorbinil Retinopathy Trial Research Group. A randomized trial of sorbinil, an aldose reductase inhibitor, in diabetic retinopathy. *Arch Ophthalmol* 1990; 108: 1234–44.
233 Kohner E, Caldwell G, Plehwe WE, Brown R, Rosen E. Ponalrestat in early diabetic retinopathy. *Diabetes* 1990; 39 (Suppl. 1): 62A.
234 van Oosterhout E, van Gerven JMA, Lemkes HHPJ, Boot JP, van Best JA. Effects of tolrestat, an aldose reductase inhibitor, on diabetic retinopathy. A six month double blind trial. *Diabetologia* 1990; 33 (Suppl.): A89.
235 Arauz-Pacheco C, Ramirez LC, Pruneda L, Sanborn GE, Rosenstock J, Raskin P. The effect of the aldose reductase inhibitor, ponalrestat, on the progression of diabetic retinopathy. *J Diab Comp* 1992; 6: 131–7.
236 Sato T, Fuji S, Yamamoto M *et al.* Effects of an aldose reductase inhibitor on urinary excretion of albumin, N-acetyl-β-D-glucosaminidase and alanine aminopeptidase in diabetic patients. In: Sakamoto N, Kinoshita JH, Kador PF, Hotta N eds. *Polyol pathway and its role in diabetic complications.* Elsevier, Amsterdam 1988: 348–53.
237 Blohme G, Smith V. Aldose reductase inhibition reduceds urinary albumin excretion rate in incipient diabetic nephropathy. *Diabetologia* 1989; 32: 467A.
238 Clarke BF, Boland O, Jenkins D, Nicole JJ, Ewing DJ. Urinary albumin and prostaglandin excretion and transcapillary protein leak are unaffected by inhibition of the polyol pathway with ponalrestat. *Diabetes* 1991; 40 (Suppl.): 442A.
239 Pedersen MM, Christiansen JS, Mogensen CE. Reduction of glomerular hyperfiltration in normoalbuminuric IDDM patients by 6 months of aldose reductase inhibition. *Diabetes* 1991; 40: 527–31.
240 Passariello N, Sepe J, Marrazzo G *et al.* Effect of aldose reductase reductase inhibitor (tolrestat) on urinary albumin excretion rate and glomerular filtration rate in IDDM subjects with nephropathy. *Diabetes Care* 1993; 16: 789–95.
241 Reichard P, Berglund B, Britz A, Cars I, Nilsson BY, Rosenqvist U. Intensified conventional insulin treatment retards the microvascular complications of insulin-dependent diabetes mellitus (IDDM): the Stockholm Diabetes Intervention Study (SDIS) after 5 years. *J Intern Med* 1991: 230: 101–8.
242 Brinchmann-Hansen O, Dahl-Jorgensen K, Sandvik L, Hanssen KF. Blood glucose concentrations and progression of diabetic retinopathy: the seven year results of the Oslo Study. *Br Med J* 1992; 304; 19–22.
243 Dvornik D. Physiopathogenesis of diabetic neuropathy. *Adv Diabetol* 1992; 5 (Suppl. 2): 70–84.

# 25 Proteinuria and Diabetic Complications

Torsten Deckert, Allan Kofoed-Enevoldsen, Pernille Mørk Hansen & Bjarne Myrup

## DEFINITION

Proteinuria is more frequently seen among patients with diabetes than among controls. When proteinuria is >0.5 g/24 h in more than two consecutive urine samples in diabetic patients without urinary infection, cardiac insufficiency or other renal diseases, the term diabetic nephropathy is used. It might be difficult to exclude other renal diseases, especially among patients with NIDDM diabetes but recent studies demonstrated that the presence of diabetic retinopathy in these patients increases the specificity of the diagnosis, whereas absence of retinopathy in NIDDM diabetic patients (fulfilling the above criteria for proteinuria) will include 30% of patients without diabetic nephropathy (1). Proteinuria in patients with diabetic nephropathy consists of many different plasma proteins (2), albumin being present in most abundant amounts. Therefore, an alternative definition of diabetic nephropathy is persistently elevated urinary albumin excretion rate (UalbV) of >200 μg/min (>300 mg/24 h) (3).

## EPIDEMIOLOGY OF DIABETIC NEPHROPATHY

Diabetic nephropathy is the most serious complication in IDDM since excess mortality from complications is nearly exclusively associated to this group of patients (Fig. 25.1). Patients without proteinuria have an excess mortality of 2–3 in comparison to age- and sex-matched non-diabetic patients, whereas patients with proteinuria have an excess mortality of about 40 (4). Death in proteinuric patients is not only due to uraemia but also due to premature atherosclerosis (5). Patients with albuminuria also have a much higher incidence of proliferative retinopathy (6) and coronary heart disease (7) than patients with normal UalbV. In fact, albuminuria is a new potent cardiovascular risk marker, not only in IDDM patients but also in patients with non-insulin-dependent diabetes (8, 9) and in controls (10, 11).

Only about 35% of patients with IDDM will ever develop diabetic nephropathy (12), and the cumulative incidence seems to be declining during the last 30 years, probably owning to better metabolic regulation and early use of antihypertensive treatment (12, 13). The incidence of diabetic nephropathy increases to a maximum after 16 years of diabetes duration and declines thereafter (4). It is higher among males than among females (4). Diabetic nephropathy is, besides albuminuria, characterised by decreasing GFR and increasing blood pressure (14). Patients with normal UalbV have normal or increased GFR. In these patients GFR does not decline

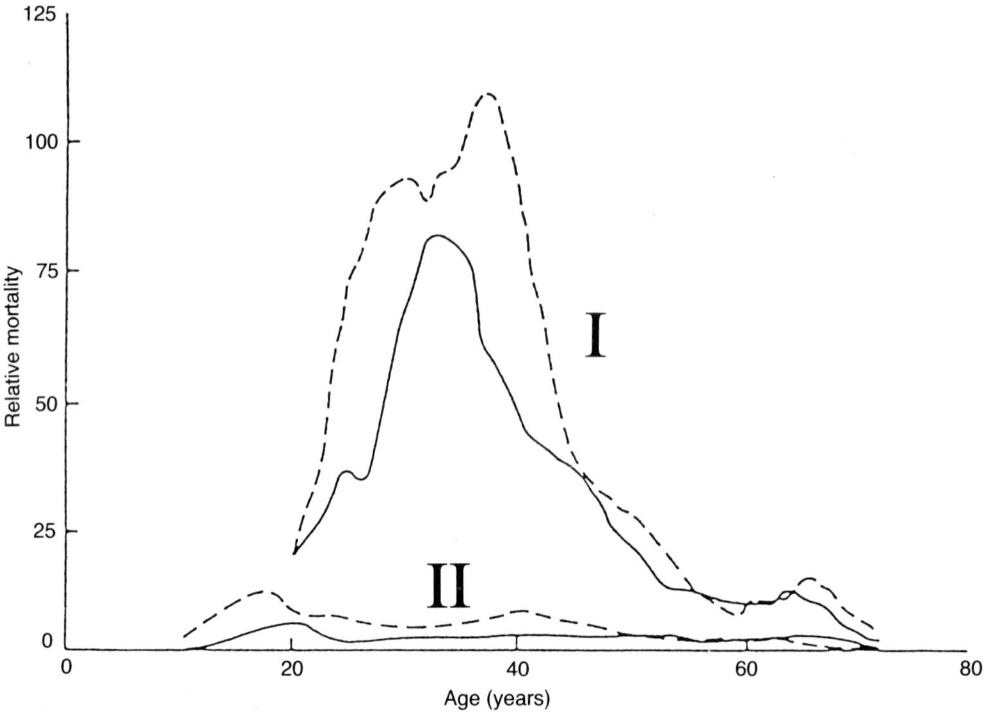


Fig. 25.1. Relative mortality of IDDM patients with (I, $n$=406) and without (II, $n$=595) persistent proteinuria in men (–) and women (---) as function of age. All patients developed IDDM before the age of 31 (from Ref. 4).

more than expected by age (15, 16). Blood pressure is increased in nearly all patients with diabetes nephropathy (17). But normoalbuminuric patients with IDDM can also have hypertension, especially in higher age groups (18). Three questions will be discussed:

1. What is the cause of albuminuria, blood pressure elevation and declining GFR?
2. Why do only a minority of patients develop diabetic nephropathy?
3. What is the cause of the association between albuminuria and premature atherosclerosis?

## ALBUMINURIA

Albuminuria is the first clinical sign of diabetic nephropathy (19). Just after the onset of IDDM, well controlled patients have normal UalbV (<30 mg/24 h) (20). Those patients who develop diabetic nephropathy (UalbV>300 mg/24 h) will pass the microalbuminuric stage where UalbV is between 30–300 mg/24 h. Not all patients with persistent microalbuminuria develop diabetic nephropathy but in those who progress to diabetic nephropathy UalbV increases in an exponential way (21). What is the cause of albuminuria?

Groups of patients with microalbuminuria demonstrate more severe glomerular morphological alterations as glomerular basement membrane (GBM) thickening and increased fractional mesangial volume, than groups of normoalbuminuric diabetic patients of similar diabetes duration (22, 23). A significant correlation exists between UalbV and glomerular alterations in diabetics with UalbV <300mg/24 h ($r$ =0.63, $p$=0.001) (22). But in spite of an association between UalbV and the quantity of morphologic glomerular alterations a plausible explanation of albuminuria has, until now, not been demonstrated by electron microscopy though several suggestions have been made (22). Changes in tubular function as a reason for albuminuria are unlikely since the excretion of two markers of tubular function such as β2 microglobulin and retinol binding protein are identical in patients with normo- and microalbuminuria and in patients with early nephropathy (24–26). The above questions can therefore be put in a more specific way. What is the reason for the increased macromolecular flow across the glomerular filtration surface, i.e. the GBM and the extracellular matrix (ECM) of the mesangium?

Dextran clearance studies and studies of the fractional clearance of IgG (molecular radius 55 Å) indicate formation of *shunt pathways* across the filtration barrier in IDDM patients with albuminuria (27). Thus, several studies have demonstrated an increased fractional clearance of large dextran molecules (>55Å radius) in patients with advanced diabetic nephropathy (24, 28). Also in patients with microalbuminuria not only is the fractional albumin clearance increased but also the fractional clearance of IgG (Fig. 25.2), suggesting formation of shunt pathways (24, 29). The formation of shunt pathways through the glomerular ECM (i.e. the thickened GBM and the expanded mesangium) reflects disruption of the macromolecular network of the ECM and is possibly reflected by the appearance of loose fluffy structures seen by electron microscopy (22). The ECM network consists of collagen IV, laminin, fibronectin and heparan sulphate proteoglycan (HS–PG) molecules (30). The cause of the formation of shunt pathways is not exactly known but increased glomerular pressure and/or qualitative alterations of the filtration barrier seem to be the main reasons.

*Intraglomerular pressure* can not be directly measured in humans but under certain conditions the filtration fraction (FF = GFR/RPF) might be used as an indicator of intraglomerular pressure. FF is significantly increased in patients with IDDM and normal UalbV (15, 31) but we do not have reasons to believe that patients with albuminuria are recruited from patients with especially high FF. Thus a follow-up study of IDDM patients with normal or slightly elevated UalbV was unable to find higher FF in patients with increasing UalbV than in patients with stable UalbV (Fig. 25.3). Also FF was not higher in patients with persistent microalbuminuria than in patients with normal UalbV (15, 24). Tooke measured capillary pressure in nail folds and found a significantly elevated capillary pressure in IDDM patients compared to controls (33). But also he was unable to find higher capillary pressure in patients with microalbuminuria compared to normoalbuminuric patients (33) though a subgroup of patients with microalbuminuria had significantly higher capillary pressure compared with well regulated long-term diabetic patients with normal UalbV (34).

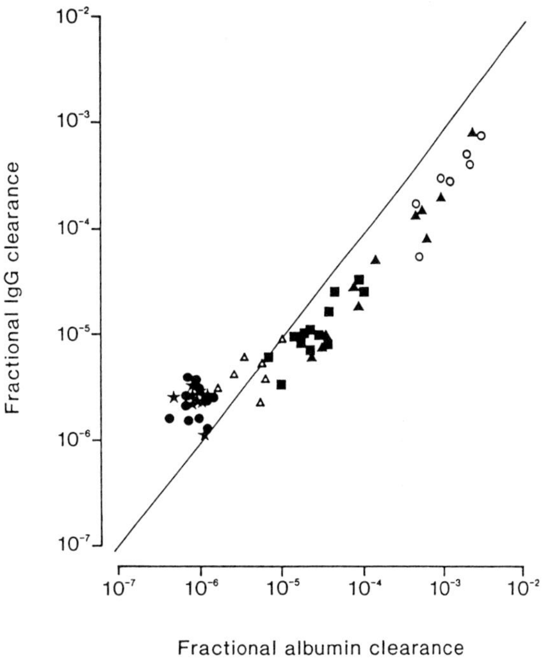


Fig. 25.2. Fractional renal clearance of albumin and IgG in controls (*) and IDDM patients of juvenile onset. ● UalbV <30 mg/24 h; △ UalbV 30–100 mg/24 h; ■ UalbV >101–300 mg/24 h; ▲ UalbV >300 mg/24 h, normal creatinine; ○ UalbV >300 mg/35 h, elevated creatinine (from Ref. 24).

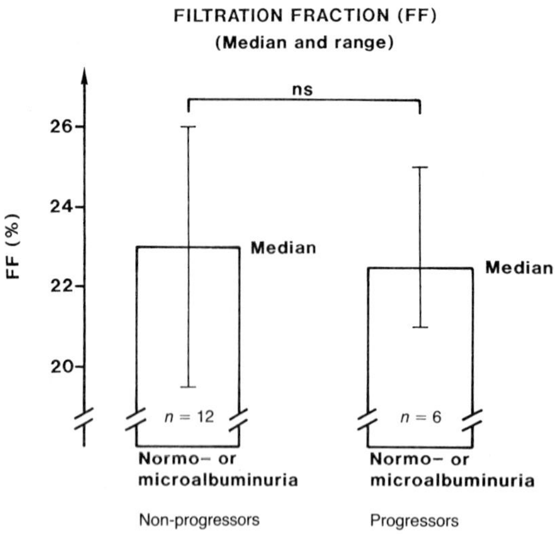


Fig. 25.3. Filtration fraction (FF) in IDDM patients of juvenile onset with normal or slightly elevated UalbV. Non-progressors demonstrated stable UalbV during the following 6 years of observation. Progressors developed clinical nephropathy. Median and range are given (from Ref. 32).

*Increased systemic blood pressure* might lead to increased intraglomerular pressure if the afferent arterioles of the glomeruli are dilated or if renal autoregulation of blood pressure is impaired. However, most studies in IDDM patients with slightly but persistently increased UalbV (30–100 mg/24 h) have found similar blood pressure as in patients with normal UalbV (35) and loss of renal autoregulation is seldom seen before diabetes nephropathy is present (36). *GFR and renal plasma flow (RPF)* are elevated in most IDDM patients with normal UalbV and it has been postulated that hyperfiltration and hyperperfusion are important contributors to the development of diabetic nephropathy (37). Thus, some follow-up studies have demonstrated that albuminuria in IDDM patients is nearly always preceded by hyperfiltration whereas patients with normal GFR rarely develop diabetic nephropathy (38). Also, animal experiments have clearly demonstrated an important role of renal haemodynamic alterations for the development of glomerular morphologic changes and albuminuria (39). From these animal and clinical studies it can be concluded that intraglomerular pressure is undoubtedly elevated in uncomplicated IDDM and that haemodynamic alterations like hyperperfusion, hyperfiltration and increased intraglomerular pressure undoubtedly contribute to the development of glomerulopathy – the characteristic morphological alterations seen in diabetes. It is likely that these haemodynamic alterations are risk factors for the development of albuminuria, however, it is questionable whether a 20–30% increase of pressure and flow in itself can lead to disruption of a normal macromolecular network within the glomerular ECM and to albuminuria. We suggest that increased glomerular pressure can only lead to formation of new shunt pathways if patients suffer from qualitative changes of the ECM. In accordance with this theory hyperfiltration does not always lead to albuminuria. Thus, a recent follow-up study demonstrated that only 40% of hyperfiltering patients developed albuminuria after 8 years of follow-up (38) and in another study over 12 years hyperfiltration was not a risk factor for the development of diabetic nephropathy (40). Also uninephrectomized patients who are suffering extreme hyperfiltration, only seldom develop albuminuria (41). Thus, hyperfiltration and/or increased intraglomerular pressure might be a contributing factor, perhaps necessary – but not sufficient – for the development of shunt pathways across the glomerular filtration barrier.

Besides haemodynamic alterations, *qualitative changes* of the filtration barrier seem to be necessary pathogenetic factors for the development of albuminuria (42). In diabetes qualitative alterations of the glomerular ECM are induced by non-enzymatic glycation and by deficient remodelling of the macromolecular network of ECM. Non-enzymatic glycation of collagen IV and laminin leads to decreased binding of heparin (43, 44) and to reduced turnover of collagen IV (45). Inhibition of the formation of the advanced glycation end products (AGE) by aminoguanidin prevents the thickening of GBM and albuminuria in diabetic rats (44). However, it is not known whether patients with microalbuminuria reveal more AGE accumulation within the glomeruli than diabetic patients without albuminuria.

Whereas non-enzymatic glycation of proteins within the ECM might contribute to the development of diabetic nephropathy, deficient remodelling of ECM seems to be another important – maybe the most important – step in the development of albuminuria (Fig. 25.4). Deficient remodelling of ECM results in an increased content of collagen IV, laminin and fibronectin (46) and decreased concentration and/or sulphation of HS – PG (47, 48) within the glomerular ECM. Among these alterations, HS–PG is of special interest because of its importance for glomerular permselectivity.

HS–PG is synthesised in the epithelial, endothelial and mesangial cells. After sulphation of the GAG side chain has taken place in the Golgi apparatus (a process initiated by the enzyme N-deacetylase) HS–PG is incorporated into the extracellular matrix of glomeruli and vessel walls, where it contributes to the structural integrity and the negative charge of the filtration barrier and vessel walls. As well as the concentration of HS–PG, the structure and sulphation of the glycosaminoglycan side chain (GAG) are of importance for the macromolecular permeability of the GBM. The density of HS–PG is highest at the lamina rara of the GBM where it forms anionic sites (49). Decrease of glomerular heparan sulphate induced by monoclonal antibodies (50), heparitinase (51) or polycations (52) will result in severe albuminuria. In contrast, ACE inhibition (53) or heparin injection (54) given to diabetic rats arrest albuminuria by increasing the content of heparan sulphate and the number of anionic sites within the glomeruli (53, 54). Decreased concentration of HS–PG in the GBM of IDDM patients with nephropathy has been described by several groups (55–57) and a negative correlation has been found between UalbV and the concentration of HS–PG (56, 156). Furthermore, diabetes reduces the activity of N-deacetylase, the key enzyme for the

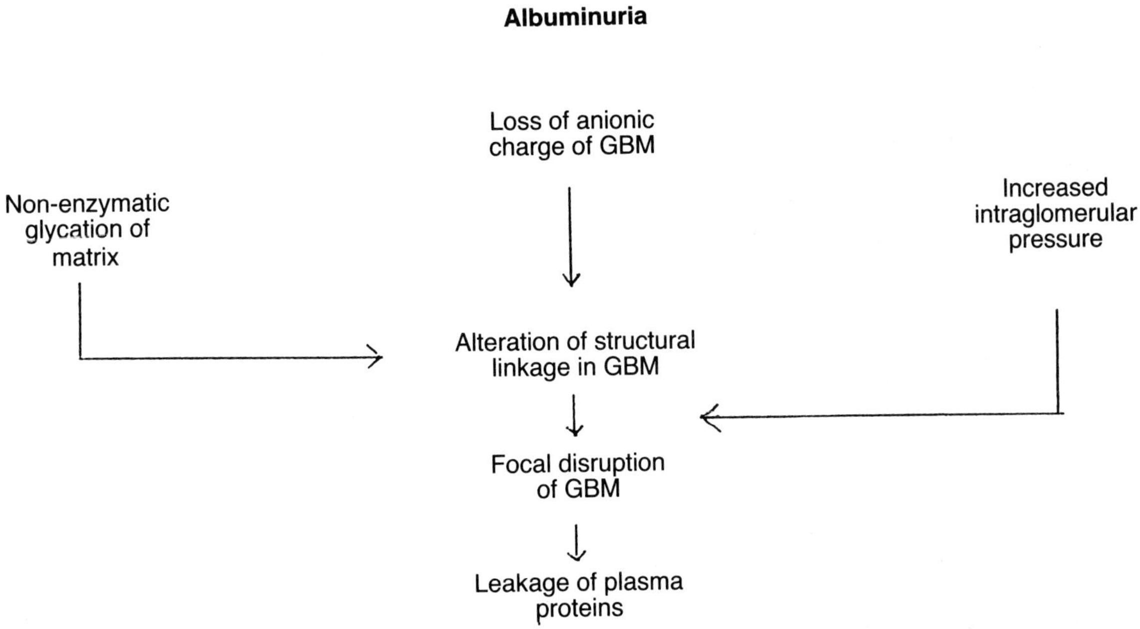


Fig. 25.4. Pathogenesis of albuminuria in IDDM.

sulphation of HS (58, 59). In accordance with this HS–PG of diabetic animals is significantly less sulphated than in non-diabetic animals (47, 60), and a significantly negative correlation has been found between the activity of N-deacetylase and albuminuria in diabetic rats (61).

Reduced density of HS–PG and/or reduced sulphation of HS will result in loss of anionic sites within the glomerular filtration barrier. In fact, a reduced number of heparitinase digestible anionic sites has recently been demonstrated in IDDM patients with albuminuria (Fig. 25.5) (57, 62, 63). Furthermore, a significant negative correlation was found between the number of anionic sites and albuminuria (57). Reduction of anionic sites is expected to lead to loss of glomerular charge selectivity. This is exactly what has been demonstrated by several authors in IDDM patients with albuminuria (24, 29, 64–66) and a negative correlation has been found between charge selectivity and fractional albumin clearance ($p$ <0.001) in albuminuric patients with IDDM (Mørk Hansen, submitted). Moreover, a highly significant loss of charge selectivity was found already in patients with slightly increased UalbV (30–100 mg/24 h) (24, 35). In these patients filtration fraction and the fractional clearance of dextran and IgG was not increased compared to normo-albuminuric diabetic patients, suggesting that loss of glomerular size selectivity (formation of shunt pathways and increased IgG clearance) is preceded by loss of anionic sites (Fig. 25.6). If loss of glomerular charge selectivity represents reduced concentration or sulphation of HS–PG within the GBM, it is fair to conclude that a reduction of HS–PG or its sulphation might well be the key event leading to albuminuria. HS–PG interacts with fibronectin, collagen IV and laminin (67, 68) and

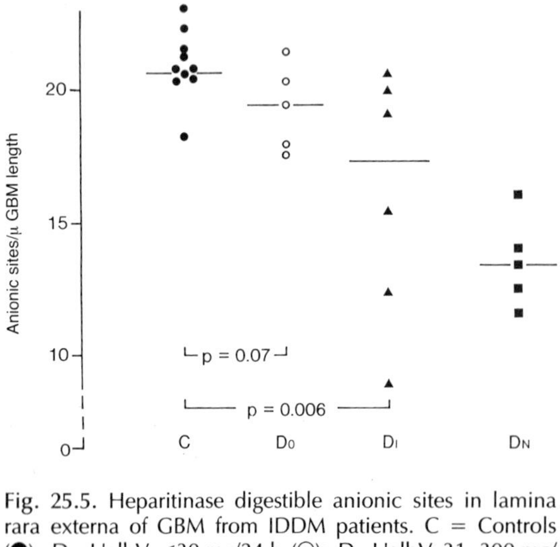


Fig. 25.5. Heparitinase digestible anionic sites in lamina rara externa of GBM from IDDM patients. C = Controls (●); $D_O$ UalbV <30 mg/24 h (○); $D_I$ UalbV 31–300 mg/24 h (▲); $D_N$ >300 mg/24 h (■). (Redrawn from Ref. 57.)

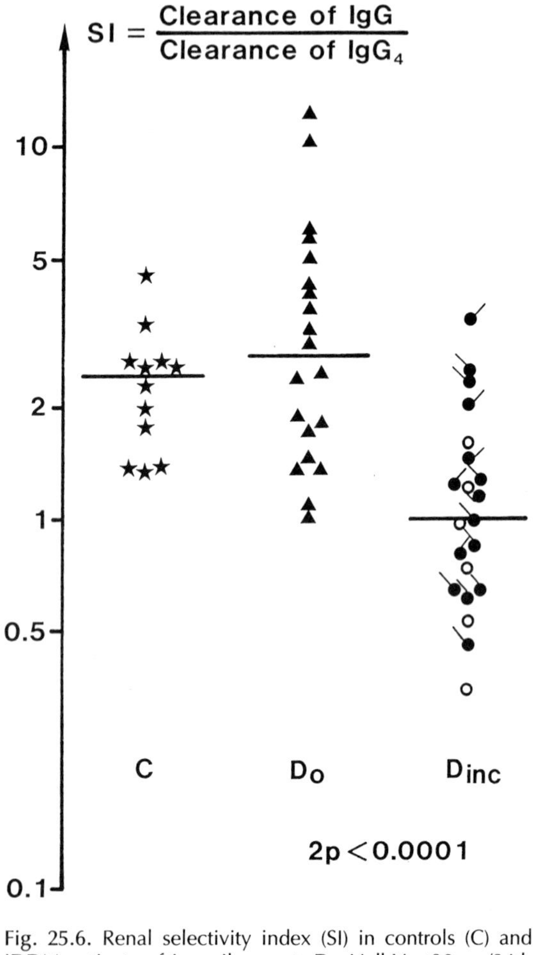


Fig. 25.6. Renal selectivity index (SI) in controls (C) and IDDM patients of juvenile onset. $D_O$ UalbV <30 mg/24 h (▲); $D_{INC}$ UalbV 31–300 mg/24 h; UalbV 31–50 mg/24 h (○); UalbV 51–100 mg/24 h (●́); UalbV 101–300 mg/24 h (●̀).

it has been demonstrated that altered cross-linking renders GBM permeable to proteins (69). It is therefore likely that reduced concentration or sulphation of HS–PG destabilises the macromolecular network of the GBM and leads to formation of shunt pathways (and increased fractional IgG clearance), especially if the intraglomerular pressure is elevated. In accordance with these observations, thickening of GBM, reduction of anionic sites and albuminuria can be totally prevented by heparin and dermatan sulphate in diabetic rats (54). Thus, decreased density or sulphation of heparan sulphate proteoglycan within the GBM and the mesangium might well be the main cause of albuminuria.

## BLOOD PRESSURE ELEVATION

Recent studies suggest that *normoalbuminuric patients* with IDDM have a slightly higher mean 24 hours systolic and diastolic blood pressure than carefully matched non-diabetic controls (70). The reason for this is not known but it might be associated with increased glucose and insulin induced tubular reabsorption of sodium (71, 72). Though the increased sodium reabsorption is outbalanced by increased GFR (71, 73), diabetic patients with normoalbuminuria have increased exchangeable total body sodium and extracellular fluid volume and a positive correlation is found between these parametes and blood pressure elevation (72, 74, 88). During the remission phase of diabetes when the insulin dose and the tubular glucose reabsorption is greatly reduced, exchangeable sodium becomes normal (74) and blood pressure decreases significantly during periods of strict metabolic control in normoalbuminuric patients (75). Thus, slightly increased blood pressure in normoalbuminuric diabetic patients might be due to metabolically and hormonally induced alterations in sodium homeostasis.

Patients with *albuminuria* have higher blood pressure than normoalbuminuric diabetic patients. The diastolic as well as the systolic blood pressure are significantly higher in patients with UalbV >100 mg/24 h (35). It is not quite clear what comes first: blood pressure elevation or increased UalbV. Some groups believe that diabetic patients with slightly elevated blood pressure or genetic disposition for hypertension are more prone to develop albuminuria (76) while other groups found blood pressure elevation to be secondary to albuminuria (77). We found most studies to be in favour of the second theory. BP was not higher in parents of patients with nephropathy than in parents of patients without nephropathy (78, 79) although Na/Li counter-transport was elevated in some studies (78) but not in others (79). Patients who later develop severe diabetic nephropathy did not have higher blood pressure before the development of albuminuria than comparable patients who escaped the development of diabetic nephropathy (80, 81) (Fig. 25.7). The prevalence of hypertension in a representative population of normoalbuminuric IDDM patients

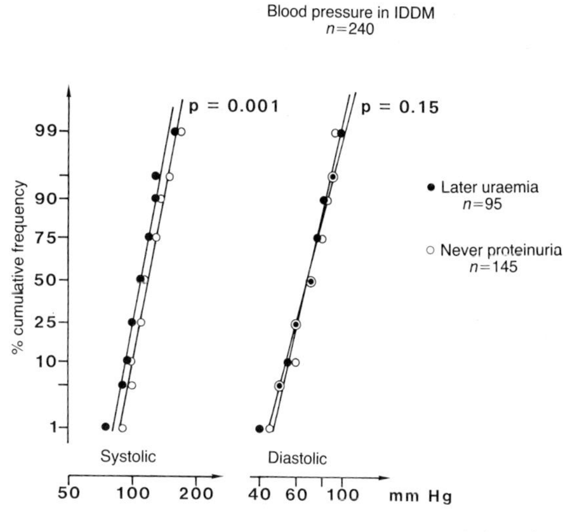


Fig. 25.7. Cumulative frequency of systolic and diastolic blood pressure in IDDM patients of juvenile onset. None of the patients had albuminuria. After blood pressure measurements with standard sphygmanometer supine in the morning after one night's rest during hospitalisation, the patients were followed for >35 years or until death: 145 patients never developed proteinuria (○), 95 patients developed clinical nephropathy with proteinuria and elevated se-creatinine (●). Blood pressure distribution was not higher in prenephropaths.

was not lower than in controls (18). Finally, two prospective studies of normoalbuminuric IDDM patients clearly demonstrated that blood pressure started to rise two years after the onset of incipient nephropathy (39, 82). Furthermore, IDDM patients can have hypertension for many years without developing elevated UalbV (83). Finally, structural renal changes clearly precede the development of hypertension (19, 84). This does not exclude the possibility that elevated blood pressure in some cases – especially in patients suffering from impaired autoregulation of blood pressure – contributes to the development of albuminuria (157, Mathiesen *et al.*, unpublished observations). However, according to the bulk of evidence the blood pressure elevation seen in IDDM patients with microalbuminuria is the consequence of renal alterations. In accordance with this, albuminuria and blood pressure increase in parallel (85) and are significantly correlated (86).

The *mechanism* by which blood pressure is increased is not totally clear. But, increased peripheral vascular resistance seems to be one responsible factor since cardiac output is decreased in IDDM patients with micro- and macro-albuminuria (87). The cause of increased peripheral resistance is likely to be associated with further accumulation of extracellular sodium and water. Thus, in microalbuminuric IDDM patients a positive correlation was found between mean blood pressure and exchangeable sodium ($p < 0.0001$) (72). Exchangeable sodium was increased in microalbuminuric patients in spite of suppressed aldosterone and angiotensin II concentration (72) and plasma volume is

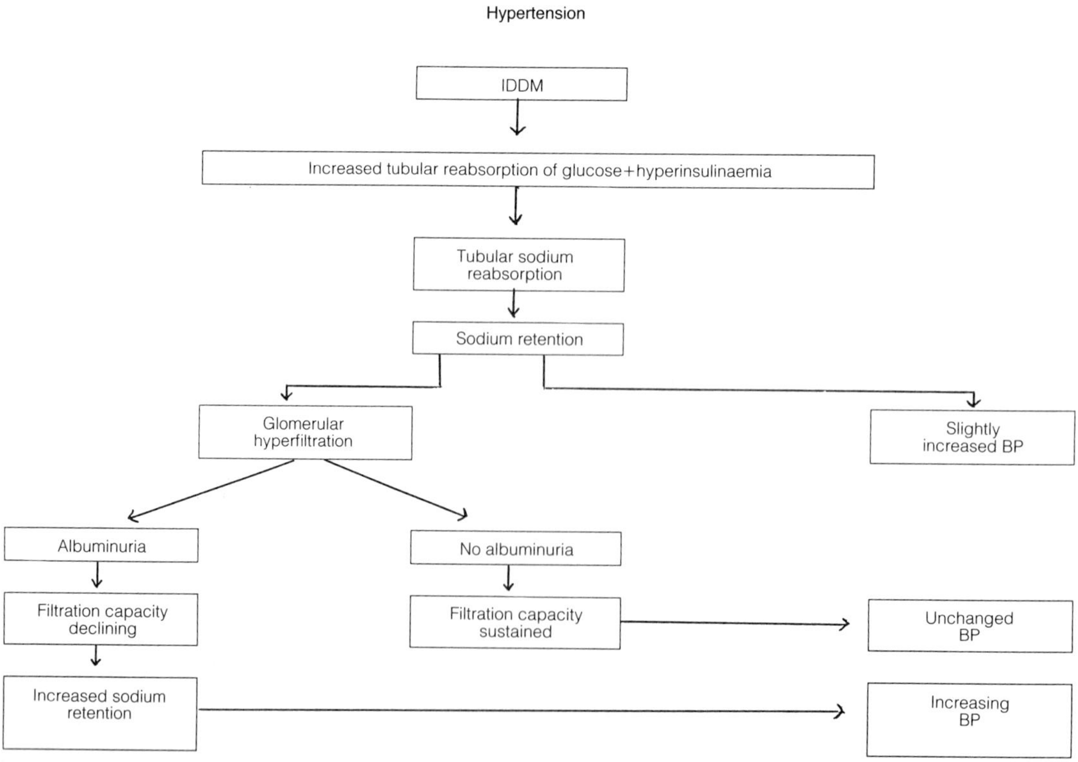


Fig. 25.8. Pathogenesis of blood pressure elevation in IDDM patients developing nephropathy.

normal or decreased (88). The overall picture is that blood pressure begins to increase when glomerular filtration capacity begins to fall and can no longer cope with the tubular reabsorption of sodium (72). This will lead to a further accumulation of exchangeable sodium and extracellular water (72, 88) and to a further blood pressure increase (Fig. 25.8). A slight increase of systemic blood pressure will help to keep total GFR at a hyperfiltering level in spite of mesangial expansion (89). This is in accordance with clinical observations which indicate albuminuria to be the first clinical sign of diabetic nephropathy followed by blood pressure elevation and, thereafter, decreasing GFR.

While UalbV can remain within normal limits for many years in IDDM patients with essential hypertension (83, 86) blood pressure elevation greatly influences UalbV in patients with persistently elevated UalbV (90, 91). As soon as the filtration barrier within the glomeruli is qualitatively altered and shunt pathways are established, variation of intraglomerular pressure has a significant impact on the degree (92) and progression (85) of albuminuria. In accordance with this, antihypertensive therapy has been shown to decrease albuminuria significantly (90).

Table 25.1. *Blood pressure (BP) and glomerular filtration rate (GFR) in IDDM patients with persistent microalbuminuria*

| UalbV | *n* | HbA1c (%) | GFR (ml/min/ 1.73 $m^2$) | Mean BP (mmHg) |
|---|---|---|---|---|
| <30 | 38 | 9.1 | $116^{ns}$ | $96^{ns}$ ]* |
| 30–100 | 32 | 9.1 | $117^{ns}$ | $99^{ns}$ ]* |
| 101–300 | 23 | 8.9 | $111^{ns}$ ]* | 103 ]* |
| >300 | 20 | 9.5 | 85 ]* | 116 ]* |

*=$P<0.01$.
UalbV=urinary albumin excretion rate (μg/min).
*n*=number of individuals.
Mean BP=diastolic+1/3 (systolic–diastolic).

## GLOMERULAR FILTRATION RATE

The decline of GFR which is so characteristic of IDDM patients with diabetic nephropathy is associated with albuminuria. Patients with normal UalbV remain normo- or hyper-filtering irrespective of diabetes duration (15). Also patients with persistent microalbuminuria in the low range (30–100 mg/24 h) show normal or elevated GFR for years (16, 21). However, when UalbV increases from 100 to >300 mg/24 h, GFR will decline usually preceded by a blood pressure increase (16, 93). Decline of GFR develops when glomerular hypertrophy can no longer cope with the process of mesangial expansion and glomerular occlusion (22) (Table 25.1). While *mesangial expansion* is an early process during the development of diabetic nephropathy, glomerular occlusion is a rather late event (94, 95). Therefore, it is likely that the initial decline of GFR is caused exclusively by the reduction of filtration surface induced by mesangial expansion (22). In accordance with this theory a significant negative correlation has been found between GFR and filtration surface on the one hand and mesangial expansion on the other (22, 96, 97). Mesangial expansion is initially caused by accumulation of ECM within the mesangium and not – or only to a minor degree – due to proliferation of mesangial cells (22).

The mechanism underlying accumulation of ECM within the mesangium is probably, in part, the same as the processes leading to GBM thickening. Thus, a highly significant correlation has been found between GBM thickness and fractional mesangial volume in normo- and microalbuminuric IDDM patients (22, 98). However, an acceleration of mesangial expansion seems to take place after the increase of UalbV has started, Whereas thickness of the GBM in IDDM patients with nephropathy is only increased by a further 10–20% compared to patients with microalbuminuria, the fractional mesangial matrix volume of the same patients is increased by a further 80–100% (22, 98). The reason for the acceleration of the mesangial expansion in albuminuric patients is not known but might well be increased *macromolecular flow across the mesangium* (19). Increased macromolecular flow across the mesangium has been discussed as a cause of mesangium expansion in other kidney disease (99), and is in accordance with the clinical experience regarding the effect of antihypertensive therapy in patients with albuminuria. When the macromolecular flow across the glomerular filtration barrier (peripheral capillary loops and mesangium) is reduced by antihypertensive therapy (indicated by reduced UalbV), the rate of GFR decline (mesangial expansion) is significantly reduced (100). This strongly indicates that increased macromolecular flow across the mesangium contributes to mesangial expansion (Fig. 25.9).

The cause of increased macromolecular flow across the mesangium might well be similar to the cause of albuminuria, i.e. increased permeability of the ECM due to decreasing concentration and/or sulphation of HS and increasing intraglomerular pressure. Decreased concentration of HS–PG within the mesangium of albuminuric patients has recently been demonstrated (56). HS also inhibits proliferation of mesangial cells (101). Decreased concentration of HS therefore most likely leads to mesangial proliferation. Thus, defect remodelling of mesangial ECM may be the main cause of the accelerated mesangial expansion seen in patients with albuminuria.

The mechanism of defect remodelling of the ECM within the glomeruli resulting in increasing amounts of collagen IV and decreased concentration and/or sulphation of HS–PG is not totally clear but until now five hyperglycaemia and/or pressure-induced processes have been identified in diabetic animals:

1. Increased gene expression and secretion of collagen IV, laminin and fibronectin but unaltered expression of HS–PG (102–105)
2. Decreased synthesis of HS–PG (47–48)
3. Decreased turnover of glycated collagen IV (44)
4. Decreased binding of HS–PG to ECM (106)
5. Decreased sulphation of HS (60, 107, 108).

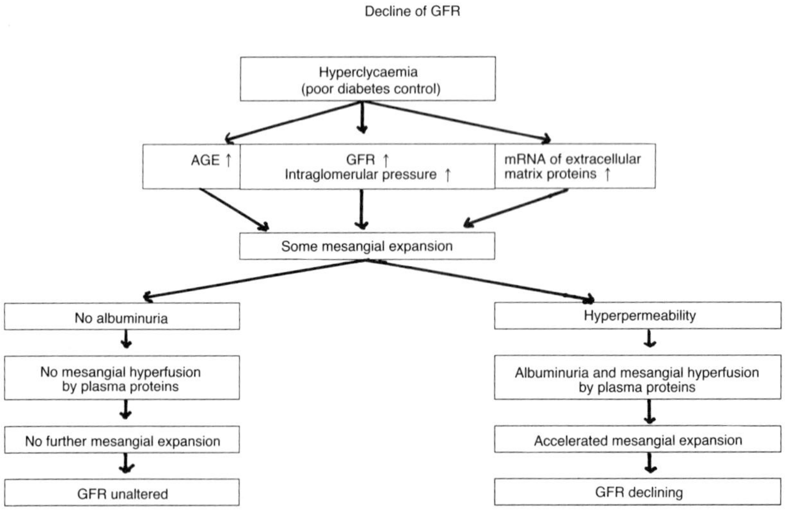


Fig. 25.9. Pathogenesis of the decline in GFR in IDDM patients developing nephropathy. AGE = advanced glycation end products.

Thus, diabetes affects the remodelling of the extracellular matrix in several ways and leads to reduced density of anionic HS–PG in the extracellular matrix. In accordance with this theory, strict metabolic control of IDDM patients with microalbuminuria seems to stop the progression of albuminuria (85) and leads to increased glomerular charge selectivity (109). Strict metabolic control also normalises the activity of N-deacetylase in diabetic rats (58). The mechanism by which poor diabetes control affects ECM-gene expression and secretion of epithelial, endothelial and mesangial cells is not totally clear but transforming growth factor-B (TGF-B) and other growth factors seems to be highly involved (154). It is to be hoped that a more specific intervention directed to increase the concentration and/or sulphation of HS–PG might be a useful way in the future to prevent diabetic nephropathy.

## WHY DO ONLY A MINORITY OF PATIENTS WITH IDDM DEVELOP ALBUMINURIA AND DIABETIC NEPHROPATHY?

Long-term poor metabolic control is the main reason for diabetic nephropathy. Usually patients developing albuminuria have higher HbA1c compared to patients with persistent normoalbuminuria, and diabetic nephropathy can be prevented by strict metabolic control (21, 155). However, in rare cases, severe diabetic nephropathy can be seen in patients with only slightly abnormal glucose tolerance. Furthermore, not all patients with poor diabetes control develop diabetic nephropathy. In a close follow-up study among 42 patients with juvenile IDDM, mean glycaemic control was identical among those who developed diabetic nephropathy and those who were protected (81). In fact, the present experience indicates that poor diabetes control is a necessary but not a sufficient precondition for the development of diabetic nephropathy. Some patients seem to be more vulnerable than others to the noxious effects of poor control. Genetic factors might be involved. Thus familial clustering of diabetic nephropathy has been demonstrated in two recent studies (110, 111). Furthermore, a comprehensive study of HLA associations in IDDM patients demonstrated clearly a higher frequency of DR4 among longterm diabetics with normal UalbV than in patients with diabetic nephropathy (112). Also, IDDM patients homozygous for class 1 alleles at the 5′ insulin gene on chromosome 11 had a higher prevalence and incidence of diabetic nephropathy than heterozygous patients (113). The familial influence in the development of nephropathy seen in Pima Indians likewise suggests genetic influence (114). Furthermore, the higher incidence of diabetic nephropathy among males compared to females (4) and the higher incidence of severe complications among Sephardic compared with Ashkenazi Jews might also indicate the involvement of genes in the development of diabetic nephropathy (115).

Genes encoding proteins regulating gomerular haemodynamic processes as ECM remodelling have been considered. Thus, glomerular hyperfiltration was found to be associated with high Na/Li countertransport, a genetic marker of essential hypertension (116). IDDM patients with albuminuria reveal higher Na/Li countertransport in erytrocytes compared to diabetic patients with normal UalbV (78). Leucocytes (117) and fibroblasts cultivated from IDDM patients with nephropathy (118) have significantly higher $H^+/Na^+$ pump activity than tissue from patients with normal UalbV. These findings indicate abnormal genetic regulation of haemodynamic processes which might be of importance for the development of diabetic nephropathy.

Besides genes encoding proteins which regulate glomerular haemodynamic alterations, genes involved in the synthesis, regulation and turnover of components of the ECM have been investigated. Thus, studies of fibroblasts have suggested that IDDM patients with nephropathy may suffer from genetic deficiencies in the regulation of the biosynthesis of glycosaminoglycans

(119) (Fig. 25.10). Also experiments in two closely related strains of rats point to the involvement of genes implicated in the synthesis of heparan sulphate proteoglycan. These studies demonstrated that the hyperglycaemia induced impairment of the activity of N-deacetylase, the key enzyme in the sulphation of heparan sulphate was significantly more pronounced in the albuminuric rat strain compared to the closely related non-albuminuric rat strain (61) (Fig. 25.11). The cDNA of HS–PG (120, 121) and of N-deacetylase (Kjellén, personal communication) has now been encoded and genetic polymorphism has recently been demonstrated in these genes by restriction fragment length polymorphism studies (120, Pernille Mørk Hansen, (personal communication). It is to be hoped that genetic markers of diabetic nephropathy will be identified soon, helping the clinicians to identify patients at risk at the onset of diabetes.

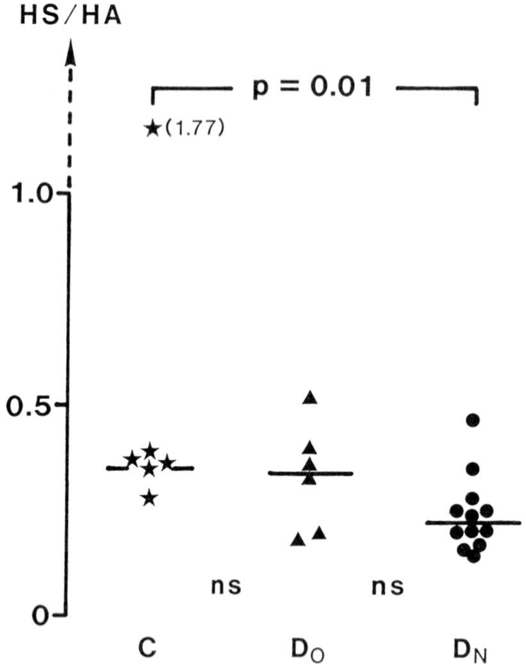


Fig. 25.10. Ratio of the incorporation of [$^3$H] glucosamine into heparan sulphate (HS) and hyaluronic acid (HA) of fibroblast cultures (cell + matrix + medium) from control subjects (C, *) and IDDM patients without ($D_O$, ▲) and with ($D_N$, ●) nephropathy.

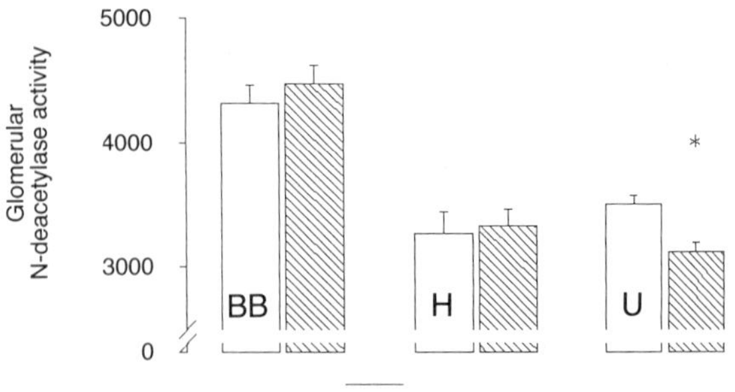


Fig. 25.11. Glomerular N-deacetylase activity in spontaneous diabetic BB rats, streptozotocin treated diabetic Sprague–Dawley rats from Hannover (H) and Sprague–Dawley diabetic rats from Uppsala (U). All rats were treated with insulin to keep blood glucose at 6–10 mmol/l □ or 15–20 mmol/l ▨. Only in U-rats a diabetes induced inhibition of N-deacetylase was seen (*, 2p <0.05).

## WHAT IS THE CAUSE OF THE ASSOCIATION BETWEEN ALBUMINURIA AND PREMATURE ATHEROSCLEROSIS?

Albuminuria is a new potent cardiovascular risk marker, not only in IDDM patients but also in patients with NIDDM and even in controls. However, the reason for this is not totally clear. One hypothesis suggests that patients with albuminuria are recruited from families characterised by a strong disposition for cardiovascular diseases which might be inherited (76). Thus, some authors found a significantly higher prevalence of cardiovascular diseases among parents of IDDM patients with nephropathy than among parents of IDDM patients with normal UalbV (76, 122). Other groups, however, were unable to confirm this observation (123). Also, blood pressure or the prevalence of hypertension was not higher among parents of patients with diabetic nephropathy than among parents of patients with normal UalbV (78, 79). The question therefore is not yet settled, but it might well be that the genetic disposition contributing to the development of albuminuria also contributes to some of the key mechanisms of premature atherosclerosis and, therefore, might be reflected in a higher morbidity from cardiovascular diseases among first degree relatives of patients with albuminuria.

Another hypothesis suggests that the high prevalence and incidence of cardiovascular complications in albuminuric patients are due to metabolic and/or haemodynamic consequences of the nephrotic syndrome and/or renal insufficiency like hyperlipidaemia and hypertension (124). In fact patients with nephropathy have significantly higher total cholesterol and blood pressure than age and sex matched diabetic patients with normal UalbV (125), independent of type of diabetes (126). However, increases in blood pressure and total cholesterol are seen already in patients with incipient nephropathy, independent of the presence of nephrotic syndrome or renal insufficiency (127). Thus, several studies have demonstrated increased concentration of total cholesterol, VLDL-cholesterol, triglycerides, fibrinogen (127–129) and apolipoprotein a (130) in diabetic patients with microalbuminuria compared to patients with normal UalbV. Also other cardiovascular risk factors like smoking (131) and hypertension (17) are more frequently seen in patients with albuminuria than in patients without albuminuria. Increases of cardiovascular risk factors in patients with early diabetic nephropathy are – though to a minor degree – contributing to the higher morbidity from coronary heart disease and cardiovascular mortality in these patients. However, an increase in plasma cholesterol by 20–25%, in fibrinogen by 20% and mean blood pressure by 10–15%, as seen in diabetic patients with nepropathy, can not explain the 10-fold higher cardiovascular mortality in these patients compared to age and sex matched diabetic patients without nephropathy (124).

In order to understand the association between albuminuria and premature atherosclerosis, it seems more fruitful to focus on the

Table 25.2. *Intimal dysfunction*

| | |
|---|---|
| p – | von Willebrand factor ↑ (132) |
| p – | thrombomodulin ↑ (133) |
| p – | angiotensin converting enzyme ↑ (72) |
| t – | plasminogen activator ↓ (135) |
| | macromolecular permeability ↑ (134) |
| | vascular charge selectivity ↓ (142) |

p =plasma.
t =tissue.
↑ ↓ =increased/decreased.

coincidence between albuminuria and intimal dysfunction. Intimal abnormalities including endothelial dysfunction are necessary steps in the pathogenesis of atherosclerotic lesions. Intimal abnormalities are closely associated with albuminuria (77). Even in patients with persistent microalbuminuria several markers of intimal and endothelial dysfunction have been demonstrated to become abnormal (Table 25.2). Thus, an increased plasma concentration of von Willebrand factor (vWf) has been demonstrated (132). Also plasma thrombomodulin (133) and angiotensin converting enzyme (ACE) (72) and the postendothelial macromolecular permeability (35, 134) are significantly increased in patients with incipient nephropathy whereas the exercise induced increase in tissue plasminogen activator activity and concentration is significantly decreased in patients with incipient nephropathy in comparison with IDDM patients with normal UalbV (135). Thus, clinical signs of intimal abnormalities are characteristic features of patients with early diabetic nephropathy. Of particular interest is the recent identification of a close coincidence between albuminuria and the increase of vWf. In a prospective study of normoalbuminuric patients with NIDDM only patients who developed persistent microalbuminuria showed a rise of vWf during the observation period and only in this group of patients was there an increase in cardiovascular morbidity (9) (Fig. 25.12). A close coincidence between the development of albuminuria and coronary heart disease was also seen in a follow-up study among patients with IDDM (7).

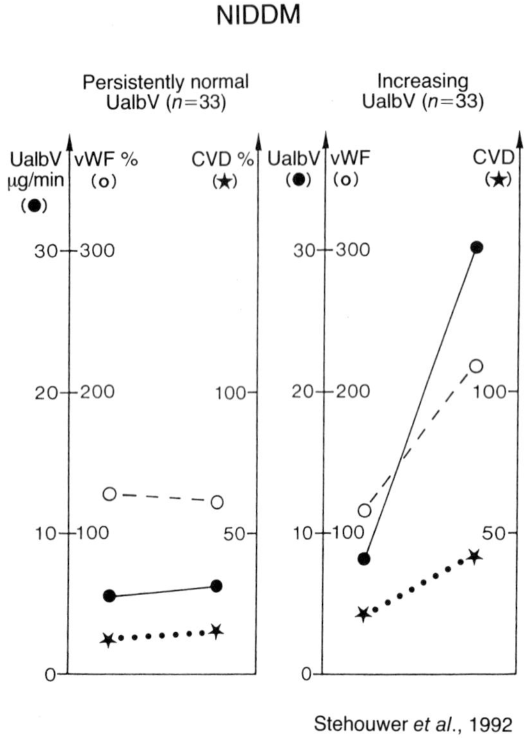


Fig. 25.12. Follow-up study (median 3 years) of NIDDM patients, age about 65 years with persistently normal UalbV (*n*=33, left panel) or developing persistent microalbuminuria (*n*=33, right panel). ● UalbV (µg/min); ○ van Willebrand factor (vWF, %); * Cardiovascular events (CVD, %). (Redrawn from Ref. 9.)

For the understanding the association between albuminuria and premature atherosclerosis also the structural similarities of the macromolecular pathways across the glomeruli and the intimal barrier could be important. The pathway for plasma proteins between capillary lumen and the urinary space in the glomeruli is the ECM of the GBM and the mesangium. The macromolecular pathways across the surface of the blood vessels are not known, but increasing evidence suggests that these pathways involve the extra-cellular matrix within the interendothelial clefts and the subendothelial space around the myomedial cells (136). Vesicular transport across the endothelial cells does not seem to play a role (137). Mesangial and arterial myomedial cells are mesanchymal cells, with contractile as well as phagocytotic properties. Both these cells can synthesise collagen IV, fibronectin, laminin and HS–PG. This is also reflected in the composition of the extracellular matrix which is quite similar in patients with albuminuria, both the glomerular accumulation of extracellular matrix and the ECM of extramural coronary vessels (138) are more pronounced than in patients without albuminuria (22). Furthermore, there are changes in the quality of the extracellular matrix (55, 56, 138) and patients with albuminuria have proliferation of mesangial cells whereas patients with atherosclerosis are characterised by proliferation of myomedial cells.

From the coincidence of albuminuria and intimal dysfunction and the structural similarities of the macromolecular pathways in the glomeruli and vessel walls it is likely that the pathogenetic event which is crucial for the development of albuminuria – decreased concentration and/or sulphation of HS–PG – plays a causative role for premature atherosclerosis in patients with albuminuria. Several studies have demonstrated a highly significant negative correlation between HS and atherosclerosis in human arteries (139, 140) (Fig. 25.13). Furthermore, in diabetic patients there is a 50%

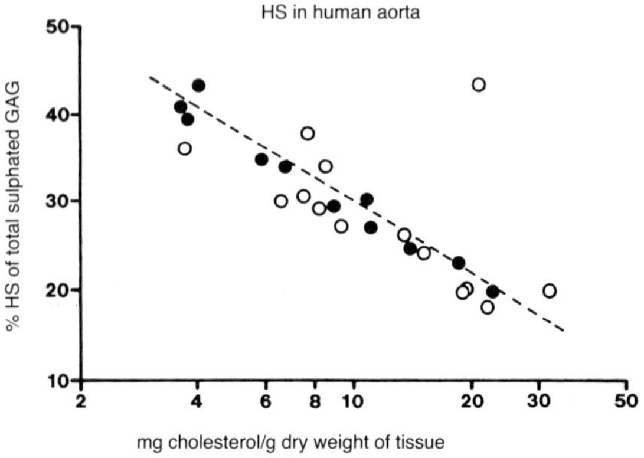


Fig. 25.13. Heparan sulphate in percentage of total sulphated GAG versus cholesterol in human aorta (intima and media): ○ grossly normal appearing areas, ● adjacent atherosclerotic areas. (From Ref. 140.)

reduction in acid glycosaminoglycans within the media of extramural coronary arteries (138). Most of these patients had diabetic nephropathy. If the concentration or the sulphation of HS–PG is reduced in the intima of large vessel walls, a reduced number of negative charges and reduced charge selectivity of vessel walls could be present in diabetic patients with nephropathy. Reduced negative surface charge on arterial endothelium of diabetic rats has been demonstrated (141) but it is not known whether the number of intimal anionic sites is reduced in patients with albuminuria in comparison to patients with normal UalbV. However, recent studies in IDDM patients with and without albuminuria indicate that the charge selectivity of vessels walls is reduced in patients with incipient and overt nephropathy (142). In these studies the transcapillary escape rate of two plasma proteins of identical size but different charges, i.e. albumin and glycated albumin, were compared. In patients with normal UalbV the transcapillary escape rate of the more negatively charged glycated albumin was significantly less than that of non-glycated albumin, indicating preserved charge selectivity (Fig. 25.14). In albuminuric patients, however, this discrimination was abolished, indicating a reduction in the number of anionic sites within the transintimal macromolecular pathways. These alterations may be due to reduced concentration or sulphation of HS–PG within the vessel wall.

HS–PG plays many important roles in the pathogenesis of atherosclerosis (143). Thus, HS–PG contributes to the anticoagulant properties of the vascular wall. Reduced density of HS within the vascular intima would lead to less binding of antithrombin III (144) and theoretically alter the coagulant balance in a procoagulant direction, resulting in greater fibrin deposition on endothelial cell surfaces (145). Deposition of fibrin in turn leads to an increased release of von Willebrand factor (145). In fact an increased concentration of von Willebrand factor is found in diabetic patients with albuminuria as mentioned above (9, 132) and increased *in vivo* platelet adhesion has also been demonstrated (125). Sulphated glycosamino glycans (GAG) are also the receptors of thrombomodulin. A decreased concentration of HS–PG within the vessel walls would be expected to lead to less binding and probably more release of thrombomodulin and, therefore, an increased plasma concentration of thrombomodulin. Such an increase is, in fact, seen in patients with incipient nephropathy (133). Furthermore, HS–PG within the vascular wall seems to play an important role in vascular permeability (Fig. 25.15). Thus, neutralisation of anionic sites on the surface of the vascular wall greatly enhances pulmonary vascular permeability of macromolecules (146). Reduced density of HS within the extracellular matrix of the intima of albuminuric diabetic patients would affect the adhesion of endothelial cells (147) and decrease the resistance of post-endothelial macromolecular flow. An increased transcapillary escape rate of plasma proteins is a characteristic abnormality in patients with incipient nephropathy (134) (Fig. 25.16) and

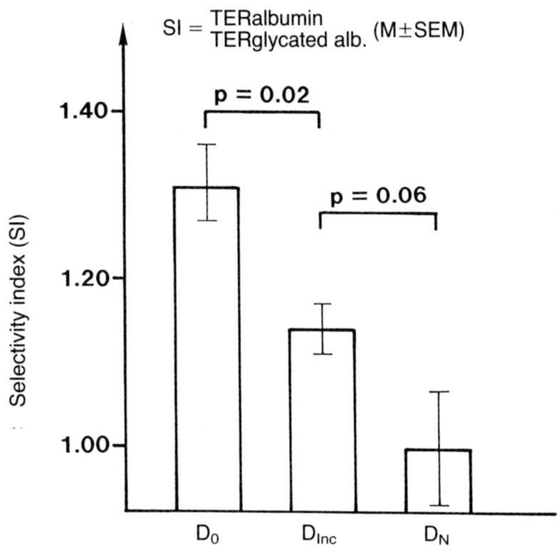


Fig. 25.14. Vascular selectivity index (SI = ratio of transcapillary escape rate (TER) of albumin/transcapillary escape rate of the more negatively charged glycated albumin) (m ± SEM) in IDDM patients with normal UalbV ($D_O$), UalbV 30–300 mg/24 h, $D_{INC}$ and UalbV >300 mg/24 h ($D_N$).

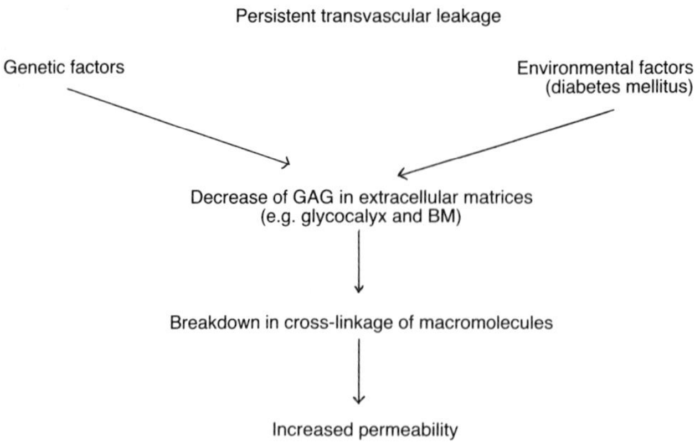


Fig. 25.15. Pathogenesis of increased transcapillary escape rate in IDDM patients with increased UalbV.

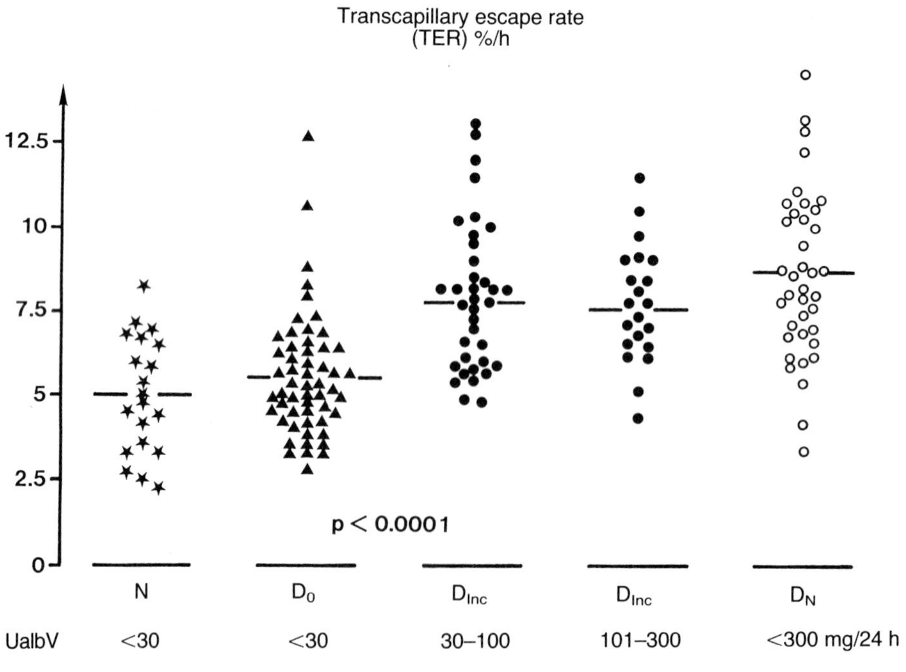


Fig. 25.16. Transcapillary escape rate of albumin (TER %/hour) in controls (N, *) and IDDM patients of juvenile onset. $D_O$ UalbV <30 mg/24 h (▲); $D_{Inc}$ incipient nephropathy, UalbV 30–300 mg/24 h (●); $D_N$ diabetic nephropathy, UalbV >300 mg/24 h (○).

macromolecular permeability is higher in atherosclerotic aorta lesions than in unaltered human aorta vessel surfaces (148). Altered resistance of macromolecular flow could also lead to an increase in the intimal transit time of LDL and an increased risk of oxidative modification, the precondition for foam cell formation (149). HS also contributes to keeping vascular smooth muscle cells in the contractile phenotype, making the cells non-responsive to mitogenes and proliferation (143, 150, 151). HS probably also helps to keep intimal LDL in the non-oxidised form, thereby preventing the uptake of LDL by scavenger receptors of monocytes and smooth muscle cells (152). HS–PG is also the receptor for lipoprotein lipase (153) on vessel walls, the key enzyme in the hydrolysis of plasma triglycerides and VLDL. It is therefore likely that reduced density or sulphation of heparan sulphate within the vessel walls would affect the clearance of triglycerides and VLDL. In fact, triglycerides and VLDL concentrations are significantly elevated in diabetic patients with albuminuria (127). Thus, the suggestion that there is a decreased concentration or sulphation of HS–PG in the intimal ECM of albuminuric patients is in accordance with most epidemiological and clinical findings and fits to the clinical observation of premature atherosclerosis.

## CONCLUSION

Defective remodelling of glomerular and intimal ECM resulting in decreased concentration and/or sulphation of HS–PG may contribute to albuminuria, mesangial expansion and intimal dysfunction.

Defective remodelling of glomerular and intimal ECM could explain the coincidence of albuminuria, mesangial expansion and intimal dysfunction and the association between albuminuria and premature atherosclerosis.

Mesangial expansion leads to declining GFR and sodium retention which in turn may lead to an increase in blood pressure. Intimal dysfunction accelerates atherosclerosis.

Defective remodelling of ECM is due to diabetes induced impaired regulation of both genetic expression and post-translational processes in the production of ECM components within the endothelial, epithelial, mesangial and myomedial cells. Thus, defective remodelling of ECM might well be the key process in the development of malignant angiopathy.

## REFERENCES


1 Parving H-H, Gall M-A, Skøtt P *et al.* Prevalence and causes of albuminuria in non-insulin-dependent diabetic patients. *Kidney Int* 1992; 41: 758–62.
2 Gerling I, Mathiesen ER, Rønn B, Deckert T. Plasma proteins in urine from insulin-dependent diabetics with different stages of diabetic nephropathy: a crossed immunoelectrophoresis study. *Diabetic Nephropathy* 1984; 3: 145–9.
3 Mogensen CE, Chachati A, Christensen CK *et al.* Microalbuminuria: an early marker of renal involvement in diabetes. *Uremia Investig* 1985–86; 9: 85–95.
4 Borch-Johnsen K, Andersen PK, Deckert T. The effect of proteinuria on relative mortality in Type 1 (insulin-dependent) diabetes mellitus. *Diabetologia* 1985; 28: 590–6.
5 Borch-Johnsen K, Kreiner S. Proteinuria: value as predictor of cardiovascular mortality in insulin dependent diabetes mellitus. *Br Med* J 1987; 294: 1651–4
6 Kofoed-Enevoldsen A, Jensen T, Borch-Johnsen K, Deckert T. Incidence of retinopathy in type 1 (insulin-dependent) diabetes: association with clinical nephropathy. *J Diabetic Complications* 1987; 3: 96–99
7 Jensen T, Borch-Johnsen K, Kofoed-Enevoldsen A, Deckert T. Coronary heart disease in young type 1 (insulin-dependent) diabetic patients with and without diabetic nephropathy: incidence and risk factors. *Diabetologia* 1987; 30: 144–8
8 Schmitz A, Vaeth M. Microalbuminuria: a major risk factor in non-insulin-dependent diabetes. A 10-year follow-up study of 503 patients. *Diabetic Med* 1988; 5: 126–34
9 Stehouwer C D A, Nauta J J P, Zeldenrust G C *et al.* Urinary albumin excretion, cardiovascular disease and endothelial dysfunction in non-insulin-dependent diabetes mellitus. *Lancet* 1992; 340: 319–23.
10 Yudkin JS, Forrest RD, Jackson CA. Microalbuminuria as predictor of vascular disease in non-diabetic subjects. *Lancet* 1988; 530–3.
11 Damsgaard EM, Frøland A, Jørgensen OD, Mogensen CE. Microalbuminuria as predictor of increased mortality in elderly people. *Br Med J* 1990; 300: 297–300.
12 Kofoed-Enevoldsen A, Borch-Johnsen K, Kreiner S, Nerup J, Deckert T. Declining incidence of persistent proteinuria in type 1 (insulin-dependent) diabetic patients in Denmark. *Diabetes* 1987; 36: 205–9.
13 Bojestig M, Arnqvist HJ, Hermansson G, Karlberg BE, Ludvigsson J. The incidence of nephropathy in juvenile type 1 diabetes has decreased. *Diabetologia* 1992; 35, suppl. 1, A69.

14 Parving H-H, Smidt UM, Andersen AR, Svendsen PA. Early aggressive antihypertensive treatment reduces rate of decline in kidney function in diabetic nephropathy. *Lancet* 1983; i: 1175–79.

15 Hansen KW, Mau Pedersen M, Christensen CK, Schmitz A, Christiansen JS, Mogensen CE. Normoalbuminuria ensures no reduction of renal function in type 1 (insulin-dependent) diabetic patients. *J Int Med* 1992; 232: 161–67.

16 Mathiesen ER, Feldt-Rasmussen B, Hommel E, Deckert T, Parving H-H. A 5-year study of glomerular filtration rate in normotensive IDDM patients with microalbuminuria. *Diabetologia* 1992; 35, suppl. 1, A60.

17 Parving H-H, Hommel E, Mathiesen ER. Prevalence of microalbuminuria, arterial hypertension, retinopathy and neuropathy in patients with insulin dependent diabetes. *Br Med J* 1988; 296: 156–60.

18 Nørgaard K, Feldt-Rasmussen B, Borch-Johnsen K, Sælan H, Deckert T. Prevalence of hypertension in type 1 (insulin-dependent) diabetes mellitus. *Diabetologia* 1990; 33: 407–10.

19 Mogensen CE, Østerby R, Würgler Hansen K, Damsgaard EM. Blood pressure elevation versus abnormal albuminuria in the genesis and prediction of renal disease in diabetes. *Diabetes Care* 1992; 15: 1192–205.

20 Lind B, Jensen T, Feldt-Rasmussen B, Deckert T. Normal urinary albumin excretion in recently diagnosed type 1 diabetic patients. *Diabetic Med* 1989; 6: 682–4.

21 Feldt-Rasmussen B, Mathiesen ER, Jensen T, Lauritzen T, Deckert T. Effect of improved metabolic control on loss of kidney function in type 1 (insulin-dependent) diabetic patients: an update of the Steno studies. *Diabetologia* 1991; 34: 164–70.

22 Østerby R. Glomerular structural changes in type 1 (insulin-dependent) diabetes mellitus: causes, consequences, and prevention. *Diabetologia* 1992; 35: 805–12.

23 Chavers BM, Bilous RW, Ellis EN, Steffes MW, Mauer SM. Glomerular lesions and urinary albumin excretion in type 1 diabetes without overt proteinuria. *N Engl J Med* 1989; 320: 966–70.

24 Deckert T, Kofoed-Enevoldsen A, Vidal P, Norgaard K, Andreasen HB, Feldt-Rasmussen B. Size- and charge selectivity of glomerular filtration in type 1 (insulin-depedent) diabetic patients with and without albuminuria. *Diabetologia* 1993; 36: 244–51.

25 Watts GF, Powell M, Rowe DJF, Shaw KM. Low molecular-weight proteinuria in insulin-dependent diabetes mellitus: a study of the urinary excretion of β-microglobulin and retinol-binding protein in alkalinized patients with and without microalbuminuria. *Diabetes Res* 1989; 12: 31–6.

26 Pontuch P, Jensen T, Deckert T, Ondrejka P, Mikulecky M. Urinary excretion of retinol-binding protein in type 1 (insulin-dependent) diabetic patients with microalbuminuria and clinical diabetic nephropathy. *Acta Diabetol* 1992; 28: 206–10.

27 Deen WM, Bridges CR, Brenner BM, Myers BD. A heteroporous model of size-selectivity: Application to normal and nephrotic humans. *Am J Physiol (Renal Fluid Electrol Physiol)* 1985; 249: F374–89.

28 Scandling JD, Myers BD. Glomerular size-selectivity and microalbuminuria in early diabetic glomerular disease. *Kidney Int* 1992; 41: 840–6.

29 Deckert T, Feldt-Rasmussen B, Djurup R, Deckert M. Glomerular size and charge-selectivity in insulin-dependent diabetes mellitus. *Kidney Int* 1988; 33: 100–6.

30 Farquhar MG. The glomerular basement membrane. A selective macromolecular filter. In: Hay ED, ed. *Cell biology of extracellular matrix*, 2nd edn. Plenum Press, New York, 1991: 365–419.

31 Christensen CK, Mogensen CE. The course of incipient diabetic nephropathy: studies of albumin excretion and blood pressure. *Diabetic Med* 1985; 2: 97–102.

32 Deckert T, Kofoed-Enevoldsen A. Pathogenesis of albuminuria in insulin-dependent diabetes mellitus. *J Diabetes Complications* 1992; 6: 266–7.

33 Sandeman DD, Shore AC, Tooke JE. Relation of skin capillary pressure in patients with insulin-dependent diabetes mellitus to complications and metabolic control. *N Engl J Med* 1992; 327: 760–4.

34 Shore AC. Jaap AJ, Tooke JE. Capillary pressure in Type 1 diabetic patients of long disease duration with and without microangiopathy. *Diabetic Med* 1992; 9 (suppl. 2) S11–12.

35 Deckert T, Feldt-Rasmussen B, Borch-Johnsen K, Jensen T, Kofoed-Enevoldsen A. Albuminuria reflects widespread vascular damage. The Steno hypothesis. *Diabetologia* 1989; 32: 219–26.

36 Parving H-H, Kastrup J, Smidt UM, Andersen AR, Feldt-Rasmussen B, Sandahl Christiansen J. Impaired autoregulation of glomerular filtration rate in type 1 (insulin-dependent) diabetic patients with nephropathy. *Diabetologia* 1984; 27: 547–52.

37 Mogensen CE. Early glomerular hyperfiltration in insulin-dependent diabetics and late nephropathy. *Scand J Lab Invest* 1986; 46: 201–6.

38 Rudberg S, Persson B, Dahlquist G. Increased glomerular filtration rate as a predictor of diabetic nephropathy – an 8-year prospective study. *Kidney Int* 1992; 41: 822–8.

39 Hostetter TH. Diabetic nephropathy. Metabolic versus hemodynamic considerations. *Diabetes Care* 1992; 15: 1205–15.

40 Lervang H-H, Jensen S, Brøchner-Mortensen J, Ditzel J. Does increased glomerular filtration rate or disturbed tubular function early in the course of childhood type 1 diabetes predict the development of nephropathy? *Diabetic Med* 1992; 9: 635–40.

41 Schmitz A, Christensen CK, Christensen T, Sølling K. No microalbuminuria or other adverse effects of long-standing hyperfiltration in humans with one kidney. *Am J Kidney Dis* 1989; 13: 131–6.

42 Ellis EN, Wiegmann TB, Savin VJ. Diminished glomerular capillary hydraulic conductivity precedes morphologic changes in experimental diabetes mellitus in the rat. *Diabetes* 1992; 41: 1106–12.

43 Tarsio JF, Reger LA, Furcht LT. Molecular mechanisms in basement membrane complications of diabetes. *Diabetes* 1988; 37: 532–9.

44 Brownlee M. Glycation products and the pathogenesis of diabetic complications. *Diabetes Care* 1992; 15: 1835–3.

45 Lubec G, Pollak A. Reduced susceptibility of nonenzymatically glycosylated glomerular basement to proteases: is thickening of diabetic glomerular basement membranes due to reduced proteolytic degradation? *Renal Pysiol* 1980; 3: 4–8.

46 Ayo SH, Radnik RA, Glass WF et al. Increased extracellular matrix synthesis and mRNA in mesangial cells grown in high-glucose medium. *Am J Physiol* 1991; 260: F 185–91.
47 Wu V-Y, Wilson B, Cohen MP. Disturbances in glomerular basement membrane glycosaminoglycans in experimental diabetes. *Diabetes* 1987; 36: 679–83.
48 Olgemöller B, Schwaabe S, Gerbitz KD, Schleicher ED. Elevated glucose decreases the content of a basement membrane associated heparan sulphate proteoglycan in proliferating cultured porcine mesangial cells. *Diabetologia* 1992; 35: 183–6.
49 Kanwar YS. Biology of disease: biophysiology of glomerular filtration and proteinuria. *Lab Invest* 1984; 51: 7–21.
50 Van Den Born J, Van Den Heuvel LPWJ, Bakker MAH, Veerkamp JH, Assmann KJM, Berden JHM. A monoclonoal antibody against GBM heparan sulfate induces an acute selective proteinuria in rats. *Kidney Int* 1992; 41: 115–3.
51 Kanwar YS, Linker A, Farquhar MG. Increased permeability of the glomerular basement membrane to ferritin after removal of glycosaminoglycans (heparan sulfate) by enzyme digestion. *J Cell Biol* 1980; 86: 680–93.
52 Hunsicker LG, Shearer TP, Shaffer SJ. Acute reversible proteinuria induced by infusion of the polycation hexadimethrine. *Kidney Int* 1981; 20: 7–17.
53 Reddi AS, Ramamurthi R, Miller M, Dhuper S, Lasker N. Enalapril improves albuminuria by preventing glomerular loss of heparan sulfate in diabetic rats. *Biochem Med Meta Biol* 1991; 45: 119–31.
54 Gambaro G, Cavazzana AO, Luzi P *et al.* Glycosaminoglycans prevent morphological renal alterations and albuminuria in diabetic rats. *Kidney Int* 1992; 42: 285–291.
55 Shimomura H, Spiro RG. Decreased levels of heparan sulfate proteoglycan and laminin. *Diabetes* 1987; 36: 374–81.
56 Nerlich A, Schleicher E. Immunohistochemical localization of extracellular matrix components in human diabetic glomerular lesions. *Am J Pathol* 1991; 139: 889–99.
57 Vernier RL, Steffes MW, Sisson-Ross S, Mauer SM. Heparan sulfate proteoglycan in the glomerular basement membrane in type 1 diabetes mellitus. *Kidney Int* 1992; 41: 1070–80.
58 Kofoed-Enevoldsen A, Eriksson UJ. Inhibition of N-acetylheparosan deacetylase in diabetic rats. *Diabetes* 1991; 40: 1449–52.
59 Kofoed-Enevoldsen A. Inhibition of glomerular glucosaminyl N-deacetylase in diabetic rats. *Kidney Int* 1992; 41: 763–7.
60 Kjellén L, Bielefeld D, Hook M. Reduced sulfation of liver heparan sulfate in experimentally diabetic rats. *Diabetes* 1983; 32: 337–42.
61 Kofoed-Enevoldsen A, Noonan D, Deckert T. Diabetes induced inhibition of glucosaminyl N-deacetylase: Effect of short-term blood glucose control. *Diabetologia* 1993: 36: 310–15.
62 Rohrbach R. Reduced content and abnormal distribution of anionic sites (acid proteoglycans) in the diabetic glomerular basement membrane. *Virchow's Arch (Cell Pathol)* 186; 51: 127–35.
63 Chakrabarti S, Ma N, Sima A A F. Reduced number of anionic sites is associated with glomerular basement membrane thickening in the diabetic BB-rat. *Diabetologia* 1989; 32: 826–8.
64 Fox JG, Quin JD, Paterson KR, O'Reilly DS, Boulton-Jones JM. Impaired glomerular charge selectivity in microalbuminuria and diabetic nephropathy. *Diabetologia* 1990; 33: suppl A67.
65 Pietravalle P, Morano S, Christina G *et al.* Charge selectivity of proteinuria in type 1 diabetes explored by immunoglobulin subclass clearance. *Diabetes* 40: Supplement 1, 552 A, 1991
66 Kverneland A, Feldt-Rasmussen B, Vidal P *et al.* Evidence of changes in renal charge selectivity in patients with type 1 (insulin-dependent) diabetes mellitus. *Diabetologia* 1986; 29: 634–9.
67 Kjellén L, Lindahl U. Proteoglycans: Structures and interactions. *Annu Rev Biochem* 1991; 60: 443–75.
68 Heremans A, De Cock B, Cassiman J-J, Van den Berghe H, David G. The core protein of the matrix-associated heparan sulfate proteoglycan binds to fibronectin. *J Biol Chem* 1990; 265: 8716–24.
69 Walton HA, Byrne J, Robinson GB. Studies of the permeation properties of glomerular basement membrane permeable to protein. *Biochim Biophys Acta* 1992; 1138: 172–83.
70 Moore WV, Donaldsen DL, Chonko AM, Ideus P, Wiegmann TB. Ambulatory blood pressure in type 1 diabetes mellitus. Comparison to presence of incipient nephropathy in adolescents and young adults. *Diabetes* 1992; 41: 1035–41.
71 Skøtt P, Mathiesen ER, Hommel E, Gall M-A, Bruun N E, Parving H-H. The increased proximal tubular reabsorption of sodium and water is maintained in long-term insulin-dependent diabetics with early nephropathy. *Scand J Clin Lab Invest* 1989; 49: 419–25.
72 Feldt-Rasmussen B, Mathiesen ER, Deckert T *et al.* Central role for sodium in the pathogenesis of blood pressure changes independent of angiotensin, aldosterone and catecholamines in type 1 (insulin-dependent) diabetes mellitus. *Diabetologia* 1987; 30: 610–17.
73 Brochner-Mortensen J, Stockel M, Sorensen PJ, Nielsen AH, Ditzel J. Proximal glomerulo-tulbular balance in patients with type 1 (insulin-dependent) diabetes mellitus. *Diabetologia* 1984; 27: 189–92.
74 Norgaard K, Feldt-Rasmussen B. Sodium retention and insulin-treatment in insulin-dependent diabetes mellitus. *Acta Diabet* 1994; 31: 19–25.
75 Mathiesen ER, Hilsted J, Feldt-Rasmussen B, Bonde-Petersen F, Christensen NJ, Parving H-H. The effect of metabolic control on hemodynamics in short-term insulin-dependent diabetic patients. *Diabetes* 1985; 34: 1301–5.
76 Viberti GC, Yip-Messent J, Morocutti A. Diabetic nephropathy. Future avenue. *Diabetes Care* 1992; 15: 1216–25.
77 Deckert T, Kofoed-Enevoldsen A, Norgaard K, Borch-Johnsen K, Feldt-Rasmussen B, Jensen T. Microalbuminuria. Implications for micro- and macrovascular disease. *Diabetes Care* 1992; 15: 1181–91.
78 Walker JD, Tariq T, Viberti GC. Sodium–lithium countertransport activity in red cells of patients with insulin dependent diabetes and nephropathy and their parents. *Br Med J* 1990; 301: 635–8.
79 Jensen JS, Mathiesen ER, Nørgaard K *et al.* Increased blood pressure and erythrocyte sodium/lithium coun-

tertransport activity are not inherited in diabetic nephropathy. *Diabetologia* 1990; 33: 619–24.

80 Jensen T, Borch-Johnsen K, Deckert T. Changes in blood pressure and renal function in patients with type 1 (insulin-dependent) diabetes mellitus prior to clinical diabetic nephropathy. *Diabetes Res* 1987; 4: 159–162.

81 Deckert T, Poulsen JE. Diabetic nephropathy: Fault or destiny? *Diabetologia* 1981; 21: 178–83.

82 Mathiesen ER, Rønn B, Jensen T, Storm B, Deckert T. Relationship between blood pressure and urinary albumin excretion in development of microalbuminuria. *Diabetes* 1990; 39: 245–9.

83 Nørgaard K, Rasmussen E, Jensen T, Giese J, Feldt-Rasmussen B. Essential hypertension and type 1 (insulin-dependent) diabetes. *Am J Hypertens* 1993; 6: 830–6.

84 Mauer SM, Sutherland DER, Steffes MW. Relationship of systemic blood pressure to nephropathology in insulin-dependent diabetes mellitus. *Kidney Int* 1992; 41: 736–40.

85 Feldt-Rasmussen B, Mathiesen ER, Deckert T. Effect of two years of strict metabolic control on progression of incipient nephropathy in insulin-dependent diabetes. *Lancet* 1986; ii: 1300–4.

86 Christensen CK, Krusell LR, Mogensen CE. Increased blood pressure in diabetes: essential hypertension or diabetic nephropathy? *Scand J Clin Invest* 1987; 47: 363–70.

87 Kelbæk H, Jensen T, Feldt-Rasmussen B *et al.* Impaired left-ventricular function in insulin-dependent diabetic patients with increased urinary albumin excretion. *Scand J Clin Lab Invest* 1991; 51: 467–73.

88 Hommel E, Mathiesen ER, Giese J, Nielsen MD, Schütten HJ, Parving H-H. On the pathogenesis of arterial blood pressure elevation early in the course of diabetic nephropathy. *Scand J Clin Lab Invest* 1989; 49: 537–44.

89 Hall JE, Guyton AC, Coleman TG, Léland Mizelle H, Woods LL. Regulation of arterial pressure: role of pressure natriuresis and diuresis. *Federat Proc* 1986; 45: 2897–903.

90 Parving H-H. Impact on blood pressure and antihypertensive treatment on incipient and overt nephropathy, retinopathy and endothelial permeability in diabetes mellitus. *Diabetes Care* 1991; 14: 260–9.

91 Nørgaard K, Feldt-Rasmussen B, Deckert T. Is hypertension a major risk factor for retinopathy in type 1 diabetes? *Diabetic Med* 1991; 8: 334–7.

92 Feldt-Rasmussen B, Baker L, Deckert T. Exercise as a provocative test in early renal disease in Type 1 (insulin-dependent) diabetes: albuminuric, systemic and renal haemodynamic responses. *Diabetologia* 1985; 28: 389–96.

93 Deckert T, Grenfell A. Epidemiology and natural history of diabetic nephropathy. In: Pickup JC, Williams G, eds. *Textbook of diabetes*, Blackwell Scientific Publications, Oxford, 1991; 651–6.

94 Frøkjær Thomsen O, Andersen AR, Sandahl Christiansen J, Deckert T. Renal changes in long-term type 1 (insulin-dependent) diabetic patients without clinical nephropathy: a light microscopic, morphometric study of autopsy material. *Diabetologia* 1984; 26: 361–5.

95 Thomsen ÅC. The kidney in diabetes mellitus. PhD Thesis, Munksgaard, Copenhagen 1965.

96 Ellis EN, Steffes MW, Goetz FC, Sutherland DER, Mauer SM. Glomerular filtration surface in type 1 diabetes mellitus. *Kidney Int* 1986; 29: 889–94.

97 Hayashi H, Karasawa R, Inn H *et al.* An electron microscopic study of glomeruli in Japanese patients with non-insulin dependent diabetes mellitus. *Kidney Int* 1992; 41: 749–57.

98 Walker JD, Close CF, Jones SL *et al.* Glomerular structure in type-1 (insulin-dependent) diabetic patients with normo- and microalbuminuria. *Kidney Int* 1992; 41: 741–8.

99 Remuzzi G, Bertani T. Is glomerulosclerosis a consequence of altered glomerular permeability to macromolecules? *Kidney Int* 1990; 38: 384–94.

100 Parving H-H, Smidt UM, Andersen AR, Svendsen PA. Early aggressive antihypertensive treatment reduces rate of decline in kidney function in diabetic nephropathy. *Lancet* 1983; i:1175–9.

101 Castellot JJ, Hoover RL, Harper PA, Karnovsky MJ. Heparin and glomerular epithelial cell-secreted heparin-like species inhibit mesangial-cell proliferation. *Am J Pathol* 1985; 120: 427–35.

102 Ledbetter S, Copeland EJ, Noonan D, Vogeli G, Hassell JR. Altered steady-state mRNA levels of basement membrane proteins in diabetic mouse kidneys and thromboxane synthase inhibition. *Diabetes* 1990; 39: 196–203.

103 Cagliero E, Roth T, Roy S, Lorenzi M. Characteristics and mechanisms of high-glucose-induced overexpression of basement membrane components in cultured human endothelial cells. *Diabetes* 1991; 40: 102–10.

104 Fukui M, Nakamura T, Ebihara I, Shirato I, Tomino Y, Koide H. ECM gene expression and its modulation by insulin in diabetic rats. *Diabetes* 1992; 41: 1520–7

105 Haneda M, Kikkawa R, Horide N *et al.* Glucose enhances type IV collagen production in cultured rat glomerular mesangial cells. *Diabetologia* 1991; 34: 198–200.

106 Klein DJ, Oegema TR, Brown DM. Release of glomerular heparan $^{35}SO_4$ proteoglycan by heparan from glomeruli of streptozotocin-induced diabetic rats. *Diabetes* 1989; 38: 130–9.

107 Unger E, Pettersson I, Eriksson UJ, Lindahl U, Kjellen L. Decreased activity of the heparan sulfate modifying enzyme glucosaminyl N-deacetylase in hepatocytes from streptozotocin-diabetic rats. *J Biol Chem* 1991; 266: 8671–4.

108 Cohen MP, Klepser H, Wu V-Y. Undersulfation of glomerular basement membrane heparan sulfate in experimental diabetes and lack of correction with aldose reductase inhibition. *Diabetes* 1988; 37: 1324–7.

109 Bangstad H-J, Kofoed-Enevoldsen A, Dahl-Jørgensen K, Hanssen K. Glomerular charge selectivity and the influence of improved blood glucose control in type 1 (insulin-dependent) diabetic patients with microalbuminuria. *Diabetologia* 1992; 35:1165–9.

110 Seaquist ER, Goetz FC, Rich S, Barbosa J. Familial clustering of diabetic kidney disease. *N Engl J Med* 1989; 320: 1161–5.

111 Borch-Johnsen K, Nørgaard K, Hommel E *et al.* Is diabetic nephropathy an inherited complication? *Kidney Int* 1992; 41: 719–22.

112 Svejgaard A, Jakobsen B K, Platz P *et al.* HLA associations in insulin-dependent diabetes: search for hetero-

geneity in different groups of patients from a homogeneous population. *Tissue Antigens* 1986; 28: 237–44.
113 Raffel LJ, Vadheim CM, Roth M-P, Klein R, Moss SE, Rotter JI. The 5′ insulin gene polymorphism and the genetics of vascular complications in type 1 (insulin-dependent) diabetes mellitus. *Diabetologia* 1991; 34: 680–3.
114 Pettitt DJ, Saad MF, Bennett PM, Nelson RG, Knowler WC. Familial predisposition to renal disease in two generations of Pima Indians with type 2 (non-insulin dependent) diabetes mellitus. *Diabetologia* 1990; 33: 438–43.
115 Kalter-Leibovici O, Van Dyk DJ, Libovici L *et al.* Risk factors for development of diabetic nephropathy and retinopathy in Jewish IDDM patients. *Diabetes* 1991; 40: 204–10.
116 Carr S, Mbanya J-C, Thomas T *et al.* Increase in glomerular filtration rate in patients with insulin-dependent diabetes and elevated erythrocyte sodium–lithium countertransport. *N Engl J Med* 1990; 322: 500–5.
117 Ng LL, Simmons D, Frighi V, Garrido MC, Bomford J, Hockaday TDR. Leucocyte Na+/H+ antiport activity in type 1 (insulin-dependent) diabetic patients with nephropathy. *Diabetologia* 1990; 33: 371–7.
118 Trevisan R, Li LK, Messent J *et al.* Na+/H+ antiport activity and cell growth in cultured skin fibroblasts of IDDM patients with nephropathy. *Diabetes* 1992; 41: 1239–46.
119 Deckert T, Horowitz IM, Kofoed-Enevoldsen A *et al.* Possible genetic defects in regulation of glycosaminoglycans in patients with diabetic nephropathy. *Diabetes* 1991; 40: 764–70.
120 Kallunki P, Tryggvason K. Human basement membrane heparan sulfate proteoglycan core protein: a 467-kD protein containing multiple domains resembling elements of the low density lipoprotein receptor, laminin, neural cell adhesion molecules, and epidermal growth factor. *J Cell Biol* 1992; 116: 559–71.
121 Murdoch AD, Dodge GR, Cohen I, Tuan RS, Iozzo RV. Primary structure of the human heparan sulfate proteoglycan from basement membrane (HSPG2/Perlecan). *J. Biol Chem* 1992; 267: 8544–57.
122 Earle K, Walker J, Hill C, Viberti GC. Familial clustering of cardiovascular disease in patients with insulin-dependent diabetes and nephropathy. *N Engl J Med* 1992; 326: 673–7.
123 Nørgaard K, Mathiesen ER, Hommel E, Jensen JS, Parving H-H. Lack of familial predisposition to cardiovascular disease in type 1 (insulin-dependent) diabetic patients with nephropathy. *Diabetologia* 1991; 34: 370–32.
124 Deckert T, Jensen T, Feldt-Rasmussen B, Kofoed-Enevoldsen A, Borch-Johnsen K, Stender S. Albuminuria a risk marker of atherosclerosis in insulin dependent diabetes mellitus. *Cardiovasc Risk Factors* 1991; 1: 347–60.
125 Valdorf-Hansen F, Jensen T, Borch-Johnsen K, Deckert T. Cardiovascular risk factors in type 1 (insulin-dependent) diabetic patients with and without proteinuria. *Acta Med Scand* 1987; 222: 439–44.
126 Mattock MB, Keen H, Viberti GC *et al.* Coronary heart disease and urinary albumin excretion rate in type 2 (non-insulin-dependent) diabetic patients. *Diabetologia* 1988; 31: 82–7.
127 Jensen T, Stender S, Deckert T. Abnormalities in plasma concentrations of lipoproteins and fibrinogen in type 1 (insulin-dependent) diabetic patients with increased urinary albumin excretion. *Diabetologia* 1988; 31: 142–5.
128 Winocour PH, Durrington PN, Ishola M, Anderson DC, Cohen H. Influence of proteinuria on vascular disease, blood pressure, and lipoproteins in insulin dependent diabetes mellitus. *Br Med J* 1987; 294: 1648–51.
129 Jones SL, Close CF, Mattock MB, Jarrett RJ, Keen H, Viberti GC. Plasma lipid and coagulation factor concentrations in insulin dependent diabetics with microalbuminuria. *Br Med J* 1989; 298: 487–90.
130 Jenkins AJ, Steele JS, Janus ED, Santamaria JD, Best JD. Plasma apolipoprotein (a) is increased in type 2 (non-insulin-dependent) diabetic patients with microalbuminuria. *Diabetologia* 1992; 35: 1055–9.
131 Telmer S, Sandahl Christiansen J, Andersen AR, Nerup J, Deckert T. Smoking habits and prevalence of clinical diabetic microangiopathy in insulin-dependent diabetics. *Acta Med Scand* 1984; 215: 63–8.
132 Jensen T. Increased plasma concentration of von Willebrand factor in insulin dependent diabetics with incipient nephropathy. *Br Med J* 1989; 298: 27–8.
133 Iwashima Y, Sato T, Watanabe K *et al.* Elevation of plasma thrombomodulin level in diabetic patients with early diabetic nephropathy. *Diabetes* 1990; 39: 983–8.
134 Feldt-Rasmussen B. Increased transcapillary escape rate of albumin in type 1 (insulin-dependent) diabetic patients with microalbuminuria. *Diabetologia* 1986; 29: 282–6.
135 Jensen T, Bjerre-Knudsen J, Feldt-Rasmussen B, Deckert T. Features of endothelial dysfunction in early diabetic nephropathy. *Lancet* 1989; i: 461–3.
136 Rippe B, Crone C. Pores and intercellular junctions. In: West JB *et al.* eds. *The lung: scientific foundations*, Raven Press Ltd., New York, 1991; 349–57.
137 Bundgaard M. Vesicular transport in capillary endothelium: does it occur? *Federation Proc* 1983; 42: 2425–30.
138 Dybdahl H, Ledet T. Diabetic macroangiopathy. Quantitative histopathological studies of the extramural coronary arteries from Type 2 (non-insulin-dependent) diabetic patients. *Diabetologia* 1987; 30: 882–6.
139 Berenson GS, Radhakrishnamurthy B, Srinivasan SR, Dalfers ER, Malinow MR. Chemical changes in the arterial wall during regression of atherosclerosis in monkeys. *Artery* 1981; 9: 44–58.
140 Hollmann J, Schmidt A, von Bassewitx DB, Buddecke E. Relationship of sulfated glycosaminoglycans and cholesterol content in normal and arterioscleroti human aorta. *Arteriosclerosis* 1989; 9: 154–8.
141 Raz I, Havivi Y, Yarom R. Reduced negative surface on arterial endothelium of diabetic rats. *Diabetologia* 1988; 31: 618–20.
142 Bent-Hansen L, Feldt-Rasmussen B, Kverneland A, Deckert T. Plasma disappearance of glycated and non-glycated albumin in type I (insulin-dependent) diabetes mellitus: Evidence for charge dependent alterations of the plasma to lymph pathway. *Diabetologia* 1993; 36: 361–3.
143 Wight TN. Cell biology of arterial proteoglycans. *Arteriosclerosis* 1989; 9: 1–20.
144 Pejler G, Bäckström G, Lindahl U *et al.* Structure and

affinity for antithrombin of heparan sulfate chains derived from basement membrane proteoglycans. *J Biol Chem* 1987; 262: 5036–43.

145 Ribes JA, Ni F, Wagner DD, Francis CW. Mediation of fibrin-reduced release of von Willebrand factor from cultured endothelial cells by the fibrin β chain. *J Clin Invest* 1989; 84: 4335–42.

146 Toyofuku T, Koyama S, Kobayashi T, Kusama S, Ueda G. Effects of polycations on pulmonary vascular permeability in conscious sheep. *J Clin Invest* 1989; 83: 2063–9.

147 Wight TN, Kinsella MG, Qwarnström EE. The role of proteoglycans in cell adhesion, migration and proliferation. *Curr Opin Cell Biol* 1992; 4: 793–801.

148 Stender S, Hjelms E. *In vivo* transfer of cholesterol from plasma into human aortic tissue. *Scand J Clin Lab Invest* 1987; 47, Suppl 1, 86: 31–9.

149 Nordestgaard BG, Hjelms E, Stender S, Kjeldsen K. Different efflux pathways for high and low density lipoproteins from porcine aortic intima. *Arteriosclerosis* 1990; 10: 477–85.

150 Pomerantz KB, Hajja DP. Eicosanoids in regulation of arterial smooth muscle cell phenotype, proliferative capacity, and cholesterol metabolism. *Arteriosclerosis* 1989; 9: 413–29.

151 Castellot JJ, Beeler DL, Rosenberg RD, Karnovsky MJ. Structural determinants of the capacity of heparin to inhibit the proliferation of vascular smooth muscle cells. *J Cell Physiol* 1984; 120: 315–20.

152 Steinberg D, Parthasarathy S, Carew TE, Khoo JC, Witztum JL. Modifications of low-density lipoprotein that increase its atherogenicity. *N Engl J Med* 1989; 320: 915–24.

153 Williams MP, Streeter HB, Wusteman FS, Cryer A. Heparan sulphate and the binding of lipoprotein lipase to porcine thoracic aorta endothelium. *Biochim Biophys Acta* 1983; 756: 83–91.

154 Yamamoto T, Nakamura T, Noble NA, Ruoslahti E, Border WA. Expression of transforming growth factor β is elevated in human and experimental diabetic nephropathy. *Proc Natl Acad Sci USA* 1993; 90: 1814–8.

155 The Diabetes Control and Complications Trial Research Group. The effect of intensive treatment of diabetes on the development and progression of long-term complications in insulin-dependent diabetes mellitus. *N Engl J Med* 1993; 329: 977–86.

156 Tamsma JT, Van Den Born J, Bruijn JA *et al.* Expression of glomerular extracellular matrix components in diabetic nephropathy. Decrease of heparan sulphate in the GBM. *Diabetologia* 1994; 37: 313–20.

157 Microalbuminuria Collaborative Study Group, UK. Risk factors for development of microalbuminuria in insulin dependent diabetic patients: a cohort study. *Br Med J* 1993; 306: 1235–9.

# 26 Pharmacological Approaches to Non-insulin-dependent Diabetes: Future Directions

Richard C. Eastman & Timothy Seaton

## INTRODUCTION

Non-insulin-dependent diabetes mellitus is a disease characterised by insulin resistance and impaired insulin secretion. In careful longitudinal studies it has been shown that insulin resistance predates the development of hyperglycaemia in some populations, and is relatively constant after diabetes develops. Impairment in insulin secretion appears to be the critical element leading to hyperglycaemia. While sulphonylureas, metformin, and insulin are the pharmacological treatments available for NIDDM at this time, numerous other approaches are under development.

Since the majority of patients with NIDDM are overweight, and since weight reduction significantly ameliorates diabetes in most of these patients, numerous pharmacological approaches to interfering with nutrient intake, uptake, and utilisation are being studied. Agents that reduce nutrient intake or digestion, such as appetite suppressants and lipase inhibitors are being targeted primarily at obese individuals, but would probably help many patients with NIDDM as well. Other agents are being targeted more specifically at individuals with diabetes, such as α-glucosidase inhibitors, agents that interfere with hepatic glucose release and gluconeogenesis, and inhibitors of fatty acid oxidation (1). These agents inhibit specific enzymes that are necessary for a given metabolic process, and do not affect the basic underlying defects in insulin secretion and action. More recently, attention has become focused on agents that enhance or mimic insulin action on target tissues. In this chapter we will review progress in three areas of current interest, namely the role of α-glucosidase inhibitors in the treatment of diabetes, and the status of agents that are insulino-mimetic, vanadium salts and the thiazolidinedione derivatives.

## ALPHA-GLUCOSIDASE INHIBITORS

A new therapeutic principle was discovered with the development of carbohydrase inhibitors (alpha-glucosidase inhibitors). Pancreatic amylase hydrolyses complex starches to oligosaccharides in the lumen of the small intestine, while alpha-glucosidases hydrolyse oligosaccharides, trisaccharides, and disaccharides to glucose and other monosaccharides in the brush border of the small intestine. Carbohydrase inhibitors, by competitive and reversible inhibition of the alpha-glucosidase enzymes, reduce or delay carbohydrate digestion. Thus, carbohydrate is digested and absorbed more slowly and the large postprandial increases in blood glucose and serum insulin levels are prevented or reduced (2). These decreases in postprandial glucose result in a long-term improvement in overall glycaemic control as measured by HbAlc.

Two alpha-glucosidase inhibitors are either approved or in large world-wide Phase III trials. Acarbose, a pseudo-oligosaccharide discovered in culture broths of Actinomycete, has received regulatory approval in 31 countries and has been marketed in 20 countries. Miglitol, a deoxynojirimycin derivative, has a similar mechanism of action and is undergoing Phase III trials in Europe and North America.

Both of these medications are taken with the first bite of each meal and decrease post-prandial glucose values by 40 to 60 mg/dl. Less consistent effects on lowering fasting glucose have been seen. Long-term (≥ six months) controlled clinical studies with acarbose have consistently demonstrated the ability of acarbose, as compared to placebo, to improve hyperglycaemia and to reduce glycated haemoglobin levels in patients with NIDDM, whether used as an adjunct to diet, sulphonylurea, metformin or insulin therapy (3–5). Furthermore, concomitantly with the reduction in glycated haemoglobin, acarbose therapy has been shown to reduce daily insulin dosage requirements as well as sulphonylurea requirements in NIDDM patients. In IDDM, acarbose has been shown to either reduce glycated haemoglobin levels or to reduce daily insulin dosage requirements (6). The magnitude of change in HbA1c from placebo ranges from 0.5–1.0% (normal HbA1c range 4.0–6.0%). Whether used in conjunction with diet, sulphonylureas or metformin. Miglitol, which is in Phase II development in Europe and North America, has been shown to have a magnitude of clinical effect similar to that of acarbose.

The most common side-effects relate to the gastrointestinal tract and include flatulence, diarrhoea or soft stools, and abdominal pain. These symptoms reflect carbohydrate maldigestion and are thereby directly attributable to the mechanism whereby carbohydrase inhibitors achieve their action. Carbohydrase inhibitors can increase the delivery of osmotically active oligosaccharides, trisaccharides, and disaccharides to the large intestine which can result in loose stools and/or diarrhoea. Most of these saccharide moieties are anaerobically metabolised by faecal flora to hydrogen and methane, which may result in abdominal pain and distension, flatulence, and/or meteorism, and to short-chain fatty acids whose absorption and metabolism prevents enteric caloric losses. There is evidence of adaption to the gastrointestinal side-effects over time similar to the adaptation that patients have with high fibre diets.

Clinically significant elevations (greater than three times the upper limit of normal) in serum transaminase levels have occasionally been seen in patients taking 200 mg tid of acarbose (SGOT: 2% for acarbose vs 0% for placebo: SGPT 2% for acarbose and 1% for placebo). These clinically significant elevations have not been seen in patients taking 50 or 100 mg tid which is the usual recommended dose of acarbose. These elevations have not been associated with any symptoms of hepatic disease and are rapidly reversible on discontinuation of the medication. The elevations have generally not been associated with other clinical or laboratory stigmata of hepatocellular inflammation or damage and are thought to be idiosyncratic in nature. An increased incidence of treatment emergent elevations in serum transaminase levels have not been seen in the Phase II studies with miglitol.

Hypoglycaemia, a common complication of tight blood sugar control with both insulin and sulphonylureas, is not seen with carbohydrase inhibitors when they are used as monotherapy. Since early control of blood glucose may be important in the prevention of complications, agents which can lower blood glucose and HbA1c without causing hypoglycaemia are important additions to the treatment regimen. The ability to lower blood glucose without causing hypoglycaemia may also have special importance in the elderly given the propensity to hypoglycaemia with sulphonylurea treatment in this group and the high mortality rate of sulphonylurea induced hypoglycaemia. Since carbohydrase inhibitors such as acarbose and miglitol primarily lower postprandial blood glucose, do not stimulate insulin secretion or cause hyperinsulinaemia, are additive to sulphonylureas, metformin and insulin in their effect on HbA1c, and do not cause hypoglycaemia, they are an important addition to the diabetic armamentarium. Finally, just as with hypertension, it may be unrealistic to expect that only one drug will control a majority of patients with NIDDM over the long term. Some patients may respond better to one regimen than another and some may require more than one agent with differing mechanisms of action. The linear relationship between HbA1c and complications shown in the Diabetes Control and Complications Trial suggests that current therapeutic approaches should be directed to combination drug therapy in order to maximally control plasma glucose in patients who respond inadequately to diet alone (7).

## VANADIUM COMPOUNDS

Since 1979 there has been considerable interest in vanadium compounds because of insulin-like effects *in vitro* and *in vivo* (8). These compounds are derived from the transition metal vanadium which is an essential trace element. Vanadium compounds are low molecular weight phosphate analogues that exist in the V+5 state as vanadate and the V+4 state as vanadyl (9). Vanadate is present extracellularly in biological systems, but is probably reduced to vanadyl intracellularly (10–12). Vanadate, but not vanadyl, is known to inhibit $Na^+$–$K^+$-ATPase, and both compounds are known inhibitors of phosphotyrosylprotein phosphatase and HMG-CoA reductase (8, 13, 14). The possibility of an insulin-like agent that can be administered orally has excited much interest in these compounds as potential therapeutic agents for human diabetes.

A number of vanadium compounds have been studied, including metavanadate, orthovanadate, and vanadyl sulphate (Table 26.1). The latter compound is the most effective as an insulin-like agent and has the least toxicity (15–17).

Table 26.1.

| Compound | Active moiety | Valence |
|---|---|---|
| Sodium metavanadate | $NaVO_3$ | $V^{+5}$ |
| Sodium orthovanadate | $Na_3VO_4$ | $V^{+5}$ |
| Vanadyl sulphate pentahydrate | $VOSO_4$-$5H_2O$ | $V^{+4}$ |

Insulin-like effects of vanadate were first demonstrated *in vivo* in streptozotocin-induced diabetes in rats in 1985 (18). Numerous other studies in animals have appeared since that time and show reasonably consistent results (8).

When administered in drinking water to non-diabetic animals, vanadium compounds have little effect on glucose homeostasis or insulin levels, although weight gain and food intake may be reduced (19). Some studies have also shown lower insulin levels during administration of vanadium compounds (17, 20, 21). Insulin levels were decreased 47% in one study of administration of vanadate to normal db/db mice (22).

Administration to diabetic animals improves or normalizes hyperglyceamia, glycosuria, and hyperlipidaemia (8).

Improvement of dyslipidaemia is seen at levels where there is no effect of glucose homeostasis (8). These effects take several days to develop and persist for days or weeks after the agent is removed from the water supply (23). In addition to correcting the metabolic abnormalities associated with diabetes, vanadium compounds have been shown to decrease renal hypertrophy and polyol accumulation (24), to decrease urine albumin and IgG excretion (25), and to ameliorate experimental nephropathy (26).

Numerous insulin-like effects of vanadium compounds have been demonstrated *in vivo* and *in vitro* in fat, liver, and skeletal muscle (14). Beta cell degeneration is prevented in some animal models (27). These effects have been observed in the streptozotocin model of diabetes in rats, as well as in mice with obesity and diabetes. It is unlikely that the mechanism of action is related to inhibition of $Na^+$–$K^+$-ATPase, since biological effects on glucose metabolism are seen at 1/100 the concentration necessary to inhibit this enzyme (14). Similarly, the effects appear not to be due to direct effects on the insulin receptor through inhibition of phosphotyrosine protein phosphatase or stimulation of tyrosine phosphorylation (8, 14). A reduction of phosphorylation of polypeptide 185, a putative mediator of intracellular insulin action, has been shown (28). An effect on calcium influx has been suggested, based on inhibition of $Ca^{2+}$–$Mg^{2+}$-ATPase activity (14). There is direct evidence of stimulation of expression of the GLUT-4 transporter gene (29) and of the GLUT-1 transporter gene (30). The latter effect is explained in part by stabilisation of messenger RNA for the transporter.

An important issue in the development of vanadium compounds as therapeutic agents for human diabetes is the potential for toxicity of these compounds. In rodents, therapeutically effective doses when given in the drinking water supply cause diarrhoea and dehydration, leading in some cases to death (31, 32). Decreased food and fluid intake and increased urea and creatinine are seen. Tissue accumulation of vanadium occurs particularly in bone, liver, and kidney; the highest accumulation is seen in rat kidney (33). Swelling of kidney epithelial cells has been observed in normal animals given vanadium compounds (34).

Vanadium compounds, particularly vanadyl sulphate, offer an interesting alternative treatment of diabetes that can ameliorate the metabolic and tissue effects of uncontrolled diabetes. The potential toxicity of long-term administration of vanadium compounds needs to be determined, and studies need to be done in humans if the animal studies prove safe. The National Institute of Diabetes and Digestive and Kidney Diseases is sponsoring a clinical trial of vanadium compounds to determine whether role for these agents in the treatment of human diabetes.

## THIAZOLIDINEDIONE DERIVATIVES

Studies of the pathogenesis of NIDDM have shown defects in insulin secretion and insulin action. The defect in insulin action precedes the development of diabetes, is familial in some populations, occurs in the absence of obesity, and is associated with hyperinsulinaemia basally and after glucose or meal challenge. Waning of insulin secretion is manifest initially as postprandial hyperglycaemia (glucose intolerance), diabetes with normal fasting blood glucose and high postprandial glucose, and subsequently fasting hyperglycaemia. Development of obesity is more common in individuals with insulin resistance, and is an important additional stressor on the baseline degree of insulin resistance.

Current therapies of NIDDM are targeted at these abnormalities. Exercise and diet increase insulin sensitivity, sulphonylureas act predominantly by stimulating endogenous insulin secretion, and exogenous insulin is given to overcome tissue insulin resistance. Agents that function at the tissue level to reduce insulin resistance could be extremely important therapeutically. They could potentially delay the onset of diabetes by decreasing the need for increased insulin secretion, could preserve beta cell function in those already having developed diabetes, and could improve glycaemic control in those with NIDDM.

In 1982, a novel class of agents was discovered that reduced insulin resistance in animal models of non-insulin-dependent diabetes (35). The agents are members of the thiazolidinedione class of drugs; the prototypical agent is ciglitazone (Fig. 26.1). Other agents in this class are pioglitazone, englitazone and CS-045.

Studies in normal animals have shown no effect of these drugs on glucose homeostasis. Unlike insulin and sulphonylureas, the thiazolidinedione derivatives do not cause hypoglycaemia in normal animals. There is also no effect in

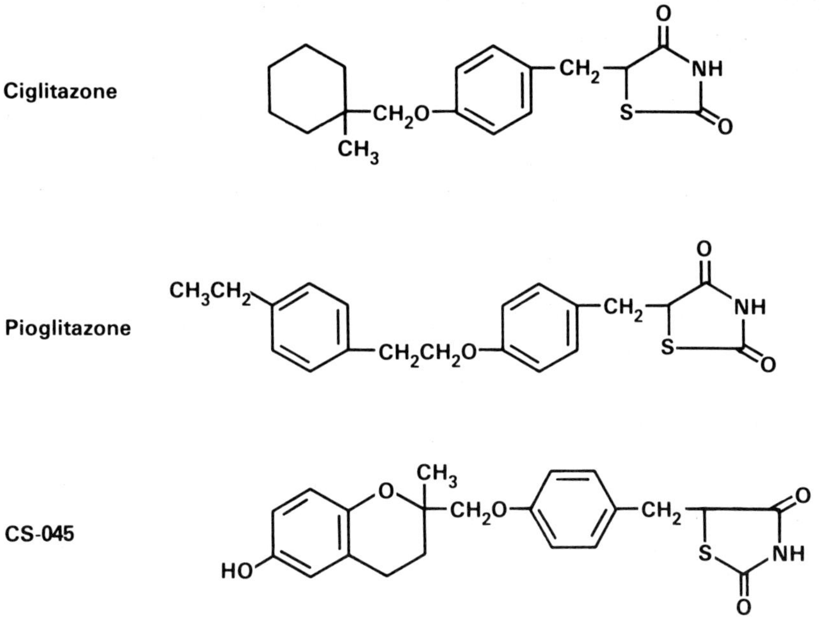


Fig. 26.1. Structures of three thaizolidinediones.

the absence of insulin. Effects on glucose metabolism are seen in obese non-diabetic animals, as well as in animal models of NIDDM. Thus the agents reduce insulin levels in Zucker fatty rats, ob/ob mice, KKAy mice, and Wister fatty rats (36). In addition to anti-hyperglycaemic effects, the agents decrease cholesterol in some animals (37).

The mechanism of action of these agents is unknown. The presence of insulin or insulin-like growth factor is required, and thus these agents potentiate insulin action. This effect is mediated distal to the initial binding of insulin to its receptor, there being no change in insulin binding or in insulin receptor affinity. Insulin stimulated autophosphorylation of the insulin receptor and of exogenous substrates is increased in obese animals but is not seen in normals (38).

Insulin-like effects are seen with these agents despite a fall in circulating insulin levels. Many of insulin's effects are seen in model systems, including stimulation of adipocyte differentiation, expression of GLUT-4 glucose transporter gene, and normalisation of increased PEPCK message and activity characteristic of uncontrolled diabetes (36). The agents stimulate glucose uptake by insulin sensitive tissues as well as decrease glucose production by the liver (39).

Early studies in humans have shown promising results. Sutter studied the effects of CS-045 in 11 subjects with NIDDM (40). Eight of eleven responded, with the non-responders having lower insulin levels. The agent decreased fasting blood glucose, decreased glycaemia after oral glucose challenge and mixed meal challenge, and lowered insulin, free fatty acid and glucagon levels. Increased glucose disposal rates were observed in all subjects, and hepatic glucose production was reduced 17% in the group as a whole.

A pilot clinical trial of CS-045 in NIDDM has also been reported (41). Little toxicity was seen in Phase I trials, and Kuzuya and co-workers studied the effect of the agent in 146 NIDDM with fasting plasma glucose greater than 140 mg/dl. Two doses (200 and 400 mg) were tested in an open label trial of 12 weeks' duration. Fasting plasma glucose fell by more than 20% in

39% of subjects. Several factors were associated with a greater response: higher dose, initial body mass index greater than 25, and initial fasting insulin >10 μU/ml.

Side-effects in the study occurred in 6% of patients and were more common at higher doses. These were predominantly gastrointestinal and included nausea, vomiting, abdominal fullness, epigastric pain and diarrhoea. Haemoglobin decreased in 3.5%, and LDH increased in 6% of patients. Rash was observed in two patients.

This new class of drugs offers promise for reversing insulin resistance in man, a defect that appears to underlie development of NIDDM. Further studies of these agents in humans with obesity, insulin resistance, glucose intolerance and diabetes are under way.

## REFERENCES


1 Bressler R, Johnson D. New pharmacologic approaches to therapy of NIDDM. *Diabetes Care* 1992; 15: 792–805.
2 Wolever TMS, Singer W, Chiasson JL, Palmasson C. Acarbose improves abnormal insulin metabolism in type 2 diabetes. *Clin Res* 1993; 41: 306.
3 Hanefeld M, Fisher S, Schulze J *et al.* Therapeutic potentials of acarbose as first-line drug in NIDDM insufficiently treated with diet alone. *Diabetes Care* 1991; 14: 732.
4 Innerfield R, Coniff RF. A multi-center, double-blind, placebo-controlled study of the long-term efficacy and safety of acarbose (BAY g 5421) in the treatment of obese patients with NIDDM treated with diet alone. *Diabetes* 1990; 39 (Suppl 1): 211.
5 Innerfield R, Coniff RF. A multi-center, double-blind, 1 placebo-controlled study of long-term efficacy and safety of acarbose (BAY g 5421) and sulfonylurea in the treatment of NIDDM inadequately controlled by maximal sulfonylurea. *Diabetes* 1990; 39 (Suppl 1): 108.
6 Hollander P, Coniff RF. Two multi-center, double-blind, placebo controlled studies of efficacy and safety of acarbose treatment of Type I diabetes. *Diabetes* 1991; 40 (Suppl 1): 307.
7 The DCCT Research Group. The effect of intensive insulin treatment of diabetes on the development and progression of long-term complications of insulin-dependent diabetes mellitus. *N Engl J Med* 1993; 329: 977.
8 Cros G, Mongold JJ, Serrano JJ, Ramanadham S, McNeill JH. Effects of vanadyl derivatives on animal models of diabetes. *Mol Cell Biochem* 1992; 109: 163–66.
9 Connor JA, Ebsworth EAV. Peroxy compounds of transition metals. Emeleus HJ and Sharpe AG, eds. *Advances in inorganic chemistry and biochemistry* New York: Academic Press, 1964; 292–9.
10 Nechay BR, Nanninga LB, Nechay PSE. Distribution of vanadium. *Federation Proc* 1986; 45: 123–32.
11 Gegani H, Gichin M, Karlish S, Schechter Y. Electron paramagnetic resonance studies and insulin-like effects of vanadium in rats adipocytes. *Biochemistry* 1981; 20: 5795–9.
12 Green A. The insulin-like effect of sodium vanadate on adipocyte glucose transport is mediated at a post-insulin-receptor level. *Biochem J* 1986; 238: 663–9.
13 Ramasarma T, Crane FL. Does vanadium play a role in cellular regulation? *Curr Topics Cell Regul* 1981; 20: 247–301.
14 Shechter Y. Insulin-mimetic effects of vanadate. Possible implications for future treatment of diabetes. *Diabetes* 1990; 39.
15 Hudson TGF, Vanadium. Toxicology and biological significance. In Ethel Browning, ed. *Elsevier monographs on toxic agents*. Amsterdam: Elsevier; 1964.
16 Llobet JM, Domingo JL. Acute toxicity of vanadium compounds in rats and mice. *Toxicol Lett* 1984; 23: 227–31.
17 Ramanadham S, Mongold JJ, Brownsey RW, Cros GH, McNeill JH. Oral vanadyl in treatment of diabetes mellitus in rats. *Am J Physiol* 1989; 257: H904–11.
18 Heyliger CE, Tahiliani AG, McNeill JH. Effect of vanadate on elevated blood glucose and depressed cardiac performance of diabetic rats. *Science* 1985; 227: 1474–7.
19 Venkatesan N, Avidan A, Davidson MB. Antidiabetic action of vanadyl in rats independent of *in vivo* insulin-receptor kinase activity. *Diabetes* 1991; 40: 492–8.
20 Pugazhenthi S, Khandelwal RL. Insulinlike effects of vanadate on hepatic glycogen metabolism in nondiabetic and streptozotocin-induced diabetic rats. *Diabetes* 1990; 39:821–7.
21 Bendayan M, Gingras D. Effect of vanadate administration on blood glucose and insulin levels as well as on the exocrine pancreatic function in streptozotocin-diabetic rats. *Diabetologia* 1989; 32:561–7.
22 Pugazhenthi S, Angel JF, Khandelwal RL. Long-term effects of vanadate treatment on glycogen metabolizing and lipogenic enzymes of liver in genetically diabetic (db/db) mice. *Metabolism* 1991; 40:941–6.
23 Ramanadham S, Brownsey RW, Cros GH, Mongold JJ, McNeill JH. Sustained prevention of myocardial and metabolic abnormalities in diabetic rats following withdrawal from oral vanadyl treatment. *Metabolism* 1989; 38:1022–8.
24 Lohr JW, Bennett MI, Pochal MA, McReynolds J, Acara M, Willsky GR. Effect of vanadate on renal hypertrophy and sorbitol accumulation in streptozotocin induced diabetes in rats. *Res Commun Chem Pathol Pharmacol* 1991; 72:191–202.
25 Nakazawa A, Igarashi K, Tani N, Momotsu T, Ito S, Shibata A. Effect of vanadate on renal function in rats with streptozotocin-induced diabetes. *J Diabet Complications* 1991; 5: 178–80.
26 Saxena AK, Srivastava P, Kale RK, Baquer NZ. Effect of vanadate administration on polyol pathway in diabetic rat kidney. *Biochem Int* 1992; 26: 59–68.
27 Mongold JJ, Cros GH, Vian L *et al.* Toxicological aspects of vanadyl sulphate on diabetic rats: effects on vanadium levels and pancreatic B-cell morphology. *Pharmacol Toxicol* 1990; 67: 192–8.

28 Meyerovitch J, Rothenberg P, Shechter Y, Bonner-Weir S, Kahn CR. Vanadate normalizes hyperglycemia in two mouse models of non-insulin-dependent diabetes mellitus. *J Clin Invest* 1991; 87: 1286–94.
29 Strout HV, Vicario PP, Biswas C *et al.* Vanadate treatment of streptozotocin diabetic rats restores expression of the insulin-responsive glucose transporter in skeletal muscle. *Endocrinology* 1990; 126: 2728–32.
30 Mountjoy KG, Flier JS. Vanadate regulates glucose transporter (Glut-1) expression in NIH3T3 mouse fibroblasts [corrected and republished article originally printed in Endocrinology 1990 Jun; 126(6): 2778–87]. *Endocrinology* 1990; 127: 2025–34.
31 Domingo JL, Gomez M, Llobet JM, Corbella J, Keen CL. Oral vanadium administration to streptozotocin-diabetic rats has marked negative side-effects which are independent of the form of vanadium used. *Toxicology* 1991; 66: 279–87.
32 Domingo JL, Gomez M, Llobet JM, Corbella J, Keen CL. Improvement of glucose homeostasis by oral vanadyl or vanadate treatment in diabetic rats is accompanied by negative side-effects. *Pharmacol Toxicol* 1991; 68: 249–53.
33 Ramanadham S, Heyliger C, Gresser MJ, Tracey AS, McNeill JH. The distribution and half-life for retention of vanadium in the organs of normal and diabetic rats orally fed vanadium (IV) and vanadium (V). *Biol Trace Elem Res* 1991; 30: 119–24.
34 Domingo JL, Sanchez DJ, Gomez M, Llobet JM, Corbella J. Administration of vanadyl sulfate by gavage does not normalize blood glucose levels in streptozotocin-induced diabetic rats. *Res Commun Chem Pathol Pharmacol* 1992; 75: 369–72.
35 Sohda T, Mizuno K, Momose Y, Ikeda H, Fujita T, Meguro K. Studies on antidiabetic agents. II. Novel thiazolidinedione derivatives as potent hypoglycemic and hypolipidemic agents. *J Med Chem* 1992; 10: 2617–26.
36 Hofmann CA, Colca JR. New oral thaizolidinedione antidiabetic agents act as insulin sensitizers. *Diabetes Care* 1992; 15: 1075–8.
37 Colca JR, Dailey CF, Palazuk BJ *et al.* Pioglitazone hydrochloride inhibits cholesterol absorption and lowers plasma cholesterol concentrations in cholesterol-fed rats. Diabetes 1991; 40: 1669–74.
38 Kobayashi M, Iwanishi M, Egawa K, Shigeta Y. Pioglitazone increases insulin sensitivity by activating insulin receptor kinase. *Diabetes* 1992; 41: 476–83.
39 Ikeda H, Taketomi S, Sugiyama *et al.* Effects of pioglitazone on glucose and lipid metabolism in normal and insulin resistant animals. *Arzneimittelforschung* 1990; 40: 156–62.
40 Sutter SL, Nolan JJ, Wallace P, Gumbiner B, Olefsky JM. Metabolic effects of a new oral hypoglycemic agent cs-045 in NIDDM subjects. *Diabetes Care* 1992; 15: 193–203.
41 Kuzuya T, Iwamoto Y, Kosaka K *et al.* A pilot clinical trial of a new oral hypoglycemic agent, CS-045, in patients with non-insulin dependent diabetes mellitus. *Diabetes Res Clin Pract* 1991; 11: 47–53.

# 27 Insulin and Insulin Analogues

R. H. Jones

## BACKGROUND

In•ulin is one of several naturally occurring peptides with shared structural and biological characteristics. Its precursor, pro-insulin and conversion intermediates from pro-insulin to insulin can be detected in the circulation and themselves possess insulin-like activity (1) (Fig. 27.1). The insulin like growth factors IGFI and IGF2, are insulin like both in terms of structural homology (2) (Fig. 27.2) and some biological effects (3). Most, if not all, forms of diabetes mellitus involve a lack of sufficient insulin at the appropriate tissue sites and with the time course required to achieve a required physiological response. In diabetes, one of many therapeutic challenges is to replace the physiological profile of insulin action either by strategies to increase insulin sensitivity by, for example, diet and exercise in NIDDM, or in profound insulin deficiency by replacement of the hormone. Such replacement is not easy to achieve. To be physiological the therapeutic regime must simulate the characteristics of timing and distribution achieved by normal pancreatic function. Fig. 27.3 illustrates the effects of hepatic extraction and of distribution and metabolism on the time course of insulin concentration following ingestion of glucose in dogs (4). Two specific points need to be noted. First the rapidity of the response, with a fourfold increase in concentration in all three vessels within the first 15 minutes and second a fourfold greater concentration in portal venous blood and hence at the surface of hepatocytes than is available to tissues solely perfused by the systemic arterial circulation. Furthermore, this ratio is maintained in the post-absorptive state. For example, after an overnight fast, the liver is continuously perfused with a gently pulsatile profile of insulin at low concentration acting to restrain hepatic glucose output and ketogenesis. Sufficient of the peptide continues to reach peripheral tissues to limit lipolysis in adipocytes and proteolysis in muscle to the low levels required to provide energy requirements for metabolism. Lack of controlled suppression of these processes as occurs in uncontrolled diabetes floods the circulation inappropriately with nutrients.

These considerations serve to establish benchmarks against which available modes of treatment can be assessed. From some perspectives insulin replacement therapy can be regarded as dramatically successful. Bliss in his history of the discovery of insulin describes how to one of the earliest recipients the effect was 'unspeakably wonderful' when compared to her previous state and as an alternative to death by inanition, the

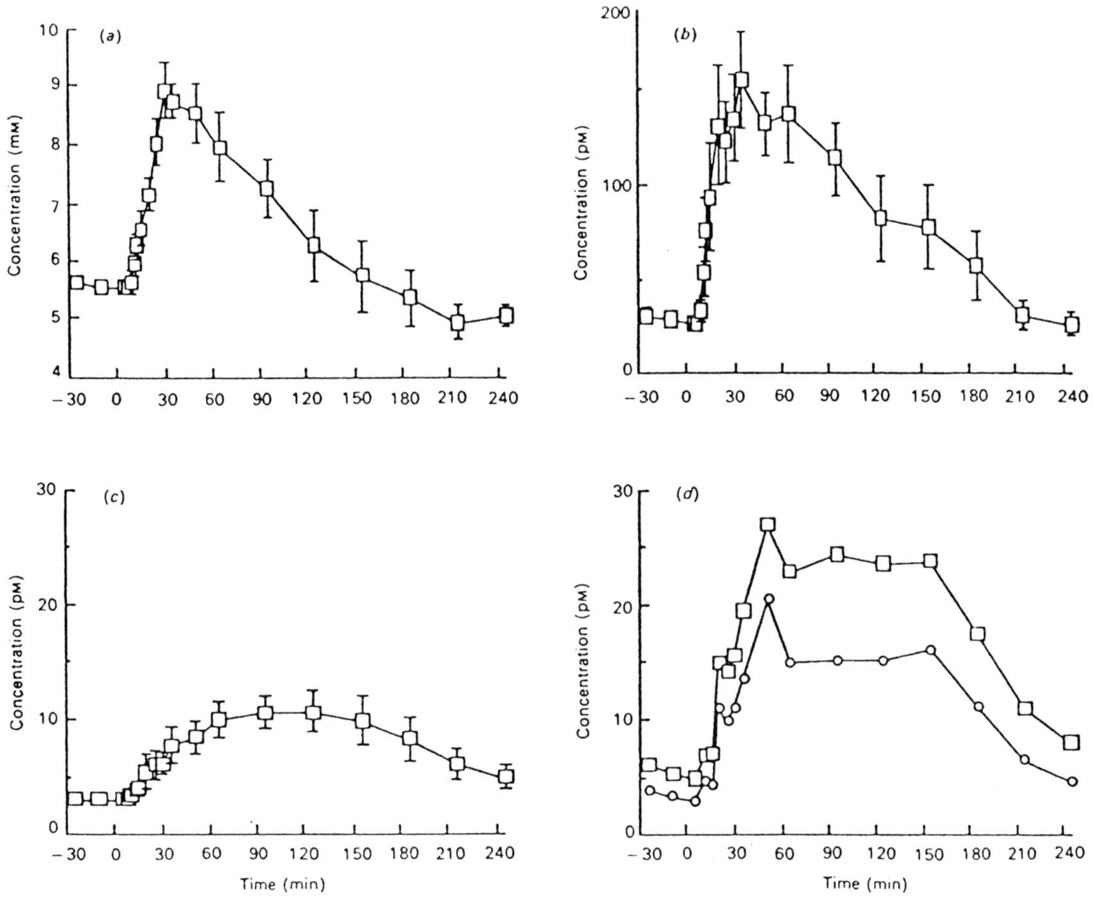


Fig. 27.1. Concentrations of (*a*) blood glucose (*b*) plasma insulin (*c*) plasma intact pro-insulin and (*d*) plasma 32–33 split pro-insulin before and following oral glucose (75 g) in non-diabetic young male subjects. In (*d*) □ represents total hormone assayed and o values corrected for cross-reaction of intact pro-insulin in the assay. From Ref. 1. (By courtesy of *Biochem J.*)

only outcome possible before the initial insulin preparations were available (5). Ever since the introduction of insulin preparations in 1923 therapeutic decisions in the management of IDDM have always been a reflection of the possible, rather than the desirable. Attempts to establish a daily pattern of insulin requirement by a diet rigid in timing and content, with occasional testing of urine or blood for glucose, is a poor replacement for the first phase insulin response to meals and the responsive and continuous glucose sensor of intact pancreatic β cells which determine insulin secretion in health (see Chapter 3).

Considerable effort has been made to devise artificial sensors for glucose in most of which enzymatic interaction with glucose is coupled electrochemically to sensitive meters for voltage or current. When the therapeutic loop can be closed by such a sensor, and its output used to compute rates of intravenous insulin infusion, very tight control of plasma glucose can be achieved. For short-term experimental purposes such an 'artificial pancreas' has been in use for many years (6). Although the technology is improving, and glucose sensors can be made

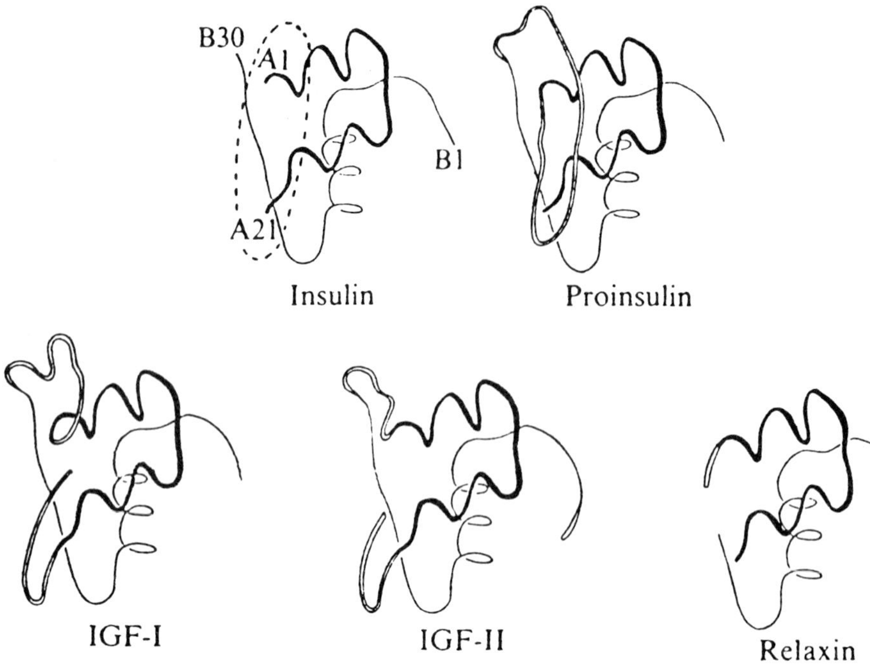


Fig. 27.2. Insulin is but one of a group of structurally related hormones. From Ref. 2. (By courtesy of *Nature*.)

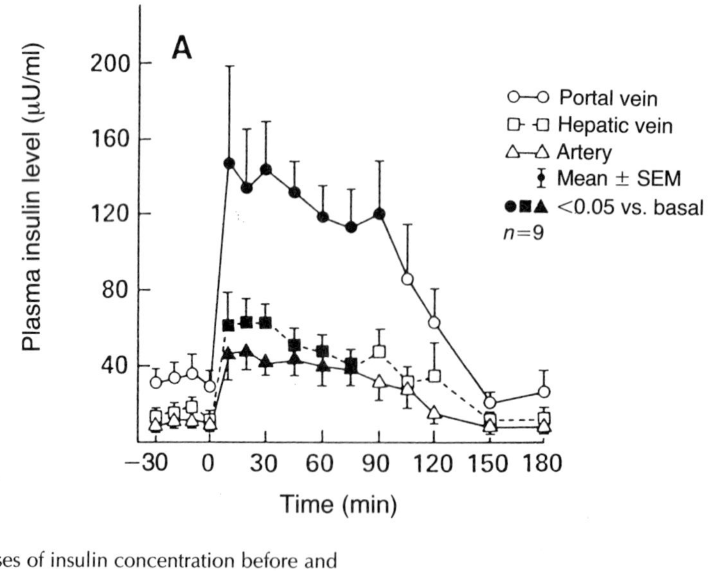


Fig. 27.3. Time courses of insulin concentration before and after oral glucose (1 g per kg body wt) in normal dogs. In the fasting state, and after ingestion, insulin levels reaching the liver via the hepatic portal vein are clearly greater than those reaching peripheral tissues supplied by systemic arteries. From Ref. 4. (Reproduced from *J Clin Invest* 1986; 78: 1355–61 © American Society for Clinical Investigation.)

small enough for subcutaneous implantation (7), anxieties concerning reliability and problems associated with intravenous cannulae are likely to preclude the widespread use of this type of closed loop in portable form for long-term insulin replacement for the foreseeable future.

## CURRENT THERAPY

For the majority of insulin-dependent diabetic individuals, treatment remains considerable dietary constraint and subcutaneous injections of insulin from one to four times every day.

Early perceptions were that available preparations of soluble insulin were too short acting or, more precisely, that they failed to last long enough. In 1936, Hagedorn described the retardation of insulin absorption produced by combining the relatively acid peptide (i.e. negatively charged at physiological pH) with basic proteins from fish sperm, the protamines (8). Modern versions of this neutral protamine Hagedorn (NPH) or isophane preparation are still a mainstay of therapy. As is now well known, retardation of insulin absorption from the subcutaneous depot can also be achieved by the addition of zinc ions which encourage aggregation of insulin into amorphous or crystalline solid phase states which dissolve slowly in subcutaneous tissue (9).

Much of the day-to-day practice of diabetes care concerns application of established knowledge of the pharmacokinetics of soluble, intermediate and long-acting insulins (10), the factors that influence their rates of absorption (10, 11), injection strategies for their use alone or as mixtures and principles of dose adjustment (12). Continuous intravenous or subcutaneous insulin infusion (CSII) from portable battery-driven pumps has reached a high level of sophistication and, in terms of achieving improved glycaemic control, can produce impressive results with adequate skilful supervision and support (13, 14).

This success has led to development of 'basal bolus' regimes in which an injection of soluble insulin before each main meal is combined with a longer-acting insulin for the hours of fasting overnight. Careful exploration of this technique has suggested that, with conventionally spaced meals, a background of continuous insulin infusion or subcutaneous depot is not required except overnight (15) (Fig. 27.4).

## INADEQUACIES OF CURRENT THERAPY

However skilfully planned and administered, currently available insulin preparations and treatment regimes cannot duplicate a normal physiological profile of insulin action.

Hagedorn succeeded in prolonging the action of insulin. Paradoxically, we now perceive even soluble preparations to be insufficiently rapid in onset after injection with an unsatisfactorily prolonged time to peak to duplicate a natural insulin profile. The rapid rise seen normally at the start of a meal cannot be achieved even when the subject remembers to administer the dose, as often instructed, about half an hour before eating. For this and other reasons, current insulin-based therapeutic regimes fail to produce the desired level of metabolic control in many cases, and always impose severe constraints on individual freedom. Further, decisions concerning the insulin regime are made solely on the bases of indices of glycaemia, i.e. self-conducted blood glucose estimates and measurement of glycosylated haemoglobin. No assessment is made of possible maladjustments of other pathways of metabolism. Disturbance of protein turnover and lipid fluxes may be subtle but are likely to contribute to long-term particularly macrovascular complications.

One contributor to this imbalance is the under-insulinisation of the liver inevitable from peripheral subcutaneous insulin administration. It follows that, to maintain euglycaemia, peripheral insulin levels need to be higher than in the non-diabetic state and systemic hyperinsulinaemia is a known associate of atherosclerotic vascular disease (16–18), although whether this

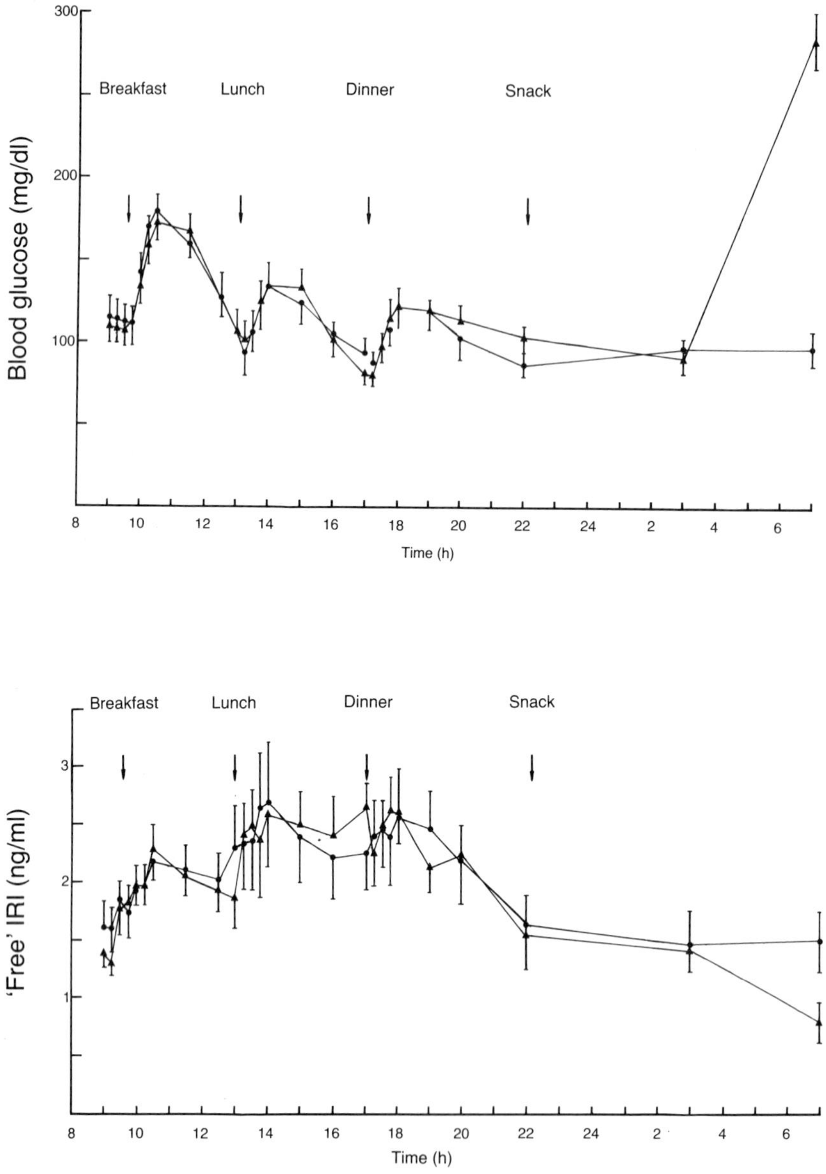


Fig. 27.4. Blood glucose and free plasma insulin concentrations over 22 h (mean values ± SEM, $n$ = 8) in nine lean type 1 diabetic subjects during subcutaneous insulin delivery by boluses alone ▲, or by boluses plus continuous infusion. Only overnight is the infusion ● required to maintain euglycaemia. From Ref 15. (By courtesy of *Lancet.*)

relationship is causal is controversial (19, 20). Possible mechanisms which remain to be explored include differential effects of hyperinsulinaemia on the two insulin receptor isoforms (Chapter 4) and possible long-term results of low grade hyperstimulation by insulin of homologous receptors, e.g. those for IGFI, thereby adding to the possible role of IGFI itself in the pathogenesis of diabetes complications (21).

In summary, control of plasma glucose concentration is maintained in IDDM by insulin regimes which are inappropriate in timing and which result in a relative understimulation of insulin receptors in the liver with inevitably fractional over-exposure of peripheral target cells. These are primarily in skeletal muscle and adipose tissue but include cells in the vascular endothelium in which abnormal metabolic activity could contribute to atherogenesis.

## ALTERNATIVE STRATEGIES

### Routes of administration

#### Intraperitoneal

At present there is no widely applied practical method of delivery of insulin directly into the portal circulation for the majority of patients. The intraperitoneal route is one option with distinct theoretical advantages. Insulin absorption through the peritoneum is more rapid and predictable than after peripheral injection with a time course better matched to physiological needs during a meal. Probably because of difficulty in achieving frequent safe and reliable access, only in end stage renal disease treated by continuous ambulatory peritoneal dialysis (CAPD) is this route in routine use. Such individuals who are clearly far from metabolically normal in view of their renal failure are unlikely to show clearly the potential benefits from the more physiological distribution of insulin which results.

It has been suggested that intraperitoneal insulin may be particularly suitable as a treatment in type II (NIDDM) diabetes in which the hyperglycaemia is predominantly due to hepatic over-production of glucose. Initial encouraging results have been reported in NIDDM with two different types of implantable insulin infusion pumps (22, 23). With these devices, intraperitoneal delivery is associated with fewer adverse mechanical difficulties, i.e. catheter occlusion or displacement than when intravenous placement is chosen. Increasing application of such pumps in both major types of diabetes may prove appropriate if current technical problems can be overcome, and already their use in other than experimental settings can be justified in the few individuals with specific clinical indications. Such situations include massive (usually unexplained) resistance to subcutaneous insulin or severely unstable 'brittle' diabetes (24, 25). It could be argued that such problems often rest with the mind rather than the metabolism and that implanted pumps are effective because they are beyond the reach of interference by the patient. If so, demonstration of their effectiveness and safety in these individuals augurs well for much wider application.

#### Oral

Taking medication by mouth is perceived as more acceptable than injections and could also potentially result in the benefits of preferential hepatic exposure. The technical problems are considerable with the need to protect the peptide from gastric proteolytic digestion an obvious priority. Some success has been achieved by inclusion of insulin in liposomes (26) or within a protective polymer coating which is degraded to release the insulin only on reaching the colon (27). However, there are major and probably insuperable obstacles in translating these technical achievements into viable options for treatment in IDDM. With increasing emphasis on normoglycaemia as a therapeutic goal, it is more and more critical to achieve precision in the delivery of insulin in this disease requiring tight control over its absorption kinetics. The time course is crucial in addition to the overall quantity absorbed. It is hard to foresee that such precision will be achieved by doses of insulin dependent on gastrio-intestinal transit for their transfer to sites of absorption.

It is perhaps more likely that oral insulin preparations could play a part in the treatment of NIDDM conceivably to provide a background suppression of hepatic glucose over-production. Both insulin resistance and β cell exhaustion in this group of patients can be at least partially reversed by normoglycaemia induced by exogenous insulin (28). One suggestion to test would be whether slow release oral insulin could 'rest the pancreas' and thereby restore meal induced endogenous insulin production potentially contributing in a major way to restoration of metabolic normality.

### Intranasal

In IDDM there is a need for a mode of administration which allows insulin levels to increase sufficiently rapidly to simulate the first phase of the normal insulin response to a meal (29) and thereby control postprandial plasma glucose concentrations.

It has been known for over 30 years that the nasal mucosa can absorb insulin. Addition of surface active reagents is required to facilitate the process and to achieve reproducible and predictable results. The time course is similar to the natural insulin response, and when combined with daily subcutaneous injection of a long-acting preparation, intranasal insulins before each main meal can achieve diabetic control for at least 4 months (30). Problems include nasal irritation caused by the surfactants and absorption of a low and somewhat variable proportion of the insufflated dose. Perhaps because of this, and because of small but significant improvements in methods of conventional treatment, intranasal insulin would seem to convey little advantage.

Conventional wisdom is clear; people do not like needles. The problem with this view is that, for most diabetic subjects, the need for injections has moved down the list of disadvantages of having the disease. Indeed, the 'basal bolus' regime using pen-like injector devices has become very popular in spite of the need for four injections per day rather than two. Patients value the increased freedom associated with multiple injection regimes, particularly the freedom to vary timing and energy content of meals. Furthermore, advances in needle technology allow predictably less painful injections. It is likely that, for the foreseeable future, the management of most individuals with IDDM will continue to includes regimes of subcutaneous injection.

## Insulin analogues

### General considerations

There is nothing new about the use of analogues in therapeutics. Indeed most endocrine replacement or treatment regimes use analogues of the natural hormone for a variety of excellent reasons. For example, a wide choice of synthetic steroid molecular structures with glucocorticoid activity is available for deliberate targeted stimulation of glucocorticoid receptors. Within the sphere of peptide hormones, the same is true.

Resistance to degradation has made desamino-8-D'arginine vasopressin (dDAVP) clearly more useful in the treatment of diabetes insipidus than vasopressin itself. Insulin has been used in its natural state because no alternative has been available until recently.

The development of recombinant DNA technology has made possible the commercial production of peptides on a large scale. These methods allow complete freedom to modify the primary amino acid sequence of the molecule at will. The power of this technique to offer therapeutic alternatives is extraordinary. It is already a routine procedure to 'design' specific insulin like molecules with specific aims in mind. The understanding of structure–function relationships of insulin which underpin these design decisions has been meticulously accumulated over the past 40 years by exploration of the properties of specifically chemically modified insulins and insulins of different species (31).

The new technology has limitations. The D-amino acid in dDAVP cannot be inserted by existing intracellular machinery, and chemical synthesis is required. Insulin structures from different species can, of course, all be manufactured biosynthetically and it is understandable, if ironic, that the first product of this technology to achieve wide therapeutic use should be human insulin; ironic because as far as human beings are concerned bovine and porcine insulins are insulin analogues. One of the marketing strategies for human insulin was to imply that finally the genuine article which had being lacking in diabetes treatment had become available. However, almost no real therapeutic advantage was discernible, particularly compared with highly purified porcine insulin which differs in structure from human by only a single amino acid. Human insulin was extensively, even exhaustively, studied in comparison with existing alternatives (32). Adverse publicity arose and continues to rumble on concerning possible links between treatment with human insulin and lack of awareness of hypoglycaemia, a well-recognised, particularly unpleasant and dangerous feature of tightly controlled or brittle diabetes or after many years of treatment in association with autonomic neuropathy. The message for the pharmaceutical industry is clear. Modern insulin treatment regimes are remarkably effective and trusted in spite of theoretical disadvantages. With human insulin, the need to emphasise subtle and questionable advantages in its marketing produced an atmosphere in which subtle and probably non-existent drawbacks could take origin and prosper.

The next generations of insulin analogues will need not only to be validated as safe by established and conscientious techniques of assessment but, in addition, should possess distinct, demonstrable and genuine advantages over currently available preparations.

## Monomeric insulin analogues

In storage form, in non-diabetic subjects, endogenous insulin molecules (monomers) are closely packed into hexamers which are themselves related to each other in crystalline structures within the pancreatic β cell granules (see Chapter 3). After release, these granules rapidly dissociate. At physiological concentrations in plasma, insulin exists predominantly as the monomer, and it is as a monomer that it reaches and binds to its receptor to elicit its action.

Insulin of pancreatic origin co-purifies with its associated zinc and at pharmaceutical concentrations exists in solution almost entirely as hexamers, of molecular weight approximately 36 000 D. This soluble preparation has been, until recently, the most rapidly absorbed available after subcutaneous injection.

Analysis of patterns of absorption of this hexameric insulin from depots under the skin has been examined by two methods. Analysis of the plasma insulin concentration profile against time, and direct assessment of rate of disappearance of radiolabelled insulin from the site of injection, have revealed an unusual pattern. Absorption directly dependent on concentration would be expected to exhibit a single exponential relationship with time, conveniently expressed as half-life or $T_{\frac{1}{2}}$. In the case of subcutaneous insulin, the profile is best described by three exponentials in sequence. The first and slowest has a $T_{\frac{1}{2}}$ of approximately 180 min and dominates the process for the first 2 h after injection. For the next 3 h, absorption is more rapid with a value of $\mathrm{T}_{\frac{1}{2}}$ about 90 min followed by an even more rapid phase $\mathrm{T}_{\frac{1}{2}} \pm 45$ min (33). Although these stages blend into each other, it is now clear that three separate states of insulin aggregation are involved in the generation of this complex time course (Fig. 27.5). At the concentrations used for injection (±0.6 mM), soluble insulin is predominantly associated into hexamers identical in structure to the natural storage state in pancreatic granules. With dilution into interstitial fluid and some

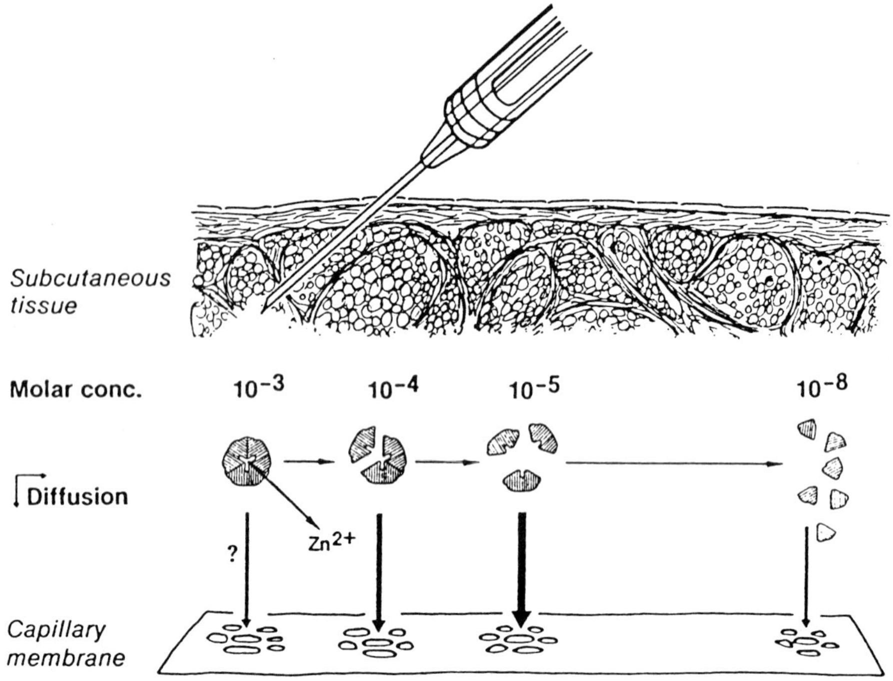


Fig. 27.5. Proposed sequence of events following subcutaneous injection of soluble insulin. Although present at the highest molar concentration, the hexamer makes little contribution to insulin absorption, because of the sieving characteristics of the capillary endothelial membrane. The monomer is rapidly absorbed, but present in such low concentration that most uptake (represented as the thickness of the vertical arrows) takes place as the insulin dimer. From Ref. 33. (By courtesy of *Diabetes Care*.)

removal from the depot through the capillary wall into the circulation, the concentration falls to the point where partial dissociation into three pairs of insulin dimers occurs. These physically smaller structures are capable of more rapid diffusion into the capillary circulation, and the second more rapid absorption phase following injection can be attributed to their absorption. Finally, as concentration falls still further complete dissociation into insulin monomers can occur even at the depot site with, as a result, the third and final rapid phase of uptake. Reference (33) describes the background and quantitation of these ideas and their elegant experimental confirmation by the biosynthetic production and study of specifically designed insulin analogues.

A number of naturally occurring insulins are themselves monomeric in solution even at high concentration. For example, the porcupine and other hystricomorph rodents have insulin amino acid sequences which differ considerably from those of other mammals. Some examples of this unusual group lack the zinc coordinating histidine residue at $B_{10}$ needed for hexamer formation (See Chapter 2), and also differ at other residues important for aggregation of dimers. In porcupine insulin, these residues are conserved, and the lack of association can be attributed to a specific change at the surface of the monomer concerned with dimerisation. In most species, the residue at $B_{22}$ is the basic amino acid arginine. In the dimer at physiological pH, the positively charged guanidium group of $B_{22}$Arg is in close proximity to the negatively charged carboxylate of $A_{21}$Asp. This attraction is one of the forces responsible for stabilisation of the monomer : monomer interface. In the porcupine, the $B_{22}$ position is occupied by aspartic acid bringing two negative charges into close proximity (34).

Others have noted that, although the growth factor IGFI shares sufficient sequence homology with insulin to adopt similar monomeric conformational structure, this member of the hormone group also fails to aggregate (35). In this case, differences in the molecular sequence homologous to the C terminus of the insulin B chain are implicated. In particular, the insulin sequence $B_{28}$Pro $B_{29}$Lys is reversed at the comparable site in the single chain of IGFI. By analogy, reversal of these two residues has been suggested as one of many possible specific sequence changes likely to interfere with aggregation of insulin itself, with the monomeric or dimeric state maintained even at high concentration.

Some of the amino acids involved in these interactions have been shown to be important for biological effect. A complete structural description of the site to site interaction of insulin and its receptors is not yet available but structure–function studies have identified conserved residues either directly involved in that interaction or concerned to maintain appropriate molecular conformation for receptor binding. Substitution of many of the residues associated with insulin dimerisation or hexamerisation also alters receptor binding affinity.

To obtain candidates for a rapidly absorbed insulin useful for treatment of diabetes, pharmaceutical companies have used site-directed mutagenesis to produce experimental quantities of many such insulin analogues potentially for clinical application. Strategies employed have included introduction of charge repulsion or steric hindrance at the aggregation interfaces, generation of hydrophilicity at sites where hydrophobic forces have been important and, as in some hystricomorphs, prevention of hexamerisation by substitution of the zinc binding histidine residue at $B_{10}$.

Some of these many analogues combine high receptor affinity with the intended low capacity for aggregation, and a few have come to clinical trial. It is not yet clear which, if any, of these preparations will achieve approval for therapeutic use. The predicted faster absorption of such analogues from porcine and more recently human subcutaneous depots has been confirmed with values for $T\frac{1}{2}$ related in a linear fashion to aggregation state at physiological pH (Fig. 27.6).

Two factors will make safety a primary concern and may delay availability. The anxieties generated about human insulin serve to

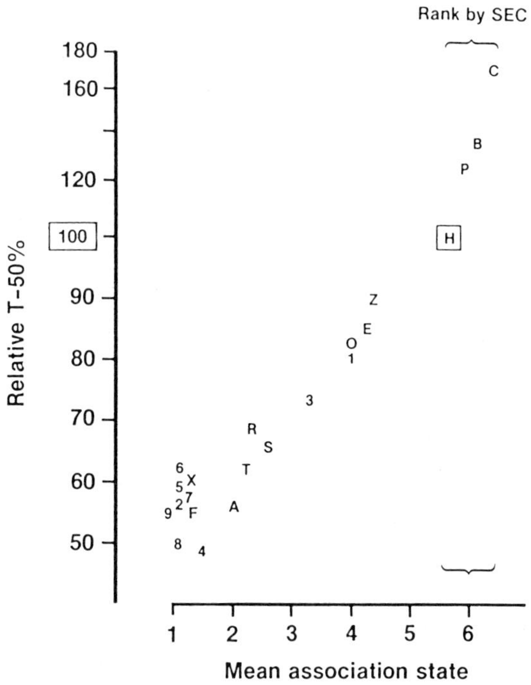


Fig. 27.6. Rates of disappearance from subcutaneous sites of injection in pigs of a wide variety of insulin formulations and insulin analogues each represented by a single numeral or letter, $T_{\frac{1}{2}}$ values are expressed as percentage values of that exhibited by human insulin[H]. Bovine and Porcine 2 $Zn^{2+}$ insulins, B and P, respectively and C a formulation of human insulin with cobalt are all more slowly absorbed. The most striking observation is, however, the linear relationship between increased absorption (reduced $T_{\frac{1}{2}}$) and mean association state at 1 mM of the insulin analogues. (For details see Ref. 33. (By courtesy of *Diabetes Care*.)

emphasise the confidence and respect held by patients and their advisers for existing regimes. A second and more substantive concern will be the need to eliminate the possibility of mitogenic effects. The $B_{28}$ Lys, $B_{29}$ Pro analogue displays no greater affinity for IGFI receptors than native insulin. However, one other mainly dimeric formulation $B_{10}$ Asp insulin has been abandoned as a therapeutic candidate because of the possibility of carcinogenesis. This analogue displays a threefold higher affinity for insulin and IGFI receptors than insulin itself, but the mitogenic activity in various cell types has been reported to be 10–20 times that of human insulin. In a study in rats, an apparently dose-dependent induction of benign and malignant mammary tumours has been observed. It has been suggested that the supraphysiological insulin receptor binding affinity exhibited by $B_{10}$Asp insulin is itself responsible or the carcinogenicity may derive from activity at other unknown cellular sites.

The generation and exploration of new insulin analogues with a range of receptor binding affinities have served to confirm one aspect of insulin physiology previously observed with chemically modified insulins (36). The insulin receptor is responsible for most insulin clearance from the circulation in addition to the initiation of an insulin like effect. High affinity analogues are more actively metabolised and therefore achieve lower concentrations in plasma than low affinity analogues given in the same dose (37, 38). The buffering effect of this phenomenon on insulin action is clearly shown in Fig. 27.7. The graphs illustrate the differences from human insulin of three insulin analogues given subcutaneously in equimolar doses. All three are more rapidly absorbed than human insulin as predicted from their reduced association states (top panels). All three reduce plasma glucose more rapidly than insulin itself and to a similar degree (lower panels). The central panels reveal the major difference between them. Asp $B_9$Gly $B_{22}$ insulin has a low receptor affinity, reduced clearance as a result and reaches high plasma immunoreactive levels (left). Asp $B_{10}$ (right panel) achieves only low plasma concentrations as expected from its high receptor binding affinity, which results in increased rates of receptor mediated removal. With Asp $B_{28}$ insulin, an analogue with similar *in vitro* characteristics to insulin, the immunoreactive levels are themselves similar in magnitude, albeit more rapidly achieved than those after insulin itself.

In summary, monomeric insulin has the potential to be synthesised commercially in quantities which could be widely available for therapeutic use. Clinical trial evidence suggests that absorption characteristics will render one or more of these analogues suitable for use as the preprandial subcutaneous preparation in insulin-treated diabetes. Reduction in postprandial glucose excursions would allow more individuals with IDDM to approach or achieve normal levels of glycosylated haemoglobin without the counterbalancing effect of low troughs of glycaemia before meals. A reduced risk of hypoglycaemia and of lack of hypoglycaemic awareness could well be an advantage of these analogues additional to their contribution to the improved overall glycaemic control. This latter is increasingly perceived to be important in the prevention of long-term diabetes complications.

## Long-acting insulin analogues

Even with conventional soluble insulin to control postprandial glycaemia, regimes of subcutaneous insulin are dependent on a longer-acting component to maintain basal insulin metabolic tone between meals and overnight. If more rapidly acting analogues supplant soluble insulin, the role of the long-acting formulations will become more, rather than less, important. The preparations in current use, isophane and insulin zinc suspension, share one major drawback, a high degree of variability in the time course of absorption, even within one individual. These preparations are 'cloudy' because their retardation depends on their remaining undissolved, i.e. in the solid state within the injected medium. Absorption is dependent on dissolution not of

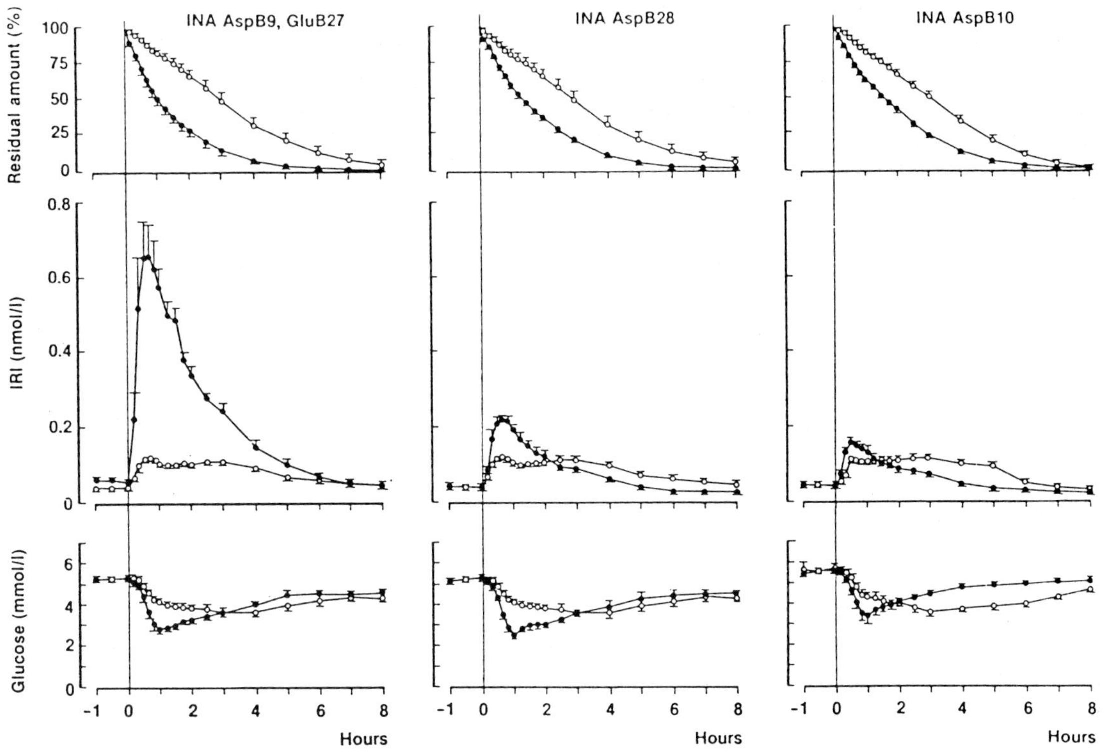


Fig. 27.7. Mean ± SE residual radioactivity at injection site and plasma immunoreactive insulin (IRI), insulin analogue (INA), and glucose concentrations after subcutaneous injection of 0.6 nmol/kg of soluble human insulin (O) or insulin analogue (●) into healthy subjects ($n$ = 7). From Ref 33. (By courtesy of *Diabetes Care*.)

soluble hexamers into smaller subunits but, even before that, of solution of crystals of variable sizes into soluble form. Variance in the effective time courses can be introduced by the impossibility of complete standardisation of crystal size between batches, and by lack of uniform mixing by the user before injection.

A need therefore exists for long-acting insulins with more tightly predictable characteristics of absorption than can be achieved by existing methods of manufacture. Several approaches are theoretically possible including delayed absorption from the injection site and retention in the circulation, for example, by binding proteins or reduction in rates of diffusion from the capillaries to tissue receptor sites. Reduced rates of metabolism can prolong pharmacological effects of active drugs of many types. For this to be successful, separation of the pathways of degradation and biological effect is important. As insulin receptors are the recognition site for pathways both of action and metabolism of the hormone there are profound theoretical difficulties in this approach for the treatment of diabetes.

Considerable progress has been made in the other proposal, namely the exploitation of properties of subcutaneous tissue to delay absorption. The principle employed is simple. In aqueous media, insulin like other peptides will precipitate and/or crystallise at its pK or isoelectric point, the pH at which the net change on the molecule is zero. Addition of positive charges to native insulin shifts the isoelectric point from 5.4 to more physiological values (Fig. 27.8). After a detailed study of the phenomenon

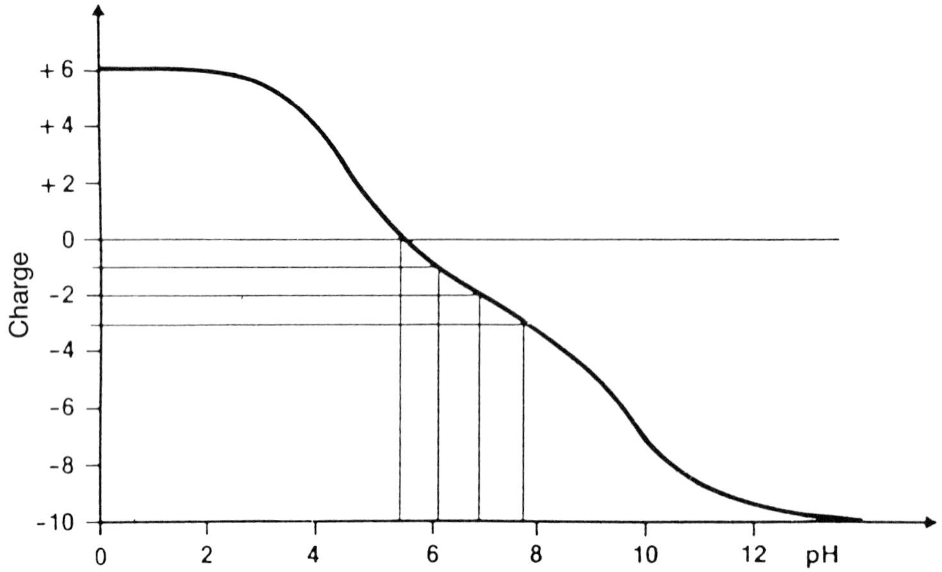


Fig. 27.8. The net molecular charge of insulin in solution as a function of pH. The isoelectric point of 5.4 is shifted to 6.2, 6.8 and 7.7 by addition of 1, 2 and 3 positive charges, respectively, to the insulin molecule. From Ref. 39. (By courtesy of Oxford University Press.)

as exhibited by chemically modified insulins (39) and analogues biosynthetically prepared (40), one specific material has been selected for potential clinical use (41). Substitution of the neutral $B_{27}$ amino acid threonine by arginine and amidation of the C terminal of the β chain have added two positive charges and increased the pK from 5.4 to 6.8. To render the molecule stable in acid solution, the asparagine at $A_{21}$ has been replaced by glycine. This analogue is soluble when buffered to pH3, but crystallises after injection as the pH increases through the isoelectric point to about 7.4. These subcutaneous crystals, remarkably uniform in size and shape, are less than 5 μm in diameter. When injected subcutaneously to diabetic subjects, the time course of absorption is much more constant in rate over many hours and subject to much greater reproducibility than the best available comparable insulin zinc suspension (Fig. 27.9). The predictability is impressive but the first-order kinetics, with a $T_{\frac{1}{2}}$ of 35 hours, is perhaps longer than ideal for most clinical applications. This elegant work has, however, clearly established the principles involved, and further examples of soluble formulations of analogues which adopt the solid state after injection are likely to offer a range of durations of action suitable for therapeutic use.

## Future possibilities

Within the foreseeable future, widespread clinical use of insulin analogues will become a reality and possibly the norm. It is unlikely that the full range of possibility has yet been addressed. Proinsulin has been shown to exhibit a relatively greater effect on hepatic glucose output than on peripheral glucose disposal although the mechanism is obscure. Human pro-insulin has been prepared and actively considered for clinical use, but abandoned after an increased frequency of acute myocardial infarction was observed in one multicentre study (42).

Other, chemically modified insulins have been observed to be relatively hepatoselective, and it seems likely that safe preparations will become available which exhibit this property. Selective

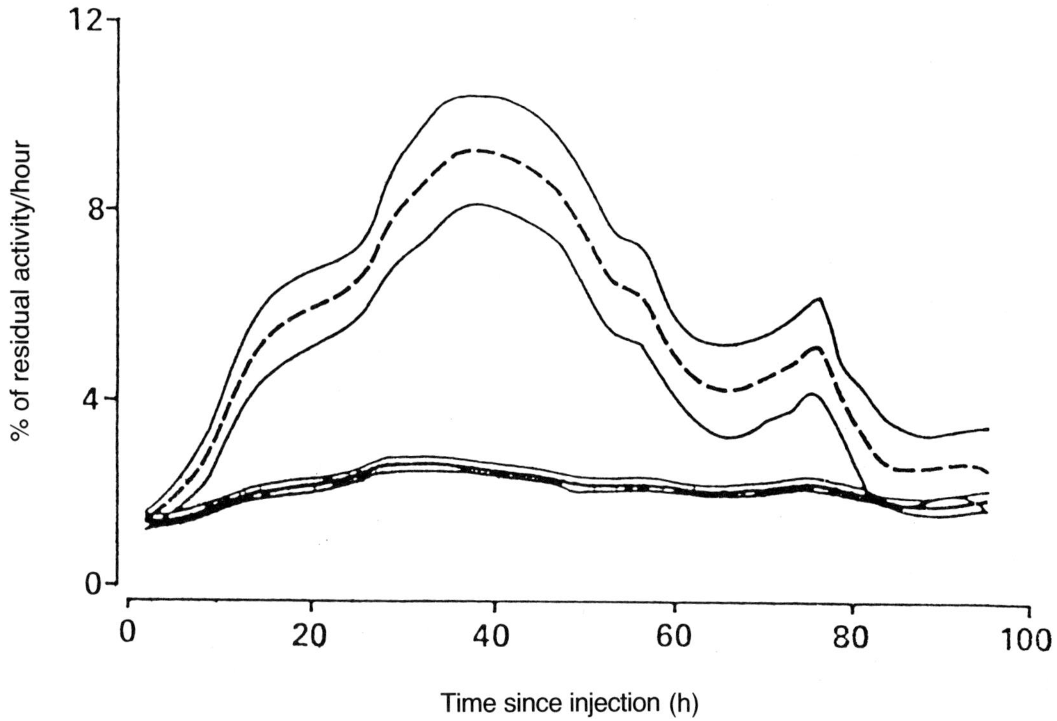


Fig 27.9. Mean ± SE rate of absorption of Gly $A_{21}$, Ang $B_{27}$, Thr $B_{30}$ – $NH_2$ human insulin (-------) with the insulin zinc suspension Ultratard HM (- - - - - -). Four injections of each preparation were injected into seven type I diabetic subjects. Two striking differences are apparent. The rate of absorption of the analogue remains proportional to the residual activity throughout the time course and variance is considerably smaller than seen with the currently available preparation. From Ref. 41. (By courtesy of *Br Med J.*)

suppression of hepatic glucose production as a means of achieving post-absorptive euglycaemia offers more advantages than the simple fact that it more closely resembles normal physiology. Reduced stimulation of peripheral metabolic pathways may result in less atherogenicity of insulin therapy. Finally, it is possible that iatrogenic hypoglycaemia induced by slight over-suppression of hepatic glucogenesis may be more easily corrected by counter-regulatory mechanisms if peripheral glucose uptake is not simultaneously stimulated. To suggest the possibility of insulin analogues which correct hyperglycaemia without risk of hypoglycaemia may stretch credibility at present, but should not be discounted for the future.

## REFERENCES

1 Sobey K, Beer SF, Carrington CA *et al.* Sensitive and specific two site immunoradiometric assays for human insulin, pro-insulin, 65–66 split and 32–33 split pro-insulins. *Biochem J* 1989; 260: 535–41.
2 Blundell TL, Humbel RE. Hormone families: pancreatic hormones and homologous growth factors. *Nature* (*Lond*) 980; 287: 781–7.
3 Zapf J, Hauri C, Waldvogel M, Froesch ER. Acute metabolic effects and half-lives of intravenously administered insulinlike growth factors I and II in normal and hypophysectomized rats. *J Clin Invest* 1986; 77: 1768–75.
4 Chap Z, Jones RH, Chou J *et al.* Effect of Dexamethasone on hepatic glucose and insulin metabolism after oral glucose in conscious dogs. *J Clin Invest* 1986; 78: 1355–61.
5 Bliss M. *The discovery of insulin.* University of Chicago Press, 1982.
6 Albisser AM, Leibel BS, Ewart TG *et al.* Clinical control of diabetes by the artificial pancreas. *Diabetes* 1974; 23: 397–404.

7 Claremont DJ, Sambrook IE, Penton C. *et al.* Subcutaneous implantation of a ferrocene-mediated glucose sensor in pigs. *Diabetologia* 1986; 29: 817–21.
8 Hagedorn HC, Jensen BN, Krarup NB *et al.* Protamine insulinate. *JAMA* 1936; 106: 177–80.
9 Chadwick T. Insulin manufacture and formulation. Pickup JC, Williams G. eds. *Textbook of diabetes.* Blackwell Scientific Publications, Oxford, 1991; 1; 357–70.
10 Binder C, Lauritzen T, Faber O, *et al.* Insulin pharmacokinetics. *Diabetes Care* 1984 7(2) 188
11 Furler SM, Kraegen EW. Quantitative aspects of subcutaneous insulin absorption. *Diabetic med* 1989; **6**: 657–65.
12 Tattersall RB. Insulin treatment. In: Besser GM, Bodansky HJ, eds. *Clinical diabetes;* Gower Medical Publishing, USA, 1988: 14.1–12.
13 Irsigler K, Kritz H. Long term continuous intravenous insulin therapy with a portable insulin dosage-regulating apparatus. *Diabetes* 1979; 28: 196–203.
14 Pickup JC, White MC, Keen H *et al.* Long-term continuous insulin infusion in diabetics at home. *Lancet* 1979; ii: 870–3.
15 Nelson JD, Marliss EB, Albisser AM *et al.* Role of continuous component in subcutaenous 'open-loop' insulin delivery. *Lancet* 1980; 1383–6.
16 Stout RW. Diabetes and atherosclerosis – the role of insulin. *Diabetologia* 1979; 16: 141–50.
17 DeFronzo RA, Ferrannini E. Insulin resistance. A multifaceted syndrome responsible for NIDDM, obesity, hypertension, dyslipidemia and atherosclerotic cardiovascular disease. *Diabetes Care* 1991; 14: (3) 175.
18 Flack JM, Sowers JR. Epidemiologic and clinical aspects of insulin resistance and hyperinsulinemia. *Am J Med* 1991; 91: (Suppl 1A): 11S–21S.
19 Sowers JR. Insulin resistance, hyperinsulinemia, dyslipidemia, hypertension, and accelerated atherosclerosis. *J Clin Pharmacol* 1991; 32: 529–35.
20 Jarrett RJ. In defence of insulin: a critique of syndrome X. *Lancet* 1992; 340: 469–71.
21 Flyvbjerg A. Growth factors and diabetic complications. *Diabetic Med* 1990; 7: 387–399.
22 Rupp WM, Barbosa JJ, Blackshear PJ *et al.* The use of an implantable insulin pump in the treatment of type II diabetes. *N Engl J Med* 1982; 307 (5): 265–70.
23 Duckworth WC, Saudek CD, Henry RR. Why intraperitoneal delivery of insulin with implantable pumps in NIDDM? *Diabetes* 1992; 41: 657–61.
24 Wood DF, Goodchild K, Guillou P *et al.* Management of 'brittle' diabetes with a preprogrammable implanted insulin pump delivering intraperitoneal insulin. *Br Med J* 1990; 301: 1143–4.
25 Paterson KR, Campbell IW, MacRury SM *et al.* Management of diabetes resistant to subcutaneous insulin with intravenous insulin via an implanted infusion pump. *Scot Med J* 1988; 33: 239–43.
26 Patel HM, Ryman BE. Oral administration of insulin by encapsulation within liposomes. *FEBS Lett* 1976; 62: 60–3.
27 Saffran M, Field JB, Peña J *et al.* Oral insulin in diabetic dogs. *J Endocrinol* 1991; 131: 267–78.
28 Garvey WT, Olefsky JM, Griffin J *et al.* The effect of insulin treatment on insulin secretion and insulin action in type II diabetes mellitus. *Diabetes* 1985; 34: 222–34.
29 Eaton RP, Allen RC, Schade DS *et al.* 'Normal' insulin secretion: the goal of artificial insulin delivery systems? *Diabetes Care* 1980; 3: 270–3.
30 Fraumann AG, Cooper ME, Parsons BJ *et al.* Long-term use of intranasal insulin in insulin-dependent diabetic patients. *Diabetes Care* 1987; 10: 573–83.
31 Gammeltoft S. Insulin receptors; binding kinetics and structure–function relationship of insulin. *Physiol Rev* 1984; 64: 1321–78.
32 Skyler JS, ed. Human insulin of recombinant DNA origin. *Diabetes Care* 1982; 5: Suppl.2: 1–186.
33 Brange J, Owens DR, Kang S *et al.* Monomeric insulins and their experimental and clinical implications. *Diabetes Care* 1990; 13: 923–4.
34 Horuk R, Blundell TL, Lazarus NR *et al.* A monomeric insulin from the porcupine (*Hystrix cristata*), an Old World hystricomorph. *Nature (Lond)*, 1980; 286: 822–4.
35 Blundell TL, Bedarkar S, Rindernecht E *et al.* Insulin-like growth factor: A model for tertiary structure accounting for immunoreactivity and receptor binding. *Biochemistry* 1978; 75(1): 180–4.
36 Jones RH, Dron DI, Ellis MJ *et al.* Biological properties of chemically modified insulins. I. Biological acitivity of pro-insulin and insulin modified at A-glycine and $B_{29}$-lysine. *Diabetologia* 1976; 12: 601–8.
37 Ribel U, Hougaard P, Drejer K, Sørensen AR. Equivalent *in vivo* biological activity of insulin analogues and human insulin despite different *in vitro* potencies. *Diabetes* 1990; 39: 1033–9.
38 Vølund Aa. Brange K, Drejer I *et al. In vitro* and *in vivo* potency of insulin analogues designed for clinical use. *Diabetic Med* 1991; 8: 839–7.
39 Markussen J, Hougaard P, Ribel U *et al.* Soluble, prolonged-acting insulin derivatives. I. Degree of protraction and crystallizability of insulins substituted in termini of the β-chain. *Protein Eng* 1987; **1** (3): 205–13.
40 Markussen J, Diers I, Engeshaard A *et al.* Soluble, prolonged-acting insulin derivatives. II. Degree of protraction and crystallizability of insulins substituted in positions A17, B8, B13, B27 and B30. *Protein Eng* 1987; 1 (3): 215–23.
41 Jørgensen S Vaag A, Langkjaer L *et al.* NovoSol Basal: pharmacokinetics of a novel soluble long acting insulin analogue. *Br Med J* 1989; 299: 415–20.
42 Galloway JA, Hooper SA, Spradlin CT *et al.* Biosynthetic human pro-insulin: review of chemistry, *in vitro* and *in vivo* receptor binding animal and human pharmacology studies, and clinical trial experience. *Diabetes Care* 1992; 15: 5; 666–92.

# 28 Hypoglycaemia

Iain C. P. Cranston & Stephanie A. Amiel

## INTRODUCTION

In diabetes mellitus, a disease state characterised by high blood glucose concentrations, it may seem paradoxical that the most feared and frequent acute complication is the exact opposite. However, hypoglycaemia, literally low blood glucose, becomes a risk as soon as treatment beyond dietary modification and exercise is introduced. Indeed, since the advent of insulin therapy, particularly with recent trends for attempting chronic 'normalisation' of blood glucose in people with diabetes, hypoglycaemia has become a fact of life for many patients. For some young patients with diabetes, iatrogenically induced hypoglycaemia imposes more limitations on life-style than the disease itself and older patients on sulphonylurea therapy may also suffer major disruption. The problem lies in the fact that glucose is the almost exclusive metabolic fuel for the brain. Since the brain can neither synthesise nor store the sugar (1), the maintenance of at least a minimum glucose concentration in the blood is critical to continued normal cerebral function. If blood glucose falls too low, irritability, confusion and even coma can result.

Defining hypoglycaemia is surprisingly difficult. A biochemical definition seems simplest but even this is complicated by differences in the samples used (2). Plasma glucose values are approximately 10% higher than whole blood glucose; arterial and capillary samples may be higher than venous samples, any biochemical description of glucose concentration must therefore state the source and nature of the sample. Clinically, it is often useful to define hypoglycaemia as a blood glucose concentration low enough to provoke a response or alteration of a glucose dependent function – a definition not so far from that attributed to Whipple (3) in 1944 when hypoglycaemia was defined by:

(*a*) symptoms or signs attributable to lack of glucose
(*b*) low measured blood glucose (by tradition <2.5 mmol/l)
(*c*) resolution of symptoms/ signs on administration of exogenous glucose.

The biochemical definition, i.e. the level at which this occurs, needs further elucidation.

In health, blood glucose concentration is maintained within very narrow limits by a combination of neurological, humoral and metabolic influences which are able to balance the rate at which glucose enters the circulation and the rate at which it leaves. This implies control at several levels over processes which can vary widely in their rates. These controls are so effective that a fall in blood glucose low enough to produce symptomatic or dysfunctional responses occurs only in the most extreme physiological situations (e.g. prolonged fast or very vigorous exercise (4–7)). Low blood glucose is extremely rare in health.

One major component of glucoregulation is the ability of the healthy pancreas to reduce insulin output as glucose levels fall (8). In diabetes, the administration of exogenous hypoglycaemic agents (sulphonylureas or insulin) unbalances this normally robust protective mechanism and relative hyperinsulinaemia may drive blood glucose down towards a level below that which is necessary for normal cerebral function. This should, and does, stimulate a neurohumoral counterregulatory response (9), with two important results; first, stimulation of glycogenolysis and gluconeogenesis (10, 11), which, together with restriction of peripheral glucose utilisation spontaneously increase blood glucose levels back towards normal, and secondly, a symptom complex is produced which the individual can recognise and respond to, by eating. Components of this part of the counterregulatory response include pancreatic glucagon, adrenaline, noradrenaline and the sympathetic nervous system, cortisol and growth hormone; the complexity of the response being a testament to the importance of maintaining adequate blood glucose concentrations.

Once the system has been overcome by excessive hyperinsulinaemia, as can occur with administration of exogenous insulin or sulphonylureas, a hypoglycaemic reaction occurs (previously 'insulin reaction', colloquially a 'hypo'). The experience of a hypo (12, 13) is one not easily described and the symptoms may be Protean. A mild episode may be felt as tingling, sweatiness, extreme hunger, palpitations, mental slowness, visual blurring, tiredness or headache (see Table 28.1). These classic symptoms may not be apparent and their recognition may depend on the circumstances in which they occur. Unusually, for some patients a hypo may present as a sudden collapse 'without warning'. To the observer, the first signs of lower than normal glucose levels may be of unusual or irrational behaviour, irritability or anger, mental slowness or vagueness. There may be few other outward signs, although more usually subjects will show evidence of adrenergic counterregulation, such as profuse sweating, pallor, agitation, and tremor. If hypoglycaemia persists, the patient may lose consciousness or suffer convulsions.

Table 28.1. *Symptoms of hypoglycaemia*

| Autonomic | Neuroglycopenic | Non-specific |
|---|---|---|
| Sweating | Double vision | Nausea |
| Tremor | Tiredness | Headache |
| Warmness | Confusion | Tearfulness |
| Pounding heart | Drowsiness | Perioral tingling |
| Shivering | Weakness | Hunger |
| Blurred vision | Dizziness | |
| Anxiety | Difficulty speaking | |
| | Inability to concentrate | |

Adapted from Ref. 73.

## THE AETIOLOGY OF HYPOGLYCAEMIA IN INSULIN-DEPENDENT DIABETES

In IDDM, individual episodes of hypoglycaemia result from a mismatch between insulin dose, carbohydrate ingestion and physical activity (14, 15). Given the pressures of modern life and the limitations of present insulin delivery systems, the occurrence of hypoglycaemia is perhaps not surprising. Studies show that up to 75% of episodes can be 'explained' on the basis of a delayed or inadequate snack (15), unexpected or inadequately compensated exercise or an 'error' in insulin dosage or timing. These factors deserve closer scrutiny.

### Exogenous insulin

It must be recognised that exogenous insulins are not the perfect replacement for normal pancreatic insulin secretion. Quite apart from problems related to delivery of insulin into the peripheral rather than the portal circulation (16), sub-cutaneously delivered soluble insulin has a duration of action considerably longer than the meal-related bursts of hyperinsulinaemia produced by the healthy pancreas (17). Adequate meal-time glycaemic control in an insulin dependent diabetic patient results in post-prandial hyperinsulinaemia. If this is not accompanied by additional carbohydrate intake (the between meals and bedtime snacks), hypoglycaemia will ensue. The absorption profiles of the 'medium acting' insulin suspensions produce a peak 6–8 hours after injection (18), which creates a risk of hypoglycaemia at lunch-time from a morning injection or during the night if sufficient insulin is to be available from an evening injection by the time the patient awakes the following morning. Despite the confidence of published predictions, absorption of subcutaneous insulin has a variability of 25–50% even for the same insulin in the same patient at the same site (19). Massage, exercise, injection technique and inadvertent intramuscular injection can all speed insulin absorption as the blood flow around the injection site is increased or the polymers in the insulin preparation are broken down (20–22). Finally, long-acting insulins can produce problems with hypoglycaemia because of their cumulative effects (beware the mid afternoon hypo in patients using long-acting insulins in the evening). In patients with insulin antibodies, immune complexes may act as an insulin reservoir, further prolonging hypoglycaemic effects (23).

### Exercise

Most people connect vigorous exercise with increased tissue consumption of glucose and anticipate hypoglycaemia during and immediately after a game of football or squash. They quickly learn to take additional carbohydrate before and during such activities and/or reduce insulin doses for the meal before. The sub-acute effects of exercise are less commonly understood, but the hypoglycaemic effect of vigorous exercise lasts 12 or even 24 hours (24, 25), and hypoglycaemia in the night (or even the following day) after strenuous physical activity is not uncommon. Reducing the overnight and background insulins after a day including vigorous exercise is a useful precaution, and essential in the well-controlled diabetic patient.

### Alcohol

Hypoglycaemia associated with alcohol excess is not unknown in the non-diabetic population (26). The suppressive effect of alcohol on gluconeogenesis (27) puts diabetic patients at particular risk for delayed hypoglycaemia – drinking in the evening may result in fasting hypoglycaemia (which must not be mistaken for drunken stupor!) the next day, as the liver switches to gluconeogenesis to maintain glucose levels. Quite moderate alcohol intake can have pharmacological effect. Recent work has highlighted another, more acute, problem – that alcohol impairs both the generation and recognition of early warning symptoms of hypoglycaemia (26, 28), putting patients at risk of more severe hypoglycaemia with neuroglycopenia as they fail to notice or respond to the onset of the problem.

## PHYSIOLOGY OF THE HYPOGLYCAEMIC RESPONSE

The brain is uniquely dependent upon circulating glucose levels to maintain its metabolism. It can neither synthesise glucose nor store more than a few minutes' supply (1) and although there is some evidence to suggest that alternative cerebral fuels (such as ketones and lactate) can be used (29–31), in normal life this does not occur to any major degree. In health, glucose supplies to the brain are threatened by reduced glucose availability as in fasting, or during accelerated peripheral glucose utilisation as in exercise. The balance is maintained by increasing glucose release from endogenous stores (primarily hepatic glycogen) and increasing synthesis of new glucose (hepatic gluconeogenesis), as well as by limiting peripheral glucose utilisation rates. Hepatic glucose production is limited by insulin (32) and stimulated by glucagon (33), both secreted directly into the portal system and its rate is controlled by a balance between the two, on which are superimposed other, primarily stimulatory, influences. Much of our understanding of the mechanisms of counterregulation has come from studies in which blood glucose is driven down artificially, usually by administration of exogenous insulin or more rarely by studies of healthy individuals undergoing prolonged fasts (34) or undertaking vigorous exercise. These studies have led to the description of a series of neurohumoral responses to a fall in blood glucose. During the initial phase of hypoglycaemic glucose counterregulation, it is hepatic glycogenolysis (35, 36) which is the main source for increased endogenous glucose production, whereas later in the response (11, 37) gluconeogenesis is recruited (hence the delayed dangers of alcohol). A reduction in endogenous insulin secretion, derepressing hepatic glucose output, and an increase in glucagon, stimulating glycogenolysis, are the primary counterregulatory humoral responses. Adrenaline, which in the absence of glucagon appears to be the most important humoral factor (38, 39), acts via beta 2 adrenergic receptors to stimulate hepatic glycogenolysis and gluconeogenesis (40); adrenaline mobilises gluconeogenic substrates from the peripheries and limits peripheral glucose utilisation (41). In addition to this, its alpha 2 actions limit insulin secretion (42). As a result of studies of acute hypoglycaemia induced by insulin injection, growth hormone and cortisol have been assigned a secondary role in counterregulation (43), predominantly related to more prolonged hypoglycaemia (44). This view has been supported by experimental observation during clamp studies, where blood glucose fall during insulin infusion is controlled by administration of exogenous glucose and the release of growth hormone and cortisol is delayed in comparison to that of glucagon and adrenaline (45, 46). Nevertheless, growth hormone and cortisol are necessary as a background and may have a substantial role in more prolonged hypoglycaemia (47). Growth hormone stimulates lipolysis and ketogenesis (48), providing gluconeogenic precursors to support hepatic glucose production, in addition, inhibits glucose oxidation. Cortisol further inhibits glucose utilisation and provides gluconeogenic precursors to the liver (49).

There is evidence for a mechanism of glucose auto-regulation independent of humoral factors, by which hepatic glucose production is found to be inversely proportional to plasma glucose concentrations (50). During low-dose insulin infusion the initial fall in blood glucose is checked despite continued hyperinsulinaemia and in the absence of any change in counterregulatory hormone levels. The higher the dose of insulin, the lower the level of the glucose plateau (51). Whilst this response is clearly protective, its mechanism and importance in the clinical setting of hypoglycaemia in diabetes remains unclear. Similarly, the role of the recently described insulin antagonist pancreatic peptide amylin, which is co-secreted with insulin rather than in response to hypoglycaemia, is not yet known (52).

In addition to their effects on glucose homeostasis, the neurohumoral responses of counterregulation contribute to another protective phenomenon. Autonomic and adrenergic stimulation during hypoglycaemia result in an increased heart rate, a rise in systolic blood pressure, a fall in diastolic blood pressure, increased left ventricular ejection fraction and therefore increased cardiac output (53, 54). These effects (which can be blocked by selective alpha or beta blockade) result in increased cerebral blood flow (55) and therefore increased nutrient supply to the brain during hypoglycaemia. There is also evidence that hypoglycaemia has effects on cerebral autoregulation, independent of the central adrenergic actions, which result in regional increases of cerebral blood flow to those areas most susceptible to hypoglycaemic damage (brainstem and thalamic areas in particular)(56).

## DEFECTIVE COUNTERREGULATORY HORMONE RESPONSES IN SUBJECTS WITH INSULIN-DEPENDENT DIABETES MELLITUS

### Persistent insulin effect

In insulin-treated diabetic patients the hypoglycaemic stimulus is exogenously administered insulin. In contrast to endogenous insulin secretion, this is not responsive to the ambient blood glucose but determined by the size, timing and pharmacokinetics of the previous insulin dose. An important part of the counterregulatory response (the reduction of insulin secretion) is thus disabled. In diabetes, well controlled by intensified insulin therapy, control of endogenous glucose production is maintained at the expense of a high peripheral : portal insulin ratio and relative peripheral hyperinsulinaemia (57). It has been suggested that this hyperinsulinaemia may contribute to both the long-term complications of diabetes and also that it may play a role in the defective counterregulation (58) seen in insulin treated diabetic patients. The 'persistent insulin effect' is more marked with the longer-acting insulin preparations, or when the duration of the insulin effect is prolonged as in the presence of circulating insulin antibodies (23). Hypothyroidism (including over-treated hyperthyroidism), renal failure or liver disease also delay insulin clearance, making hypoglycaemia more of a risk.

### Defects in counterregulatory hormone responses

Patients with insulin-dependent diabetes mellitus lose the ability to secrete glucagon in response to hypoglycaemia (59). Some studies have demonstrated a loss of glucagon responses in newly diagnosed patients (60, 61) but this phenomenon may be transient. A more established defect is seen in patients with a diabetes duration of 5 years or more, in whom full glucagon responses to insulin-induced hypoglycaemia are not seen (62). This does not seem to be recoverable. In the absence of a glucagon response, adrenaline and the sympathetic nervous system assume a critical role in recovery from hypoglycaemia. However, patients with IDDM may also develop defects in these components of the response (62).

Impaired adrenaline responses to hypoglycaemia have been documented in patients with long duration of disease. Adrenaline responses to hypoglycaemia are also reduced in patients with autonomic neuropathy (63); the clinical relevance of this is disputed, since a small study has suggested that increased beta adrenergic sensitivity may augment the effects of the residual response (64). Loss of adrenaline responses usually coincide with loss of the response of pancreatic polypeptide to hypoglycaemia, the importance of which is uncertain but has been suggested to reflect a loss of vagal innervation of the pancreas (63, 65). This loss of the catecholamine response to hypoglycaemia is a further reduction in the potential for spontaneous recovery of blood glucose, as well as being intimately related to a loss of awareness of early hypoglycaemia.

Recently it has been shown experimentally that adrenaline responses to hypoglycaemia in both normal subjects and diabetic patients are diminished in the 24 hours following a previous hypoglycaemic event (66, 67). It is likely that there is more than one explanation for the defective adrenergic responses to hypoglycaemia associated with diabetes. In some cases the deficient adrenaline response to subsequent hypoglycaemia, particularly for those subjects in whom defective counterregulation has been induced by prior hypoglycaemia, may be reversible (68, 69).

In the presence of excessive exogenous insulin and multiple defects of the counterregulatory response, insulin-treated diabetic patients are at risk from hypoglycaemic events that can be prolonged and severe. It is likely that over time the responses to hypoglycaemic episodes are diminished and that awareness of symptoms related to them can be reduced, further increasing the risk of severe neuroglycopenic episodes.

## THE HYPOGLYCAEMIA SYMPTOM COMPLEX

Notwithstanding the importance of endogenous mechanisms of recovery from hypoglycaemia, in daily life subjective recognition of the associated symptoms and the ability to make an appropriate response to them (i.e. eat) provide the major protection against hypoglycaemia deep enough to impair cognitive function. There is still a lack of knowledge of the precise mechanisms generating the various symptoms of hypoglycaemia but they have traditionally been divided into two groups, those assumed to be related to activation of the sympathoadrenal pathway (adrenergic or autonomic) and those that occur through the direct effect of glucose deprivation on higher cerebral function (neuroglycopenic). There is also a group of symptoms whose aetiology is probably mixed and which are therefore non-specific markers of hypoglycaemia.

The conventional doctrine is that the autonomic symptoms occur first (i.e. at a higher blood glucose level) and warn of impending brain dysfunction from neuroglycopenia, allowing avoiding action to be taken. Unfortunately the situation is not as simple as this. The relationship between adrenaline secretion and 'adrenergic' symptoms is not firm – patients with adrenalectomy for example may still experience some of the symptoms of hypoglycaemia (70) and 'adrenergic' symptoms during controlled experimentally induced hypoglycaemia may precede detectable rise in circulating adrenaline (71). Even the link between the adrenergic symptoms and the autonomic nervous system is not a simple one. In studies of patients with cervical spinal cord transsection (and therefore no autonomic nervous control), in whom catecholamine responses to hypoglycaemia are absent, symptoms attributed to the adrenergic pathway can still be experienced (72). As will be discussed in detail below, it is likely that all counterregulatory responses are triggered from the brain, suggesting that a local lack of cerebral glucose is a primary event. The term 'neurogenic' has been mooted to replace 'autonomic'.

More recently, statistical approaches have been applied to the constellation of symptoms that occur during hypoglycaemia. This has led to the grouping of the symptoms into three categories within each of which the symptoms may be assumed to have common aetiologies (Table 28.1). Reassuringly, these do broadly conform to the older classifications (73).

In experimentally induced hypoglycaemia in non-diabetics (and indeed in most people with diabetes), autonomic symptoms do precede significant loss of cerebral function as blood glucose falls (71), thus affording warning of and protection against severe neuroglycopenia. However, early experience of insulin use indicated that symptoms may be idiosyncratic for individual subjects and vary in prominence, intensity and heirachy between patients (74).

## COGNITIVE DYSFUNCTION DURING HYPOGLYCAEMIA

### Incidence of hypoglycaemic events in insulin-treated diabetes mellitus

Mild (self-treated) hypoglycaemia is almost certainly under-reported but it is conservatively estimated that patients on conventional insulin therapy suffer an average of one episode of mild (self-treated) hypoglycaemia each week (75). The frequency is tripled in patients aiming for chronic normoglycaemia with intensified insulin therapy (76). This makes hypoglycaemia easily the most frequent acute morbid event in IDDM. In surveys of patients, hypoglycaemia is one of the most feared complications (77), ranking alongside fear of blindness and renal failure.

Severe hypoglycaemia (by definition that

requiring external assistance) occurs less often but is probably better documented. Published studies document that about 10–25% of patients on conventional therapy will experience an episode requiring outside assistance (glucagon or glucose administration) for recovery, or associ ated with a fit (75). The incidence may rise each year three- to six-fold during intensified insulin therapy (78).

Estimates of hypoglycaemia are rendered inaccurate even in prospective studies by failure of recall (79), difficulties in definition and episodes of hypoglycaemia without subjective awareness. Hypoglycaemia at night particularly may occur without awareness. During nocturnal monitoring, glucose concentrations below 2.5 mmol/l will occur in as many as 30% of conventionally controlled diabetic patients and 50% of patients on intensified therapeutic regimen (80, 81).

## EXPERIMENTAL INVESTIGATION OF HYPOGLYCAEMIA

Detailed study of the hypoglycaemic physiological responses and the factors influencing them poses several practical difficulties. Hypoglycaemia induced in the laboratory setting is a far cry from hypoglycaemia occurring as a result of a late snack or excess effort during a hectic day at work. It has been shown that the method of achieving hypoglycaemia can affect the responses to it (8), making this a particularly important point to consider when extrapolating experimental findings to the clinical situation. Nevertheless, the mechanisms underlying the responses to hypoglycaemia can only be examined in controlled circumstances. The information gained in such controlled studies can be applied to the clinical situation in qualitative terms but caution must be exercised in extrapolating quantitative data.

The simplest experimental method of inducing hypoglycaemia (and that used in much of the original work on the subject) is to give a single intravenous injection of insulin. This has the advantage that it resembles 'wild-type' hypoglycaemia (particularly if physiological doses of insulin are used), allows counterregulatory ability to be examined and enables the study of the effects of hypoglycaemia *per se* (10, 11). However, even if standardised doses of insulin are used, the variability of the resultant hypoglycaemia makes direct comparisons of responses between individuals, groups or even studies impossible except in terms of the glucose profiles themselves.

A modification of the insulin clamp technique allows the degree of hypoglycaemia to be controlled and therefore standardised. This method of investigation has been used in much recent work (82, 83). Hyperinsulinaemia is produced by a continuous (primed) fixed-rate insulin infusion and blood glucose levels are then controlled by a variable rate glucose infusion, adjusted on the basis of frequent accurate estimates of arterial or arterialised venous blood glucose. This allows the blood glucose to be manipulated precisely, resulting in a reproducible hypoglycaemic stimulus. Using a series of insulin-clamped glucose steps gradually proceeding to a nadir, the glucose levels at which various aspects of the counterregulatory responses begin can be measured. This tool has contributed much to present day understanding of the mechanisms of human counterregulatory physiology but here it is particularly true that quantitative extrapolation to the clinical situation must be done with caution. The degree of hyperinsulinaemia may affect responses to hypoglycaemia (8, 58) and it is possible that giving glucose during hypoglycaemia may affect responses. Furthermore, hypoglycaemic 'clamps', because they control blood glucose, cannot be used to examine overall ability to counterregulate. A combination of methods is therefore needed.

The mechanisms of counterregulation itself have been examined by using tracer methods to follow glucose kinetics during insulin infusion (35). These methods allow semi-quantitative estimates of hepatic glucose production, gluconeogenesis and peripheral glucose uptake. Recent work has raised questions about the mathematical models used to calculate such kinetic data (84, 85), especially during clamp studies, where unlabelled glucose has been used to control blood glucose causing changes in specific activities of the circulating tracer which may invalidate the calculations. Nevertheless, useful information has been acquired in this way.

### The acute hypoglycaemic event

Brain function is dependent upon a nutrient – generally glucose – supply. As glucose falls below a critical level defective cognitive function can be detected. In research studies a variety of techniques – trail making, simple reaction times, four choice reaction times, measurement of evoked potentials and electroencephalography – have been used to measure higher cerebral function. With the exception of the electrophysiological tests, in clamp studies performance deteriorates as blood glucose falls below 2.8 mmol (71). Deterioration may occur earlier during hypoglycaemia induced by unopposed insulin infusion (86). In life, the ability to perform complex tasks may deteriorate before the patient is aware of malaise. As glucose continues to fall, conscious level is impaired, leading eventually to loss of consciousness and coma. Transient focal neurological deficits may follow a severe hypoglycaemic episode (sometimes mistaken for a transient ischaemic attack) and may take up to 24 hours to resolve. Severe neuroglycopenia can cause grand mal seizures. These should not be diagnosed as epilepsy as they may occur in anyone if blood glucose is driven low enough. In the most profound hypoglycaemia, tissue damage may occur within the brain. Obvious permanent neurological sequelae are rare, although they have been reported, usually after massive insulin overdoseage (87). Physical damage during hypoglycaemia is more likely to result from confusion or decreased conscious level during a potentially hazardous activity that requires good concentration and co-ordination, such as driving or operating machinery.

## CONSEQUENCES OF HYPOGLYCAEMIA

### Metabolic

The response to hypoglycaemia includes stimulated release of the hormones of insulin antagonism. Relative insulin resistance may follow a hypoglycaemic episode – in the immediate post-hypoglycaemic phase (88), this can be obliterated by adrenergic blockade (89) and is likely to be due to catecholamines, but the effects of growth hormone (and perhaps cortisol) are delayed and prolonged and may underlie post-hypoglycaemic insulin resistance hours after the event (90). These phases of relative insulin resistance may contribute to the extreme lability of diabetes control in some adolescents, insulin resistant because of the hormonal changes of puberty. With the vigorous counterregulatory responses of youth, quite a moderate hypo may result in marked exacerbation of insulin resistance later (91, 92). It should be said, however, that much post-hypoglycaemic hyperglycaemia results from over-treatment of the original hypo. For a long time it was believed that the stress response to hypoglycaemia could induce severe hyperglycaemia and ketosis (the Somogyi effect) and that such an effect may underlie the cause of fasting hyperglycaemia. The mechanism just described might provide an explanation for this phenomenon but, in fact, fasting hyperglycaemia with or without ketosis almost certainly requires waning of the previous night's insulin at least as much as any endogenous endocrine response to a hypo in the night (93–96).

### Cognitive function

Following induced hypoglycaemia, cognitive function can be shown to return to baseline within 30–45 minutes (71). However, some patients describe a period of impaired concentration and lethargy following a clinical episode of hypoglycaemia which may last for many hours. This may represent the effects of counterregulatory hormones on cognitive function, but, since experimentally, the onset of cognitive dysfunction and hormone responses are independent, it is more likely that it represents a recovery period for cognitive function. Recovery of cognitive function after an episode of hypoglycaemia in a clinical, as opposed to an experimental, setting has not been examined in detail, but initial studies have not shown a major effect on performance the morning after a nocturnal hypoglycaemic event (97).

### Long-term cognitive effects

The long-term consequences of repeated hypoglycaemic episodes remain uncertain. Early studies suggested that children with poorly controlled diabetes performed worse than children with better-controlled hypoglycaemia-prone diabetes when IQ tested in adolescence (98). Studies are complicated by the difficulties of determining cause and effect. If a coincidence between frequent hypoglycaemia and poor achievement is noted, is it simply that the poor achiever is less able to control his/her regimen to avoid hypoglycaemia, or are the two causally related?

Two retrospective studies of data looking for an effect of recurrent hypoglycaemia on cognitive function seem to suggest that a significantly greater IQ drop is experienced over time (particularly non-verbal IQ) in the groups with recurrent severe hypoglycaemia whose prediabetic IQs were similar to other diabetic controls (99, 100). The under five age group may be particularly at risk. The published prospective study, to date, comparing cognitive function in patients on conventional and intensified insulin regimens (and therefore groups with different rates of hypoglycaemic experience) was not able to detect any such relationship between hypoglycaemia experience and IQ or other cognitive / neuropsychological measures (101), although the time scale of the study may not have been adequate. This area is clearly important and requires further investigation.

Table 28.2. *Glucose levels at which counterregulatory responses occur*

| | Non-diabetic | Diabetic | Intensive Rx |
|---|---|---|---|
| Symptoms | 3.0–3.4 | 3.2–4.3 | 2.4 |
| Adrenaline | 3.3–3.5 | 3.4–3.9 | 2.6 |
| EEG | <2.0 | <2.0 | 2.0 |
| Cognition | 2.8 | 2.8 | 2.8 |

Composite data.

## WHAT TRIGGERS THE COUNTERREGULATORY RESPONSE?

It is the absolute blood glucose concentration which stimulates counterregulation, rather than the rate or magnitude of the glucose fall (102–104). However, the glucose level associated with a given response may not be fixed – it varies between individuals and with different circumstances in any one individual. There is also variation between the glucose levels required to produce different aspects of the response within an individual, and the order in which responses occur is not fixed (105) (Table 28.2).

The site of a 'glucose sensor' that recognises a falling blood glucose and initiates the counterregulatory response has been the subject of intense debate and research.

There is evidence that the body's glucose sensor is situated in the brain (more specifically that part of the brain supplied by the posterior circulation) (106, 107) and responds to a falling blood glucose level. In man, subtle electrophysiological changes can be detected in the cerebral cortex (brain stem) at very minor degrees of hypoglycaemia (108), leading to suggestions that asymptomatic, or at least regional, neuroglycopenia is a trigger for counterregulation. The evidence for a cerebral site for the glucose sensor stems from animal studies using selective catheterisation techniques to isolate certain parts of the cerebral circulation during hypoglycaemia. Using these techniques, it has been demonstrated that peripheral hypoglycaemia does not produce counterregulation if the brain glucose supply is maintained (106, 107).

The putative cerebral glucose sensor responds to glucose deficiency. It is probable that the signal is a fall in the cellular metabolic rate (109). Providing non-glucose fuels to support metabolism during hypoglycaemia attenuates the counterregulatory response to hypoglycaemia in studies in dogs, thus indirectly identifying cerebral metabolic rate as the trigger to counterregulation. Similar work in humans has been less conclusive (110) but, both ketone and lactate infusions have been shown to attenuate the counterregulatory response to hypoglycaemia suggesting a similar mechanism may operate in man (29, 31). The invasive animal studies of cerebral metabolism/blood flow are not reproducible in man; however, recent advances in non-invasive 'functional imaging' techniques (such as magnetic resonance imaging, SPECT and positron emission tomography) allow regional cerebral glucose metabolism to be measured *in vivo*. As studies using these techniques become more sophisticated, a definitive answer to the question of 'the glucose sensor' in man may be found.

## Severe hypoglycaemia and loss of warning of hypoglycaemia

Severe hypoglycaemia with neuroglycopenia occurs when counterregulatory responses fail and blood glucose falls so low that normal cerebral function cannot be maintained. Occasionally this is the result of overwhelming hypoglycaemic drive – massive insulin overdosage or very vigorous exercise in association with artificially maintained hyperinsulinaemia and a failure to eat. In general, however, some further failure of counterregulation is required since the normal recovery mechanisms are so powerful.

There have been several attempts to characterise diabetic patients who are particularly prone to severe hypoglycaemia. In children, there is an association with the use of single or multiple (as opposed to two) daily insulin injections (14) and, in some studies, there is a relationship with lower HbA1. The incidence is not dissimilar from that seen in adults, although severe hypoglycaemia is less common in children with a disease duration of less than five years. In adults, the best predictor for severe hypoglycaemia is a history of previous episodes of it (111). In small studies, patients with a history of severe hypoglycaemia have longer disease duration. In one very large study, 'improving' glycaemic control with intensified insulin therapy was associated with a three- to six-fold increase in the incidence of severe hypoglycaemia (78).

One recent study (112) demonstrated that patients with a history of severe hypoglycaemia had defective counterregulation. In the face of a fixed insulin infusion, patients with a history of recurrent severe hypoglycaemia became obviously obtunded and/or had glucose falls to below 2 mmol/l, whereas patients without a history of severe hypoglycaemia (including some with documented autonomic neuropathy) maintained blood glucose in excess of 2.7 mmol/l without confusion in the same protocol. Patients with long duration diabetes, the group most susceptible to severe hypoglycaemia, are prone to defective counterregulatory responses to hypoglycaemia (113). Intensified insulin therapy, with the risk of severe hypoglycaemia, could induce defects in counterregulatory responses. Patients who had defective counterregulation before undertaking intensified insulin therapy are exceptionally prone to severe hypoglycaemia once it has been started (114).

Intensified insulin therapy, aimed at avoiding all hyperglycaemia in an attempt to reduce the risk of the microvascular complications of diabetes, is associated with a three-fold increase in the incidence of asymptomatic or biochemical hypoglycaemia, i.e. blood glucose measurements of 2.8 mmol/l or less recorded at times when the patient feels fine (115). The increased incidence of severe hypoglycaemia during this therapy has been mentioned (78). It is likely that this syndrome is due to a lowering of the glucose level at which counterregulatory responses are triggered, i.e. the glucose level at which cognitive function deteriorates remains the same (116, 117). This results in cognitive dysfunction occurring before any autonomic responses (118) – by the time these occur, cerebral function is so impaired that a rational response cannot be made.

Impairment of responses to experimental hypoglycaemia is very similar to that found in diabetic patients on intensified insulin therapy and can be induced in healthy subjects both with and without diabetes by inducing hypoglycaemia in the 12 hours before the test (66, 67). It is suggested that recurrent and perhaps quite mild hypoglycaemia during daily life, which becomes much more frequent as a patient strives for normoglycaemia, induces a tolerance of hypoglycaemia. This tolerance is manifested as a lowering of the glucose level which is recognised as abnormal, triggering a protective response. If brain dysfunction occurs at a higher glucose level than do the 'warning' symptoms, the scene is set for severe hypoglycaemia to occur. Counterregulatory failure and loss of warning of hypoglycaemia seem to coincide and a history of recurrent hypoglycaemia may underlie many cases. There may be many mechanisms underlying the triad of asymptomatic hypoglycaemia (119), increased risk of severe hypoglycaemia and defective counterregulation, with different causes in different people. However, for those in whom a history of recurrent hypoglycaemia seems to be the cause as well as the effect, there is some early experimental evidence to suggest that total elimination of hypoglycaemia for a period may restore a degree of counterregulatory competence as well as warning for future episodes (69). In clinical practice, this may require a redefining of glucose aims in a particular patient. In all patients, sub-normal glucose readings should be avoided, and aims for therapy should not be set at less than 4 mmol/l.

Warning of hypoglycaemia may be impaired by mechanisms other than failure of endogenous counterregulation. Alcohol, for example, in addition to its propensity for causing delayed hypoglycaemia by its suppression of gluconeogenesis, diminishes appreciation of warning symptoms and predisposes to severe hypoglycaemia (26). Non-selective beta blockade also interferes with some elements of the autonomic responses to hypoglycaemia and may interfere with glucose recovery (120–124), although whether this effect is clinically important is uncertain. Certainly, patients with diabetes should not be denied cardioselective beta blockers for ischaemic heart disease, although the use of other agents preferentially for hypertension may be sensible. Whether conversion to the use of human insulin encourages loss of warning of hypoglycaemia is controversial.

There is no evidence that hypoglycaemia induced experimentally with human insulin produces major differences in neurohumoral responses (71, 125, 126), although minor differences, usually at mild hypoglycaemic levels, in some components have been reported (127–129). Prospective clinical studies have failed to find a difference in the presentation or frequency of hypoglycaemia, although one group in Switzerland recently found that loss of concentration became a more prominent symptom of episodes of hypoglycaemia when well-controlled patients were given, in double blind fashion, human insulin (58, 130). Despite the experimental evidence, there are patients who associate loss of warning of hypoglycaemia with conversion to the use of human insulin and, although it is essential that other known causes of recurrent hypoglycaemia are rigorously sought and treated, such patients should not remain on an insulin they distrust (131). Pharmacokinetic differences or even differences in counterregulation too small to be detected on formal testing may be clinically relevant to susceptible patients, and the anticipated theoretical advantages of human over purified pork insulins have not been realised in clinical practice.

## Management of hypoglycaemia

### The acute event

Most hypoglycaemia is detected by the patient and self-treated. Over-treatment is common because the symptoms are unpleasant and the consequences of under-treatment frightening and because symptomatic relief, though fast, is not instantaneous. It is said that Eliot Joslin recommended an orange as treatment of a hypoglycaemic event because, in the time taken to peel the fruit, the patient could decide whether the symptoms were truly those of hypoglycaemia or not! This tale may be apocryphal but the orange and its juice continue to be regarded as useful therapy.

Mild hypoglycaemia is best treated by a combination of rapidly available carbohydrate (132) (half a glass of orange juice, 100 ml Lucozade or two glucose tablets) to arrest the glucose fall and provide rapid relief, followed by a more slowly absorbed carbohydrate such as two semi-sweet biscuits or a piece of bread. This second intake will maintain the recovery until the next meal. The rapidly available carbohydrate is repeated if no improvement is detected within 10 minutes. Glucose tablets are more convenient to carry than liquids and can be substituted by confectionery. The quantities should be noted. A whole standard size Mars bar may be enjoyable but is usually surplus to requirement!

If conscious level is impaired, it is dangerous to administer glucose drinks. Glucose gels (e.g. Hypostop – available from Bio Diagnostics) or honey can be placed inside the buccal cavity. Commercially available gels are favoured by some patients and their families. However, if conscious level is significantly impaired, parenteral therapy is necessary; 1 mg glucagon given intramuscularly will produce recovery in all but the very malnourished in approximately 10 to 15 minutes. It is almost as quick as intravenous glucose and much more readily given. Parents, spouses and friends can be taught to administer it at home, avoiding the need to call emergency services and speeding recovery. Nausea and vomiting may follow glucagon administration. Intravenous administration of 50% glucose is also effective: 25 ml is a good starting dose, repeated after 10 minutes if no recovery occurs; it is, however, very hypertonic and must be given into a large vein without extravasation. 20% glucose may be as effective as 50%, with less risk of phlebitis.

Once the patient is conscious, he/she must eat to prevent immediate recurrence. Hypoglycaemia, if due to sulphonylurea therapy or substantial insulin overdose, may be very prolonged and merits in-patient monitoring. Glucose infusion may be required. It is essential to consider the cause of an individual episode of severe hypoglycaemia and look at ways of preventing repetition.

## Prevention of recurrent hypoglycaemia

The timing and possible precipitating factors of individual episodes of hypoglycaemia should be examined. Consideration should be given to reducing insulin or drug doses, increasing (or introducing) snacks, making greater compensation for exercise or changes in activity levels or alcohol consumption. Patient fears of weight gain and subsequent reluctance to take snacks must be addressed (133) and overcome to ensure compliance with dietary regimens. It is worthwhile remembering that increased calorie intake during hypos does not help with weight loss! In a patient with multiple episodes of severe hypoglycaemia, his/her warning symptoms should be considered. There is some evidence that patients can be trained to recognise extremes of blood glucose more effectively, and this is worth considering. Recognition of new symptoms may be necessary as the presenting symptoms of hypoglycaemia change with time (134). Finally, goals of treatment may need reassessment. The relationship between recurrent hypoglycaemia and loss of warning symptoms of hypoglycaemia has been discussed above. If a patient is running very close to non-diabetic glucose levels, the risks of blood glucose levels being very low without recognition or awareness of intellectual dysfunction are great and relaxation of glucose control may be necessary.

### Hypoglycaemia in non-insulin-dependent diabetes mellitus

Although we have concentrated on hypoglycaemia in IDDM, it is also a major potential risk for patients with non-insulin dependent diabetes mellitus, once they are started on oral hypoglycaemic agents, where there is some evidence that counterregulatory deficiencies also exist (135). The risk is greatest with the sulphonylureas, which act by stimulating endogenous insulin responses to glucose, and thus create an artificial hyperinsulinaemia which may be excessive. Drugs with long half-lives, such as chlorpropamide, are particularly likely to cause hypoglycaemia, and there is evidence to suggest that the incidence of hypoglycaemia with glibenclamide, which is also long acting and remains bound to the β-cell for a prolonged period (136, 137) may be similar. The actions of drugs cleared largely by the kidney will be prolonged by renal impairment and insulin is therefore usually preferable in such patients.

In terms of presentation, treatment and avoidance, there are no major differences between IDDM and NIDDM, although it must be remembered that the hypoglycaemia of sulphonylurea therapy can be very protracted and inpatient monitoring is necessary after severe acute episodes. Neuroglycopenia is often unrecognised in elderly patients who may be particularly prone to confusion if diet is poor and long-acting sulphonylureas are used. Cessation, or at least reduction, of the oral agent responsible should be considered in all NIDDM patients who experience a hypoglycaemic event.

There has been considerably less research into the mechanisms of counterregulation in NIDDM although recent work seeks to correct this lack. The effects of ageing have also escaped definitive study, perhaps owing to the practical difficulties of studying the condition in the elderly. However, it is known that the counterregulatory response in adolescents is particularly brisk, and early work in the elderly suggests that the counterregulatory responses are blunted in a universal fashion independent of any specific disease process (138).

## CONCLUSION

Hypoglycaemia is a common consequence of pharmacological therapy designed to normalise blood glucose in diabetic patients. It carries serious risks for the patient. Over time, either related to an effect of the disease process itself on normal counterregulatory responses or to an effect of frequent hypoglycaemic events on subsequent reactions, symptoms warning of impending hypoglycaemia can be lost. Patients with this hypoglycaemic unawareness are at much greater risk of frequent and severe hypoglycaemia, with its inherent problems. The physiological responses to a hypoglycaemic event are now clearly documented, however, the mechanisms by which the body recognises blood glucose levels, and methods of enhancing hypoglycaemic awareness or preventing hypoglycaemia *per se* remain elusive. They are, and will continue to be, the subjects of intense research interest.

## REFERENCES


1 Sokoloff L. Metabolism of the central nervous system *in vivo*. In: *Handbook of physiology*. Section 1. Neurophysiology. Waverly Press Inc Baltimore, 1960; 1843.
2 Marks V. The measurement of blood glucose and the definition of hypoglycemia. *Horm Metabol Res* 1986; Suppl 6: 1–6.
3 Whipple AO. Hyperinsulinism in relation to pancreatic tumor. *Surgery* 1944; 16: 289–98.
4 Bolli G, Gottesman I, Cryer P, Gerich J. Glucose counterregulation during prolonged hypoglycemia in normal humans. *Am J Physiol* 1984; 247: E206–14.
5 Hirson IB, Marker JC, Smith LJ *et al*. Roles of insulin and glucose in the prevention of hypoglycaemia during exercise in humans. *Am J Physiol* 1990.

6 Merimee TJ, Tyson JE. Stabilization of plasma glucose during fasting. Normal variation in two separate studies. *N Engl J Med* 1974; 291: 1275–8.
7 Simonson DC, Koivisto V, Sherwin RS *et al.* Dannfelt A, DeFronzo RA. Adrenergic blockade alters glucose kinetics during exercise in insulin dependent diabetics. *J Clin Invest* 1984; 73: 1648–58.
8 Service FJ, Nelson RL, Rubenstein AH, Go VLW. Direct effect of insulin on secretion of insulin, glucagon, gastric inhibitory polypeptide, and gastrin during maintenance of normoglycemia. *J Clin Endocrinol Metab* 1978; 47: 488–93.
9 Sacca L, Sherwin RS, Hendler R, Felig P. Influence of continuous physiologic hyperinsulinemia on glucose kinetics and counterregulatory hormone responses in normal and diabetic humans. *J Clin Invest* 1979; 63: 849–57.
10 Garber AJ, Cryer PE, Santiago JV, Haymond MW, Pagliara AS, Kipnis DM. The role of adrenergic mechanisms in the substrate and hormonal response to insulin-induced hypoglycemia in normal man. *J Clin Invest* 1976; 58: 7–15.
11 Gerich J, Cryer PE, Rizza R. Hormonal mechanisms in acute glucose counterregulation: the relative roles of glucagon, epinephrine, norepinephrine, growth hormone and cortisol. *Metabolism* 1980; 29: 1164–75.
12 Darley J. Hypos from hell. *Balance* 1992/3; 132: 33.
13 Hallett L. Loss of hypo warning signs. *Balance* 1991; 125 :20–21.
14 Bhatia V, Wolfsdorf JI. Severe hypoglycaemia in youth with insulin dependent diabetes mellitus: frequency and causative factors. *Paediatrics* 1991; 88.6: 1187–93.
15 Caspari AF, Ewing LD. Severe hypoglycemia in diabetic patients: frequency, causes prevention. *Diabetes Care* 1985; 8: 141–5.
16 Pickup J. The pursuit of perfect control; better insulin better delivered. *BMJ* 1988; 297: 929–30.
17 Owens DR, Jones MK, Birtwell AJ *et al.* Hayes TM, Heding LG. Pharmacokinetics of subcutaneously administered human, porcine and bovine neutral insulin to normal men. *Horm Metabol Res* 16 supp: 195–199.
18 Botterman P, Gyaram H, Wahl K *et al.* Pharmacokinetics of biosynthetic human insulin and characteristics of its effect. *Diabetes Care* 1982; 5 supplement 2: 168–9.
19 Gallway JA, Spradlin CT, Nelson RL, Wentworth SM, Davidson JA, Swarner JL. Factors influencing absorption, serum insulin concentration and blood glucose responses after injections of regular insulin and various insulin mixtures. *Diabetes Care* 1981; vol 4: 366–76.
20 Dandona P, Hooke D, Bell J. Exercise and insulin absorption from subcutaneous tissue. *BMJ* 1978; 1: 479–80.
21 Hildenbrandt P, Sestoft L, Nielsen SL. The absorption of subcutaneously injected short acting soluble insulin; the influence of injection technique and concentration. *Diabetes Care* 1983; 6: 459–462.
22 Linde B, Philip A. Massage enhanced insulin absorption – increased distribution or dissociation of insulin? *Diabetes Res* 1989; 11: 191–194.
23 Greenbaum CJ, Palmer JP. Insulin antibodies and insulin autoantibodies. *Diabetic Med* 1991; 8: 97–105.
24 Arlasian S, Nixon PA, Becker D, Drash A. Impact of physical fitness and glycaemic control on *in vivo* insulin action in adolescents with IDDM. *Diabetes Care*; vol 13: 9–10.
25 Berger M, Berchtold P, Cuppers HJ *et al.* Metabolic and hormonal effects of muscular exercise in juvenile type diabetics. *Diabetologia* 1977; vol 13: 355–65.
26 Kerr D, Macdonald IA, Heller SR, Tattersall RB. Alcohol causes hypoglycaemic unawareness in healthy volunteers and patients with Type 1 (insulin-dependent) diabetes. *Diabetologia* 1990; 33: 216–21.
27 Field JB, Williams HE, Mortimer GE. Studies on the mechanism of ethanol-induced hypoglycaemia. *J Clin Invest* 1963; 42: 497–506.
28 Frienkel N, Singer DL, Arky RA, Bleicher SJ, Anderson JB, Silbert CK. Alcohol Hypoglycaemia. *J Clin Invest* 1963; vol 42: 1112–1133.
29 Amiel SA, Archibald HR, Chusney G, Williams AJK, Gale EAM. Ketone infusion lowers hormonal responses to hypoglycaemia – evidence for acute cerebral utilisation of a non-glucose fuel. *Clin Sci* 1991; 81: 189–194.
30 Avogaro A, Nosadini R, Doria A *et al.* Substrate availability other than glucose in the brain during euglycaemia and insulin-induce hypoglycaemia in dogs. *Metabolism* 1990; 39(1): 46–50.
31 Maran A, Cranston I, Lomas J, Macdonald IA, Amiel SA. Protection by lactate of cerebral function during hypoglycaemia. *Lancet* 1994; 343: 16–20.
32 Ferrannini E, DeFronzo RA. Insulin actions *in vivo*: glucose metabolism. In: Alberti KGMM, Keen H, DeFronzo RA, Zimmet P. eds. *International textbook of diabetes mellitus.* John Wiley and Sons; England, p 421.
33 Cherrington AD, Williams PE, Shulman GI, Lacy WW. Differential time course of glucagon's effect on glycogenolysis and gluconeogenesis in the conscious dog. *Diabetes* 1980; 30: 180–7.
34 Owen OE, Morgan AP, Kemp HG, Sullivan JM, Herrara HG, Cahill GF. Brain metabolism during fasting. *J Clin Invest* 1967; 46: 1590–5.
35 Caprio S, Sacca L, Tamborlane WV, Sherwin RS. Relationship between changes in glucose production and gluconeogenesis during mild hypoglycaemia in humans. *Metabolism* 1988; 37: 707–10.
36 LeCavalier L, Bolli G, Cryer P, Gerich J. Contribution of gluconeogenesis and glycogenolysis during glucose counterregulation in normal man. *Am J Physiol* 1989; 256: E844–51.
37 Lager I, Atvall S, Eriksson BM, Von Schenk H, Smith U. Studies on the insulin antagonistic effect of catecholamines in normal man. *Diabetologia* 1986; 29: 409–16.
38 Rizza RA, Haymond MW, Cryer PE, Gerich JE. Differential effects of physiologic concentrations of epinephrine on glucose production and disposal in man. *Am J Physiol* 1979; 237: E356–62.
39 Sacca L, Vigorito C, Cicala M, Ungaro B, Sherwin RS. Mechanisms of epinephrine-induced glucose intolerance in normal humans. *J Clin Invest* 1982; 69: 284–93.
40 Sacca L, Vigorito C, Cicala M, Corso G, Sherwin RS. Role of gluconeogenesis in epinephrine-stimulated hepatic glucose production in humans. *Am J Physiol* 1983; 247: E294–304.
41 Sacca L, Gelfand RA, Sherwin RS. Epinephrine–insulin

interactions in humans: dissociation of glucose and branched chain amino acid uptake by skeletal muscle. *Diabetes* 1986; 35 (Suppl 1): 83A.
42 Porte D, Graber Al, Kuzuya T, Williams RH. The effect of epinephrine on immunoreactive insulin levels in man. *J Clin Endocrinol Metab* 1973; 37: 479–86.
43 Shamoon H, Hendler R, Sherwin RS. Synergistic interactions amoung anti-insulin hormones in the pathogenesis of stress hyperglycemia in humans. *J Clin Endocrinol Metab* 1980; 52: 1236–41.
44 Boyle PJ, Cryer PE. Roles of growth hormone and cortisol in defense against prolonged hypoglycemia. *Diabetes* 1990; 39 Suppl 1: 5A.
45 DeFeo P, Perriello G, DeCosmo S *et al.* Comparison of glucose counterregulation during short term and prolonged hypoglycemia in normal man. *Diabetes* 1986; 35: 563–9.
46 Rizza RA, Cryer PE, Gerich JE. Role of glucagon, catecholamines and growth hormone in human glucose counterregulation. *J Clin Invest* 1979; 64: 62–71.
47 DeFeo P, Perriello G, Torlone E *et al.* Demonstration of a role for growth hormone in glucose counterregulation. *Am J Physiol* 1989; 256: E835-43.
48 MacGorman L, Rizza R, Gerich JE. Physiologic concentrations of growth hormone exert insulin-like and insulin antagonist effects on both hepatic and extrahepatic tissues in man. *J Clin Endocrinol Metab* 1981; 53: 556–9.
49 Rizza RA, Mandarino L, Gerich JE. Cortisol induced insulin resistance in man. *J Clin Endocrinol Metab* 1981; 54: 131–8.
50 Hansen I, Firth R, Haymond M, Cryer P, Rizza R. The role of autoregulation of the hepatic glucose production in man's response to a physiological decrement in plasma glucose. *Diabetes* 1986; 35: 186–91.
51 Diamond MP, Hallarman L, Zych K *et al.* Insulin *per se* suppresses counterregulatory hormone responses to hypoglycemia. *Diabetes* 1990; 39 Suppl 1: p4a, 15.
52 Edwards BJA, Morley JA. Amylin. Mini Review. Life Sci 1993; 51: 1899–912.
53 Fisher BM, Gillen G, Dargie HJ, Inglis GC, Frier BM. The effects of insulin-induced hypoglycaemia on cardiovascular function in normal man: studies using radionuclide ventriculography. *Diabetologia* 1988; 30: 841–5.
54 Fisher BM, Gillen G, Hepburn DA, Dargie HJ, Frier BM. Cardiac responses to acute insulin-induced hypoglycemia in humans. *Am J Physiol* 1990; 258: H1775–9.
55 Neil HAW, Gale EAM, Hamilton SJC, Lopez-Espinoza L, Kaura R, McCarthy ST. Cerebral blood flow increases during insulin induced hypoglycaemia in Type 1 (insulin dependent) diabetic patients and control subjects. *Diabetologia* 1987; 30: 305–9.
56 Sieber FE, Koehler RC, Derrer SA, Saudek CD, Traystman RJ. Hypoglycemia and cerebral autoregulation in anaesthetized dogs. *Am J Physiol* 1990; 258: H1714–21.
57 Bergenstal I, Dupre J, Lawson PM, Rizza R, Rubenstein AH. Observations on C-peptide and free insulin in the blood during continuous subcutaneous insulin infusion and conventional insulin therapy. *Diabetes* 1985; 34 suppl 3: 31–6.
58 Egger M, Smith GD, Teuscher AU, Teuscher A. Influence of human insulin on symptoms and awareness of hypoglycaemia; a randomised double blind trial. *BMJ* 1991; 303: 622–6.
59 Gerich JE, Langloisd M, Noacco C, Karam JH, Forsham PH. Lack of a glucagon response to hypoglycemia in diabetes: evidence for an intrinsic pancreatic alpha-cell defect. *Science* 1973; 182: 171–3.
60 Lalic NM, Zamaklar M, Simonson DC, Jackson R, Dordevic PB. Impairments in glucose disposal in patients with recent-onset type 1 (insulin dependent) diabetes. *Diabetologia* 1992; 35 (1): A106; 405
61 Singer-Granick C, Hoffman RP, Becker DJ *et al.* Glucagon responses to hypoglycaemia in children and adolescents with IDDM. *Diabetes Care* 1988; 11: 643–9.
62 Bolli GB, Dimitraidis GD, Pehling GB *et al.* Abnormal glucose counterregulation after subcutaneous insulin in insulin-dependent diabetes mellitus. *N Engl J Med* 1984; 310: 1706–11.
63 Hilstead J, Madsbad S, Karaup T *et al.* No response to pancreatic hormones to hypoglycemia in diabetic autonomic neuropathy. *J Clin Endocrinol Metab* 1982; 54: 815–19.
64 Berlin I, Grimaldi A, Landault C *et al.* Lack of hypoglycaemic symptoms and decreased beta adrenergic sensitivity in insulin dependent diabetic patients. *J Clin Endocrinol Metab* 1987 66 (2): 273–8.
65 Hilstead J, Madsbad S, Krarup T *et al.* Hormonal, metabolic and cardiovascular responses to hypoglycemia in diabetic autonomic neuropathy. *Diabetes* 1981; 30: 626–33.
66 Heller SR, Cryer PE. An antecedent episode of hypoglycemia reduced neuroendocrine and symptomatic responses to subsequent hypoglycemia after 1 episode of hypoglycaemia in non-diabetic humans. *Diabetes* 1991; 40; 223–6.
67 Widom B, Simonson DC. Intermittent hypoglycaemia impairs glucose counterregulation. *Diabetes* 1992; 41 (12): 1597–603.
68 Fanelli C, Rambotti AM, Epifano L *et al.* Short-term reversibility of hypoglycaemia unawareness in type 1 (insulin dependent) diabetes mellitus. *Diabetologia* 1992; 35 (1): A 42, 156.
69 Cranston I, Lomas J, Maran A, Macdonald IA, Amiel SA. Restoration of hypoglycaemia awareness in patients with long-duration insulin-dependent diabetes. *Lancet* 1994; 344: 283–7.
70 Ginsberg J, Paton A. Effects of insulin after adrenelectomy. *Lancet* 1956; 15: 491–494.
71 Maran A, Lomas J, Archibald H, Macdonald IA, Gale EAM, Amiel SA. Double blind clinical and laboratory study of hypoglycaemia with human and porcine insulin in diabetic patients reporting hypoglycaemia unawareness after transferring to human insulin. *BMJ* 1993; 306: 167–2.
72 Palmer JP, Henry DP, Benson JW, Johnson DG, Ensinck JW. Glucagon response to hypoglycaemia in sympathectomised man. *J Clin Invest* 1976; 57: 522–5.
73 Dary IJ, Hepburn DA, MacCleod KM, Frier BM. Symptoms of hypoglycaemia: validation of a three factor model in two large samples of patients with insulin treated diabetes. *Diabetic Med* 1992; 9 suppl: A 30
74 Lawrence RD. Insulin hypoglycaemia. Changes in nervous manifestations. *Lancet* 1941; ii: 602.
75 Potter J, Clarke P, Gale EAM, Dave SH, Tattersall RB. Insulin-induced hypoglycaemia in an accident and emergency department: the tip of an iceberg? *Br Med J* 1982; 285: 1180–2.

76 Tang Fui SN, Pickup JC, Bending JJ, Collins ACG, Keen H, Dalton N. Hypoglycemia and counterregulation in insulin dependent diabetic patients: a comparison of continuous subcutaneous insulin infusion and conventional insulin injection therapy. *Diabetes Care* 1986; 9: 221–7.

77 Cox DJ, Irvine A, Gonder-Frederick L, Nowacek G, Butterfield J. Fear of hypoglycaemia: quantification validation and utilization. *Diabetes Care* 1987; 10: 617–21.

78 The DCCT research group. Epidemiology of severe hypoglycaemia in the diabetes control and complications trial. *Am J Med* 1991; 90: 450–9.

79 Heller SR, Chapman JE, McCleod JM, Parnell L, Ward JD. A failure to question patients partners underestimates the clinical problems of hypoglycaemia. *Diabetic Med* 1992; 9 suppl: 77.

80 Bendtson I, Gade J, Wildschicettz G, Rosenfalck A, Binder C. Non-invasive detection of nocturnal hypoglycaemia in Type 1 diabetic patients. *Diabetologia* 1990; 33: A121.

81 Shalwitz RA. Prevalence and consequences of nocturnal hypoglycemia in conventionally treated children with diabetes mellitus. *J Pediatr* 1990; 116: 685–9.

82 Amiel SA, Tamborlane WV, Simonson DC, Sherwin RS. Defective glucose counterregulation after strict control of insulin-dependent diabetes mellitus. *N Engl J Med* 1987; 316: 1376–3.

83 Simonson DC, Tamborlane WV, DeFronzo RA, Sherwin RS. Intensive insulin therapy reduces the counterregulatory hormone responses to hypoglycemia in patients with Type 1 patients. *Ann Int Med* 1985; 103: 184–90.

84 Finegood DT, Bergman RN, Vranic M. Estimation of endogenous glucose production during hyperinsulinaemic-euglycaemic glucose clamps: comparison of unlabelled and labelled exogenous glucose infusates. *Diabetes* 1987; 36: 914–24.

85 Finegood DT, Bergman RN, Vranic M. Modelling error and apparent isotope discrimination confound estimation of endogenous glucose production during euglycaemic glucose clamps. *Diabetes* 1988; 37: 1025–4.

86 Pramming S, Thorsteinsson B, Theilgaard A, Pinner EM, Binder C. Cognitive function during hypoglycaemia in type 1 diabetes mellitus. 1986 *BMJ*; 292:

87 Lawrence RD. Hemiplegia in a diabetic producing unilateral peripheral neuritis and hypoglycaemic attacks. *Lancet* 1967; i: 1321–2.

88 Clare JN, Brennan JR, Gebhart SP, Newsome HH, Nestler JE, Blackard WG. Prolonged insulin resistance following insulin induced hypoglycaemia. *Diabetologia* 1987; 30: 851–8.

89 Attvall S, Ericksson BM, Fowelin J, von Schenk H, Lager I, Smith U. Early post-hypoglycemic insulin resistance in man is mainly an effect of β adrenergic stimulation. *J Clin Invest* 1987; 80: 437–2.

90 Metcalfe P, Johnson DG, Nosadini R, Orksov H, Alberti KGMM. Metabolic effects of acute and prolonged growth hormone excess in normal and insulin deficient man. *Diabetologia* 1981; 20: 123–8.

91 Amiel SA, Sherwin RS, Simonson DC, Lauritano AA, Tamboriane WV. Impaired insulin action in puberty: a contributing factor to poor glycemic control in adolescents with diabetes. *N Engl J Med* 1986; 315: 215–19.

92 Amiel SA, Caprio S, Sherwin RS, Plewe G, Haymond WV, Tamborlane WV. Insulin resistance of puberty: a defect restricted to peripheral glucose metabolism. *J Clin Endocrinol Metab* 1991; 72:

93 Gale EAM, Kurtz AB, Tattersall RB. In search of the Somogyi effect. *Lancet* 1980; ii: 279–82.

94 Havlin CE, Cryer PE. Nocturnal hypoglycemia does not commonly result in major morning hyperglycemia in patients with diabetes mellitus. *Diabetes Care* 1987; 10: 141–7.

95 Hirsch IB, Smith LJ, Havlin CE, Shah SD, Clutter WE, Cryer PE. Failure of nocturnal hypoglycemia to cause daytime hyperglycemia in patients with IDDM. *Diabetes Care* 1990; 13: 133–42.

96 Periello G, DeFeo P, Torone E *et al.* The effect of asymptomatic nocturnal hypoglycemia on glycemic control in diabetes mellitus. *N Engl J Med* 1988; 319: 1233–9.

97 Bendtson I, Gade J, Theilgaard A, Binder C. Cognitive function in type 1 (insulin dependent) diabetic patients after nocturnal hypoglycaemia. *Diabetologia* 1992; 35: 898–903.

98 Ryan C, Vega A, Drash A. Cognitive defects in adolescents who developed diabetes in early life. *Pediatrics* 1985; 75: 921–7.

99 Langan SJ, Deary IJ, Hepburn DA. Cumulative cognitive impairment following recurrent severe hypoglycaemia in adult patients with insulin-treated diabetes mellitus. *Diabetologia* 1990; 34: 337–44.

100 Wredling R, Levander S, Adamson U *et al.* Permanent neuropsychological impairment after recurrent episodes of severe hypoglycaemia in man. *Diabetologia* 1990; 33: 152–7.

101 Reichard P, Britz A, Rosenqvist U. Intensified conventional insulin treatment and neuropsychological impairment. *BMJ* 1991; 303: 1439–42.

102 Amiel SA, Simonson DC, Tamborlane WV, DeFronzo RA, Sherwin RS. The rate of glucose fall does not affect the counterregulatory hormone responses to hypoglycemia in normal and diabetic man. *Diabetes* 1987; 36: 518–22.

103 DeFronzo RA *et al.* A test of the hypothesis that the rate of glucose fall triggers a counterregulatory hormone response to hypoglycaemia. *Diabetes* 1977; 26: 445–52.

104 Gale EAM, Bennet T, Macdonald IA, Holst JJ, Matthews JA. The physiological effects of insulin-induced hypoglycaemia in man: responses at differing levels of blood glucose. *Clin Sci* 1983; 65: 263.

105 Boyle PJ, Schwartz NS, Shah SD, Clutter WE, Cryer PE. Plasma glucose concentrations at the onset of hypoglycemic symptoms in patients with poorly controlled diabetes and in non-diabetics. *N Engl J Med* 1988; 318: 1487–92.

106 Biggers DW, Myers SR, Neal D *et al.* Role of the brain in counterregulation of insulin induced hypoglycemia in dogs. *Diabetes* 1989; 38: 7–16.

107 Cane P, Haun CK, Evered J, Joun JH, Bergman RN. Response to deep hypoglycaemia does not involve glucoreceptors in carotid perfused tissue. *Am J Physiol* 1988; 255: E680–7.

108 DeFeo P, Gallal V, Mazzotta G *et al.* Modest decrements in plasma glucose concentration causes early impairment in cognitive function and later activation

of glucose counterregulation in the absence of hypoglycemic symptoms in normal man. *J Clin Invest* 1988; 82:
109 Nagy RJ, O'Connor A, Boyle PJ. Modest hypoglycaemia impairs brain glucose utilisation before the onset of symptoms. *Diabetes* 1992; 41: 69A, 253.
110 FrolundJ, Kerult H, Christiansen NJ, Alberti KGMM. Effect of ketone body infusion on plasma catecholamine and substrate concentrations during acute hypoglycaemia in man. *J Clin Endocrinol Metab* 1980; 50: 557–1.
111 Clausen Sjobom N, Adamson U, Lins PE. The prevalence of impaired glucose counterregulation during an insulin infusion test in insulin-trested diabetic patients prone to severe hypoglycaemia. *Diabetologia* 1989; 32: 818–52.
112 Ryder RJ, Owens DR, Hayes TM, Ghatei MA, Bloom SR. Unawareness of hypoglycaemia and inadequate hypoglycaemic counterregulation: no causal relationship with diabetic autonomic neuropathy. *Br Med J* 1980; 301: 783–7.
113 Hepburn DA, Patrick AW, Eadington, DW, Ewing DJ, Frier BM. Unawareness of hypoglycaemia in insulin treated diabetic patients: prevalence and relationship to autonomic neuropathy. *Diabetic Med* 1990; 7: 711–17.
114 White NH, Skor D, Cryer PE, Bier DM, Levandoski L, Santiago JV. Identification of type 1 diabetic patients at increased risk for hypoglycemia during intensive therapy. *N Engl J Med* 1983; 308: 485–91.
115 Lager I, Atvall S, Blohme G, Smith U. Altered recognition of hypoglycaemic symptoms in Type 1 diabetes during intensified control with continuous subcutaneous insulin infusion. *Diabetic Med* 1986; 3: 322–5.
116 Amiel SA, Pottinger R, Cunnah DC *et al.* Effect of antecedent glucose control on cerebral function during hypoglycaemia. *Diabetes Care* 1991; 14: 109–18.
117 Widom B, Simonson DC. Glycaemic control and neurophysiologic function during hypoglycaemia in patients with insulin dependent diabetes mellitus. *Ann Int Med* 1990; 112: 904–12.
118 Maran A, Macdonald I, Lomas J, Archibald H, Amiel SA. Cerebral function during hypoglycaemia in type 1 diabetic patients with hypoglycaemia unawareness: is the brain protected? *Diabetic Med* 1992; 9 suppl: A 29.
119 Clarke WL, Gonder-Frederick LA, Richards FE, Cryer PE. Multifactorial origin of hypoglycaemic symptom unawareness in IDDM. Association with defective glucose counterregulation and better glycaemic control. *Diabetes* 1991; 40: 680–5.
120 Frier BM, Corrall RJM, O'Brien IAD, Lewin IG, Hay ID, Roland J. Hypoglycemia during adrenergic betablockade: evidence against mediation via a deficiency of lactate for gluconeogenesis. *Metabolism* 1985; 34: 1039–43.
121 Hirsch IB, Boyle PJ, Craft S, Cryer PE. Does beta-adrenergic blockade mask the symptoms of hypoglycemia in IDDM? *Diabetes* 1990; 39 Suppl 1: 6A.
122 Macdonald IA, Bennett T, Gale EAM, Walford S. The effect of propranolol or metoprolol on thermoregulation during insulin induced hypoglycaemia in man. *Clin Sci* 1982; 63: 301–10.
123 Molner GW, Read RC. Propranolol enhancement of hypoglycaemic sweating. *Clin Pharmacol Ther* 1974; 15: 490–6.
124 Popp DA, Tse TF, Shah S, Clutter WE, Cryer PE. Oral propranolol and metoprolol both impair glucose recovery from insulin induced hypoglycemia in insulin dependent diabetes mellitus. *Diabetes Care* 1984; 7: 243–7.
125 Anderson JH, Holcombe JH, Grimes JA, Galloway JA. Hypoglycaemia unawareness and human insulin. *Diabetologia* 1990; 33: A122
126 Mülhauser I, Berger M, Heinemann L, Fritsche E, Lennep K. Hypoglycaemic warning symptoms and incidence of severe hypoglycaemia during treatment with human and animal insulin. *Diabetologia* 1990; 33: A122.
127 Berger W, Keller U, Henegger B, Faggi E. Warning symptoms of hypoglycaemia during treatment with human and porcine insulin in diabetes mellitus. *Lancet* 1989; i: 1041–4.
128 Heine RJ, Van Der Heyden EAP, Van der Veen EA. Responses to human and porcine insulin in healthy subjects. *Lancet* 1989; ii: 946–8.
129 Lingenfelser T, Maassen H, Overtcamp D, Glück H, Eggstein M, Jakober B. Changes of mood and psychomoter function during human and porcine insulin induced hypoglycaemia. *Diabetologia* 1990; A123.
130 Egger M, Smith GD, Imhof H, Teuscher A. Risk of severe hypoglycaemia in insulin dependent diabetic patients transferred to human insulin. *BMJ* 1991; 303: 617–21.
131 Pickup J. Human insulin. *BMJ* 1989; 299: 991–3.
132 Collier A, Steedman DJ, Patrick AW *et al.* Comparison of intravenous glucagon and dextrose in the treatment of severe hypoglycaemia in the accident and emergency department. *Diabetes Care* 1987; 10: 712–15.
133 The DCCT Research Group. Weight gain associated with intensive therapy in the diabetes control and complications trial. *Diabetes Care* 1988; 11: 567–573.
134 Cryer PE, Binder C, Bolli GB, Cherington AD, Gale EAM, Gerich JE, Sherwin RS. Hypoglycaemia in IDDM. *Diabetes* 1989; 38: 1193–9.
135 Bolli GB, Tsalikian E, Haymond MW, Cryer PE, Gerich JE. Defective glucose counterregulation after subcutaneous insulin in non-insulin dependent diabetes mellitus. *J Clin Invest* 1984; 73: 1532–41.
136 Asplund K, Wilholm BE, Lithner F. Glibenclamide-associated hypoglycaemia: a report on 57 cases. *Diabetalogia* 1983; 24: 412–17.
137 Clarke BF, Campbell IW. Long-term comparative trial of glibenclamide and chlorpropamide in diet-failed, maturity onset diabetics. *Lancet* 1975; i: 246–8.
138 Marker JC, Cryer PE, Clutter WE. Attenuated glucose recovery from hypoglycaemia in the elderly. *Diabetes* 1992; 41: 671–8.

# 29 Strategies for Prevention of Insulin-dependent Diabetes

Paolo Pozzilli

## PATHOGENIC NOTES RELEVANT FOR IDDM PREVENTION

Type I (insulin-dependent) diabetes (IDDM) is probably caused by an autoimmune destruction of insulin-producing cells mediated by cytotoxic cells recognising specific antigens associated with beta cells (1 and Chapter 10). A variety of mononuclear cells including T lymphocytes and macrophages have been implicated in the islet beta cell destruction associated with the disease. However, how these cells mediate their islet beta cell destructive effect is still a matter for discussion. Effective mechanisms mediating islet beta cell injury involve direct contact between immunological cells (effectors) and beta cells (targets) and result in the release of soluble mediators by the effector cells (2). Cytokines, in particular interleukin 1 (IL-1), tumour necrosis factor (TNF) and interleukin 6 (IL-6), are secreted by activated T cells and are candidates for the initiation of islet beta cell damage (3). It has yet to be ascertained how these cytokines induce beta cell destruction, but recent data suggest that the participation of free oxygen radicals in cytokine-mediated islet beta cell destruction, together with hyper-expression of HLA class II by beta cells, could be a major event in the pathogenesis of IDDM (4). It is also known that islet cells produce cytokines themselves if infected by viruses. This effect has been observed in insulinoma beta cells infected *in vitro* with measles and mumps viruses (5). Under such circumstances, beta cells are able to release cytokines, in particular IL-1 and IL-6, thereby expanding the autoimmune response towards the beta cells by committed T lymphocytes which are represented in the islet cell infiltrative process in susceptible prediabetic subjects. This observation could explain how a viral infection can precipitate predisposed individuals towards the onset of clinical IDDM.

The possibility that nitrogen free oxygen radicals may be involved in cytokine action on islet cells is supported by a recent report that IL-1 and TNF induced blockade of insulin released from islets *in vitro* involving the free radical, nitric oxide (6). However, it is not known how cytokines and, in particular, IL-1 and TNF, stimulate oxygen free radical production in pancreatic islets. Current data available on nitric oxide do not provide a complete picture. This radical product acts as a neurotransmitter, prevents platelet aggregation and, more importantly in this context, is a major defence molecule against tumour cells and intracellular bacteria (7). Nitric oxide, secreted in high quantities by activated macrophages, represents a major cytotoxic effector molecule and its role in non-specific immune defence is well established. Evidence is accumulating to suggest that the lysis of pancreatic islet cells by activated macrophages may play a major role in the pathogenesis of IDDM. Indeed, recent data suggest that the lysis of islet cells by activated macrophages is mediated by nitric oxide (8). Cultivation of islets with chemicals which spontaneously release nitric oxide also leads to beta cell death. These data suggest that nitric oxide could contribute to autoimmune destruction in IDDM but the mechanism involved in this process is still being debated. A simple impairment of mitochondrial respiration should be excluded, since nicotinamide, an inhibitor of poly (ADP-ribose) synthetase, protects islet cells from macrophage cytotoxicity and nitric oxide damage (9). Whatever the mechanism, the possibility that nitric oxide may represent an unrecognised factor in tissue destruction cannot be ruled out, and this should be considered when strategies to prevent IDDM are taken into account. Since IL-1, IL-6 and TNF are potent inducers of nitric oxide secretion, some of the pathogenic effect mediated by these cytokines could be a direct consequence of nitric oxide action.

## PREVENTION OF IDDM: GENERAL GUIDELINES

In theory, three types of preventive approaches can be used to target any given disease condition: *primary prevention*, understood as intervention among the normal population, with the aim of targeting the aetiological or risk factors associated with a specific disease; *secondary prevention*, that is the early identification of a disease and/or the relevant risk factors and how to intervene in order to interrupt or slow down the process. Finally, there is *tertiary prevention*, which investigates the various clinical complications associated with disease onset and ways to prevent them (Table 29.1).

For a chronic-degenerative disease such as IDDM, primary prevention entails identifying possible risk factors while secondary prevention is dependent on early diagnosis. Tertiary prevention is not really a genuine preventive technique as it focuses on preventing complications associated with clinical onset and may reduce long-term diabetic complications by preserving residual beta cell function.

Table 29.1. *Prevention of IDDM*

*Primary prevention*
Intervention at birth in normal populations by:
*Removal of aetiological factors*
- diabetogenic viruses
- other environmental factors, i.e. dietary restrictions/changes in diet

*Removal of risk factors*
- diabetes genes: too widespread among the general population to be effective

*Secondary prevention*
- Intervention during the latency phase in subjects with a positive marker for the disease

*Tertiary prevention*
- Intervention at early diagnosis of the disease to protect residual beta cell mass and function

Given that there is no prevention without prediction, preventive attempts should only be tested on those subjects identified as being susceptible to the disease.

### Prediction requirement for preventive strategies

Several aspects concerning IDDM aetiology have yet to be clarified, including the possible role of various unidentified environmental factors (see Chapter 10). Such factors, which some authors tend to link with viruses, could lead to the establishment of a model for the aetiopathological characteristics of the disease including a primary event of beta cell insult and subsequent chronic disease evolution. This model may be useful for designing preventive strategies at different levels.

*Primary prevention* of IDDM is currently impractical since the aetiological agents involved in the disease process are unknown. Furthermore, no genetic investigation is feasible in susceptible subjects for the disease, even though

Table 29.2. *Secondary prevention (guidelines)*

*Condition for a screening programme in relation to:*

*Disease*

global relevance of the disease (prevalence, severity, social impact, morbidity, mortality, etc.)

- identification at pre-clinical stage
- effect of treatment at time of diagnosis

*Screening test*

- sensitivity, specificity, positive predictive value
- technical procedures involved, consistency of results
- degree of invasiveness
- cost

*Screening programme*

- study population and disease prevalence
- feasibility and cost of programme
- follow-up of subjects with positive markers
- psychological implications of false positive diagnosis

*Possible tests for screening IDDM pre-diabetes*

- immunoserological tests: ICA, IAA, anti-64k/GAD
- genetic tests: HLA typing

such individuals are thought to be distributed fairly evenly throughout the general population. However, at this stage it should be pointed out that the first attempt at primary prevention of the disease is currently being carried out in Finland on a national scale. The rationale underlying this project is based on the possible role various proteins in the diet (and, in particular, milk protein) may play in triggering disease onset. Crucial evidence in support of this theory is represented by the high prevalence of anti-bovine albumin antibodies in diabetic children, a protein normally found in cow's milk (10). This primary prevention venture aims to evaluate the effect that a diet deficient in this protein may have on IDDM incidence in young diabetic children and to compare the resulting data with the effects of a diet where this milk protein is included.

As a first step, *secondary prevention* of IDDM requires the implementation of a screening programme to identify individuals at risk. The feasibility of such a screening campaign is detailed in Table 29.2. The natural history of IDDM makes it a suitable candidate for the implementation of a screening campaign as part of a secondary prevention programme. However, it is more difficult to evaluate whether such a screening programme, while allowing the identification of susceptible subjects, subsequently results in accurate prevention of this disease. Among the markers reported in Table 29.2, the most valuable in terms of sensitivity (percentage of positive subjects among affected individuals), specificity (percentage of negative subjects among non-affected individuals), consistency and relative ease of procedure is represented by the islet cell antibodies (ICA). However, the high positive predictive value (reflecting a strong probability of the disease occurring in individuals who test positively) of this serological specificity has only been demonstrated within the framework of family studies. Since any intervention programme proposing to significantly reduce the incidence of IDDM needs to be carried out among the general population, it is of crucial importance, as with other markers, to identify the predictive value of ICA antibodies in such a general population, particularly when implementing a large-scale prevention programme. Only recently has this problem been confronted, producing results which, initially at least, do not appear to be very promising. It is in fact a well-established principle of statistical epidemiology (Bayes' Theorem) that the sensitivity and specificity of tests are not influenced by variations in disease prevalence. However, it would seem that this is not the case when evaluating the positive predictive value of such tests, which do seem to be influenced by disease prevalence in the group under investigation. None the less, providing sensitivity and specificity are equal, it has been established that the positive predictive value of a given test will be much higher, when disease prevalence is very high. In principle, if such theories are applied to IDDM and ICA, it would seem realistic to assume that the predictive value of ICA may be notably lower in the general population where disease prevalence is relatively low.

Experimental verification of such hypotheses is now possible thanks to a study being carried

Table 29.3. *Screening programme using ICA to identify subjects at risk for IDDM (comparison between two European regions)*

| | General population | | Brothers and sisters of IDDM patients | |
|---|---|---|---|---|
| | Oxfordshire (%) | Lombardy (%) | Oxfordshire (%) | Lombardy (%) |
| Type 1 diabetes prevalence | 0.21 | 0.09 | 2.8 | 2.1 |
| ICA prevalence >4 JDF units | 2.8 | 2.7 | 6.6 | 6.2 |
| ICA prevalence >20 JDF units | 0.8 | 0.3 | 2.2 | 4.1 |
| PV(+) ICA >4 JDF units | 8.7 | 3.9 | 56.7 | 48.9 |
| PV(+) ICA>20 JDF units | 33.9 | 18.0 | 87.5 | 83.6 |

PV=Positive predictive value.

out in the Oxford region in England among an extensive sample of school-aged children (11) (see Chapter 10). Similar data were reported for a similar study being carried out in Italy. The following factors have been observed in both regions:

i) Higher prevalence rates for ICA than IDDM have been observed among both the general population and families.
ii) The positive predictive value of ICA was notably lower in the general population in comparison with family groups (Table 29.3). In the study conducted in Lombardy, Italy, where other markers, such as anti-insulin antibodies (IAA) or genetic markers such as the HLA-DQβ57-Asp/negative and the DQα52-Arg/positive were used, the predictive value for them in the general population was even lower than the value obtained using ICA. Therefore, since the maximum positive predictive value of ICA is 34%, no screening campaign relying on a single test of ICA to identify subjects at risk for IDDM is likely to be implemented.

## Multiple screening tests for diabetes prediction

The use of multiple screening tests seems a more appropriate tool for IDDM prediction. Since no test, no matter how accurate it may be, can achieve 100% sensitivity or specificity, it follows that no screening programme aimed at targeting a relatively low frequency disease and relying on a single test, will be satisfactory from the point of view of predictive ability. This problem, as far as IDDM is concerned, can be overcome by using multiple screening tests (see Chapter 10). These tests can be carried out using a system of parallel procedure or a series of tests. The latter seems more appropriate for use in screening campaigns for IDDM, where a relatively simple initial screening test can be followed up by a series of more investigative as well as more costly (such as genetic phenotyping) investigations, which are none the less inappropriate for mass screening analysis and would appear to be more realistic for use in pre-selected campaigns.

An important point to keep in mind when implementing a multi-screening test programme, is that any new data arising from individual tests must first be evaluated independently of existing data; in other words, it is necessary to use tests which have the potential to illustrate specific pathogenic conditions at different time points and, finally, care must be taken to ensure that existing data on IDDM is not duplicated. However, it is possible that ICA, IAA and anti-GAD/64 kD antibodies reflect aspects or different degrees of the same phenomenon which, when combined, may be quite valuable in terms of improving disease prediction (12). Furthermore, although it has yet to be demonstrated, the use of HLA typing in association with ICA or other antibody measurement could result in more accurate disease prediction.

One advance in terms of IDDM prediction has been the so-called dual parameter model proposed by Eisenbarth and co-workers (13). By combining insulin antibodies (IAA) evaluation with insulin response during an *in vivo* glucose tolerance test (IVGTT, insulinaemia 1 + 3 min) in a group of first degree relatives of diabetic children with ICA, and assuming that there is a linear progression in beta cell mass destruction (a hypothesis still awaiting experimental verification), these authors have defined an accurate predictive model for the clinical onset of IDDM. However, this model can only be used in the final stage of pre-IDDM when beta cell function is impaired. In this context, the IVGTT can no longer be viewed as a screening test, but must be seen rather as a diagnostic test which allows the early diagnosis of a disease, as opposed to facilitating the identification of possible risk factors.

### Early diagnosis, accurate prediction, effective prevention

We now need to consider the link between early diagnosis, predictive accuracy and disease prevention effectiveness. In IDDM, the use of available markers in conjunction with new and more accurate techniques in disease prediction (increased sensitivity in testing has been achieved by combining multiple tests) has meant that the disease is being diagnosed at a much earlier stage than 20 years ago (14). This observation may have important implications for preventive therapy which should be implemented at the right time and not too early on in the disease process; otherwise it may target too many 'false positives' (individuals who test positively for the disease but who never go on to develop the overt form). On the other hand, if such procedures are implemented at a later stage in disease development they would certainly target a larger proportion of high risk groups. However, the latter approach may prove to be less effective if implemented at too late a stage in the natural history of the disease when therapeutic efficacy in preventing beta cell destruction is difficult to achieve. In Table 29.4, the requirements necessary for the use of specific drugs for intervention in pre-IDDM are illustrated.

Table 29.4. *Intervention in Type 1 pre-diabetes: selection criteria for drugs to be considered for preventive trials*

- disease prevention in animal models of IDDM
- no reduction in insulin secretion or increase in insulin resistance
- no reduction in growth or reproductive capacity
- no significant side-effects

## SECONDARY PREVENTION

### Free oxygen radical scavengers and their potential to protect beta cells

Since oxygen free radicals are involved in the process of immune-mediated damage to islet beta cells (4), free oxygen scavengers have been proposed for use in IDDM prevention. Thus, a large body of data has accumulated to suggest that free oxygen radical scavengers can prevent the spontaneous development of the disease in experimental animal models (15). Dexferioxamine, an inhibitor of hydroxide radical formation, and nicotinamide have been found to protect islet cells from immune destruction in islet graft rejection and subsequent disease recurrence (16). More recently, a potent antioxidant (Probucol) protects rat islets from the cytotoxic effects of cytokines and also prevents diabetes development in NOD mice (17). It is still not known whether the protective effect of this compound is caused by the reduction of cytokine-induced oxygen free radical production and lipid peroxidation in islet cells. In theory, all compounds capable of inhibiting oxygen free radical activity can be tested to prevent the development of IDDM at any stage before the clinical onset of acute hyperglycaemia. Such treatment is expected to be most valuable if therapy is started well before the formation of lymphocytic infiltration in the islets. It has already been ascertained that when massive lymphocytic infiltration is present (i.e. at the time of onset of hyperglycaemia), beta cell cytotoxicity is at its highest level. Thus, any beneficial effects of treatment with free oxygen radical scavengers may be limited at this stage of the disease process.

## Nicotinamide

We have seen that agents with a particular tropism for pancreatic beta cells or other cytotoxic factors can induce DNA damage either directly or via the generation of free oxygen radicals. Chemical compounds and physical factors which induce islet-DNA breaks could be aetiological factors in IDDM. Together with DNA breaks, there is also an increase in the activity of poly (ADP-ribose) polymerase which uses NAD for DNA repairing processes, thus reducing the intra-β cell NAD content required for insulin synthesis. As a NAD precursor, nicotinamide (NCT) increases insulin synthesis, thereby reducing the hyperglycaemia caused by partial pancreatectomy (18). Furthermore, the fact that poly (ADP-ribose) polymerase inhibitors induce pancreatic β-cell regeneration indicates that this enzyme may play a role in restricting β-cell replication. This concept is supported by the observation that poly-ADP-ribosylation suppresses DNA replication in rat nuclei and that NCT stimulates DNA synthesis in HeLa cells (19). Therefore IDDM is theoretically preventable through inhibiting poly (ADP-ribose) polymerase activity (20).

From a practical point of view, strategies for influencing the replication of islet β-cells and growth of the β-cell mass for IDDM may be important. By screening the regenerating islet-derived cDNA library, a novel gene expressed in regenerating islets was identified (21). The cDNA has one large open reading frame encoding for a 165-amino acid protein. This novel gene was called reg 1, i.e. regenerating gene, with the implication that the gene may be involved in islet regeneration. Reg 1 is, indeed, expressed in human and rat regenerating islets but not in normal islets. The increase in reg 1 gene expression is temporarily correlated with an increase in the number of β-cells in the regenerating islets.

The observation that the addition of NCT to a standard insulin regimen is able to increase β-cell function, which in turn could induce better metabolic control, may also be relevant in attempts to prevent the disease (9). Thus, treatment with NCT might be used safely in the early phases of the disease in susceptible individuals with immunological and metabolic markers suggestive of a progressive β-cell destruction.

The experience of Elliot in New Zealand has been crucial in determining that NCT is a favourable substance to use in controlled clinical trials to prevent IDDM; immunologically susceptible but still non-diabetic first degree relatives of IDDM probands, were apparently protected from developing IDDM by NCT (22). However, pilot studies conducted in the United States suggest that intervention with oral NCT may be ineffective in individuals with measurably impaired first phase insulin response (23). This suggests that NCT, if capable of preventing IDDM, may do so only when administered when there are no signs of metabolic impairment. Although the protective properties of NCT on beta cells can be envisaged at all ages, different autoimmune mechanisms of beta cell destruction may operate in the various phases of childhood and later life. Furthermore, it is generally accepted that IDDM develops faster in children compared with adults (24). Therefore, clinical trials aimed at evaluating the administration of NCT in the prevention of IDDM in children should reveal the relative effectiveness of the substance over a shorter observation time compared with adult subjects. For this reason the German Nicotinamide Intervention Trial (DENIS), for example, focuses on children below 12 years of age. Other studies, such as the European Nicotinamide Diabetes Intervention Trial (ENDIT), which include subjects up to the age of 40 who are at risk of developing the disease, address the question of the effectiveness of NCT at various ages.

Nicotinamide, which is essentially a vitamin, seems to be safer than most, if not all, of the immunomodulants tested to date, although its efficacy is still debated. Whether it is able to prevent overt IDDM when administered early enough can only be evaluated by a well-designed and sufficiently large multicentre project. Properly undertaken, the project should comprise a double-blind placebo, randomised, long-term prospective trial in first degree relatives with positive immune markers of the disease.

The dose of NCT to be adopted in trials for diabetes prevention may be one of the major problems that investigators dealing with this compound need to solve before embarking on the long perspective clinical enterprise which awaits them. When administered in solution in two separate doses for 14 days at 25 mg/kg/day to normal subjects, NCT had no effect on basal insulin levels, acute or total glucose stimulated release, glucose disposal and fasting or stimulated glucose insulin ratios (25). Furthermore, we did not observe any acute effect of NCT on insulin and C-peptide secretion in normal subjects within 1 hour following the administration of 25 mg/kg/body weight of NCT (26). Data in animal models have shown that the dose of NCT capable of preventing diabetes in the NOD mouse is at least 20 times higher than the dose that has been used in newly diagnosed IDDM.

Our work with the NOD mouse indicates that NCT doses need to be carefully considered. We investigated the effect of NCT in NOD mice from weaning to 30 weeks of age and found a similar incidence of diabetes in both control and experimental groups receiving a dose of 125 mg/kg/day body weight in their diet (27). Other studies have shown a reduction in the incidence of diabetes in NOD mice with a dose of 450 mg/kg/day body weight (28). In comparison, it should be noted that the dose normally administered in human trials is 25–50 mg/kg/day orally. Critical factors which determine whether NCT might prevent IDDM in humans should include, according to animal models, the dose, route of administration, and time of intervention in the pre-diabetic phase. Long-term trials in humans should therefore seriously consider not only the route of administration and the time of intervention, but also the effective dose that needs to be employed. Interestingly NCT may be available in the future in the form of slow release which could be a great advantage especially for patient compliance. So, when considering the possible effect of NCT either as a poly (ADP-ribose) polymerase inhibitor or as a free oxygen radical scavenger (the two effects may be dependent upon different doses), the dose used must be carefully evaluated and should be the first item to be widely discussed among researchers and investigators involved in trials of IDDM.

### Insulin

There is a great deal of interest in the use of insulin itself as a means to halt the progression of diabetes. Insulin therapy has been shown to delay the appearance and progression of insulitis in animal models of IDDM. Injection of young, pre-diabetic BB rats or NOD mice with insulin has been shown to inhibit the development of diabetes and the lymphocytic infiltration of the islet cells (insulitis) that precedes diabetes (29). Insulin therapy has also been shown to prevent the adoptive transfer of diabetes in the NOD mouse (30). Insulin may act either as an immune modulator (31), as an agent inducing tolerance or to temporarily block or 'rest' beta cell activity, thus making such cells less susceptible to immune attack (32). The beta cell rest hypothesis is that, by giving insulin before the development of overt disease, it is possible to reduce antigen expression associated with endogenous insulin secretion. *In vitro*, stimulated beta cells are more susceptible to immune attack, including cytotoxic actions of cytokines, than are resting beta cells.

In contrast to other interventions, which have generalised effects on the immune system, insulin has the advantages of being beta cell specific, not affecting other aspects of the immune

Table 29.5. *Insulin therapy in the prevention of IDDM*

*Rationale:*
- prevention of IDDM in animal models (only if given at weaning)
- reduction in the antigenicity associated with endogenous insulin secretion
- reduction in the expression of ganglioside antigens on beta cells
- induction of beta cell rest favouring possible beta cell regeneration
- similarity with the mechanism operating in autoimmune thyroid disease where thyroxine treatment reduces thyroid autoimmunity

*Against:*
- no evidence of a preventive effect is given close to the time of diabetes onset in animal models
- possible boost on insulin antibody production
- induction of hyperinsulinaemia in normal children
- ethical consideration
- difficulty of acceptance by the potential patient

system, well documented, with clearly defined side-effects which can be controlled. Table 29.5 summarises the *pros* and *cons* of the insulin approach in preventing Type 1 diabetes. This preventive attempt is currently under way in the form of a double blind trial in the USA (see list of ongoing trials).

## Monoclonal antibodies

The evidence that the immunological destruction of beta cells is mediated by activated T-lymphocytes supports a potential role for anti-T-lymphocyte therapy in the treatment of early IDDM diabetes. Monoclonal antibodies (MoAb) have been used in patients with newly diagnosed IDDM and some of these may be envisaged for use in subjects at risk for the disease.

### Anti-blast MoAb

Culler *et al.* (33) used the antiblast MoAb CBL1 within 1 month of diagnosis in four subjects (aged 4–13 years) without any apparent benefits being observed.

### Anti-CD3 MoAb

Cyclosporin plus either azathioprine and/or the anti-T-lymphocyte MoAb OKT3 are still being tested at the diagnosis of IDDM stage (34). The preliminary study was discontinued due to the severity of adverse effects of this treatment, including fever, headaches, arthralgia, and skin rash.

### Anti-CD5 immunoconjugate with ricin A chain

In an open-label, uncontrolled multi-centre pilot study, a MoAb anti-CD5 antigen has been used (35). The Moab antibody consists of a murine IgG directed against the CD5 antigen (which is present on the majority of mature lymphocytes).

### IL-2 conjugates with diphtheria toxin

An IL-2 receptor-targeted fusion protein, consisting of a diphtheria toxin-related protein, linked to IL-2 ($DAB^{486-}$ IL-2), conferred protection against diabetes induced by the adoptive transfer of diabetic spleen cells in NOD mice (36). Based on these results an open-label pilot study was initiated in patients with recent-onset IDDM (36). Patients were treated with 0.025–0.075 $mg/kg^{-1}/day^{-1}$ for 7 days followed by a tapering dose of cyclosporin. Preliminary data in 18 subjects showed a decrease in insulin dosage, good metabolic control, and preservation of beta cell function. The results are sufficiently promising to warrant initiation of a randomised controlled clinical trial.

## Photophoresis

The phototherapy procedure entails extracorporeal irradiation with ultraviolet-A light of lymphocytes treated with 8-methoxypsoralen. The treated cells are reinfused into the subject. The procedure lasts 4 to 5 hours. Harrison *et al.* (37) have used photophoresis in a pilot study in 17 subjects with recent onset IDDM and 3 with pre-diabetes. In the newly diagnosed IDDM patients, insulin requirement and HbA1c were stable over the first year and then deteriorated. Some patients showed a decrease in their *in vitro* T-lymphocyte response to specific and non-specific islet antigens, including GAD65 suggesting an immunomodulatory effect of this treatment. In combination with free oxygen radical scavengers, photophoresis is currently being used in recent onset IDDM and it may be considered for use in pre-diabetes in a larger trial.

## Oral antigen therapy

The idea that orally induced antigenic tolerance might be useful to interfere in autoimmune states has been proposed (38). In animals, ingestion of soluble, T-lymphocyte-dependent antigens usually establishes immunological tolerance whereas intradermal injection of these same antigens in a lipid adjuvant causes sensitization. This immunological dichotomy provides a mechanism to give protection from invading organisms, while at the same time preventing sensitisation by ingested foreign antigens particularly component food proteins.

Antigen-driven peripheral immuno-tolerance is a possible means of producing tolerance and immunological hypo-responsiveness (39). Oral administration of autoantigens suppresses autoimmunity, including experimental encephalomyelitis (40) and collagen induced arthritis (41). More recently a reduction in diabetes incidence in the NOD mouse was obtained by oral administration of insulin (42). However, protection from diabetes was not complete and the mechanism underlying the reduction in incidence has not been clarified, although a hypothesis of antigen-driven bystander suppression was proposed in an attempt to explain the mechanism of oral induced tolerance (43). In preliminary studies intragastric recombinant human GAD65 also resulted in less diabetes in NOD mice (personal communication).

A multicentre, double-blind, randomised controlled trial is being planned to determine whether induction of orally induced tolerance to islet cell antigens can delay and/or prevent the clinical onset IDDM. These studies seek to test the feasibility of abrogating the immune responses to endogenous insulin or GA65 through the oral administration of recombinant human insulin and/or human GAD65.

Table 29.6. *Main ongoing trials in IDDM pre-diabetes*

| Agent | Type of study | Responsible |
|---|---|---|
| Nicotinamide | open randomised | P Vague |
| Nicotinamide | open randomised | R Elliot |
| Nicotinamide | double blind | ENDIT Group |
| Nicotinamide | double blind | DENIS Group |
| Nicotinamide | double blind | CANADIAN Group |
| Insulin | pilot trial | A Ziegler |
| Insulin | placebo controlled | GS Eisenbarth |
| Cyclosporin | open trial | P Bougneres |
| Ketotifen | double blind | H Kolb |
| FK-506 | pilot trial | D Becker |
| DAB-486-IL2 | pilot trial | C Boitard |
| Photophoresis | open randomised | L Harrison |

Table 29.6 reports on the main trials currently under way for second prevention of IDDM.

## Beta cell growth and regeneration

Islet cell replication should be taken into account when partial beta cell damage has occurred, as in the case of subjects with immune markers of IDDM. Therapies aimed at blocking the autoimmune beta cell destructive process are being assessed, however stimulating replication and growth of beta cells may be an important option. In animal models, islet cell regeneration can be evaluated by using bromodeoxyuridine to measure the capacity of islet beta cells to replicate. In our experience, the proliferation of islet parenchymal cells within infiltrated islets during the pre-diabetic phase is comparable to non-infiltrated islets, indicating that the destructive process caused by infiltrating lymphocytes and their products does not promote regeneration of the islet parenchymal cells. Furthermore, there is no information regarding the influence of genetic background on beta cell regeneration. Although it is known that islet cell proliferation is genetically determined, the description of a gene expressed in regenerating rat islets coding for a 165 amino acid protein, has been a major step forward (21). However, this gene is only expressed in rats with 90% pancreatectomy or following therapy in animals with a poly ADP ribose polymerase inhibitor, such as nicotinamide. These data are encouraging and may prove an interesting approach.

However, the limitation of the total regenerative capacity, as indicated by the size of the proliferative compartment, determines whether compensatory growth of the remaining beta cells could be successful in IDDM prevention. There is no question that this capacity depends on a preset genetic factor and on the age of the individual at the time of beta cell failure.

Up to this point we have not included the genetic background in the preventive therapeutic strategy though the response of beta cells to an autoimmune attack may depend upon the HLA background of affected subjects. This theory is supported by the observation that differences in the capacity for islet cell replication have been demonstrated in rats of different strains. Since certain HLA haplotypes are associated with the development of IDDM (22), it would appear that the capacity of islet cells to proliferate is only partially determined by the development of autoimmune diabetes. We should conclude by saying that the early insurgence of beta cell growth and development confers a lifelong limitation in the ability to increase beta cell mass and insulin production in response to diabetogenic stimuli. This opens up new perspectives for investigation, focusing in particular on the identification of subjects who are prone to develop the disease and therefore promoting implementation of earlier treatment.

## TERTIARY PREVENTION: IMMUNOINTERVENTION AT THE TIME OF CLINICAL DIAGNOSIS

Data from the Eurodiab subarea A study on the incidence and mode of presentation of childhood IDDM in Europe (44) confirm that IDDM is currently diagnosed at a stage when some beta cell function is still preserved. This is particularly true in patients over 15 years of age at diagnosis.

Based on our present knowledge of the pathogenesis of the disease, administration of an immuno-toxin or an immunosuppressive agent to T-lymphocyte subsets involved in beta cell killing may be considered in the last phase of the pre-diabetic process and at the time of clinical diagnosis. Immunotoxins, known as conjugates of a toxin by an enzymatic method to monoclonal antibodies, are directed towards antigens expressed on the cell surface and, at present, are used mainly in tumour therapy. The use of monoclonal antibody anti-T lymphocytes (CD5) conjugated with ricin in early phases of IDDM has already been proposed at diagnosis (35). A serious limitation to the use of immunotoxins is that foreign proteins induce the formation of neutralising antibodies, thus precluding prolonged and repeated treatment. This may significantly limit the duration of therapy, but the use of chimeric monoclonal antibodies and a panel of immunologically irrelevant toxins may resolve some of the inherent difficulties.

A short course of immunosuppressive therapy combined with agents capable of beta cell regeneration may be adopted at the time of clinical diagnosis. During the course of the cytotoxic process, the capacity of beta cells to regenerate may be limited by persistence of the autoimmune process. Therefore, therapy in the early stages of overt IDDM, when some beta cell mass is still present, could involve suppressing the immune response over a short term with immunosuppressive therapy, while at the same time facilitating the replication of beta cells using a compound such as nicotinamide. The addition of nicotinamide in insulin therapy at diagnosis reduces the insulin dose required to normalise blood glucose levels and may even preserve residual beta cell function (45). Not only is it clinically easier to control the disease with small insulin doses but a low incidence of microvascular complications is usually reported in patients with some residual beta cell function; this encourages the adoption of some sort of adjunct therapy to insulin at clinical diagnosis of IDDM.

Interesting observations in animal models of IDDM, in particular the NOD mouse, indicate that free oxygen radical scavengers may be useful even if given in the late phase of beta cell destruction because of their effect in protecting beta cells from cytokine-mediated cytotoxicity. Compounds worth mentioning in this respect are acetylcysteine, glutathione and vitamin E since they produce no side-effects.

In summary, earlier diagnosis of IDDM coupled with short-term immunosuppressive therapy and agents capable of protecting residual beta cell function are the tools which are currently available as adjuncts to intensified insulin therapy for tertiary prevention.

Results from the two most well-known IDDM immunotherapy studies, both of which were multi-centre and double blind (46, 47), have shown that when used in the initial phase of the disease, the immunosuppressive approach is capable of extending clinical remission by as much as 20 to 30 % (suspension of insulin treatment). However, it has also been observed that, within two years of clinical diagnosis (after suspension of adjuvant therapy), the percentage of clinical remission observed does not differ substantially from that recorded for patients treated with insulin only (rarely more than 2%). Furthermore, the fact that this treatment yields very poor results on a long-term basis, together with the added danger of renal complications, have understandably raised some doubts as to the value of cyclosporin in the treatment of IDDM at diagnosis. None the less, the adoption of immunotherapy in the treatment of this disease has proved to be particularly effective. Further studies should be based on a specific pathogenic hypothesis with a clear goal.

Table 29.7. *Recommendations of the International Diabetes Immunotherapy Group for trials in the prevention of IDDM*

- definition of the pre-clinical stage (ICA, IAA, HLA, metabolic changes)
- definition of objectives (these may not be limited to simple prevention of the disease)
- informed consent even when studies with vitamins are being carried out
- trials to be conducted only in Centres with experience in the field of diabetes prevention and immunotherapy

One of the most debated aspects concerning immunotherapy trials has been the standardisation of the parameters for measuring remission data and issuing recommendations for those conducting trials (Table 29.7). The International Diabetes Immunotherapy Group (IDIG) has been instrumental in bringing about a final agreement on the reporting of remission data (48). The term clinical remission is now used to define the suspension of insulin therapy for at least 4 weeks, maintaining normal blood glucose values before, and 2 hours after meals, and in particular, normal levels of glycated haemoglobin. The term partial remission has now been abolished and replaced by integrated parameters of metabolic control so as to reflect the partial therapeutic effect this form of therapy can achieve. The term encompasses the calculation of insulin requirements (Units/kg body weight), measurement of glycated haemoglobin and evaluation of beta cell function by measuring baseline and stimulated C peptide. Depending on the study hypothesis proposed, other clinical and immunological parameters (e.g. ICA, anti GAD antibodies, etc.) can be evaluated and should therefore be included in the study protocol. Given that comparison of results from various trials is essentially dependent on a uniform procedure for evaluating control parameters, it seems practical to aim towards standardisation of methods used to measure beta cell function and peripheral insulin sensitivity, and IDIG are currently working towards this goal.

Finally, it must be stressed that immunotherapy treatment in IDDM at diagnosis remains an experimental approach to be used only in those research centres with a well-established background in the use of such therapy and with experience of immunological studies. This is a particularly relevant factor when subjects at risk for the disease are being considered for treatment. It is clear therefore that trials which do not implement IDIG guidelines should be actively discouraged.

## REFERENCES


1 Atkinson M, Maclaren NK. What causes diabetes? *Sci Am* 1990; 262: 61–71.

2 Wilson K, Eisenbarth GS. Immunopathogenesis and immunotherapy of type 1 diabetes. *Ann Rev Med* 1990; 41: 497–508.

3 Campbell IL, Harrison LC. Molecular pathology of type 1 diabetes. *Mol Biol Med* 1990; 7: 299–309.

4 Nerup J, Mandrup-Poulsen T, Molvig J, Helqvist S, Wogensen L, Egeberg J. Mechanisms of pancreatic β-cell destruction in type 1 diabetes. *Diabetes Care* 1990; 11 (Suppl. 1): 16–23.

5 Cavallo MG, Baroni MG, Toto A *et al.* Viral infection induces cytokine release by beta cells. *Immunology* 1992; 75: 664–8.

6 Mandrup-Poulsen T, Helqvist S, Wogensen LD *et al.* Cytokines and free radicals as effector molecules in the destruction of pancreatic beta cells. *Curr Top Microbiol Immunol* 1990; 164: 169–93.

7 Oberley LW. Free radicals and diabetes. *Free Radical Biol Med* 1988; 5: 113–24.

8 Kolb H, Kolb-Bachoen V. Type 1 (insulin-dependent) diabetes mellitus and nitric oxide *Diabetologia* 1992; 35: 796–7.

9 Pozzilli P, Andreani D. Nicotinamide, a vitamin with the potential to prevent type 1 diabetes *Diab Metab Rev* 1993; 9: 219–30.

10 Karjalainen J, Martin JM, Knip M *et al.* A bovine albumin peptide as a possible trigger of insulin dependent diabetes mellitus, *N Engl J Med* 1992; 327: 302–7.

11 Bingley PJ, Bonifacio E, Shattock M. *et al.* Can islet cell antibodies predict insulin dependent diabetes in the general population? *Diabetes Care* 1993; 16: 45–50.

12 PJ Bingley, Christie MR, Bonfanti R *et al.* Combined analysis of autoantibodies enhances prediction of IDDM in islet cell antibody (ICA) positive relatives, *12th International Immunology Diabetes Workshop: American Diabetes Association*, Orlando 15–18 April, 1993, p. 76 (Abstract).

13 Ziegler AG, Ziegler R, Vardi P, Jackson RA, Soeldner JS, Eisenbarth GS. Life-table analysis of progression to diabetes of anti-insulin autoantibody-positive relatives of individuals with type 1 diabetes. *Diabetes* 1989; 38: 1320–5.

14 Pozzilli P, Andreani D. Type 1 diabetes at presentation, the scene changes. *Diab Med* 1990; 7: 762–3.

15 Boitard C, Timsit J, Sempe P, Back JF. Experimental immunoprevention of type 1 diabetes mellitus. *Diab Metab Rev* 1991; 7: 15–33.

16 Nomikos IN, Prowse SJ, Carotenuto P, Lafferty KJ. Combined treatment with nicotinamide and desferrioxamine prevents islet allograft destruction in NOD mice. *Diabetes* 1986; 35: 1302.

17 Fukada M, Ikegami H, Kawaguchi Y, Fujioka Y, Tahara Y, Hattori M, Ogihara T. Probucol inhibits generation of free radical oxygen in islet cells and prevents cyclophosphamide induced diabetes in NOD mice. *Diab Res Clin Pract* 14(1): W1-P26, 1991 (Abstract).

18 Yonemura Y, Takashima T, Miwa K, Miyazaki I, Yamamoto H, Okamoto H. Amelioration of diabetes mellitus in partially depancreatized rats by poly (ADP-ribose) synthetase inhibitors. *Diabetes* 1984; 33: 401–3.

19 Okamo H. The role of poly (ADP-ribose) synthetase in the development of insulin-dependent diabetes and islet B-cell regeneration. *Biomed Biochim Acta* 1985; 44: 15–20.

20 Okamato H. In: Okamoto H, ed. *Molecular biology of the islets of Langerhans*. Cambridge University Press, Cambridge, 1990; 209–231.

21 Terazono K, Yamamoto H, Takasawa S *et al.* A novel gene activated in regenerating islets. *J Biol Chem* 1988; 263: 2111–14.

22 Elliot RB, Chase HP. Prevention or delay of type 1 (insulin-dependent) diabetes in children using nicotinamide. *Diabetologia* 1991; 34: 362–6.

23 Herskowitz RD, Jackson RA, Soeldner JS, Eisenbarth GS. Pilot trial to prevent type 1 diabetes: progression to overt IDDM despite oral nicotinamide. *Autoimmun* 1989; 2: 733–7.

24 Palmer JP, McCulloch DK. Prediction and prevention of IDDM. *Diabetes* 1991; 40: 943–7.

25 Bingley PJ, Calsa G, Bonfanti R, Gale EAM. Nicotinamide and insulin secretion in normal subjects. *Diabetologia* 1992; 35: A217, 838.

26 Pozzilli P, Boccuni ML, Visalli N. Nicotinamide does not change acutely C-peptide and insulin secretion in normal subjects. *Diab Nutr Metab* 1993; 6: 159–61.

27 Beales P, Xu S, Williams A. Nicotinamide dose and protection from diabetes in: *Diabetes prevention and therapy*, John Wiley and Sons, Chichester, 1992; 6: 18–19.

28 Reddy S, Bibby NJ, Elliott RB. Early nicotinamide treatment in the NOD mouse: effects on diabetes, insulitis suppression and autoantibody levels. *Diabetes Res* 1990; 15: 95–102.

29 Vlahos WD, Seemayer TA, Yale JF. Diabetes prevention in BB rats by inhibition of endogenous insulin secretion. *Metabolism* 1991; 40:825–9.

30 Atkinson MA, Maclaren NK, Luchetta R. Insulitis and insulin dependent diabetes in NOD mice reduced by prophylactic insulin therapy. *Diabetes* 1990; 39: 933–7.

31 Peakman M, Hussain MJ, Millward BA, Leslie RDG, Bargani D. Effect of initiation of insulin therapy on T-lymphocyte activation in type 1 diabetes. *Diab Med* 1990; 7:327–30.

32 Aaen K, Rygard J, Josenson K, Petersen H, Brogren CH, Horn T, Buschard K. Dependence of antigen expression on functional state of cells. *Diabetes* 1990; 39:697–701.

33 Culler FL, O' Connor R, Kaufmann S, Jones KL, Roteh JC. Immunospecific therapy for type 1 diabetes mellitus. *N Engl J Med* 1985; 313:695–6.
34 Bach JF, Feuteren G, Boitard C. Immunoprevention of insulin-dependent diabetes by cyclosporin. In: Andreani D, Kolb H, Pozzilli P, eds. *Immunotherapy of Type 1 diabetes*. Chichester, John Wiley & Sons Ltd, 1989.
35 Skyler JS, Byers V, Einhorn D *et al.* Effects of an anti-CD5 immunoconjugate (H65-RTA) on pancreatic islet beta cell function in type 1 diabetes mellitus. *Diabetes Res Clin Prac* 1991; 14 (Suppl. 1):S54 (Abstract).
36 Boitard C, Timsit J, Assan *et al.* Treatment of type 1 diabetes mellitus with $DAB_{486}$-IL-2, a toxin conjugate which targets activated T-lymphocytes. *Diabetologia* 1992; 35 (Suppl. 1):A218 (Abstract).
37 Harrison LC, Honeyman M, Steele C, Graham M. Photophoresis trial in IDDM: an interim report. *Proc Aust Diabetes Soc* 1992: 91.
38 Thompson HSG, Staines NA. Could specific oral tolerance be a therapy for autoimmune disease? *Immunol Today* 1990; 11:396–9.
39 Shizuru JA, Edwards-Taylor C, Banks B, Gregory AK, Fathman CG. Immunotherapy of the non-obese diabetic mouse: treatment with an antibody to T-helper lymphocytes. *Science* 1988; 240:659–66.
40 Lider O, Santos LMB, Lee CSY, Higgins PJ, Weiner HL. Suppression of experimental autoimmune encephalomyelitis by oral administration of myelin basic protein. II. Suppression of disease and of immune responses are mediated by antigen-specific CD8+ T lymphocytes. *J Immunol* 1989; 142:748–52.
41 Zhang ZJ, Davidson L, Eisenbarth G, Weiner HL. Suppression of adjuvant arthritis in Lewis rats by oral administration of type II collagen. *J Immunol* 1990; 145: 2489–93.
42 Zhang ZJ, Davidson L, Eisenbarth G, Weiner HL. Suppression of diabetes in non obese diabetic mice by oral administration of insulin. *Proc Natl Sci USA* 1991; 88: 10252–6.
43 Miller AM, Lider O, Weiner HL. Antigen-driven bystander suppresion after oral administration of antigens. *J Exp Med* 1991; 174: 791–8.
44 Green A, Gale EAM, Patterson CC, for the EURODIAB ACE Study Group. Incidence of childhood onset insulin-dependent diabetes mellitus: the EURODIAB ACE Study. *Lancet* 1992; 339: 905–9.
45 Pozzilli P, Visalli N, Ghirlanda G, Manna R, Andreani D. Nicotinamide increases C-peptide secretion in patients with recent onset type 1 diabetes. *Diabetic Med* 1989; 6: 568–72.
46 Feutren G, Assan R, Karsenty G *et al.* Cyclosporin increases the rate and length of remission in insulin-dependent diabetes of recent onset. *Lancet* 1986; 2: 119.
47 Canadian European Randomized Control Trial Group (CERCTG). Cyclosporin induced remission of IDDM. *Diabetes* 1988; 37: 1574.
48 Kolb H, Bach JF, Eisenbarth GS *et al.* Criteria for immune trials in Type 1 diabetes, *Lancet* 1989; ii: 686 (Letter).

# 30 Treatment of Early Diabetic Renal Disease, with Special Reference to Antihypertensive Therapy

Carl Erik Mogensen

Early renal disease in diabetes is frequently associated with elevated blood pressure, which is usually moderate, but sometimes there is only minor increase which is only detectable by careful monitoring, e.g. 24 h ambulatory recordings (1). The elevation of blood pressure is found in both types of diabetes, but there seem to be several differences in the aetiology of hypertension, comparing IDDM patients with NIDDM patients. Some of the differences are clearly explained by the different aetiology and nature of the diabetic state (2). Obviously, in NIDDM patients, greater age, increased body weight, as well as insulin resistance and related hyperinsulinaemia may be important factors. Also hypertension related to renal impairment is often seen in NIDDM patients. However, the renal genesis of hypertension is much more predominant in the usually relatively young IDDM patients (3).

In recent years there has been a growing interest in the nature of renal disease and blood pressure elevation in diabetes (4–8). The reason is obvious: usually two or more risk factors must co-exist to provoke serious organ damage. One risk factor may not be sufficient, and translated into diabetes this means that some degree of poor glycaemic control may not always be deleterious, unless another risk factor is present, e.g. elevated blood pressure. Many other risk factors may compete also in the diabetic patient to provoke vascular damage, e.g. lipid abnormalities, smoking, obesity, overeating. This means that the metabolic syndrome, or syndrome X, is important (9, 10). Also a high protein intake may play a role as an aggravating factor. A clustering of genetic factors is also likely to be involved. Importantly, diabetic renal disease tends to accumulate in families (11) possibly related to poor metabolic control clustering in certain families (12).

Comparing the different risk factors, in addition to poor metabolic control, blood pressure elevation seems to be not only the most important factor related to organ damage, but also the most easily measurable and modifiable factor. Almost all studies agree that standard medical antihypertensive treatment is able to reduce blood pressure in diabetes (13). Many studies (4, 14) have confirmed the original observation of a beneficial impact of antihypertensive treatment on diabetic renal disease (15, 16), also with combination therapy (17).

A striking similarity exists between the consequences of blood pressure elevation and hyperglycaemia. The degree of hyperglycaemia and elevated blood pressure we observe in most of our patients does not cause significant symptoms. Rather the two risk factors produce long-term vascular damage, both in the microvasculature and in large vessels, and, importantly, they may act in a synergistic way to produce vascular damage. There are several proposed mechanisms of elevated blood pressure in diabetic patients but it is important to stress the renal hypertension, which is so common in diabetes. Sodium retention induced hypertension may be an important factor, related to both renal abnormalities as well as hyperinsulinaemia, of endogenous or exogenous origin. Thus the insulin-related mechanisms (related to the kidney) will also be discussed briefly. It is important to note that isolated systolic hypertension is not uncommon in older diabetic patients, often associated with macrovascular disease of arteriosclerotic nature. The question of dietary protein in the genesis and in particular in the treatment of early renal disease will also be discussed.

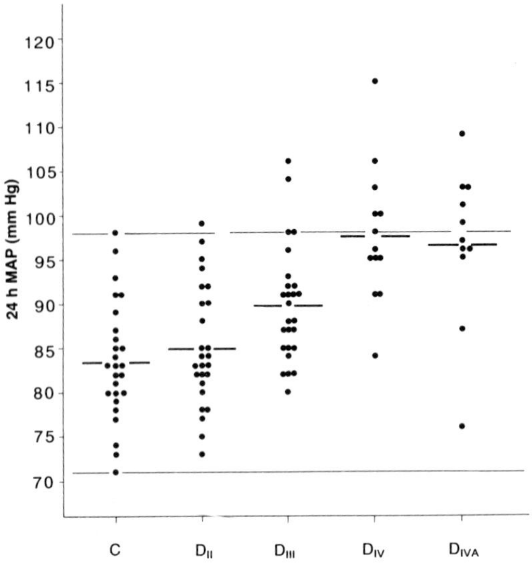


Fig. 30.1. 24 h mean blood pressure in healthy controls (C, $n = 26$), normoalbuminuric IDDM patients ($D_{II}$, $n = 26$), microalbuminuric patients ($D_{III}$, $n = 6$), patients with overt nephropathy without antihypertensive treatment ($D_{IV}$, $n = 13$) and patients with overt nephropathy and antihypertensive treatment ($D_{IVA}$, $n = 11$). Horizontal lines indicate range for healthy controls. (Provided by K. W. Hansen, M.D.)

## EXTENT OF THE PROBLEM

### Degree of blood pressure elevation in diabetes

Very high blood pressure levels are very rarely observed in diabetic patients, and would be mostly recognised in populations where no structured care for hypertension in diabetic patients exists. An increase in blood pressure is a self-perpetuating process, not only in diabetic but also non-diabetic individuals. Interestingly, in diabetes renal damage, as evidenced by abnormal albuminuria, also seems to be a self-perpetuating process. It is suggested that increased traffic of plasma proteins (3, 18), e.g. albumin, may produce vascular damage in glomeruli, especially in the mesangial regions, thereafter resulting in elevated blood pressure. This hypothesis remain to be tested in humans.

However, with proper antihypertensive programmes the extent of elevation of blood pressure is not as pronounced as in earlier years (19). Thus in studies where 24-hour blood pressure recordings in diabetic patients are compared to levels in non-diabetic patients (1, 20), the blood pressure is only elevated by about 5 mmHg on average in microalbuminuric patients (Fig. 30.1). Obviously such data are biased, because patients already on treatment are excluded. On the other hand, even minor blood pressure elevation may produce vascular damage, especially when co-existing with another risk factor, e.g. hyperglycaemia. A correlation exists between albuminuria and blood pressure (see Fig. 30.2) and the association is much stronger when 24 ambulatory blood pressure values are used rather than ordinary clinic based blood pressures (1). Diabetic patients may be particularly sensitive to systemic blood pressure elevation, because the normal protection exerted by the renal arteriolar vasculature is likely to be disturbed in them.

On considering previous data, it is clear that blood pressure elevation used to be higher (19,

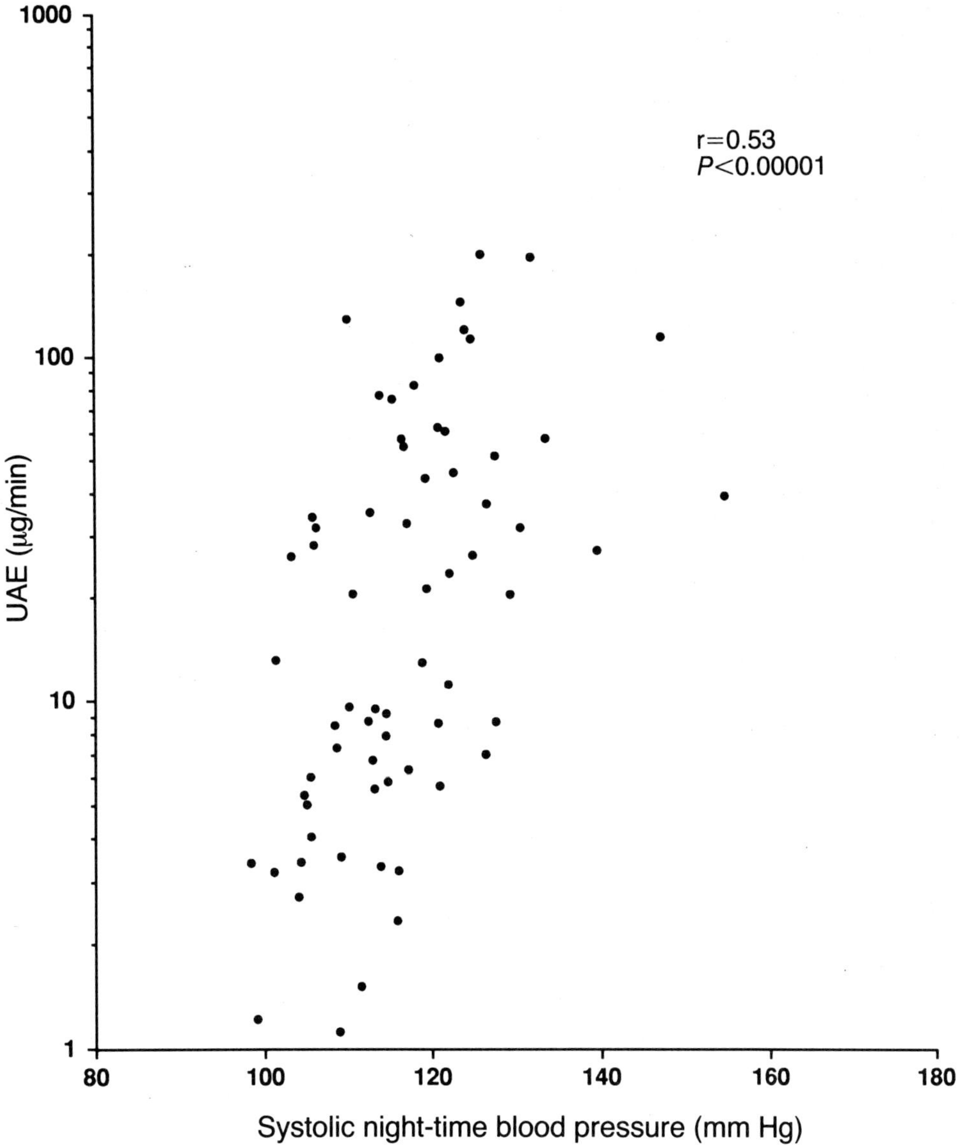


Fig. 30.2. Correlation between overnight UAE (log scale) and systolic night time value (r = 0.53, *P* <0.00001) in IDDM patients (*n* = 68). (Provided by K. W. Hansen, M.D.)

21). Thus, a pronounced fall in recorded blood pressure has been observed during the last decade, which is also evident from a study from the Steno Diabetes Center, where blood pressure levels in cohorts of patients from the 1960s were compared to those in the 1980s (19). A pronounced reduction could be found, which could be explained by the availability today of effective antihypertensive agents without serious side-effects. Importantly, all evidence suggests that survival has also been greatly improved by modern antihypertensive intervention (19).

### Prevalence of hypertension

Interesting differences exist between the two types of diabetes: in IDDM, the prevalence of hypertension is clearly associated to the degree of abnormal albuminuria (Table 30.1) (22). With normal albumin, excretion rate is close to the prevalence of hypertension in that of a normal population, which is also observed in recent studies using 24-hour blood pressure recording (see Fig. 30.1). Once microalbuminuria is detected there is a dramatic increase in the prevalence of elevated blood pressure (see Table 30.1), and even more marked changes are seen with overt diabetic nephropathy. Thus, a clear relationship exists in IDDM between hypertension and renal disease.

In NIDDM the picture is more complex, although there is usually an association between the degree of abnormal albuminuria and blood pressure (23). However, this correlation is weaker than in IDDM. The prevalence of blood pressure elevation is high in the elderly NIDDM patients, even at clinical diagnosis, about 30–40% of such patients show an elevated blood pressure or receive antihypertensive treatment (24, 25). In a control population without diabetes this figure may be 20% (23). The rate of blood pressure elevation increases with an increase in duration of diabetes and higher age frequency (23–25). Interestingly the blood pressure elevation in NIDDM patients is usually systolic (26) and may be in part related to the metabolic syndrome.

There is a continual increase in elevated blood pressure with time in IDDM patients in particular in association with microalbuminuria or overt proteinuria (27–29), supporting the idea that this is a self-perpetuating process. This increase in hypertension rates with time is mainly observed in IDDM patients though data are difficult to obtain in NIDDM as many patients are treated and discontinuation of treatment is not advisable. In IDDM, rates of hypertension may increase by 2–3% per year in microalbuminuria (27), and about 6% per year in overt renal disease (28). Such data may be difficult to reproduce today, simply because so many patients are early and effectively treated.

Table 30.1. *Prevalence of hypertension (%) in IDDM patients aged 30–39 years*

| | Women | Men |
|---|---|---|
| Background population | 1.7 | 3.1 |
| Normoalbuminuria | 2.2 | 3.1 |
| Microalbuminuria | 26.7 | 15.4 |
| Proteinuria | 85.5 | 77.8 |

Hypertension, blood pressure ≥160/95 mmHg or receiving antihypertensive therapy, possibly started at level <160/95 (Nørgaard *et al.*, 1990) (22).

## ENDPOINTS IN RENAL DISEASE AND DIABETES AS RELATED TO HYPERTENSION AND DIETARY PROTEIN INTAKE

A key question in diabetic nephrology is to define parameters that can be considered important intermediary or final endpoints, indicating disease activity and poor outcome (see Table 30.2). This is of special importance in intervention trials and in the daily treatment of patients, where results from trials are quickly reflected in clinical management. An outline of the natural history of renal disease in IDDM patients is given in Fig. 30.3.

It has been known for many years that hypertensive proteinuric diabetic patients carry a poor prognosis (30–32). It has also become clear that abnormal albuminuria in the microalbuminuric range (20–200 μg/min) is an important long-term predictor for poor outcome (3, 33, 34). Another important parameter is the rate of fall of GFR as measured by exact and reproducible techniques (36). Either end-stage renal failure (ESRF) or death are clear endpoints, but in patients with early clinical proteinuria or advanced microalbuminuria, this would be a very distant endpoint since the time to develop-

Table 30.2. *The solid endpoint: GFR fall rate related to intermediary endpoints in diabetic patients*

| Intermediary endpoints | GFR fall (Young IDDM patients) | GFR fall (Middle-aged NIDDM patients) |
|---|---|---|
| Microalbuminuria (20–200 µg/min) | Fall in GFR only seen with progression to proteinuria | Fall rate of GFR not significantly different from normoalbuminuria |
| Proteinuria (macroalbuminuria, >200 µg/min) | Clear fall in GFR (Reduced by antihypertensive treatment) | Clear fall in GFR High mortality |
| Elevated blood pressure or hypertension | Controversy exists, but a clear risk factor with co-existing abnormal albuminuria | Risk factor along with proteinuria Controversy exists, but a clear risk factor with co-existing abnormal albuminuria |

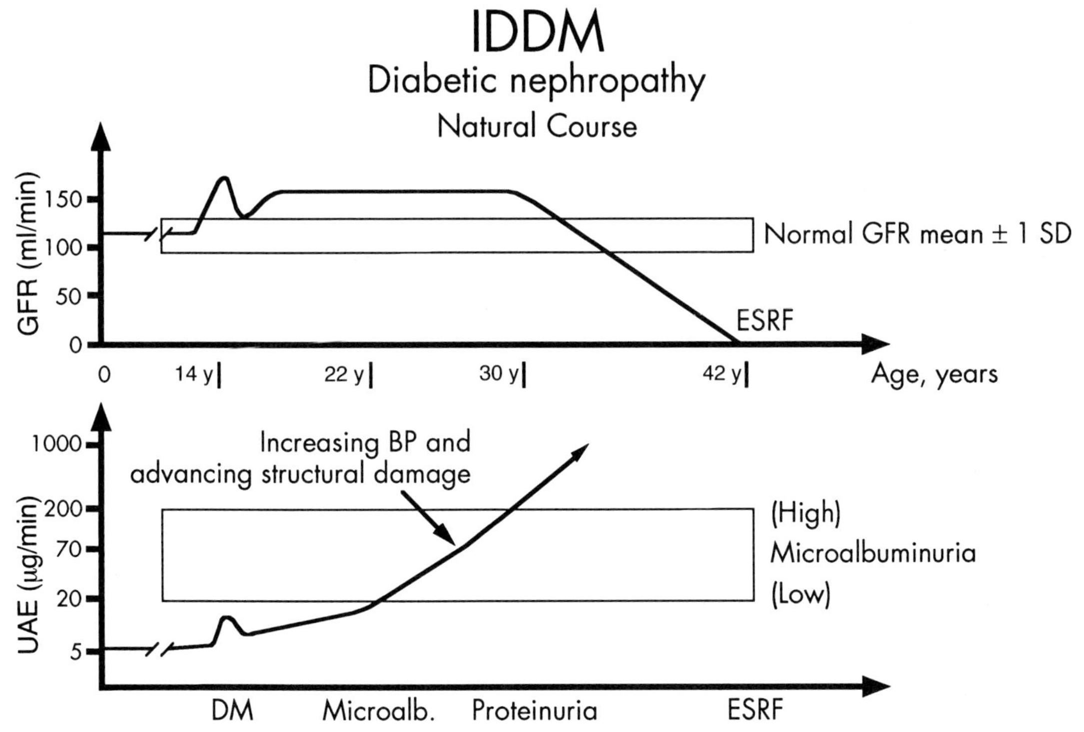


Fig. 30.3. Natural history of renal changes in IDDM patients.

ment of ESRF may last one or two decades, especially with antihypertensive treatment (19). Blood pressure elevation may be an endpoint, but it is likely that this factor is more an effect parameter, although there is an intriguing relationship between elevated blood pressure and abnormal albuminuria, both of which probably relate to rates of fall of GFR (19, 35).

Evidence suggests that abnormal albuminuria is a key parameter and an important intermediary end-point in the follow-up of all diabetic patients, not only because it is closely related to the more final endpoints, but also because this parameter can be used in treatment strategies

Table 30.3. *Stability or change in GFR and albuminuria in IDDM (without antihypertensive treatment)*

| Reference and designation in Fig. 30.4 | Number of patients | Mean diabetes duration (years) | Follow-up period (month) | Albumin excretion mean of period μg/min (geometric mean ×/÷ confidence factor | GFR (ml/min) Initial→follow-up | Blood pressure (mean of period) |
|---|---|---|---|---|---|---|
| From Christensen *et al.*, 1987) (A) | 12 | 8 | 24 | 4.8×/÷1.3 | 138→139* | 113/77 |
| Mau Pedersen [unpublished] ($B_1$) | 7 | 21±6 | 14 | 29.9×/÷1.4 | 147→146* | 121/80 |
| From Christensen & Mogensen, 1987 ($B_2$) | 6 | 20 | 78 | 84.5×/÷1.5 | 142→141* | 134/87 |
| From Feldt-Rasmussen *et al.*, 1991*a* ($C_1$) | 15 | 15 | ≈78 | ≈36 | 116→116** | 128/82 |
| From Mathiesen *et al.*, 1991 ($C_2$) | 16 | 17 | 48 | 55.6×/÷1.2 | 117→114** | 125/76 |
| From Mathiesen *et al.*, 1991 ($C_3$) | 7 | 17 | 48 | 268.7×/÷1.1 | Fall in GFR** 0.33 ml/min/month | 127/80 |
| From Mogensen, 1976 (D) | 7 | 18±2 | 28 | 2689.7×/÷1.3 | Fall in GFR* 0.96 ml/min/month | 161/101 |

* Constant infusion technique for GFR determination.
** Single-sheet procedure for GFR determination.

for controlled clinical trials, as well as in the day-to-day management of patients.

## RESULTING ACUTE SYMPTOMS AND LONG-TERM ORGAN DAMAGE

Acute symptoms related to elevated blood pressure in diabetes are extremely rare. Usually the blood pressure elevation is totally asymptomatic and only observed because it is routine to record blood pressure in diabetic patients. Blood pressure elevation could be considerable (21), and used to be found in conjunction with a nephrotic syndrome (19). Oedema is extremely rare today because of effective diuretic treatment. Still, many patients may exhibit asymptomatic sodium retention.

The main interest in blood pressure elevation in diabetes relates to the long-term effect of elevated blood pressure on the micro- and macro-vasculature. Thus, lesions may develop over many years, eventually resulting in severe organ dysfunction or total failure, e.g. uraemia, blindness related to diabetic retinopathy or heart failure where hypertension also may also be a promoting factor.

### Diabetic nephropathy: relationship between abnormal albuminuria/blood pressure elevation and decline in GFR in IDDM

Table 30.3 and Fig. 30.4 summarise data from several studies (15, 36–40) where the relationship between albuminuria and rate of change in GFR was examined in 70 patients studied for a mean of 3.3 years. It is clear that patients with normal albumin excretion rate preserve intact renal function even in long-term studies ($\approx$ 12 y) (3), although with extremely long follow-up ($\approx$ 20 y) there may be a small, probably age-related, reduction in GFR (33). Patients with persistent microalbuminuria usually maintain intact renal function (see Table 30.3), but then a subsequent fall in GFR can be predicted. Thus, with the development of proteinuria there is a significant decline in GFR (39, 40). Feldt-Rasmussen *et al.* (39) also observed a significant drop in GFR with the development of clinical nephropathy (UAE $>$ 300 mg/24 h) but most of their patients received antihypertensive treatment which modifies the level of UAE and GFR. In patients with more advanced renal disease a very significant rate of fall in GFR is seen of an average 10 ml/min/year (see Fig. 30.3) (15). This same study also showed glomerular hyperfiltration in microalbuminuric patients without a time-dependent decline in GFR (15).

In IDDM patients with elevated blood pressure, but normal albumin excretion rate, Nørgaard *et al.* (41) documented well-preserved renal function. These patients may have essential hypertension and diabetes; in them the level of elevated blood pressure *per se* ($\approx$ 150/95) is not an immediate risk factor for decline in GFR, unless patients show microalbuminuria or overt diabetic nephropathy. It should be noted that most hypertensive patients in this study were under treatment which was discontinued 4 weeks before the investigations (41) and that there are certain differences in GFR values as measured by different techniques. It is likely that the single-shot-procedure systematically underestimates GFR by 10–15%, while the constant infusion technique provides a more correct value.

In conclusion, it is likely that abnormal albuminuria is the main marker, or even risk determinant, of a decline in renal function, although the nature of the initial permeability defect is not yet explained. As discussed by Remuzzi established albuminuria in itself may promote renal damage (18), either by increased transglomerular traffic of proteins leading to further glomerular damage or increased tubular reabsorption rate of albumin. The latter may cause interstitial damage, which could lead to structural damage in glomeruli. Another hypothesis to explain this self-perpetuating process involves glomerular hyperfiltration. Patients with some decline in GFR due to nephron closure are likely to show single nephron hyperfiltration in their remaining glomeruli. On the

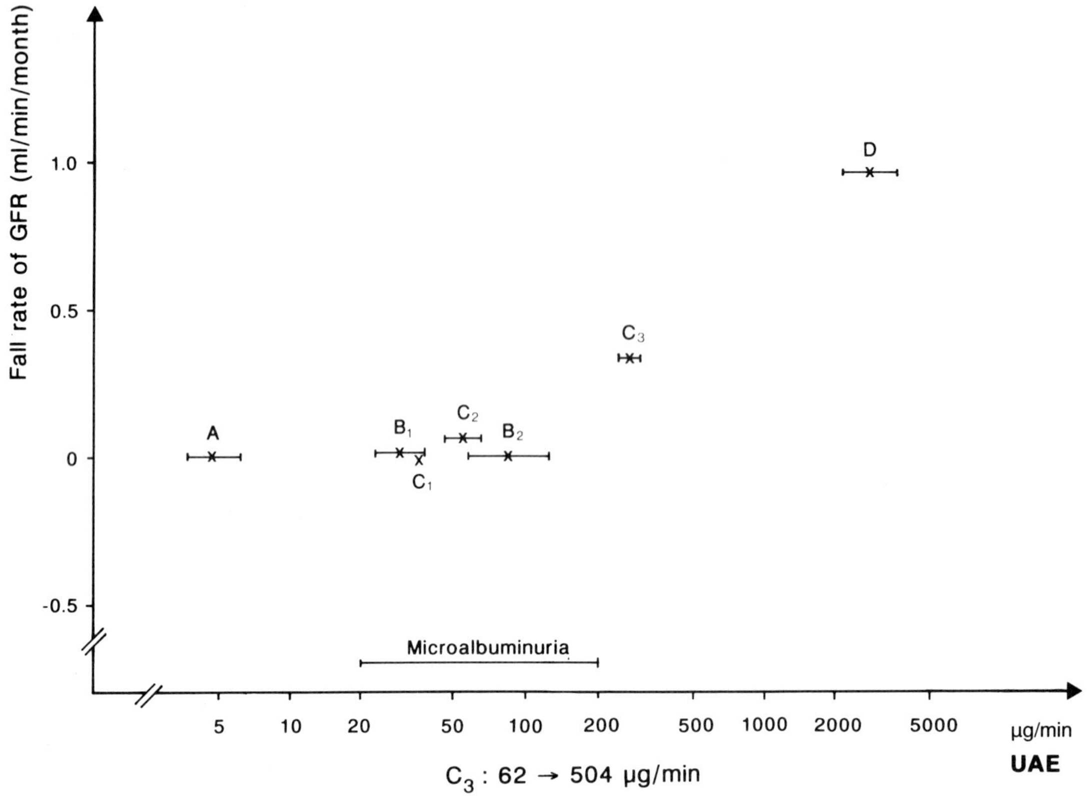


Fig. 30.4. Fall rate in glomerular filtration rate (GFR) compared with different levels of urinary excretion rate (UAE) in IDDM patients without antihypertensive treatment. UAE as geometric mean is shown in the groups from Table 30.3 ($n$ = 70).

other hand, patients with microalbuminuria usually do not exhibit decline in GFR but instead show some compensatory hyperfunction in addition to the usual diabetic hyperfiltration. Microalbuminuric IDDM patients do show total kidney hyperfiltration, and the two processes may also work in combination, even aggravated by systemic blood pressure elevation, which is to some extent transmitted to glomeruli (3).

## Diabetic retinopathy: organ damage and albuminuria/blood pressure elevation

It was documented some years ago that microalbuminuria strongly predicts proliferative diabetic retinopathy (42). However, in this study it was not possible to separate clearly the effect of increasing blood pressure, because the patients with progression in albumin excretion rate and development of proliferative retinopathy both initially and at follow-up 12 years later had clearly elevated blood pressure (138/91 → 156/105 mmHg). Studies by Klein *et al.* (43) provided detailed data relating to blood pressure elevation; clinical proteinuria (>0.3 g/l) clearly increased the incidence of proliferative diabetic retinopathy by a factor 2.3 in a 2–4 year prospective study. This observation was further substantiated by Nørgaard *et al.* (44). In a cross-sectional study, patients were divided according to blood pressure elevation and normoalbuminuria versus overt nephropathy. The patients with normal albumin excretion rate and elevated blood pressure (diabetic patients with essential hypertension) did not show significantly more advanced retinal changes. In NIDDM patients

(Pima Indians) Knowler *et al.* (45) found that elevated blood pressure (systolic > 145 mmHg) increased the risk of exudates in a six-year follow-up study.

Taken together, it can be concluded that abnormal albuminuria is a stronger risk factor for proliferative diabetic retinopathy than blood pressure elevation, but clearly hypertension superimposed on nephropathy-associated factors is associated with an increase in the severity of retinopathy.

### Left ventricular hypertrophy: related to abnormal albuminuria and blood pressure

In essential hypertension, hypertrophy of the left ventricle is associated with increased cardiovascular morbidity and mortality (46). Early echocardiographic studies showed increased left ventricular wall thickness in hypertensive diabetic patients with a high prevalence of microvascular complications (47). Later studies have shown normal cardiac wall thickness in short-term uncomplicated diabetes (47), but increased wall thickness seems to be an early and prevalent finding in hypertensive microalbuminuric and proteinuric diabetic patients (48, 49). Thuesen *et al.* (47) related the wall thickness and the wall mass of the left ventricle to the blood pressure, the UAER and the disease duration. By multiple regression analysis the blood pressure was found to be the most important determinant of hypertrophy of the left ventricular wall.

## ORIGIN OF BLOOD PRESSURE ELEVATION IN DIABETES

### Relation to kidney function

There is overwhelming evidence that elevated blood pressure in IDDM is related to impaired renal function. Blood pressure starts to rise in the microalbuminuria stage. There is some controversy regarding the transition from normo- to micro-albuminuria. Some groups suggests that elevated blood pressure is important in this transition process (6), while other studies suggest that blood pressure increases only after the occurrence of microalbuminuria (5). However, it is clear that blood pressure elevation tends to increase with increasing microalbuminuria and with overt proteinuria a clear elevation in blood pressure can be documented. The exact mechanism behind the increase in blood pressure as related to renal impairment is not clear. It is well established that blood pressure increases with a reduction of GFR, but elevated blood pressure is seen before this reduction in renal function in diabetic patients. It is possible that the mesangial expansion documented in diabetic nephropathy from the microalbuminuria stage is important (50). The blood pressure elevation may also relate to sodium excess associated with renal disease (51). The degree of abnormal albuminuria is clearly related to structural renal change (50).

In NIDDM the relationship between an increase in blood pressure and impaired renal function is also present, but less clear, due to confounding factors; usually there is some correlation between blood pressure elevation and degree of abnormal albuminuria (26).

### Sodium excess mechanisms

There is a correlation between exchangeable sodium and the elevated blood pressure in microalbuminuria patients suggesting that sodium excess may play a role in elevating blood pressure (51). The sodium excess may be explained by an increased tubular reabsorption of sodium, possibly stimulated by exogenous or endogenous insulin (52). However, the association is merely empiric and there may be other underlying mechanisms that explain both sodium excess and elevated blood pressure.

### Cardiac function, hyperperfusion and local pressures

There is some evidence of an increased cardiac contractility in diabetes, which may produce increased cardiac output and contribute to vascular hyperperfusion in diabetes (53). Interestingly, there is in IDDM a correlation between cardiac contractility and the degree of microalbuminuria. However, with the transition to overt proteinuria there is a decrease in cardiac contractility (53). Besides generalised hyperperfusion, there may be evidence of increased localised pressure not only in the kidney, but also in the peripheral circulation as recently demonstrated by Sandeman *et al.* (54). This may possibly parallel the increase of glomerular pressure in the kidney.

## Large vessel disease

In NIDDM there is evidence of increased arterial stiffness (26) which may explain why the blood pressure elevation is mostly of systolic nature (26). Diastolic pressure is usually also elevated in NIDDM, but often to a minor extent unless clear renal damage is present.

## Insulin-related mechanism

Patients with essential hypertension do show insulin resistance and hyperinsulinaemia (55). Since insulin resistance is involved in the pathogenesis of NIDDM, insulin resistance may also contribute to blood pressure elevation in diabetes. Indeed, elevated blood pressure is found in NIDDM at diagnosis (24, 25), when insulin resistance may be important. However, there is some controversy regarding this concept, because insulin itself does not necessarily produce hypertension (56) and also the correlation between insulin resistance and elevated blood pressure is relatively imprecise, probably because multiple factors are involved.

Other abnormalities may be involved in the genesis of hypertension in diabetes, such as increased sympathetic nervous activity producing increased vascular reactivity (58). This increased nerve activity may also be related to obesity; however, since these phenomena do not point to specific modalities of treatment, they will not be discussed in this paper.

## Mechanisms of blood pressure elevation and choice of therapy

Based upon the known mechanisms operating in the genesis of hypertension interesting concepts have been developed regarding selection of antihypertensive treatment. Abnormalities in renal function including hyperperfusion, hyperfiltration and increased glomerular pressure may be important and point to the use of ACE-inhibitors in diabetes, since these agents tend to reduce efferent glomerular resistance (57). The effect of these agents reducing glomerular pressure, may even act independently of systemic hypertension or systemic blood pressure level (3). The observed sodium retention observed in NIDDM but also in IDDM, may point to the use of diuretics or sodium restriction in antihypertensive programs in diabetes (51, 52). The early cardiac hyperfunction in microalbuminuric patients may also point to the use of cardioselective $\beta_1$-blockers particular in diabetic patients (see Tables 30.4 and 30.5).

Obviously, from a theoretical point of view, potential additional beneficial effect should be considered (see Table 30.5). For example, ACE-inhibitors may specifically reduce the increased localised pressures seen in these patients. (57). The occurrence of oedema, of course, favours the use of diuretics. It is suggested that arrythmias may play a role in the early mortality, especially in NIDDM patients, and the observation that in post-myocardial infarction trials, β-blockers are especially effective in diabetic patients (59), points to the additional beneficial effects of β-blockers in the management of hypertension and diabetes.

Obviously, side-effects are important and these are usually dose related. For example, the well-known diabetogenic effect of diuretics may be clearly dose dependent with sufficient blood pressure reduction without the diabetogenic effect or adverse lipid effect at small doses (60). Potassium loss is important and can clearly be restored by potassium supplementation. Potassium supplementation may in itself reduce blood

Table 30.4. *How antihypertensive agents may be combined in diabetes*

| | | | | |
|---|---|---|---|---|
| β-blockers | Yes (diuretics often required) | | | |
| ACE-inhibition | Yes (diuretics often required) | Yes | Yes (theoretically interesting combination, preliminary results promising) | |
| Nifedipine (or other Ca-blocker) | Yes | Yes (rare) | Yes (rare) | Yes (pronounced blood pressure drop may occur) |
| | Diuretics | β-blockers | β-blockers+diuretics | ACE-inhibition |

Careful clinical metabolic and blood pressure monitoring always required, including control of serum electrolytes and serum creatinine or GFR index.

pressure. One side-effect that has caused some concern in patients on insulin treatment is hypoglycaemic unawareness. This is typically found with unselective β-blockers and only to a limited extent with cardio-selective β-blockers, when used in appropriate doses. ACE-inhibitors do not appear to have any diabetogenic effect. Thus there seems on balance to be no effect on glucose or lipid metabolism. This neutral pattern may therefore favour the use of ACE-inhibitors in diabetic patients. Cough as a side-effect is surprisingly rare in diabetic patients, maybe due to diabetic neuropathic changes.

## ANTIHYPERTENSIVE TREATMENT WITH FOCUS ON EARLY ACE-INHIBITION IN DIABETIC NEPHROPATHY

Evaluation of treatment effect has to be differentiated according to degree of abnormal albuminuria. IDDM-patients with normoalbuminuria rarely need antihypertensive treatment. With microalbuminuria there is well-preserved renal function and thus the target is simply reduction of albuminuria, but with long-term follow-up the target may be the prevention of a fall in GFR. In patients with overt nephropathy the main target is to reduce the rate of fall of GFR, with reduction of albuminuria as a secondary target (61).

### Incipient diabetic nephropathy

Several intervention studies have been published, some with self-controlled or cross-over design, some double-blinded, but not long-term, some long-term and randomised but not blinded as outlined in Table 30.6 (5, 17, 38, 40, 62–70). The table provides information on data of 12 trials, including a recent randomised double-blinded large-scale placebo-controlled study (70). The effect of Captopril was investigated in this multicentre study with respect to progression to clinical nephropathy in normotensive IDDM patients with microalbuminuria. The study endpoints were the progression to persistent proteinuria (UAE $>$ 200 μg/min). The total number of treated patients was 88:12 patients in the placebo group (44 patients) and 4 patients in the Captopril group (44 patients) progressed to clinical proteinuria (Fisher's exact test, $p=0.05$) (70). Thus treatment with Captopril in this study delayed the progression to overt renal disease in normotensive, IDDM patients with microalbuminuria.

Interestingly, in all the studies from 1985 to 1992, indicated in Table 30.6, patients were included purely on the basis of microalbuminuria, patients with overt hypertension were generally excluded. Clearly, in most studies blood pressure was close to normal, and in some of the patients the blood pressure was in the middle of

Table 30.5. *Diabetes-related side-effects and favourable effects related to antihypertensive treatment in diabetics (mainly IDDM)*

| | Diuretics (Thiazide or loop) | Non-cardioselective β-blockers | Cardioselective β-blockers | ACE-inhibitors | Triple treatment: diuretic $\beta_1$-blockers/ ACE-inhibitors | Calcium blockers |
|---|---|---|---|---|---|---|
| Glucose intolerance | Yes (NIDDM, but related strongly to hypokalaemia) | No problem | Limited problem | No side-effects | Limited (with small dosages) | No |
| Hypoglycaemic masking | No | Yes, mainly in IDDM | A problem, but limited, seen in few patients | Not seen | Limited (with small dosages) | No |
| Unfavourable lipid profits | Yes | Likely | Limited | No side-effects | ? | No |
| Other unfavourable effects | May cause sodium depletion | Less physical exercise capacity | Less physical exercise capacity | Cough and drug-related side-effects | Limited (with small dosages) | Foot oedema seen in few patients |
| Favourable effects (apart from blood pressure reduction) | Elimination of oedema | Reduction of cardiovascular morbidity/mortality? Normalisation of cardiac arrhythmias | Reduction of cardiovascular morbidity/mortality? Normalisation of cardiac arrhythmias | Elimination sodium excess and possibly restoration of glomerular pressure gradients | Probably also combination of favourble effects (stable GFR?) | Effect on certain arrhythmias? No potentiation of peripheral ischaemia? |
| Effect on abnormal albuminuria | Not well documented | Not well documented | Yes, but relatively few studies exist | Very consistent finding | Addition of ACE-inhibition reduces abnormal albuminuria | Not a consistent finding |
| Reducing fall rate of GFR | Not documented | Not documented | Yes | Yes, good results | GFR possibly stable on this programme | Not documented long term |

Table 30.6. *Trial in young non-hypertensive microalbuminuric IDDM patients (resulting in slightly reduced blood pressure)*

| | Nature of trial | Intervention | n and duration of treatment | Microalbuminuria | Remarks |
|---|---|---|---|---|---|
| Christensen & Mogensen, 1985+1987 | Self-controlled Open | $\beta_1$-blocker + diuretics | ($n$=6) 5 yr | Reduced | Gradual reversal by antihypertensive treatment |
| Marre *et al.*, 1988 | Double-blinded Randomised with parallel controls | ACE-inhibition | ($n$=20) 1 yr | Reduced by ACE-inhibition | Untreated patients showed rapid increase in UAE |
| Brichard *et al.*, 1989 | Open | ACE-inhibition | ($n$=7) 1 yr | Reduced by ACE-inhibition | Open study |
| Rudberg *et al.*, 1990 | Open | ACE-inhibition | ($n$=12) $\frac{1}{2}$ yr | Reduced by ACE-inhibition | Young patients |
| Cook *et al.*, 1990 | Cross-over, double-blinded | ACE-inhibition | ($n$=12) $\frac{1}{4}$ yr | Reduced by ACE-inhibition | Children |
| Melbourne Diabetic Nephropathy Study Group, 1991 | Open, randomised with parallel controls | ACE-inhibition versus calcium blocker | ($n$=43) 1 yr | Reduced by ACE-inhibition and by calcium blocker | Effect mostly seen with elevated blood pressure |
| Mathiesen *et al.*, 1991 | Open, randomised with parallel controls | ACE-inhibition | ($n$=44) 4 yr | Reduced by ACE-inhibition | First study to indicate preservation of GFR. Proteinuria prevented |
| Marre *et al.*, 1991 | Double-blinded Randomised with parallel controls | ACE-inhibition | ($n$=16) 6 weeks | Reduced | Effect not dose dependent |
| Mau Pedersen *et al.*, 1991 | Open Cross-over | $\beta_1$-blocker thiazide + ACE-inhibition | ($n$=8) $\frac{1}{4}$ yr | Albuminuria reduced | Triple treatment may be useful (early nephropathy) |
| Mau Pedersen *et al.*, 1992 | Cross-over Double-blinded | $\beta_1$-blocker thiazide + ACE-inhibition | ($n$=10) $\frac{1}{3}$ yr | Albuminuria reduced | Triple treatment may be useful (early nephropathy) (similar results as in open study (69)) |
| Hallab *et al.*, 1993 | Randomised with parallel controls | ACE-inhibition versus thiazide | ($n$=21) 1 yr | Reduced by ACE-inhibition | ACE-inhibition more efficient than thiazide |
| Viberti, Mogensen *et al.*, 1994 | Multicentre Double-blinded Randomised with parallel controls | ACE-inhibition | ($n$=92) 2 yr | Reduced by ACE-inhibition | First large-scale double-blind study Increase in albuminuria and proteinuria significantly prevented |

the range seen in healthy young individuals (with a mean arterial pressure of ≈90 mmHg) (71). There does seem to be a correlation between the reduction in blood pressure and the reduction in albuminuria. A recent analysis (3) concluded that about 50% of the antialbuminuric effect in one study (40) could be caused by blood pressure reduction alone.

The clinical consequence of these observations is that antihypertensive treatment is indicated for microalbuminuria (as in the clinical trials) rather than elevation of blood pressure. Obviously elevation of blood pressure would further strengthen the indication for treatment (because there is a correlation between rate of progression of microalbuminuria and blood pressure), but the conclusion from the studies in Table 30.6 would be to start antihypertensive treatment when microalbuminuria is found consistently. A more cautious view would be to start antihypertensive treatment if microalbuminuria is increasing, but the variability in UAE makes this approach somewhat difficult. As seen from Table 30.6 all studies document a reduction in microalbuminuria, irrespective of the treatment used. However, most studies were conducted with ACE-inhibitors as a principal agent, with few or no side-effect, though diuretics were added in one important study. Thus the criteria for antihypertensive treatment, in particular ACE-inhibitors, are changing from an elevated blood pressure to increased or increasing UAE. An outline of the result of intervention in microalbuminuric IDDM patients is shown in Fig. 30.5.

As discussed in this paper abnormal albuminuria correlates more closely with organ damage (in the kidney and elsewhere) than blood pressure elevation. This concept would further strengthen the view that microalbuminuria could be an independent indicator to start antihypertensive treatment, in particular ACE-inhibitors, often combined with a small dose of diuretics. This idea was proposed in 1984, using a $\beta_1$-blocker as principal agent (+diuretic later) (62). New studies show that addition of ACE-inhibitors to $\beta_1$-blockers and diuretics may be beneficial (36). The risk with this approach is limited or non-existent (and the treatment is not costly), the potential benefit enormous (increasing life-expectancy by postponing end-stage renal failure) (19).

## Overt diabetic nephropathy

In untreated patients there is a correlation between their rate of fall of GFR and blood pressure (15), but interestingly the correlation between rate of fall of GFR and albuminuria is equally strong (15). Recently it has been suggested (61) that a pronounced fall in proteinuria after the start of antihypertensive treatment predicts a more benign course of renal disease in IDDM patients. Several studies have documented that antihypertensive treatment clearly reduces rate of fall of GFR (see Fig. 30.4). This is always accompanied by a reduction in albuminuria (14, 16, 72, 73). Therefore antihypertensive treatment is the major therapeutic option for these patients. The use of ACE-inhibitors (with diuretics) is clearly popular, but also antihypertensive programs with $\beta_1$-blocker seems to be effective, but possibly with more side-effects (61). A low protein diet may also reduce the rate of fall of GFR in these patients (74). Recently a large-scale study confirmed the positive effect of ACE-inhibitors with an effect on ESRF (75).

In NIDDM patients it has also been shown that during treatment there is a correlation between blood pressure elevation and rate of decline in GFR (76–78), suggesting that in NIDDM patients an elevated blood pressure is also important for the rate of progression in renal disease. These studies included patients with overt proteinuria, generally with a poor prognosis. An important long-term intervention trial has been conducted in NIDDM with index of GFR as an end-point (79). Microalbuminuria is reduced by the use of ACE-inhibitors (67, 79).

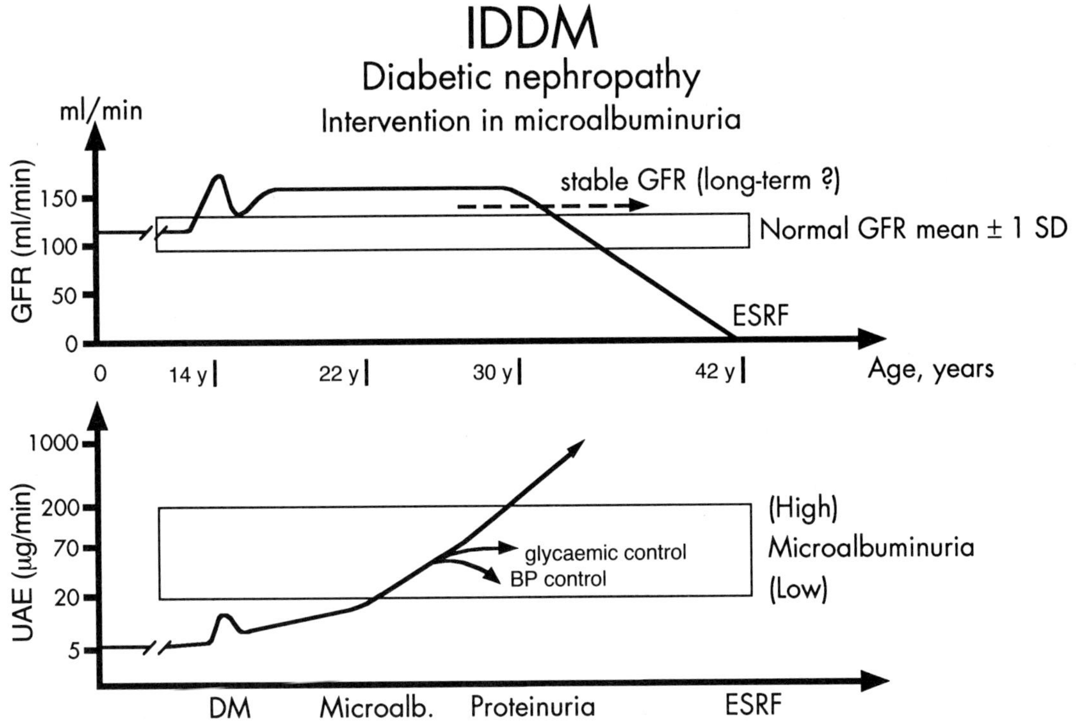


Fig 30.5. Outline of effect of antihypertensive treatment and optimised metabolic control in microalbuminuric patients.

## Triple treatment using diuretics, β-blockers, and ACE-inhibitor in early nephropathy

As mentioned this treatment modality has a clear pathophysiological rationale. ACE-inhibition has shown promising results in diabetic nephropathy, but long-term results on survival are not available, in contrast to data on $\beta_1$-blockers (19). In a cohort of patients receiving antihypertensive treatment predominantly consisting of β-blockers in combination with diuretics, support for an improved survival has been presented (19). Addition of ACE-inhibition to such a combination treatment may be favourable both due to the suggested renoprotective effects of ACE-inhibitors and because diuretics activate the renin–angiotensin system. In IDDM patients with early diabetic nephropathy (UAE <1000 µg/min), who were receiving continuous therapy with metoprolol and bendroflumethiazide, a double-blind cross-over study with four months, addition of ramipril 5 mg and placebo was conducted (17). UAE and fractional albumin excretion were significantly reduced after the four months of ramipril administration. Renal plasma flow tended to increase, while GFR ($^{125}$I-iothalamate clearance) stayed unchanged (121 ± 8 vs. 120 ± 9 ml/min/1.73 m$^2$). Mean arterial pressure during clearance studies fell moderately (95 ± 3 vs. 101 ± 1 mmHg, $2p < 0.05$) and correlated with the change in UAE. Renal resistance was decreased. ACE-activity was suppressed in all patients. Surprisingly, twenty-four-hour ambulatory blood pressure measurements were not significantly different after the two periods. It can be concluded that addition of an ACE-inhibitor reduces UAE in patients on ongoing antihypertensive therapy. Qualitatively the renal response to ACE-inhibition in the patients on β-blocker and thiaz-

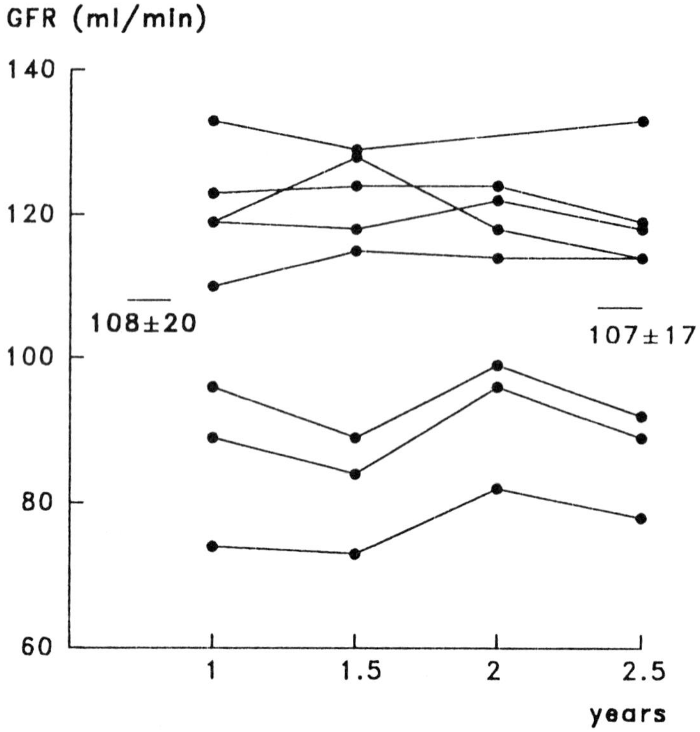


Fig. 30.6. GFR in 8 diabetic patients with early nephropathy. Note stability of GFR on triple-treatment ($\beta_1$-blocker/diuretic/ACE-inhibitor, namely Metoprolol/Bendroflumethiazide/Ramipril).

ide treatment corresponds to the haemodynamic effects observed in previously untreated diabetic patients. Importantly, GFR continues to be stable long term using this therapy as seen in Fig. 30.6. The figure shows data after 1 year of treatment as it is important to exclude GFR-values during initial treatment, because of a potential acute haemodynamic effect (36).

## LOW PROTEIN DIET

### Microalbuminuria

An important study suggests that microalbuminuria can be reduced by a low protein diet (80) but, so far, no long-term results are available. Progression was also correlated to blood pressure level.

### Overt nephropathy

In diabetic nephropathy new data have recently been published indicating that the rate of decline of GFR can be reduced by a low protein diet (74). Patients were monitored on their usual dietary intake of proteins and thereafter patients were put on a low protein diet. A remarkable reduction in the fall rate of GFR was observed, although the response varied considerably. The mean fall rate of GFR was reduced from 0.61 to 0.14 ml/min/month. Patients served as their own controls without a parallel untreated group and the possibility that late or long-term action of antihypertensive treatment may explain at least part of observed beneficial effect cannot be excluded. In another randomised study also documented the beneficial effect on the fall rate of GFR in these patients (74).

Dietary advice over recent years has resulted in a high protein intake, and it cannot be excluded that such a dietary program may contribute to the development of renal disease. There has been considerable debate regarding a protein-reduced diet in non-diabetic nephropathy, but protein restriction now seems to be effective in some patients also in hormoalbuminuria (81, 82).

## OPTIMISED INSULIN TREATMENT

Some evidence suggests that optimised insulin treatment will stabilise or reduce microalbuminuria and may in the long run prevent reduction in GFR (see Fig. 30.5) (39). Insulin treatment will, however, be discussed elsewhere in this volume. Microalbuminuria was not affected in the DCCT-Study (M.Steffes, pers. comm.).

## CONCLUDING REMARKS

This review documents that abnormal albuminuria related to increased blood pressure is associated with actual or subsequent organ damage, not only in the kidney but also in other organs, especially the eyes and the heart. In the kidney abnormal albuminuria, starting from the microalbuminuric range, is a reflection of more advanced glomerular structural lesions, although the exact location of the permeability defect has not been defined at an ultrastructural level. Poor metabolic control is important for transition from normo- to microalbuminuria (5). Blood pressure elevation may not initiate the glomerular permeability defect but high systemic blood pressure aggravates the course of established lesions (5). Transition from micro- to macro-albuminuria is associated with a reduction in GFR, the key parameter in the evaluation of renal function.

Biochemical and haemodynamic hypotheses have been put forward supported by animal models, but these ideas are difficult to substantiate in humans, where phenomena cannot be studied in isolation, nor with direct measurement, e.g. of glomerular wall charge and intraglomerular pressure. A unifying concept would be attractive, comprising biochemical aberrations, such as charge defects (83), changes in enzymatic activities (84) and glycation phenomena (85) as well as haemodynamic changes such as hyperfiltration with elevated glomerular pressure, aggravated by an early rise in systemic blood pressure (29). These changes may be seen along with vascular and endothelial changes, reflected by increases in von Willebrand factor (86, 87), circulating prorenin (88) as well as increased transcapillary escape rate of albumin (89). A common pathway explaining all or most of these abnormalities should be searched for, with the basis in prolonged hyperglycaemia and related chemical changes, characteristic the diabetic state (90).

However, when diabetic complications are evolving an increase in blood pressure remains a major factor in promoting organ damage in the kidney. Conversely antihypertensive treatment may be the major therapeutic element in ameliorating deterioration in organ function. A low protein diet may also reduce albuminuria and the rate of fall in GFR. However, strict antihypertensive therapy (91–95) may limit the need for a very pronounced reduction in the protein content of the diet to achieve a beneficial effect (72, 73).

## REFERENCES


1 Hansen KW, Poulsen PL, Mogensen CE. Ambulatory blood pressure and abnormal albuminuria in type 1 diabetic patients. *Kidney Int* 1994; 45: suppl. 45: S134–40.

2 Schmitz A. The kidney in non-insulin-dependent diabetes. Studies on glomerular structure and function and the relationship between microalbuminuria and mortality. *Acta Diabetologia* 1992; 29: 47–69.

3 Mogensen CE, Osterby R, Hansen KW, Damsgaard EM. Blood pressure elevation versus abnormal albuminuria in the genesis and prediction of renal disease in diabetes. *Diabetes Care* 1992*b*; 15: 1192–204.

4 Parving H-H. Impact of blood pressure and antihypertensive treatment on incipient and overt nephropathy, retinopathy, and endothelial permeability in diabetes mellitus. *Diabetes Care* 1991; 14: 260–9.

5 Mogensen CE, Poulsen PL. Epidemiology of microalbuminuria in diabetes and in the background population. *Curr Opin Nephrol Hypertens* 1994; 3: 248–56.

6 Viberti GC, Messent J. Introduction: hypertension and diabetes. Critical combination for micro- and macrovascular disease. *Diabetes Care* 14: suppl 1991; 4: 4–7.

7 Mogensen CE, Poulsen PL, Heinsvig EM. Abnormal albuminuria in the monitoring of early renal changes in diabetes. In: Mogensen CE, Standl E, ed. *Concepts for the*

*ideal diabetes clinic*, Berlin, New York, Walter de Gruyter, 1993; 289–313.
8 Baba T, Ishizaki T. Recent advances in pharmacological management of hypertension in diabetic patients with nephropathy. Effects of antihypertensive drugs on kidney function and insulin sensitivity. *Drugs* 1992; 43: 464–89.
9 DeFronzo RA, Ferrannini E. Insulin resistance. A multifaceted syndrome responsible for NIDDM, obesity, hypertension, dyslipidemia, and atherosclerotic cardiovascular disease. *Diabetes Care* 1991; 14: 173–94.
10 Reaven GM. Insulin resistance, hyperinsulinemia, hypertriglyceridemia, and hypertension. Parallels between human disease and rodent models. *Diabetes Care* 1991; 14: 195–202.
11 Seaquist ER, Goetz FC, Rich S, Barbosa JJ. Familial clustering of diabetic kidney disease. *N Engl J Med* 1989; 320: 1161–5.
12 Borch-Johnsen K, Nørgaard K, Hommel E, Mathiesen ER, Jensen JS, Deckert T, Parving H-H. Is diabetic nephropathy an inherited complication? *Kidney Int* 1992; 41: 719–22.
13 Mogensen CE. Pharmacology of the kidney in IDDM patients. In: Mogensen CE, Standl E, eds. *Pharmacology of diabetes. Present practice and future perspective*, Berlin, New York, Walter de Gruyter, 1991; 263–81.
14 Mogensen CE. Angiotensin converting enzyme inhibitors and diabetic nephropathy (editorial). *Br Med J* 1992*a*; 304: 227–8.
15 Mogensen CE. Progression of nephropathy in long-term diabetics with proteinuria and effect of initial antihypertensive treatment. *Scand J Clin Lab Invest* 1976; 36: 383–8.
16 Mogensen CE. Long-term antihypertensive treatment inhibiting progression of diabetic nephropathy. *Br Med J* 1982; 285: 685–8.
17 Mau Pedersen M, Hansen KW, Schmitz A, Sørensen K, Christensen CK, Mogensen CE. Effect of ACE-inhibition supplementary to beta-blockers and diuretics in early diabetic nephropathy. *Kidney Int* 1992; 41: 883–90.
18 Remuzzi G, Bertani T. Is glomerulosclerosis a consequence of altered glomerular permeability to macromolecules? *Kidney Int* 1990; 38: 384–94.
19 Mathiesen ER, Borch-Johnsen K, Jensen DV, Deckert T. Improved survival in patients with diabetic nephropathy. *Diabetologia* 1989; 32: 884–6.
20 Hansen KW, Mau Pedersen M, Marshall SM, Christiansen JS, Mogensen CE. Circadian variation of blood pressure in diabetic nephropathy. *Diabetologia* 1992*b*; 35: 1074–9.
21 Viberti GC, Keen H, Wiseman MJ. Raised arterial pressure in parents of proteinuric insulin-dependent diabetics. *Br Med J* 1987; 295: 515–17.
22 Nørgaard K, Feldt-Rasmussen B, Borch-Johnsen K, Sælan H, Deckert T. Prevalence of hypertension in Type 1 (insulin-dependent) diabetes mellitus. *Diabetologia* 1990; 33: 407–10.
23 Damsgaard EM, Mogensen CE. Microalbuminuria in elderly hyperglycaemic patients and controls. *Diabetic Med* 1986; 3: 430–5.
24 United Kingdom Prospective Diabetes Study. A Multicenter Study. III. Prevalence of hypertension and hypotensive therapy in patients with newly diagnosed diabetes. *Hypertension* 1985; 7: suppl. II: II–8–13.
25 de Fine Olivarius N, Andreasen AH, Keiding N, Mogensen CE. Renal involvement in newly diagnosed middle-aged and elderly diabetics. *Diabetologia* 1993; in press.
26 Schmitz A, Mau Pedersen M, Hansen KW. Blood pressure by 24 h ambulatory recordings in Type 2 (non-insulin dependent) diabetics. Relationship to urinary albumin excretion. *Diabetic Metab* (*Paris*) 1991; 17: 301–7.
27 Feldt-Rasmussen B, Mathiesen ER, Deckert T. Effect of two years of strict metabolic control on the progression of incipient nephropathy in insulin-dependent diabetes. *Lancet* 1986; ii: 1300–4.
28 Parving H-H, Smidt UM, Andersen AR, Svendsen PAa. Early aggressive antihypertensive treatment reduces rate of decline in kidney function in diabetic nephropathy. *Lancet* 1983; I: 1175–9.
29 Mogensen CE. Hyperfiltration, hypertension, and diabetic nephropathy in IDDM patients. *Diab Nutr Metab* 1989; 2: 227–44.
30 Borch-Johnsen K, Andersen PK, Deckert T. The effect of proteinuria on relative mortality in Type 1 (insulin-dependent) diabetes mellitus. *Diabetologia* 1985; 28: 590–6.
31 Borch-Johnsen K, Kreiner S. Proteinuria – value as predictor of cardiovascular mortality in insulin-dependent diabetes mellitus. *Br Med J* 1987; 294: 1651–4.
32 Borch-Johnsen K, Nissen H, Henriksen E, Kreiner S, Salling N, Deckert T, Nerup J. The natural history of insulin-dependent diabetes in Denmark: 2. Long-term survival – Who and why? *Diabetic Med* 1987; 4: 211–16.
33 Mau Pedersen M, Christensen CK, Mogensen CE. Long-term (18 year) prognosis for normo- and microalbuminuric type 1 (insulin-dependent) diabetic patients (abstract). *Diabetologia* 1992; 35: A60.
34 Messent JWC, Elliott TG, Hill RD, Jarrett RJ, Keen H, Viberti GC. Prognostic significance of microalbuminuria in insulin-dependent diabetes mellitus: A twenty-three year follow-up study. *Kidney Int* 1992; 41: 836–9.
35 Mogensen CE, Mau Pedersen M, Hansen KW, Christensen CK. Micro-albuminuria and the organ-damage concept in antihypertensive therapy for patients with insulin-dependent diabetes mellitus. *J Hypertens* 10: suppl. 1992a; 1: S43–51.
36 Mogensen CE, Hansen KW, Nielsen S, Mau Pedersen M, Rehling M, Schmitz A. Monitoring diabetic nephropathy: glomerular filtration rate and abnormal albuminuria in diabetic renal disease: reproducibility, progression studies and efficacy of antihypertensive intervention. *Am J Kidney Dis* 1993; 22: 174–87.
37 Christensen CK. The pre-proteinuric phase of diabetic nephropathy. *Dan Med Bull* 1991; 38: 145–59.
38 Christensen CK, Mogensen CE. Antihypertensive treatment: long-term reversal of progression of albuminuria in incipient diabetic nephropathy. A longitudinal study of renal function. *J Diab Compl* 1987; 1: 45–52.
39 Feldt-Rasmussen B, Mathiesen ER, Jensen T, Lauritzen T, Deckert T. Effect of improved metabolic control loss of kidney function in Type 1 (insulin-dependent) diabetic patients: an update of the Steno studies. *Diabetologia* 1991*a*; 34: 164–70.
40 Mathiesen ER, Hommel E, Giese J, Parving H-H. Efficacy of captopril in postponing nephropathy in normo-

tensive insulin-dependent diabetic patients with microalbuminuria. *Br Med J* 1991; 303: 81–7.
41 Nørgaard K, Rasmussen E, Jensen T, Giese J, Feldt-Rasmussen B. Essential hypertension and type 1 diabetes (abstract). *Diabetologia* 1992; 35: A144.
42 Mogensen CE, Vigstrup J, Ehlers N. Microalbuminuria predicts proliferative diabetic retinopathy. *Lancet* 1985; ii: 1512–13.
43 Klein R, Moss SE, Klein BEK. Gross proteinuria predicts the incidence of proliferative diabetic retinopathy. *Diabetes* 41: suppl. 1992; 1: abstract no. 129.
44 Nørgaard K, Feldt-Rasmussen B, Deckert T. Is hypertension a major independent risk factor for retinopathy in Type 1 diabetes? *Diabetic Med* 1991; 8: 334–7.
45 Knowler WC, Bennett PH, Ballintine EJ. Increased incidence of retinopathy in diabetics with elevated blood pressure. A six-year follow-up study in Pima Indians. *N Engl J Med* 1980; 302: 645–50.
46 Casale PN, Devereux RB, Milner M. Value of echocardiographic measurement of left ventricular mass in predicting cardiovascular morbid events in hypertensive men. *Ann Int Med* 1986; 105: 173–8.
47 Thuesen L, Christiansen JS, Mogensen CE, Henningsen P. Echocardiographic-determined left ventricular wall characteristics in insulin dependent diabetic patients. *Acta Med Scand* 1988*b*; 224: 343–8.
48 Sampson MJ, Chambers JB, Sprigings DC, Drury PL. Interventricular septal hypertrophy in type 1 diabetic patients with microalbuminuria or early proteinuria. *Diabetic Med* 1990; 7: 126–32.
49 Sampson MJ, Chambers JB, Sprigings DC, Drury PL. Regression of left ventricular hypertrophy with 1 year of antihypertensive treatment in type 1 diabetic patients with early nephropathy. *Diabetic Med* 1992; 8: 106–10.
50 Østerby R. Glomerular structural changes in Type 1 (insulin-dependent) diabetes mellitus: causes, consequences, and prevention. *Diabetologia* 1992; 35: 803–12.
51 Feldt-Rasmussen B, Nøgaard K, Jensen T, Deckert T. Microalbuminuria, clinical nephropathy and hypertension in diabetes. *J Human Hypertens* 1991*b*; 5: 255–263.
52 Weidmann P, Ferrari P. Central role of sodium in hypertension in diabetic subjects. *Diabetic Care* 1991; 14: 220–32.
53 Thuesen L, Christiansen JS, Mogensen CE, Henningsen P. Cardiac hyperfunction in insulin-dependent diabetic patients developing microvascular complications. *Diabetes* 1988*a*; 37: 851–6.
54 Sandeman DD, Shore AC, Tooke JE. Relation of skin capillary pressure in patients with insulin-dependent diabetes mellitus to complications and metabolic control. *N Engl J Med* 1992; 327: 760–4.
55 Ferrannini E, Buzzigoli G, Bonadonna R, Giorico MA, Oleggini M, Graziadei L et al. Insulin resistance in essential hypertension. *N Engl J Med* 1987; 317: 350–7.
56 Gans ROB, Bilo HJG, Nauta JJP, Heine RJ, Donker AJM. Acute hyperinsulinemia induces sodium retention and a blood pressure decline in diabetes mellitus. *Hypertension* 1992; 20: 199–209.
57 Anderson S. Pathogenesis of diabetic glomerulopathy: hemodynamic factors. In: Brenner BM, Stein JH, ed. *The kidney in diabetes mellitus*, New York, Edinburgh, London, Melbourne, Churchill Livingstone, 1989; 67–85.
58 Daly PA, Landsberg L. Hypertension in obesity and NIDDM. Role of insulin and sympathetic nervous system. *Diabetic Care* 1991; 14: 240–8.
59 Kjekshus J, Gilpin E, Cali G, Blackey AR, Henning H, Ross J Jr. Diabetic patients and α-blockers after acute myocardial infarction. *Eur Heart J* 1990; 11: 43–50.
60 Carlsen J, Køber C, Torp-Pedersen C, Johansen P. Relation between dose of bendrofluazide antihypertensive effect and adverse biochemical effect. *Br Med J* 1990; 300: 975–8.
61 Parving H-H, Rossing P. The use of antihypertensive agents in prevention and treatment of diabetic nephropathy. *Curr Opin Nephrol Hypertens* 1994; 3: 292–300.
62 Christensen CK, Mogensen CE. Effect of antihypertensive treatment on progression of incipient diabetic nephropathy. Hypertension 1985; 7: suppl. II: II-109–13.
63 Marre M, Chatellier G, Leblanc H, Guyenne T-T, Ménard J, Passa Ph. Prevention of diabetic nephropathy with Enalapril in normotensive diabetics with microalbuminuria. *Br Med J* 1988; 297: 1092–5.
64 Brichard SM, Santoni JPh, Thomas JR, van de Voorde K, Ketelslegers JM, Lambert AE. Long term reduction of microalbuminuria after 1 year of angiotensin converting enzyme inhibition by perindropil in hypertensive insulin-treated diabetic patients. *Diab Metab* (Paris) 1989; 1992; 16: 30–6.
65 Rudberg S, Aperia A, Freyschuss U, Persson B. Enalapril reduces microalbuminuria in young normotensive type 1 (insulin-dependent) diabetic patients irrespective of its hypotensive effect. *Diabetologia* 1990; 33: 470–6.
66 Cook JJ, Daneman D, Spino M, Sochett E, Perlman K, Balfe JW. Angiotensin converting enzyme inhibitor therapy to decrease microalbuminuria in normotensive children with insulin-dependent diabetes mellitus. *J Pediat* 1990; 117: 39–45.
67 Melbourne Diabetic Nephropathy Study Group. Comparison between perindopril and nifedipine in hypertensive and normotensive diabetic patients with microalbuminuria. *Br Med J* 1991; 302: 210–6.
68 Marre M, Hallab M, Billiard A, Le Jeune JJ, Bled F, Girault A, Fressinaud Ph. Small doses of ramipril to reduce microalbuminuria in diabetic patients with incipient nephropathy independently of blood pressure changes. *J Cardiovasc Pharmacol* 18: suppl. 1991; 2: S165–8.
69 Hallab M, Gallois Y, Chatellier G, Rohmer V, Fressinaud P, Marre M. Comparison of reduction in microalbuminuria by enalapril and hydrochlorothiazide in normotensive patients with insulin dependent diabetes. *Br Med J* 1993; 306: 175–82.
70 Viberti GC, Mogensen CE, Groop L, Pauls JF for the European Microalbuminuria Captopril Study Group. Effect of captopril on progression to clinical proteinuria in patients with insulin-dependent diabetes mellitus and microalbuminuria. *JAMA* 1994; 271: 275–9.
71 Mogensen CE, Hansen KW, Mau Pedersen M, Christensen CK. Renal factors influencing blood pressure threshold and choice of treatment for hypertension in IDDM. *Diabetic Care* 14: suppl 1991; 4: 13–26.
72 Parving H-H, Andersen AR, Smidt UM, Hommel E, Mathiesen ER, Svendsen PAa. Effect of antihypertensive treatment on kidney function in diabetic nephropathy. *Br Med J* 1987; 294: 1443–7.

73 Björck S, Mulec H, Johnsen SA, Nordén G, Aurell M. Renal protective effect of enalapril in diabetic nephropathy. *Br Med J* 1992; 304–43.

74 Walker JD. Non-glycaemic intervention in diabetic nephropathy: the role of dietary protein intake. In Mogensen CE, ed. *The kidney and hypertension in diabetes mellitus*, 2nd ed. Boston, Dordrecht, London, Kluwer Academic Publishers, 1994; 369–79.

75 Lewis EJ, Hunsicker LG, Bain RP, Rohde RD, for the Collaborative Study Group. The effect of angiotensin-converting-enzyme inhibition on diabetic nephropathy. *N Engl J Med* 1993; 329: 1456–62.

76 Baba T, Murabayashi S, Tomiyama T, Takebe K. Uncontrolled hypertension is associated with rapid progression of nephropathy in type 2 diabetic patients with proteinuria and preserved renal function. *Tohokn J Exp Med* 1990; 161: 741–8.

77 Gall M-A. The course of kidney function in Type 2 (non-insulin-dependent) diabetic patients with diabetic nephropathy. *Diabetologia* 1993; in press.

78 Nielsen S, Schmitz A, Mogensen CE. Rate of progression of nephropathy in normo and microalbuminuric type 2 diabetic patients (abstract). *Diabetologia* 1991; 34: A144.

79 Ravid M, Savin H, Jutrin I, Bental T, Katz B, Lishner M. Long-term stabilizing effect of angiotensin-converting enzyme inhibition on plasma creatinine and on proteinuria in normotensive type II diabetic patients. *Ann Intern Med* 1993; 118: 577–81.

80 Dullaart RPF, Beusekamp BJ, Meijer S, van Doormaal JJ, Sluiter WJ. Long-term effects of protein-restricted diet on albuminuria and renal function in IDDM patients without clinical nephropathy and hypertension. *Diabetes Care* 1993; 16: 483–92.

81 Mau Pedersen M, Winther E, Mogensen CE. Reducing protein in the diabetic diet. *Metabolism (Paris)* 1990; 16: 454–9.

82 Mau Pedersen M, Mogensen CE, Jørgensen FS *et al.* Renal effects from limitation of high dietary protein in normoalbuminuric insulin-dependent diabetic patients. *Kidney Int* suppl. 1989; 27: S115–21.

83 Deckert T, Feldt-Rasmussen B, Borch-Johnsen K, Jensen T, Kofoed-Enevoldsen A. Albuminuria reflects widespread vascular damage. The Steno hypothesis. *Diabetologia* 1989; 32: 219–26.

84 Cohen MP. General aspects of aldose reductase inhibition. In Mogensen CE, Standl E, ed. *Pharmacology of diabetes. Present practice and future perspectives*, Berlin New York, Walter de Gryter, 1991; 181–91.

85 Giardino I, Brownlee M. Glycosylatin inhibition. In: Mogensen CE, Standl E, eds. *Pharmacology of diabetes. Present practice and future perspectives*, Berlin, New York, Walter de Gruyter, 1991; 211–20.

86 Stehouwer CDA, Nauta JJP, Zeldenrust GC, Hackeng WHL, Donker AJM, den Ottolander GJH. Urinary albumin excretion, cardiovascular disease, and endothelial dysfunction in non-insulin-dependent diabetes mellitus. *Lancet* 199; 340: 319–23.

87 Stehouwer CDA, Stroes ESG, Hackeng WHL, Mulder PGh, den Ottolander GJH. Von Willebrand factor and development of diabetic nephropathy in IDDM. *Diabetes* 1991; 40: 971–6.

88 Franken AAM, Derkx FHM, Man in't Veld AJ *et al.* High plasma prorenin in diabetes mellitus and its correlation with some complications. *J Clin Endocrinol Metab* 1990; 71: 1008–15.

89 Feldt-Rasmussen B. Increased transcapillary escape rate of albumin in type 1 (insulin-dependent) diabetic patients with microalbuminuria. *Diabetologia* 1986; 29: 282–6.

90 The Diabetes Control and Complications Trial Research Group. The effect of intensive treatment of diabetes on the development and progression of long-term complications in insulin-dependent diabetes mellitus. *N Engl J Med* 1993; 329: 977–86.

91 Molitch ME. ACE inhibitors and diabetic nephropathy. *Diabetes Care* 1994; 17: 756–60.

92 Mogensen CE. Renoprotective role of ace-inhibitors in diabetic nephropathy. *Br Heart J* 1994; in press.

93 Mogensen CE. Management of the diabetic patient with elevated blood pressure or renal disease. Early screening and treatment programs: albuminuria and blood pressure. In: Laragh JH, Brenner BM, eds. *Hypertension: pathology, diagnosis and management*. 2nd ed. New York; Raven Press Ltd. 1995, in press.

94 Mogensen CE. Systemic blood pressure and glomerular leakage with particular reference to diabetes and hypertension. *J Intern Med* 1994; 235: 297–316.

95 Mogensen CE (ed). *The kidney and hypertension in diabetes mellitus*, 2nd ed. Boston, Dordrecht, London, Kluwer Academic Publishers, 1994.

# 31 Pancreatic Transplantation in Humans with Diabetes Mellitus

David M. Kendall, Adrian U. Teuscher & R. Paul Robertson

In the seven decades since its discovery, insulin has been used to treat diabetes mellitus and has provided marked improvements in glycaemic control, quality of life and survival of diabetic patients. None the less, despite these successes, insulin therapy has fallen short of providing *sustained euglycaemia* in Type I diabetic patients. At the same time, prolonged survival of patients with diabetes has resulted in an increased incidence of renal, retinal, neurological, and macrovascular complications.

A major question in diabetes research is whether transplanted pancreatic tissue can be used successfully for the treatment of diabetes mellitus in humans. Pancreatic and islet cell transplantation has successfully restored and maintained normoglycaemia in diabetic animals. Pancreas transplantation in diabetic humans can maintain normoglyceamia, but it is accompanied by significant financial cost and patient morbidity. In contrast, islet transplantation has yet to achieve predictable, long-term success in human recipients. In this chapter, we review the current status of pancreas transplantation and summarise both the benefits and risks associated with this procedure. A brief overview of islet transplantation will be included, emphasising both the potential advantages of this procedure, and the possible reasons for its lack of success.

## PANCREAS TRANSPLANTATION

Pancreas transplantation was first performed at the University of Minnesota in 1966. Kelly and Lillehei (1) transplanted pancreases in two patients with long-standing diabetes and far advanced secondary complications. Only one had satisfactory graft function, and this patient remained normoglycaemic for only 6 months. These early efforts were plagued by numerous technical problems. Serious infection, graft thromboses, and rejection prevented long-term graft survival in nearly all patients. Overall, patient and graft survival was disappointingly low with no patient remaining insulin independent for more than one year.

Beginning in the late 1970s, transplantation of whole and hemi-pancreas grafts was performed with increased frequency. Significant advances in surgical technique and immunosuppression combined with improved patient monitoring resulted in improvements in both patient and graft survival. This progress has been thoroughly reviewed in numerous reports by Sutherland *et al.* from the University of Minnesota (2) as well as in reports of the International Pancreas Transplant Registry (3). To date, over 3000 pancreas transplants have been performed world-wide and, since 1990, over 1000 transplants have been performed. Current success rates are comparable to those of other whole organ allografts, including liver and heart transplantation (4,5). Since 1987, one-year graft and patient survival rates are 72% and 91%, respectively, while three-year graft and patient survival rates are 57% and 80%.

## THE TECHNIQUE OF PANCREAS TRANSPLANTATION

Currently, most pancreatic grafts are transplanted in diabetic patients with end-stage renal disease (ESRD), either simultaneously with, or following, kidney transplantation. Both whole and hemi-pancreas grafts are used. The donor organ and splenic vessels are isolated and prepared for transplantation. The graft is placed into the iliac fossa and vascular anastomoses are made with the recipient's iliac vessels. In the majority of cases, pancreatic exocrine secretions are drained via an anastomosis of the pancreatic duct with the urinary bladder or (less commonly) via a segment of jejunum. Efforts to eliminate pancreatic exocrine secretions by duct obliteration with prolene, or free intraperitoneal drainage of inactive exocrine enzymes, are alternate approaches. The use of bladder drainage avoids possible enteric contamination during surgery and allows monitoring of urinary amylase excretion as a measure of pancreatic graft function. A decrease in urinary amylase is taken as an early marker of graft rejection, and signals the need to begin anti-rejection therapy.

Immunosuppressive regimens have greatly improved in the past decade. Following the introduction of cyclosporin A, multi-drug regimens were begun. These allow for lower dosages of each component drug which minimises the negative side-effects of each. A typical immunosuppressive regimen includes cyclosporin, azathioprine and glucocorticoids. Combinations of anti-lymphocyte globulin and high-dose glucocorticoids are used to induce immunosuppression as well as to treat acute rejection.

The majority of pancreas grafts are obtained from donors who have recently died. From 1977 to 1992, investigators at the University of Minnesota also utilised hemi-pancreas grafts from living-related donors. Seventy such donors underwent 50% pancreatectomy, and the donor tissue was transplanted into a diabetic relative. Although graft survival rates for organs from living-related donors were initially better, the current success of cadaveric grafts approaches that of the living donor grafts. Consequently, the use of living donors has declined precipitously, and is presently limited to cases of high-titre cytotoxic antibodies in potential recipients.

Despite loss of 50% of their pancreas, donors have been able to maintain normal or near-normal glucose levels. However, Kendall *et al.* reported that oral glucose tolerance tests were abnormal in a seven of 28 donors studied one year after hemi-pancreatectomy (6). Subsequently, Seaquist and Robertson reported that hemi-pancreas donors have defective insulin secretion in response to intravenous glucose and have overall diminished insulin secretory reserve (7). These studies suggest that hemi-pancreatectomy may increase the risk of development of hyperglycaemia. Hence, use of living-related hemi-pancreas donors requires the consideration that glucose intolerance or frank diabetes may be induced in the donor.

## EFFECTS OF PANCREAS TRANSPLANTATION ON CARBOHYDRATE AND LIPID METABOLISM

Successful pancreas transplantation results in the normalisation of blood glucose in both the fed and fasting states (8–14). Haemoglobin A1c (glycosylated haemoglobin) levels are consistently normalised. However, the metabolic effects of successful transplantation extend beyond normalisation of blood glucose and include beneficial effects on both counter-regulation of hypoglycaemia and plasma lipoproteins.

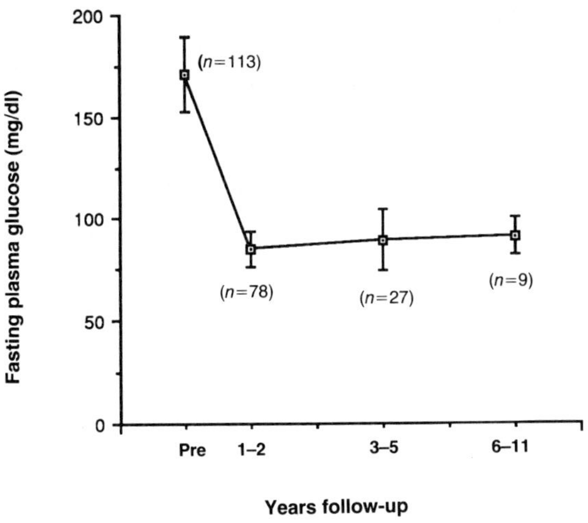


Fig. 31.1. Mean (± SD) fasting plasma glucose (mg/dl) in 113 recipients of successful pancreas transplants at the University of Minnesota between 1978 and 1992.

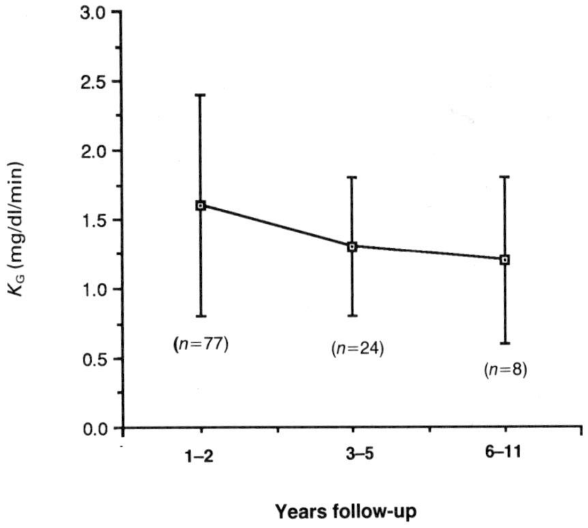


Fig. 31.3. Mean (± SD) glucose disposal rate ($K_G$) during intravenous glucose tolerance test (mg/dl/min) in 113 recipients of pancreas transplants at the University of Minnesota between 1978 and 1992.

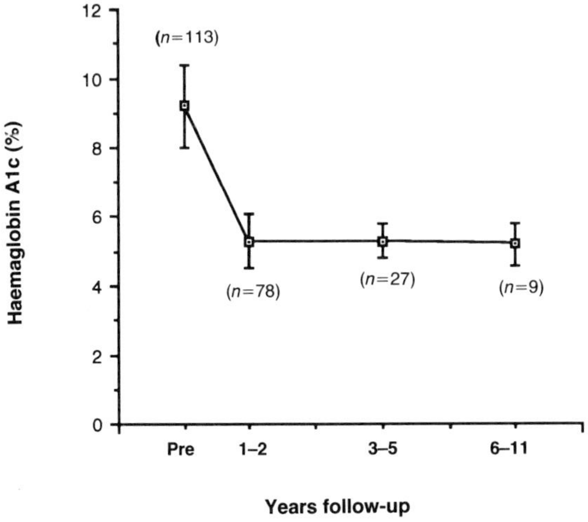


Fig. 31.2. Mean (± SD) per cent haemaglobin Alc in 113 recipients of successful pancreas transplants at the University of Minnesota between 1978 and 1992.

## Glucose metabolism

After successful pancreas transplantation, glucose levels during 24-hour periods of normal diet and activity, as well as during oral and intravenous glucose tolerance testing, are normal. Current cross-sectional data from successful transplant recipients at our institution demonstrate fasting plasma glucose levels of 91±4 (mean±SEM) in 9 patients up to 11 years following transplantation (Fig. 31.1). HbAlc levels declined from a pretransplant levels of 9.2±0.3 (*n*=113) to 5.2±0.2 (*n*=9) six to eleven years after the procedure (Fig. 31.2). Rates of glucose disposal (kg) during intravenous glucose tolerance testing are restored to normal and maintained within the normal range (greater than 1.0%/minute) throughout the period of follow-up (Fig. 31.3).

## Insulin secretion

Basal insulin levels and insulin response to intravenous and oral glucose following successful pancreas transplantation are increased two to three fold compared to normal non-diabetic control subjects. This basal and stimulated hyperinsulinaemia following transplantation results in part from insulin resistance which develops during treatment with glucocorticoids (15), but as shown by Diem *et al.* the routine use of systemic (rather than portal) venous drainage of the pancreatic graft plays the dominant role (16). Systemic venous drainage bypasses the usual first pass hepatic metabolism of insulin that occurs when the hormone is secreted by the native pancreas. Portal venous drainage of the native pancreas normally results in 50–90% degradation of insulin. Acute insulin responses to both intravenous glucose and arginine are restored and maintained up to 11 years following successful transplantation of either whole or hemi-pancreatic grafts (Fig. 31.4).

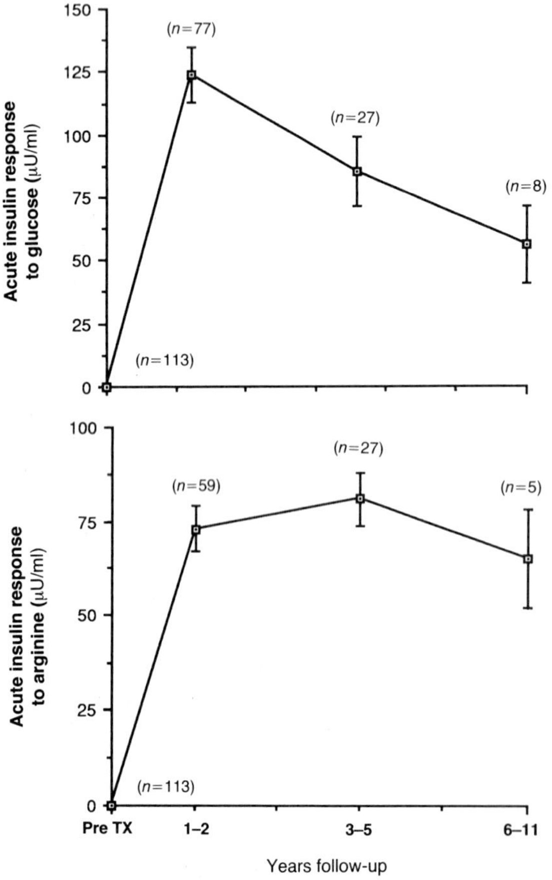


Fig. 31.4. Mean (± SE) acute insulin response to intravenous glucose and arginine in recipients of successful pancreas transplants at the University of Minnesota between 1978 and 1992.

## Counterregulation of hypoglycaemia

Counterregulation of insulin-induced hypoglycaemia is favourably affected by transplantation (17, 18). Defective counterregulation of hypoglycaemia in patients with long-standing Type I diabetes is a well-described entity (19, 20). Such diabetic patients consequently have significantly increased risk for insulin-induced hypoglycaemia. To make matters worse, recent data suggest that short-term, mild hypoglycaemia itself further impairs the ability to correct hypoglycaemia (21). Markedly decreased or absent glucagon responses play the major role in this defective counter-regulation of hypoglycaemia (19, 20). Studies by Diem *et al.* have shown that glucose recovery after insulin-induced hypoglycaemia is improved by pancreas transplantation owing, in great part, to a restoration of the glucagon response (17). Our recent data from hypoglycaemic clamp studies done between 2 and 6 years after successful pancreas transplantation demonstrate normalisation not only of glucagon secretion but also hepatic glucose production during the recovery phase after insulin-induced hypoglycaemia (22).

## Lipid metabolism

The effects of glucose normalisation on lipid metabolism are well known. Poor glucose control is associated with elevations of fasting lipids – particularly triglycerides and low density lipoprotein (LDL) cholesterol (23). Pancreas transplantation, with its positive effects on glucose control, would be expected to favourably influence serum lipids. On the other hand, elevated serum insulin has potential adverse effects on circulating triglyceride levels and the development of artherosclerosis (24). The results of studies in pancreas transplant recipients indicate that transplantation is associated with decrements in circulating triglyceride and LDL-cholesterol levels and increments in high density lipoprotein (HDL)-cholesterol levels (25, 26).

## IMPACT OF PANCREAS TRANSPLANTATION ON DIABETIC COMPLICATIONS

The microvascular complications of diabetes have long been associated with poor glycaemic control (27), leading to the hope that more precise control of blood glucose might decrease the incidence of diabetic complications, or at least slow their rate of progression.

### Kidney

Bohman *et al.* first reported data suggesting that simultaneous transplantation of kidney and pancreas grafts prevented the development of nephropathy in the kidney grafts (28). Bilous and coworkers at the University of Minnesota (29) have since published that successful pancreas transplantation is accompanied by a slowing in the rate of change of specific microscopic abnormalities of diabetic renal disease (32). This study prospectively examined kidney biopsy material of renal transplants in diabetic patients both with and without pancreas transplantation. Rates of glomerular basement membrane thickening and mesangial expansion were slowed by successful pancreas transplantation. However, these data have not demonstrated a significant functional advantage in the pancreas transplant group, perhaps because the recipients use cyclosporin for immunosuppression which decreases glomerular filtration rates.

### Retina

The impact of glycaemic control on the development and rate of progression of retinopathy has been reported in several studies (28, 30–33, 34). A few have utilised pancreas transplantation as the method of improved glycaemic control. Ramsay *et al.* evaluated the rates of progression of diabetic retinopathy in patients following successful pancreas transplantation (33). These patients were compared to a group of similarly affected diabetic patients who had undergone pancreas transplantation, but had subsequently lost graft function. The results showed no difference in the rate of progression of diabetic eye disease within the first 4 years after transplantation. The potential impact of successful transplantation on patients who had no previous retinal changes could not be assessed since all patients included in the study had evidence of at least background retinal disease prior to pancreas transplantation. These observations raise the issue of whether earlier pancreas transplantation might effectively retard the development of eye disease.

### Nerves

The impact of pancreas transplantation on the development and progression of diabetic neuropathy has also been the subject of intense interest. Kennedy *et al.* compared both motor and sensory nerve function following transplantation (34). Eleven recipients of successful grafts were compared to 12 patients whose grafts had failed shortly after transplantation. The authors concluded that successful transplantation may halt the progression of motor and sensory neuropathy. Other studies have confirmed these findings, but the clinical impact of these changes is not clear, since only a minority of patients report a significant subjective change in their neuropathic symptoms (35–38). A report by Navarro *et al.* examined the impact of pancreas transplantation on the association between diabetic autonomic neuropathy and early mortality (39). They concluded that successful transplantation may offer a survival advantage in patients with autonomic neurological complications. This report, as with many others, was weakened because no randomised control group was studied simultaneously.

### Macrovascular disease

Large vessel disease, whether involving coronary, cerebral or peripheral arteries, contributes more than any other complication to premature mortality in Type 1 diabetic patients. This effect is increased in patients who develop end-stage renal disease such that cardiovascular mortality accounts for one-year patient survival rates of less than 50% (40). Beneficial changes in the lipid profile of patients who have undergone pancreas transplantation might provide benefits in terms of prevention of macrovascular disease. However, no studies have been reported which address morbidity and mortality related to the development of macrovascular disease in patients who have received pancreas transplantation.

## EFFECT OF PANCREAS TRANSPLANTATION ON QUALITY OF LIFE

Successful pancreas transplantation eliminates the need for exogenous insulin and provides normalisation of blood glucose. Additional benefits are the freedom from insulin-induced hypoglycaemia and the standard dietary restrictions of the diabetic patient. Freedom from exogenous insulin, in turn, eliminates the need for frequent monitoring of blood glucose. However, the risks of the operative procedure and lifelong immunosuppression seriously offset these advantages. Two recent studies have demonstrated improved quality of life in recipients of successful pancreas transplants. They took into account features such as ability to return to work, perceived sense of health, and freedom from hospitalisation (41, 42). As with many other studies, however, these compared only patients with either failed or successful pancreas transplants. None has compared a control group of insulin-treated patients matched to a group undergoing pancreas transplantation.

## CONSIDERATION OF HEALTH CARE COSTS

Whole organ transplantation is expensive, and pancreas transplantation is no exception. Current estimates place the cost of pancreas transplantation at approximately £41 000–£54 000 ($60–80 000). Moreover, the expense of immunosuppression approaches £2041 ($3000) per year. No data are currently available to compare the cost of pancreas transplantation with the maintenance costs for non-transplanted diabetic patients. This further underscores the need for controlled studies using all endpoints noted above to clearly assess the utility of pancreas transplantation.

## ISLET CELL TRANSPLANTATION

While virtually all of the success with transplantation emanates from the use of whole or segmental pancreatic grafts, the use of pancreatic islets for transplantation continues to be looked to as the future option of choice. If this approach becomes feasible, islet cell transplantation should provide several advantages over organ transplants, including relative technical simplicity, the ability to transplant tissue from more than one donor source, and lesser morbidity and financial cost of the procedure.

Islet cell transplants became a theoretical possibility with the successful isolation of viable islet tissue in 1967 (43). Reports several years later demonstrated that successful islet transplantation could partially correct experimental forms of diabetes in rodents (44). Islet cell transplantation is technically less complex than organ transplantation. Donor pancreases are digested with protease enzymes and islet cells are isolated by differential centrifugation. Following isolation, the islets are infused into the portal vein and implant in the liver parenchyma. Extensive experimental efforts are under way to transplant islets in immunologically protected sites (45). In addition, many investigators are presently attempting to modulate the immunogenicity of islets by various pretransplant immunomodulation techniques (46) or by using islet allo- and xeno-grafts within isolated diffusion chambers. These topics are discussed elsewhere in this book.

## Islet transplantation in humans

Islet transplantation in humans is rarely successful. This procedure is plagued by numerous technical problems including difficulty with islet isolation and purification, and extremely high degrees of early rejection. Within the past decade, however, several case reports of insulin independence after islet cell transplantation have been published (47, 48). These successes have rekindled enthusiasm for islet transplantation, and have raised hopes that this procedure may prove effective in treating Type I diabetes. Still, the fact remains that, to date, only a single patient has demonstrated insulin independence for more than two years following islet transplantation (48).

While the ultimate success or failure of islet *allo*transplantation is yet unknown, recently published data have demonstrated preservation of normal phasic insulin secretion and carbohydrate tolerance following islet *auto*transplantation. Pyzdrowski *et al.*(49) evaluated five non-diabetic patients with chronic pancreatitis who had undergone total pancreatectomy because of chronic, severe pain. Their own islets were harvested and autotransplanted via portal vein infusion within hours of isolation. After transplantation, the patients had demonstrable phasic insulin and glucagon secretion in response to intravenous injections of glucose or arginine, and four of the five were able to maintain normoglycaemia without exogenous insulin treatment. These data suggested that as few as 265 000 islets can provide adequate beta cell mass to provide for normal glucose tolerance.

The reasons for the lack of success of islet *allo*-transplantation remain obscure. The experience with autotransplantation suggests that current techniques of isolation and implantation are effective. Islet number should not be limiting as 250 000–500 000 islets can usually be obtained from donor pancreases. One consideration is that the immunosuppressive drugs used may harm the transplanted islets. Combined therapy with cyclosporin and glucocorticoids is associated with changes in glycaemic control following transplantation (50), and cyclosporin itself has been shown to decrease insulin secretion in response to intravenous glucose (51). That these immunosuppressive agents are currently used successfully in whole graft transplant but fail to protect islet transplants remains a perplexing puzzle. Is the isolated islet somehow more sensitive to the immune rejection phenomenon? Does removal of the islet from its normal site within the pancreas render it more susceptible to damage by macrophages, cytokines, or drugs used for immunosuppression? If the technical problems with islet allografts can be overcome, islet transplantation should receive widespread use in the treatment of IDDM and ultimately replace whole organ pancreas transplantation.

## FUTURE DIRECTIONS

Pancreas transplantation as a treatment for diabetes has overcome most of the technical roadblocks faced during the early years of this procedure. Current patient and graft survival data suggest that the operative procedure is sound and achieves similar survival rates when carried out in the many institutions with extensive experience in the procedure (3). A recently published position paper (52) and technical review (53) from the American Diabetes Association (ADA) discussed the current status of pancreas transplantation in patients with diabetes mellitus. This document suggested limiting pancreatic transplantation to individuals with end-stage renal disease who have undergone or will undergo renal transplantation. The ADA position paper emphasised the relative risks of immunosuppression and suggested that pancreas transplant alone is not warranted, since available data suggest that the risks of immunosuppression may be greater than that of conventionally treated Type I diabetes. This same review considered islet cell transplantation a hopeful but experimental procedure at this time. The results of islet transplantation continue to improve and provide hope that it may achieve widespread success in the treatment of diabetes.

At this point in the greater than 25-year history of pancreatic transplantation, however, randomised studies to assess the relative benefits and risks of this procedure are still lacking. Data relating the correction of hyperglycaemia to prevention of progression of diabetic complications have been either retrospective or derived from unrandomised and/or uncontrolled trials. Only appropriately controlled studies can reveal the true impact of pancreas transplantation on secondary complications and compare these outcomes to the potential risks of surgery and the effects of long-term immunosuppression in the diabetic patient.

Whether to offer this procedure to patients prior to the onset of complications is a very difficult question. Restoration and maintenance of euglycaemia through transplantation early in the disease would by itself be beneficial to the patient's sense of well-being. Glycaemic control may reduce the development of complications if normoglycaemia is re-established prior to the initial onset of complications. However, since prediction of secondary complications prior to their onset is not possible, pancreas transplantation with its associated surgical risks and immunosuppression is difficult to justify for patients in whom standard insulin treatment is adequate to provide reasonable glycaemic control. Further data which demonstrate a reduction in complication rates must first be obtained. Again, only with the completion of appropriately controlled studies can the benefits and risks of pancreas transplantation be fully understood.

## ACKNOWLEDGEMENT

This work was supported by NIH grant R01 DK 39994 and the General Clinical Research Center Program (M01 RR 00400).

## REFERENCES

1 Kelly WD, Lillehei RC, Merkel FK, Idezuki Y, Goetz FC. Allotransplantation of the pancreas and duodenum along with the kidney in diabetic nephropathy. *Surgery* 1967; 61: 827–37.

2 Sutherland DER, Dunn DL, Goetz FC *et al.* A 10-year experience with 290 pancreas transplants at a single institution. *Ann Surg* 1989; 210: 274–88.

3 Sutherland DER, Gruesner A, Moudry-Munns K. Report on results of pancreas transplantation in the United States October 1987 to October 1991 from the United Network for Organ Sharing Registry. In Terasaki P, ed. *Clinical transplants.* Los Angeles, CA, UCLA Press, 1991; Chapter 3: 31–8.

4 Evans RW, Dong FB, Manninen DL. The center effect in heart transplantation. *Clin Transpl* 1991; 45–9.

5 Detre KM, Belle SH, Beringer KC, Murphy JB, Vaughn WK. Pitt-UNOS Liver Transplant Registry. *Clin Transpl* 1989; 9–18.

6 Kendall DM, Sutherland DER, Najarian JS, Goetz FC, Robertson RP. Effects of hemipancreatectomy on insulin secretion and glucose tolerance in healthy humans. *N Engl J Med* 1990; 322: 898–903.

7 Seaquist ER, Robertson RP. Effects of hemipancreatectomy on pancreatic alpha and beta cell function in healthy human donors. *J Clin Invest* 1992; 89: 1761–6.

8 Robertson RP. Seminars in Medicine of the Beth Israel Hospital, Boston. Pancreas transplantation for diabetes: cures or curiosities? *N Engl J Med* 1992; 327: 1861–9.

9 Osei K, Henry ML, O'Dorisio TM, Tesi RJ, Sommer BG, Ferguson RM. Physiological and pharmacological stimulation of pancreatic islet hormone secretion in Type I diabetic pancreas allograft recipients. *Diabetes* 1990; 39: 1235–42.

10 Robertson RP, Diem P, Sutherland DER. Time-related, cross-sectional and prospective follow-up of pancreatic endocrine function after pancreas allograft transplantation in Type I (insulin-dependent) diabetic patients. *Diabetologia* 34 (Suppl 1): 1991; S57–60.

11 Landgraf R, Nusser J, Riepl RL *et al.* Metabolic and hormonal studies of Type I (insulin-dependent) diabetic patients after successful pancreas and kidney transplantation. *Diabetologia* 34 (Suppl 1): 1991; S61–7.

12 Secchi A, Dubernard JM, La Rocca E *et al.* Endocrinometabolic effects of whole versus segmental pancreas allotransplantation in diabetic patients – a two-year follow-up. *Transplantation* 1991; 51: 625–9.

13 Holdaas H, Brekke IB, Hartmann A *et al.* Long-term metabolic control in recipients of combined pancreas and kidney transplants. *Diabetologia* 1991; 34 (Suppl 1): S68–70.

14 Katz, Homan M, Velosa J, Robertson P, Rizza R. Effects of pancreas transplantation on postprandial glucose metabolism. *N Engl J Med* 1991; 325: 1278–83.

15 Luzi L, Secchi A, Facchini F *et al.* Reduction of insulin resistance by combined kidney-pancreas transplantation in Type I (insulin-dependent) diabetic patients. *Diabetologia* 1990; 33: 549–556.

16 Diem P, Abid M, Redmon JB, Sutherland DER, Robertson RP. Systemic venous drainage of pancreas allografts as independent cause of hyperinsulinemia in Type I diabetic recipients. *Diabetes* 1990; 39: 534–40.

17 Diem P, Redmon JB, Abid M *et al.* Glucagon, catecholamine and pancreatic polypeptide secretion in

Type I diabetic recipients of pancreas allografts. *J Clin Invest* 1990; 86: 2008–13.
18 Bolinder J, Wahrenberg H, Linde B, Tyden G, Groth CG, Ostman J. Improved glucose counterregulation after pancreas transplantation in diabetic patients with unawareness of hypoglycemia. *Transpl Proc* 1991; 23: 1667–9.
19 Gerich JE, Langlois M, Noacco C, Karam JH, Forsham PH. Lack of glucagon response to hypoglycemia in diabetes: evidence for an intrinsic alpha cell defect. *Science* 1973; 182: 1271–3.
20 Benson JW Jr, Johnson DG, Palmer JP, Werner PL, Ensinck JW. Glucagon and catecholamine secretion during hypoglycemia in normal and diabetic man. *J Clin Endocrinol Metab* 1997; 44: 459–64.
21 Widom B, Simonson DC. Intermittent hypoglycemia impairs glucose counterregulation. *Diabetes* 1992; 41: 1597–602.
22 Barrou Z, Seaquist ER, Robertson RP. Pancreas transplantation in diabetic humans normalizes hepatic glucose production during hypoglycemia. *Diabetes* 1994; 43: 661–6.
23 Reaven GM, Greenfield MS. Diabetic hypertriglyceridemia: evidence for three clinical syndromes. *Diabetes* 1981; 30: 66–75.
24 Fontbonne AM, Eschwege EM. Insulin and cardiovascular disease. Paris prospective study. *Diabetes Care* 1991; 14: 461–9.
25 Larsen JL, Stratta RJ, Ozaki CF, Taylor RJ, Miller SA, Duckworth WC. Lipid status after pancreas–kidney transplantation. *Diabetes Care* 1992; 15: 35–42.
26 La Rocca E, Secchi A, Parlavecchia M *et al.* Lipid metabolism after successful kidney and pancreatic transplantation. *Transpl Proc* 1991; 23: 1672–3.
27 Pirart J. Diabetes mellitus and its degenerative complication: a prospective study of 4,400 patients observed between 1947 and 1973. *Diabetes Care* 1978; 1(3): 168–88 and 1978; 1(4): 252–63.
28 Bohman S-O, Tyden G, Wilczek H *et al.* Prevention of kidney graft diabetic nephropathy by pancreas transplantation in man. *Diabetes* 1985; 34: 306–8.
29 Bilous RW, Mauer SM, Sutherland DER, Najarian JS, Goetz FC, Steffes MW. The effects of pancreas transplantation on the glomerular structure of renal allografts in patients with insulin-dependent diabetes. *N Engl J Med* 1989; 321: 80–5.
30 Kroc Collaborative Study Group. Blood glucose control and the evolution of diabetic retinopathy and albuminuria. *N Engl J Med* 1984; 311: 365–72.
31 Lauritzen T, Larsen H-W, Frost-Larson K, Deckert T and the Steno Study Group. Effect of 1 year of near-normal blood glucose levels on retinopathy in insulin-dependent diabetics. *Lancet* 1983; i: 200–3.
32 Engerman RL, Kern TS: Progression of incipient diabetic retinopathy during good glycemic control. *Diabetes* 1987; 36: 808–12.
33 Ramsay RC, Goetz FC, Sutherland DER *et al.* Progression of diabetic retinopathy after pancreas transplantation for insulin-dependent diabetes mellitus. *N Engl J Med* 1988; 318: 208–4.
34 Kennedy WR, Navarro X, Goetz FC, Sutherland DER, Najarian JS. Effects of pancreatic transplantation on diabetic neuropathy. *N Engl J Med* 1990; 322: 1031–7.
35 Secchi A, Martinenghi S, Galardi G, Comi G, Canal N, Pozza G. Effects of pancreatic transplantation on diabetic polyneuropathy. *Transpl Proc* 1991; 23: 1658–9.
36 Aridge D, Reese J, Niehoff M *et al.* Effect of successful renal and segmental pancreatic transplantation on peripheral and autonomic neuropathy. *Transpl Proc* 1991; 23: 1670–1.
37 Calder R, Sanseverino R, Lefrancois N, Martin X, Martinenghi S, Dubernard JM. Pancreas transplantation: long term results. *Clin Transpl* 1991; 5: 260–4.
38 Gaber AO, Cardoso S, Pearson S, *et al.* Improvement in autonomic function following combined pancreas-kidney transplantation. *Transpl Proc* 1991; 23: 1660–2.
39 Navarro X, Kennedy WR, Loewenson RB, Sutherland DER. Influence of pancreas transplantation on cardiorespiratory reflexes, nerve conduction, and mortality in diabetes mellitus. *Diabetes* 1990; 39: 802–6.
40 Bennett WM, Kloster F, Rosch J, Barry J, Porter GA. Natural history of asymptomatic coronary arteriographic lesions in diabetic patients with end-stage renal disease. *Am J Med* 1978; 65: 779–84.
41 Zehrer CL, Gross CR. Quality of life of pancreas transplant recipients. *Diabetologia* 1991; 34 (Suppl 1): S145–9.
42 Piehlmeier W, Bullinger M, Nusser J *et al.* Quality of life in Type I (insulin-dependent) diabetic patients prior to and after pancreas and kidney transplantation in relation to organ function. *Diabetologia* 1991; 34 (Suppl 1): S150–7.
43 Lacy PE, Kostianovsky M. Method for the isolation of intact islets of Langerhans from the rat pancreas. *Diabetes* 1967; 16: 35–9.
44 Ballinger WF, Lacy PE. Transplantation of intact pancreatic islets in rats. *Surgery* 1972; 72: 175–86.
45 Posselt AM, Barker CF, Tomaszewski JE, Markmann JF, Choti MA, Naji A. Induction of donor-specific unresponsiveness by intrathymic islet transplantation. *Science* 1990; 249: 1293–5.
46 Weber C, Krekun S, Koschitzky T *et al.* Prolonged functional survival of rat to NOD mouse islet xenografts by ultraviolet-B (UV-B) irradiation plus microencapsulation of donor islets. *Transpl Proc* 1991; 23 (1 Part 1): 764–6.
47 Scharp DW, Lacy PE, Santiago JV *et al.* Insulin independence after islet transplantation into Type I diabetic patients. *Diabetes* 1990; 39: 515–18.
48 Warnock GL, Kneteman NM, Ryan E, Seelis REA, Rabinovitch A, Rajotte RV. Normoglycemia after transplantation of freshly isolated and cryopreserved pancreatic islets in Type I (insulin-dependent) diabetes mellitus. *Diabetologia* 1991; 34: 55–8.
49 Pyzdrowski KL, Kendall DM, Halter JB, Nakhleh RF, Sutherland DER, Robertson RP. Preserved insulin secretion and insulin independence in human islet autograft recipients. *N Engl J Med* 1992; 327: 220–6.
50 Yamamoto H, Akazawa S, Yamaguchi Y *et al.* Effects of cyclosporin A and low dosages of steroid on post-transplantation diabetes in kidney transplant recipients. *Diabetes Care* 1991; 14: 867–70.
51 Alejandro R, Feldman EC, Bloom AD, Kenyon NS. Effects of cyclosporin on insulin and c-peptide secretion in healthy beagles. *Diabetes* 1989; 38: 698–703.
52 American Diabetes Association. Position statement on pancreas transplantation for patients with diabetes mellitus. *Diabetes Care* 1992; 15: 1673.
53 American Diabetes Association. Technical review on pancreas transplantation for patients with diabetes mellitus. *Diabetes Care* 1992; 15: 1668–72.

# 32 Rational Insulin Management of Insulin-dependent Diabetes

Robert E. Ratner

> Insulin is a remedy primarily for the wise and not for the foolish, be they patients or doctors. Everyone knows it requires brains to live long with diabetes, but to use insulin successfully requires more brains.
>
> *Elliot P. Joslin,* in *The Treatment of Diabetes Mellitus,* 1923(1).

The isolation of the pancreatic extract in 1921 by Banting and Best which effectively lowered blood glucose levels in pancreatectomised dogs initiated the modern age of clinical care for individuals with insulin-dependent diabetes. After first observing the effects of injected insulin on himself, Banting undertook the treatment of Leonard Thompson, a 14-year old boy with diabetes, on January 11, 1922. Only a slight fall in blood glucose was observed, while abscesses occurred following six of the first seven injections(2). Improved extraction techniques resulted in greater potency and a more purified preparation which was reported by Macleod.

> Thus, it caused the blood sugar to return to the normal level, the sugar of the urine to disappear, acetonuria to vanish and the respiratory quotient to rise to its usual level. Not alone were the objective symptoms relieved, but the well-being of the patients definitely improved. . . . In agreement with observations of other investigators on laboratory animals, it has been found that without careful control, severe toxic reactions may be encountered and this will undoubtedly be a factor in the evaluation of the ultimate therapeutic utility of the method(3).

With this landmark discovery, the debate and disagreement concerning the appropriate form of insulin to use, its frequency of administration, and its ultimate ability to stave off the long-term sequelae of diabetes was presaged in the original description of its clinical use over 70 years ago.

## PHARMACOLOGY OF INSULIN

The original water soluble, animal insulin had a short (4 to 6 hour) duration of action and was significantly contaminated by a multitude of pancreatic peptides, including pro-insulin and insulin degradation products. Progressive purification techniques have now yielded insulins of 99.9% purity with addition of a variety of retarding agents to slow absorption from the subcutaneous depot and prolong the activity. In the early 1980s, human insulin was introduced into clinical practice with much initial excitement, followed by scepticism and some concern.

At the present time, two basic techniques are utilised for manufacturing human insulin. Semisynthetic conversion of porcine insulin by threonine for alanine transpeptidation at the B-30 position results in insulin structurally indistinguishable from cadaveric human insulin. Biosynthetic human insulin is made by recombinant DNA technology employing a variety of transfecting vectors, host cells, and DNA templates. The initial commercial product of biosynthetic human insulin utilised *E. coli* as the host cell with two separate transfected batches. One strain secreted pure A-chain while the second strain made pure B-chain. An extra biochemical fermentation was required to join the two polypeptides to form the well-known double-chain insulin polypeptide with two interchain disulphide bridges. This complex process was required because current recombinant techniques are able to produce only a single polypeptide per transfected cell. Because insulin is synthesised as a pro-hormone in the islet cell, the use of a pro-insulin DNA template was attempted. Unless the pro-hormone is protected, however, post-translational proteolysis occurs which alters the ultimate three-dimensional structure of insulin. As a result, it is necessary to modify the insulin precursor. Two mechanisms are currently utilised to accomplish this task. In one, pro-insulin is protected by binding it to tryptophan synthetase, causing intracellular accumulation of the complex. The *E. coli* are lysed and the pro-insulin cleaved from the carrier. Subsequent cleavage of the pro-insulin to insulin and C-peptide with purification to its final commercial product are performed. A second technique for manufacturing genetically engineered human insulin has recently been perfected. In this process, baker's yeast (*Saccharomyces cerevisiae*) is utilised as the host cell rather than *E. coli*. Baker's yeast can be made to secrete insulin precursor directly into the medium for rapid isolation and purification and makes no pyrogens or toxins which could contaminate the medium, or ultimately, the insulin. The DNA template has a modified, shortened C-peptide which facilitates the folding of the molecule to achieve the correct tertiary structure, but prevents intracellular proteolysis. The secreted product has the correct disulphide bridges and simply requires cleavage of the modified C-peptide by trypsin in the presence of threonine–ester to form human insulin ester. Three purification steps result in a product which is greater than 99% pure human insulin.

Previous studies revealed immunological differences between human insulins made by various manufacturers (4). The difference appeared to result from variable degrees of self-aggregation into high molecular weight insulin aggregates among the different manufacturers. Differing concentration of these high molecular weight aggregates in the insulin preparations themselves translated into a greater blast transformation response in lymphocytes from individuals with documented insulin allergy.

More recent studies have revealed improved stabilisation of the insulin products, with less than 2% of the insulin existing in high molecular weight aggregate form (5). Cross-over study of the therapeutic effects and complications of insulins from two major manufacturers has shown no difference in insulin requirement, glycaemic control, insulin or high molecular weight insulin aggregate levels in the serum, insulin antibodies, thresholds or frequency of hypoglycaemia (6). It now appears that, unlike other hormones such as L-thyroxine or conjugated equine oestrogens, insulin therapy is interchangeable between major brands of commercial preparations. We are fortunate, indeed, to have a potentially unlimited supply of pure, high quality human insulin for therapeutic use.

With 70 years' experience with animal source insulins and their therapeutic use, the availability of human insulin raised the critical question of why use a human insulin preparation? Commercial human insulin is structurally identical to cadaveric human insulin, relatively free of contaminants from the manufacturing process, and has comparable receptor binding. The ability of human insulin to stimulate peripheral glucose uptake and suppress hepatic glucose production is consistent with porcine insulin (7). Absorption characteristics appear to be somewhat faster than porcine, being more pronounced with regular insulin and varying somewhat between intermediate acting preparations depending upon the manufacturer (8). Early reports of potentially serious nocturnal hypoglycaemia due to supper time human NPH therapy appeared to have been resolved by moving the dose to bedtime.

These minor changes in pharmacodynamics are sometimes noted in cross-over studies comparing porcine and human insulin and result in slight changes in insulin requirement or glycaemic control. The observed complications of animal insulin therapy (including lipoatrophy, immunological resistance, and allergy) are relatively rare and insufficient to justify a wholesale transfer of patients over to the then new, more expensive human preparations. None the less, in the absence of any demonstrable disadvantages to the use of human insulin, the small clinical benefits together with the psychological advantage of treating 'human insulin deficiency' with human insulin, resulted in a widespread shift to both semisynthetic and biosynthetic human insulins in the 1980s. Cost has now become a reason to use human insulin, as animal insulins have risen in retail price to first match and now surpass the cost of human insulin. In a small survey of retail pharmacies in the metropolitan Washington, DC area, human and mixed beef/pork insulins were comparably priced, while purified pork was 38% more expensive (personal observation). In the United States, the phasing out of animal insulin preparations has already begun, with human insulin now accounting for over two-thirds of insulin sales; and one can anticipate that human insulin will be the only readily available preparation within five years.

The initial introduction of human insulin held great hope for the resolution of antibody generation mediating both allergy and insulin resistance. But, subsequent discovery of insulin autoantibody formation in IDDM mitigated much of the enthusiasm. None the less, formation of both IgG and IgE antibodies is less in patients treated with human insulin as compared to porcine or beef (9, 10). Patients with neutralising insulin antibodies on animal insulin therapy demonstrate a profound fall in insulin binding capacity upon transfer to human insulin (11). Although all of these data are statistically significant, much debate exists concerning their clinical significance. Both insulin allergy and immunological insulin resistance are rare observations, and though they remain firm indications for the use of human insulin, their potential occurrence alone cannot justify its exclusive clinical use. A fascinating recent observation has been the correlation of insulin antibody levels with macrosomia in infants of diabetic mothers (12). This finding substantiates the current recommendation that only human insulin be used to treat pregnant women requiring insulin.

Hypoglycaemia – its frequency, severity, and recognition – remains the greatest concern following initiation of insulin therapy. A great deal has been made of the initial anecdotal reports of severe hypoglycaemia without warning which occurred following patient transfer from animal to human insulin. Surveys performed in the United Kingdom after the introduction of human insulin suggested that as many 30% of patients lost awareness of hypoglycaemic symptoms when using human insulin(13). Methodological problems and lack of uniform definitions have rendered these data highly suspect. Many studies, including five within the last three years, have examined the relationship between hypoglycaemia and insulin species. In a cross-sectional, prospective analysis of over 500 patients, Muhlhauser *et al.* found no differences in the incidence of severe hypoglycaemia (defined as loss of consciousness) between patients treated with human vs animal insulins (0.46 vs 0.45 cases/patient–year, respectively) (14). According to the patients in both groups, trembling and sweating were the most common initial warning symptoms and a similar percentage reported impaired awareness of hypoglycaemia. In a case-control trial of patients admitted to the hospital for hypoglycaemia or diabetic coma, Egger *et al.* found the use of human insulin increased the relative risk of hypoglycemia by three-fold, although this was overshadowed by the role of a previous history of hypoglycaemic coma as a risk factor(15). This study also

Table 32.1. *Indications for human insulin use*

| |
|---|
| Cost savings compared to animal insulins |
| Insulin treatment during pregnancy |
| Lipoatrophy |
| Documented insulin allergy |
| Documented immunological insulin resistance |
| Intermittent insulin therapy |

uncovered a 2.5-fold greater rate of previous hypoglycaemia in the human insulin group, which may explain the indication for its use in the first place.

In a subsequent randomised, double-blind cross-over study by the same authors, two episodes of coma occurred while on porcine as compared to only one on human insulin (16). The only difference in warning signs was an increased frequency of restlessness and lack of concentration described by those on human insulin, although the overall frequency of hypoglycaemia (defined as capillary glucose < 50 mg/dl) was no different. Patients specifically complaining of altered perception of hypoglycaemia while on human insulin were challenged in a blinded fashion to either porcine or human insulin; however, there were no subjective (i.e. symptom score and perception of hypo-glycaemia) or objective (i.e. tachycardia, sweating or cognitive dysfunction) differences noted following IV infusion to achieve a glucose nadir of 30 mg/dl (17). Furthermore, counter-regulatory hormone responses to hypoglycaemic challenge have been repeatedly shown to be unchanged by the species of insulin used (18).

Human insulin is a useful clinical advance in the treatment of diabetes, providing pure insulin preparations at stable cost, with unlimited supply potential. Like all insulin preparations, it lowers plasma glucose levels by suppressing hepatic glucose production and stimulating peripheral glucose uptake. When used in excessive doses, it results in progressive hypoglycaemia which leads to activation of counter-regulatory hormones, adrenergic and neuro-glycopaenic symptoms. Lowering of serum glucose is the action of insulin and *not* a complication; if hypoglycaemia occurs, it is an indication to modify the timing or dosage, not the species of insulin. There are no convincing data to support the use of animal insulins preferentially to human, and there are several firm indications for the particular use of human insulin (see Table 32.1).

## PHARMACODYNAMICS OF INSULIN

The rational use of insulin in the treatment of IDDM requires the firm understanding of the absorption characteristics and potential complicating variables of administered insulin. Unlike the normal physiological state, therapeutic insulin administration is clearly backwards. In the intact organism, insulin is secreted into the portal system in response to a stimulus of carbohydrate and protein absorption from the GI tract. The magnitude of insulin secretion is dependent upon the rapidity and magnitude of the bolus absorbed. In contrast, therapeutic insulin is traditionally introduced via the systemic circulation in anticipation of the ingestion of a caloric load. If the patient and physician have guessed right in the timing, injection site, insulin type and dose together with the caloric intake, then euglycaemia is achieved. More commonly, if any of these variables are not perfectly predicted and anticipated, then either clinically significant hyper- or hypoglycaemia will ensue. Overcoming the problems inherent in this backwards approach to insulin therapy is the ultimate goal of the rational insulin management of IDDM.

At the present time, subcutaneous administration of insulin is the only realistic clinical delivery system. Absorption from this subcutaneous depot is dependent upon local blood flow which may vary according to site and depth of the injection, or exercise or massage of the injection site. Volume of the injection together with the physical state of the insulin molecule further modifies absorption rates (19). Even when site and volume of injection are held constant, clinical responses vary enormously within individual patients. Peak insulin levels may vary by 20 to

30% while time to peak insulin concentration demonstrates a coefficient of variation as high as 50% within individuals (20).

In addition, the plasma insulin response to subcutaneous insulin injection differs markedly from that seen in response to a glucose challenge in a non-diabetic subject. The rate of increase of insulin in plasma is considerably slower and plateaus rather than peaking following systemic injection. The portal/systemic insulin concentrations are equal rather than demonstrating the 2.5 to 1 gradient seen in non-diabetic subjects. Finally, exogenous insulin therapy results in prolonged elevations of plasma insulin levels well beyond the timing of a glucose challenge (19). As a result, early portal hypo-insulinaemia results in unrestrained hepatic glucose production with early hyperglycaemia, while persistent late hyperinsulinaemia both suppresses hepatic glucose production and stimulates peripheral glucose uptake resulting in late hypoglycaemia.

Ideally, glycaemic control will be improved by removing as many of these potential variables as possible. The traditional recommendation for rotation of insulin injection sites is an important means of avoiding lipohypertrophy and its subsequent erratic insulin absorption (21). Absorption from the abdomen has been found to be faster and more predictable than either the arm, leg or buttock (22). Thus, exclusive use of the abdomen as an injection site during the day is preferable. Rotation about the umbilicus will minimise the risks of lipohypertrophy forming while providing a greater degree of predictability in insulin absorption. Utilisation of the arm, leg or buttock should be limited to bedtime doses of intermediate acting insulin preparations, minimising the potential impact of exercise on insulin absorption rates. In addition, the delayed absorption of subcutaneous insulin mandates injection 20 to 60 minutes prior to ingestion of a caloric load. This latency period is dependent upon the source of calories being ingested (liquid versus solid, or carbohydrate versus a mixed meal) as well as the intrinsic functioning of the GI tract. Autonomic dysfunction resulting in gastroparesis diabetocorum may markedly slow gastric emptying and subsequent GI absorption requiring a marked alteration in timing of the insulin injection. Even before considering dietary intake or insulin dosing, it is not surprising that clinical glucose control is so poor in our patients with IDDM.

Efforts to improve glycaemic control have historically centred around manipulation of the insulin molecule rather than the more difficult patient management strategies of diet, monitoring and exercise. The original water soluble, animal insulin preparation of Banting and Best had a duration of action of 4 to 6 hours. Thus, patients were required to administer 4 to 6 shots daily in an effort to maintain adequate circulating plasma insulin levels. The introduction of a stable form of protamine zinc insulin (PZI) in the 1930s and the subsequent introduction of NPH and Lente insulins in the 1950s were hailed as monumental breakthroughs for patients with IDDM. By combining insulin with retarding agents, the circulating half-life of injectable insulin was extended to as long as 36 hours. Treatment with one and sometimes two injections daily was considered to be a profound advance in the quality of life for patients with IDDM. Predicting the latency phase for peak insulin action, together with the duration allowed greater predictability for timing of insulin injections and intake of calories. Integrated analysis of carbohydrate handling, such as 24 h urine glucose excretion, could be improved by utilisation of these longer-acting insulin preparations. Hypoglycaemia could be minimised by the ingestion of snacks or meals at the time of anticipated insulin peak action, but postprandial hyperglycaemia was unaffected (see Table 32.2).

Rough predictions of insulin pharmacodynamics as shown in Table 32.2 have been incorporated into numerous insulin regimens in an effort to achieve glycaemic control. By examining 24-hour plasma glucose and free insulin levels in non-diabetic individuals (23) (Fig. 32.1) one can immediately see why a single injection

Table 32.2. *Insulin preparations*

| | Duration (hours) of action[a] | | |
|---|---|---|---|
| | Onset | Peak | Duration |
| *Rapid-acting* | | | |
| Regular (soluble) | 0.25–0.5 | 1–3 | 4–6 |
| *Intermediate-acting* | | | |
| Isophane (NPH) | 2–4 | 6–8 | 12–16 |
| Lente | 2–4 | 6–8 | 12–16 |
| *Long-acting* | | | |
| Protamine–zinc (PZI) | 3–4 | 14–20 | 24–36 |
| Ultra-lente | 3–4 | 14–20 | 24–36 |

[a] Values for onset, peak and duration of action are approximate and vary with dose and with individual patient response.

of intermediate-acting insulin in the morning is incapable of achieving glycaemic control in a patient with IDDM. One can progressively move from a simple single daily injection to more complex regimens including split dose regimens, mixed dose regimens, and split-mixed regimens (Fig. 32.2). Most interesting is the realisation that a basal–bolus (most reminiscent of the multiple injections used in the early days of insulin therapy) would appear to most closely mimic the insulin profile of the non-diabetic subjects (24). In essence, we have come full circle.

## INSULIN REGIMENS

Rational insulin therapy of the patient with IDDM requires close co-operation between patient, physician, and diabetes educator. Any regimen prescribed by the physician must fit within the lifestyle of the patient, and be acceptable to him/her. Non-adherence, in fact, is a major source of brittle diabetes. The use of intermediate and long-acting forms of insulin significantly improved patient compliance and treatment with insulin therapy. Patients frequently prefer administration of one or at most

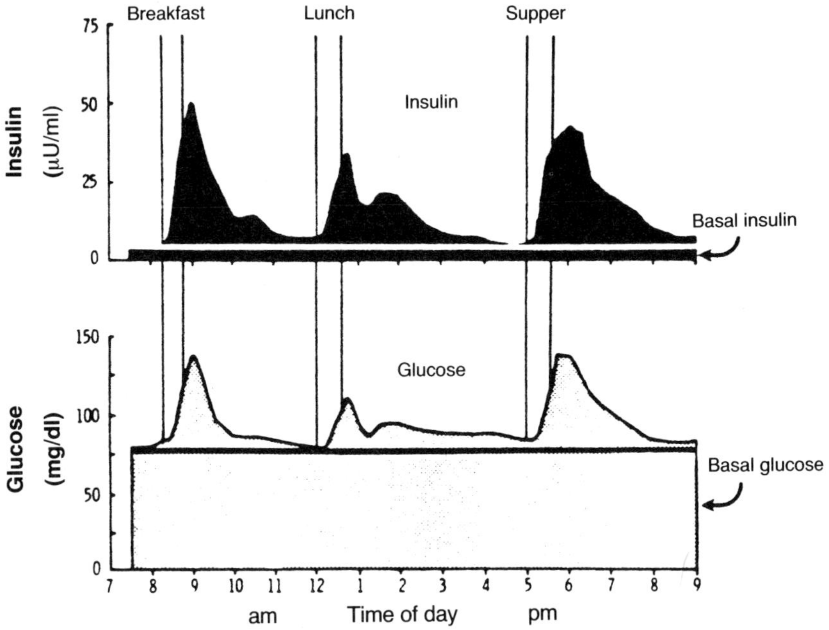


Fig. 32.1. Mean 24-hour insulin and glucose profiles in non-diabetic subjects. (Adapted from Ref. 23.)

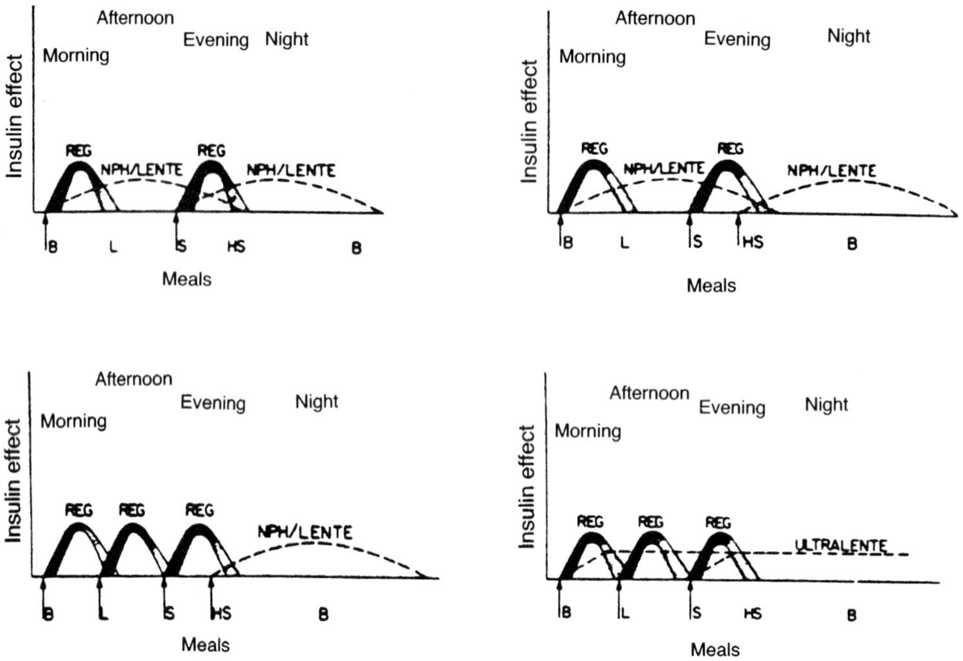


Fig. 32.2. Intensified insulin regimens. Upper panels represent split, mixed regimens, while lower panels are examples of basal–bolus regimens. Insulin effect is idealised and may be affected by site, volume and depth of injection. (Adapted from Ref. 23.)

two injections daily to the need of taking four to six shots. Traditional approaches to insulin therapy have included the utilisation of one or two injections of intermediate acting insulin, sometimes in combination with regular insulin with the subsequent modification in dietary caloric intake (25). Efficacy of such therapy was usually determined by assessment of patient's symptoms of hyper and hypoglycaemia, office glucose determination, and 24-hour urine glucose excretion (26). Monitoring of urine glucose excretion, initially with Benedict's solution and subsequently with strips capable of semi-quantitative measurement of reducing substances in the urine, added additional information for the regulation of so-called conventional insulin therapy.

More precise insulin management required more timely and accurate assessment of circulating plasma glucose levels. Development of capillary blood glucose monitoring devices which could be utilised by patients in their homes ushered in a new age of insulin therapy (27). In retrospect, it is now apparent that this is the single most important technological development in the care of patients with diabetes since the isolation and purification of insulin. However, as recently as 1983, the utilisation of self-monitoring of blood glucose by patients with IDDM was not universally accepted. In fact, it was felt to be of utility limited to those individuals with brittle diabetes or during pregnancy (28).

The efficacy of conventional insulin therapy was assessed in a wide variety of epidemiologic and prospective studies (26, 29). In general, the limited parameters of 24-hour urine glucose excretion, hospitalisation rates, frequency of hypoglycaemia, and development of late complications suggested that some individuals with diabetes were able to adequately control plasma glucose levels and minimise their development of late complications to some degree.

Not surprisingly, conventional insulin therapy has changed dramatically over the last decade. Even within the Diabetes Control and Complications Trial (DCCT), the conventionally treated group moved from mandatory urine glucose testing with optional self-monitoring of blood glucose (SMBG) to almost universal SMBG. An increase in the number of insulin injections with modifications of insulin therapy based upon these findings have also become standard in conventional insulin management.

The progression from conventional insulin therapy to intensified conventional therapy goes far beyond the simple number of insulin injections taken daily. Although intensified conventional therapy implies three to four injections of insulin per day, the more important aspect is the utilisation of SMBG in the context of a firm understanding of insulin action, diet and exercise effects to allow the patient to adjust insulin doses and timing in an effort to approach normoglycaemia. Diabetes patient education becomes an integral part of such therapy, as the individual with diabetes is placed in the primary decision-making position.

In general, intensified conventional insulin therapy implies the utilisation of at least two forms of insulin (short and intermediate or long-acting) given in various combinations three to four times daily. As previously described, a single injection of intermediate-acting insulin daily is incapable of providing the insulin profile necessary to approach normoglycaemia. Even the use of the conventional split, mixed regimen of regular plus intermediate-acting insulin twice daily is sub-optimal. This regimen provides improved insulin coverage during the day, but because the intermediate-acting insulin is given prior to the evening meal, its peak action tends to occur during sleep and it is dissipated by breakfast time (Fig. 32.2). As a result, fasting hyperglycaemia is the natural consequence unless insulin doses are pushed higher and higher at the risk of nocturnal hypoglycaemia.

A more intensified regimen would begin with the utilisation of mixed regular and intermediate-acting insulin in the morning in order to provide adequate insulin coverage for the breakfast and midday meal together with a dose of regular insulin prior to supper and movement of the intermediate-acting insulin to bedtime. This adjustment alters the time action characteristics of the PM dose of intermediate-acting insulin to avoid nocturnal hypoglycaemia and provide better control of the fasting blood glucose level – but only at the expense of a 50% increase in the number of insulin injections. This three-shot regimen can be effective for a large number of patients with IDDM as long as daytime activities and timing of meals are predictable. The latency and prolonged action of the morning dose of intermediate-acting insulin demands dietary and exercise compliance at the risk of midday hypo- or hyper-glycaemia. For those individuals with erratic eating schedules or very active lifestyles, improved flexibility can be achieved by moving to one of several so-called basal-bolus regimens. Implied in this description is the presence of an intermediate or long-acting form of insulin given in low dose in order to provide a background basal level of circulating insulin. The intent of the basal dose of insulin is to maintain euglycaemia in the fasting state. Superimposed upon this basal level of insulin, bolus injections are taken shortly before the ingestion of carbohydrate in order to mimic the postprandial rise in endogenous insulin secretion. As a result, meals are more flexible in timing because the bolus injection is taken shortly before the meal is ingested and the dose may be adjusted according to the anticipated caloric load. Implementation of the basal–bolus regimens typically consists of regular insulin taken approximately 30 minutes prior to meals together with either NPH insulin at bedtime or *ultra-lente* insulin taken either in the morning or at bedtime.

The utility of intensified conventional therapy in achieving near normoglycaemia is absolutely dependent upon patient modification of the insulin dose according to data obtained by

SMBG. Regardless of the number of insulin injections taken daily, it is the modification of the necessary dose which achieves the desired glycaemic effect. Frequency of SMBG and utilisation of this information is critically important and has been shown to independently determine the level of glycaemic control (30).

Efforts to carry the basal–bolus concept further led to the development of continuous subcutaneous insulin infusion (CSII) systems utilising portable pumps. The initial description (31) described a mechanical syringe system capable of injecting extremely small volumes of diluted insulin into the subcutaneous space on a continuous basis. In addition, boluses could be provided by holding down an injection button to provide larger quantities of insulin. Despite the need to dilute insulin, wear a bulky contraption on one's belt, and endure the placement of a subcutaneous catheter, the concept of 'insulin-pump' therapy was rapidly popularised. Patients viewed the insulin pump as a space-age solution to glycaemic control. And, in fact, multiple investigators were able to demonstrate that CSII was able to achieve stable and reproducible glucose control over time (32, 33).

As with most technological developments, initial enthusiasm fades with the report of limitations and complications. The presence of an indwelling subcutaneous catheter together with reliance on continuous mechanical infusion of very small quantities of insulin predisposes insulin pump therapy to multiple potential complications. Pump malfunction, tubing occlusion, battery failure, and catheter disconnection result in rapid disappearance of circulating plasma insulin with subsequent rapid increase in plasma glucose levels. Deterioration to diabetic ketoacidosis may occur in a matter of hours, as there is no depot insulin for delayed absorption and attenuation of ketosis. In addition, infusion site infections and inflammation may occur unless meticulous care and technique are employed (34). The use of continuous subcutaneous insulin infusion systems requires patients to frequently assess their metabolic state and make appropriate adjustments. In combination with literally wearing their disease on their belt, psychosocial adjustments and behavioural abnormalities may ensue. Selection of patients for CSII must be carefully initiated, assessing patient expectations of pump therapy, willingness to undergo the appropriate instruction and education, and psychosocial stability and support systems for pump operation. With the initiation of insulin pump therapy, one-year attrition rates for discontinuation of therapy were as high as 75% because of the inappropriate application of the technology. Now, improved diabetes education and patient selection has resulted in better acceptability of the technology; however, even in the DCCT where pump therapy and multiple daily injection therapy were interchangeable, pump therapy was utilised by only 59% of intensively treated patients and accounted for only 34% of the treatment time (35).

The efficacy of CSII in achieving glycaemic control in appropriately instructed patients has been confirmed in numerous studies. Comparisons of intensified conventional therapy utilising three more injections of insulin daily versus CSII have uniformly shown equivalence of the regimens (33, 36). In all circumstances, the critical variable in achieving glycaemic control remains the patient's willingness to perform self-monitoring of blood glucose and utilisation of this information in making appropriate insulin adjustments (30). Newer insulin pumps have improved both compliance as well as glycaemic control by improving insulin delivery at very low volumes, integrating multiple basal rates, and miniaturisation.

Intrinsic to the concept of intensive management of IDDM, is the inclusion of appropriate education and support systems to inform and empower the individual with IDDM to care for their own disease. Selection of patients for intensive therapy is thus a critical component determining both safety and efficacy (37). Patients must be both motivated to enter into the education process and adherent to the intensified demands of the regimen. There must be adequate support systems within the home, school, or workplace to ensure safety of the application of the regimen. Because of the frequent SMBG, as well as the costs of insulin pump therapy, financial support must also be forthcoming.

In addition, it is now clear that some patients are at increased risk of complications stemming from intensified insulin regimens. Severe hypoglycaemia originally identified in association with CSII (34) underlines the altered counterregulatory response present in IDDM. Subsequent findings of marked increased incidence of severe hypoglycaemia in the experimental group of the DCCT further emphasises the implicit risk of hypoglycaemia associated with attempts to achieve normoglycaemia (38). Efforts to identify individuals at increased risk for hypoglycaemia during intensive therapy are both cumbersome and insensitive (39). Some have even suggested that individuals with a history of severe hypoglycaemia not be enrolled in intensive treatment regimens (40). Rather, it is important to emphasise that intensified management of IDDM implies the efforts employed to achieve an established glycaemic goal rather than the glycaemic goal itself. Patients with histories of severe hypoglycaemia may still be managed in intensive regimens by simply establishing goals of therapy somewhat higher than usual in an effort to avoid hypoglycaemia stemming from minor variations in timing or quantity of food or exercise.

The emphasis required to institute intensified management of IDDM must be placed on diabetes education. Patients must be instructed not only in the traditional survival techniques associated with diabetes treatment, but also in more sophisticated techniques of self-monitoring of blood glucose, utilisation of CSII, interaction of stress, diet, and exercise in glucose control, and in sophisticated insulin adjustment algorithms. A team approach consisting of patient, physician, nurse educator, nutritionist, and behaviouralist are essential to ensuring both safety and efficacy of intensified management (41). Once again, the DCCT has emphasised the critical importance of the educator components of the team in achieving the implied goal of normoglycaemia associated with intensified therapy regimens.

One of the critical roles of the educators is to instruct patients in any one of a variety of insulin adjustment algorithms. Approaches to insulin adjustment are as numerous as physicians and educators utilising them. However, inherent in all is the concept of utilising SMBG data together with anticipated diet and exercise to determine subsequent insulin doses. Because of the inherent variability in predicting GI absorption, glucose needs, and timing of absorption of injected insulin, insulin algorithms are as much art as they are science. Two basic approaches have been utilised in attempts to achieve improved glycaemic control with the use of insulin algorithms. Traditionally, sliding scale insulin regimens have been used to prevent rapid deterioration in glycaemic control. Supplemental doses of short-acting insulin are administered depending upon the blood glucose determinations at that moment. Although extremely useful in preventing serious metabolic deterioration in the setting of systemic illness, they may be of limited value in an everyday setting. The concept underlying sliding scale insulin is the immediate response with an injection of insulin to remedy a miscalculation in a previous insulin requirement. Given the delayed action of the sliding scale insulin, the response is frequently too little too late. In essence, an effort is being made to make insulin work backwards (42). When sliding scale insulin is utilised as the only means of insulin adjustment, the patient is constantly in a situation of playing catch up with their altered blood glucose. Sliding scale insulin does not imply remedying the underlying error in insulin dosage which resulted in hyperglycaemia in the first place. Frequently, sliding scale insulin results in over-insulinisation and subsequent so-called brittle diabetes (43).

A second common approach to insulin adjustment involves utilisation of pattern recognition and anticipatory insulin adjustments. In such a protocol, patients monitor their blood sugars looking for patterns of highs and lows that are recurrent and unexplainable on the basis of alterations in diet, exercise or illness. Adjustments in the insulin are made in the insulin dose responsible for glycaemic control during that time of day (see *Appendix*). In addition, this type of anticipatory insulin adjustment would encourage patients to alter their insulin prior to changes in diet or exercise. For example, increased regular insulin might be taken prior to a meal which would be expected to increase plasma glucose in excess of what is typically achieved. Likewise, reduction of insulin may be employed in anticipation of expected exercise and its attendant increased glucose disposal following injection of the insulin. A variety of insulin adjustment algorithms have been published and can be utilised according to both patient and physician acceptance (24, 44).

This type of pattern recognition and response has lent itself very nicely to efforts to develop computerised systems for determining insulin requirements. Pioneering work by Albisser provides computer-generated analysis of glucose trends as well as insulin responses to determine future insulin requirements (45). Further refinement in the development of expert systems capable of 'learning' individual responses to both insulin and glucose have also been undertaken (46). Both approaches allow for a systematic analysis of data with appropriate calculation of caloric needs, caloric expenditure, and insulin requirements. The results obtained are dependent upon the quality of the data entered. Not only is increased patient compliance necessary for data entry, but therapeutic recommendations are qualified by the limitations of our own knowledge and prediction of insulin absorption and effect as previously discussed. None the less, the development of computerised algorithms and expert systems may have important contributions to current efforts of intensified diabetes management today and are critical for the development of closed loop systems for the future.

## FUTURE CONSIDERATIONS

With presentation of the results of the Diabetes Control and Complications Trial (DCCT) in June of 1993, the clear mandate for treatment of IDDM is the achievement of near normoglycaemia without complications of hypoglycaemia. Intensive therapy, consisting of multiple daily injections of insulin or CSII, frequent self-monitoring of blood glucose, intensive education, and frequent insulin adjustments was capable of achieving mean glycated haemoglobin levels of 7.2%. This remains far above the mean for a non-diabetic population, and so future therapies will demand closer linkage between circulating plasma glucose levels and subsequent insulin infusion.

For over 10 years, efforts to develop closed loop insulin infusion systems have been undertaken. The concept of an implantable insulin infusion pump could potentially provide for portal delivery of insulin in a continuous manner, thus circumventing the vagaries of subcutaneous absorption. The convenience to the patient of not requiring daily injections of insulin must be balanced by the potential dangers of pump malfunction, catheter obstruction, and problems associated with refilling the insulin reservoir. Current experience with these implantable pump systems has demonstrated the capacity to achieve near normoglycaemia in a research setting (47). Limitations of the current technology, however, include problems associated with catheter migration, pocket infections, and rare pump malfunction. None the less, the technology is severely limited by the lack of ability to close the loop.

Current implantable pump technologies continue to require the patient to monitor capillary blood glucose and adjust insulin infusion rates and determine bolus needs according to insulin adjustment algorithms. A functional, implantable glucose sensor has remained an elusive goal for ultimately closing the loop. Despite extensive research, we do not appear to be any closer to the development of an *in vivo* continuous glucose sensor than we were a decade ago (48).

Manipulation of the human insulin molecule to achieve altered absorption characteristics more closely mimicking normal insulin dynamics provides an alternative therapeutic approach. Insulin analogues, which fail to undergo non-covalent binding into hexamers, are rapidly absorbed from the subcutaneous depot, offer a rapid onset of cellular activity, and are then quickly cleared. These rapid acting insulin monomers bind avidly to the insulin receptor and are bioactive (49). Early efforts to develop analogues for clinical use were side tracked by development of mammary tumours in test animals, presumably due to augmented mitogenic activity of the insulin analogue itself (50). Current clinical trials are ongoing world-wide with an insulin analogue in which lysine and proline have been transposed in the B chain of the molecule. This transposition renders the insulin stable in a monomeric form giving a peak activity within 20 minutes and a duration of action of approximately 40 minutes following subcutaneous injection. Thus, rapid acting insulin analogues serve as a more appropriate bolus therapy to provide adequate insulinisation immediately following caloric ingestion to suppress hepatic glucose output and stimulate peripheral glucose uptake. The short duration of action should prevent the development of late postprandial hypoglycaemia frequently seen in today's basal–bolus regimens.

Similarly, modifications of the insulin molecule to provide a true long-acting insulin preparation with no peak would facilitate basal insulin administration. An extremely long-acting basal insulin would be added to bolus injections of rapid-acting insulin to provide the ultimate basal–bolus regimen. As of yet, these extremely long-acting insulin analogues have not been tested in clinical trials.

Alternate delivery systems for insulin, bypassing subcutaneous injection routes, would also be of clinical importance. Intranasal administration of aerosolised insulin has been actively pursued for a decade. Employing a variety of surfactants to promote absorption through the nasal mucosa, intranasal insulin was utilised to provide premeal, bolus therapy in several clinical trials. Absorption characteristics reveal a nadir in plasma glucose approximately 45 minutes following administration (51). A typical dose–response curve was noted both in rise in serum insulin and fall in plasma glucose with increasing doses. Unfortunately, low bioavailability (approximately 20%) requires large volume administrations of the nasal insulin preparations (52). Subsequent nasal irritation from both the concentrated insulin and the utilised surfactant limit the applicability and efficacy of this approach.

Oral delivery of insulin has been limited by the proteolytic destruction of insulin by gastrointestinal enzymes. Ideally, oral administration would provide the more appropriate portal delivery of insulin in conjunction with a carbohydrate load. By coating insulin with an impermeable polymer film, proteolytic digestion in the stomach and small intestines can be avoided, and insulin absorption via the colonic mucosa achieved. Portal delivery of insulin results in a nadir in plasma glucose occurring 4 to 8 hours following ingestion (53). Once again, variable absorption rates associated with gastric motility and intestinal flora have precluded the general application of this technology.

The ultimate closed loop system for insulin delivery remains the intact beta cell. Despite the rapid advances in transplant technology and the marked increase in the number of whole organ pancreas transplants, this technique cannot be currently viewed as generally clinically applicable. Isolated pancreas transplantation suffers from an unacceptably high rate of rejection episodes (96% of patients) with graft loss in as many as 42% of cases in the first year (54). Isolated islet cell transplants have been hampered by lack of availability of human islets, the continued need for immunosuppressive therapy, and the apparent 3 to 4 month lifespan of transplanted islets (55). Promising techniques of immuno-isolation in biohybrid devices or of antigen masking provide hope that a true closed loop system may be clinically available in the new future (56, 57).

Finally, future considerations for IDDM include the identification of individuals in a prediabetic state with subsequent intervention to prevent the progression to full blown IDDM. Through the work of Soeldner, Eisenbarth, and MacLaren, it is now clear that IDDM is an autoimmune disease with its onset occurring many years before clinical hyperglycaemia (58, 59). The development of predictors of clinical onset, including islet cell antibodies, insulin autoantibodies, and first phase insulin secretion in response to an IV glucose tolerance test provide insight into both the progression of disease and efficacy of interventions. Previous trials of cyclosporin within two weeks of presentation in hyperglycaemia revealed only a modest response when measured by insulin independence and normoglycaemia (60). Current trials are under way in which individuals with evidence of β-cell attack, but still normoglycaemic, are being treated with a variety of immunomodulating agents. We currently await reports of controlled trials utilising imuran, nicotinamide, and oral insulin. The future is bright for the ultimate prevention of IDDM.

## CONCLUSION

No discussion of the rational management of IDDM would be complete without emphasising the importance of diet, exercise, and patient education. Clinical experience has taught us that glycaemic control is impossible without appropriate meal planning, self-monitoring of blood glucose, and appropriate insulin adjustments. Appropriate care of the patient with IDDM demands utilisation of diabetes educators for implementation of all of the necessary tools to achieve glycaemic control. It is quite clear that the primary care provider in the treatment of IDDM is the patient himself. Appropriate knowledge and motivation inspired by aggressive medical, nursing, and nutritional care is imperative for the rational management of the patient with IDDM.

> Insulin does not cure diabetes. Insulin does not allow a diabetic to eat anything he desires. It is a potent preparation alike for evil and for good. Insulin has revolutionized diabetic treatment in more ways than one: (1) It can give more food, strength, and weight, but, (2) to do this it demands not only a knowledge and respect for the diabetic diet on the part of the doctor and patient, but adherence to the same if the diabetic wishes to get his money's worth for the insulin he injects.(1)

## REFERENCES


1 Joslin EP. *The treatment of diabetes mellitus with observations based upon 3000 cases.* 3rd ed. Lea and Febiger, Philadelphia; 1923: 38–9.

2 Burrow GN, Hazlett BE, Phillips MJ. A case of diabetes mellitus. *N Eng J of Med* 1982; 306: 340–3.

3 MacLeod, JJR. Pancreatic extract and diabetes. *Can Med Assoc J* 1922; 12: 423–5.

4 Ratner RE, Phillips TS, Steiner ML. Persistent cutaneous insulin allergy resulting from insulin aggregates. *Diabetes* 1990; 39: 728–33.

5 Robbins DC, Mau M, Pic L, Parentesis G, Shen C. Covalent aggregates of insulin in the blood of Type I diabetic patients: a cross over study comparing two contemporary insulin brands. *Diabetes* 1993; 42 (Suppl 1): 205A.

6 Mau M, Robbins DC, Pic L, Ratner RE. What happens when patients change insulin brands? A control crossover study. *Diabetes* 1993; 42 (Suppl 1): 205A.

7 DeMeyt P, Halban P, Hepp KD. *In vitro* studies on biosynthetic human insulin: an overview. *Diabetes Care* 1981; 4 (Suppl 2): 144–6.

8 Clark AJ, Wiles PG, Leiper JM *et al.* A double-blind crossover trial comparing human insulin (recombinant DNA) with animal insulins in the treatment of previously insulin-treated diabetic patients. *Diabetes Care* 1982; 5 (Suppl 2): 129–4.

9 Schernthaner G, Borkenstein M, Fink M *et al.* Immunogenicity of human insulin (novo) or pork monocomponent insulin in HLA-DR typed insulin dependent diabetic individuals. *Diabetes Care* 1983; 6 (Suppl 2): 43–8.

10 Fireman P, Fineberg SE, Galloway JA. Development of IgE antibodies to human (recombinant DNA), porcine, and bovine insulins in diabetic patients. *Diabetes Care* 1982; 5 (Suppl 2): 119–25.

11 Fineberg SE, Galloway JA, Fineberg NS, Rathbun MJ. Immunologic improvement resulting from the transfer of animal insulin treated diabetic subjects to human insulin (recombinant DNA). *Diabetes Care* 1982; 5 (Suppl 2): 107–13.

12 Menon RK, Cohen RM, Sperling MA *et al.* Transplacental passage of insulin in pregnant women with insulin dependent diabetes mellitus, its role in fetal macrosomia. *N Engl J Med* 1990; 322: 309–15.
13 Gale EAM. Hypoglycemia and human insulin. *Lancet* 1989; ii: 1264–6.
14 Muhlhauser I, Heinemann L, Fritsche E *et al.* Hypoglycemic symptoms and frequency of severe hypoglycemia in patients treated with human and animal insulin preparations. *Diabetes Care* 1991; 14: 745–9.
15 Egger M, Smith GD, Imhoof H, Teuscher A. Risk of severe hypoglycemia in insulin-treated diabetic patients transferred to human insulin: a case control study. *Br Med J* 1991; 303: 617–21.
16 Egger M, Smith GD, Teuscher AU, Teuscher A. Influence of human insulin on symptoms and awareness of hypoglycemia: a randomized double-blind crossover study. *Br Med J* 1991; 303: 622–6.
17 Patrick AW, Bodmer CW, Tieszen KL *et al.* Human insulin and awareness of acute hypoglycemic symptoms in insulin-dependent diabetes. *Lancet* 1991; 338: 528–32.
18 Jones TW, Caprio S, Diamond MP *et al.* Does insulin species modify counter-regulatory hormone response to hypoglycemia? *Diabetes Care* 1991; 14: 728–31.
19 Bolli GB. The pharmacokinetic basis of insulin therapy in diabetes mellitus. *Diabetes Res Clin Pract* 1989; 6: S3–16.
20 Galloway JA, Spradlin CT, Howey DC, Dupre J. Intra subject differences in pharmacokinetics and pharmacodynamic responses: the immutable problem of present day treatment? *Diabetes*, 1985: Proc 12th Cong Int Diabetes Federat Madrid, 23–28, September 1985. International Congress Series No. 700. Excerpta Medica, Amsterdam, 1986; 877–886.
21 Young RJ, Hannan WJ, Frier BM *et al.* Diabetic hypertrophy delays insulin absorption. *Diabetes Care* 1984; 7: 479–80.
22 Koivisto VA, Felig P. Alterations in insulin absorption and in blood glucose control associated with varying insulin injection sites in diabetes patients. *Ann Int Med* 1980; 92: 59–61.
23 Schade DS, Santiago JV, Skyler JS, Rizza RA eds. *Intensive insulin therapy*, Excerpta Medica, Princeton, 1983; 23–5 and 209–23.
24 Skyler J, Skyler D, Seigler D, O'Sullivan M. Algorithms for adjustment of insulin dosage by patients who monitor blood glucose. *Diabetes Care* 1981; 4: 311–18.
25 Galloway JA, Bressler R. Insulin treatment in diabetes. *Med Clin N Am* 1978; 62: 663–80.
26 Pirart J. Diabetes mellitus and its degenerative complications: a prospective study of 4400 patients observed between 1947 and 1973. *Diabetes Care* 1978; 1: 169–88.
27 Tattersal LR, Gale EAM. Patients self-monitoring of blood glucose and refinements of conventional insulin treatment. *Am J Med* 1981; 70: 177–82.
28 Health and Public Policy Committee, American College of Physicians. Selected methods for the management of diabetes mellitus. *Ann Int Med* 1983; 99: 272–4.
29 Knowles HC. The problem of the relation of the control of diabetes to the development of vascular disease. *Trans Am Clin Climatol Assoc* 1964; 76: 142–7.
30 Schiffrin A, Belmonte M. Daily self-glucose monitoring: its essential role in long-term glucose control in insulin-dependent diabetes patients treated with pump and multiple subcutaneous injections. *Diabetes Care* 1982; 5: 479–84.
31 Pickup JC, Keen H, Parsons JA, Alberti KGMM. Continuous subcutaneous insulin infusion: an approach to achieving normal glycemia. *Br Med J* 1978; i: 204–7.
32 Tamborlane WV, Sherwin RS, Genel M, Felig P. Reduction to normal plasma glucose in juvenile diabetes by subcutaneous administration of insulin with a portable infusion pump. *N Engl J Med* 1979; 300: 573–8.
33 Reeves ML, Seigler DE, Ryan EA, Skyler JS. Glycemic control and insulin-dependent diabetes mellitus: comparison of outpatient intensified conventional therapy with continuous subcutaneous insulin infusion. *Am J Med* 1982; 72: 673–80.
34 Mecklenberg RS, Benson EA, Benson JW *et al.* Acute complications associated with insulin infusion pump therapy, report of experience with 161 patients. *JAMA* 1984; 252: 3265–9.
35 The Diabetes Control and Complications Trial Research Group. The effect of intensive treatment of diabetes on the development and progression of long-term complications in insulin-dependent diabetes mellitus. *N Engl J Med*, 1993; 329: 977–86.
36 Shiffrin A, Belmonte MM. Comparison between continuous subcutaneous insulin infusion and multiple injections of insulin: a one-year prospective study. *Diabetes* 1982; 31: 255–64.
37 Gerich JE. Selection of patients for intensive insulin therapy. *Arch Int Med* 1985; 145: 1383–4.
38 The DCCT Research Group. Epidemiology of severe hypoglycemia on the Diabetes Control and Complications Trial. *Am J Med* 1991; 90: 450–59.
39 White NH, Skor DA, Cryer PE *et al.* Identification of Type I diabetic patients with increased risk for hypoglycemia during intensive therapy. *N Engl J Med* 1983; 308: 485–91.
40 Boden G, Hoeldtke RD. Making intensified insulin treatment Safer. *Ann Int Med* 1983; 99: 268–69.
41 Flavin K, White NH. The intensive insulin therapy team. *Diabetes Educ* 1989; 15: 249–52.
42 Shagan BP. Does anyone here know how to make insulin work backwards? Why sliding-scale insulin coverage doesn't work. *Pract Diab* 1990; 9: 1–4.
43 White NH and Santiago JV. Clinical features and natural history of Brittle diabetes in children. In: Pickup JC, ed. *Brittle diabetes*, Blackwell Scientific Publications, Oxford, 1985; 19–28.
44 Hirsch IB, Farkas-Hirsch R, Skyler JS. Intensive insulin therapy for treatment of Type I diabetes. *Diabetes Care* 1990; 13: 1265–83.
45 Albisser, AM, Six generations of the insulin dosage computer: a new clinical device for diabetes self-management through specialized centers. *Horm Metabol Res* 1990; 24 (suppl): 140–4.
46 Hauser T, Kraegen EW, Campbell LV *et al.* Assessment of expert's approach to insulin therapy and development of a simulator for diabetes insulin adjustment. *Diabetes Care* 1992; 15:221–31.
47 Selam J-L, Micossi P, Dunn FL, Nathan DM. Clinical trial of programmable implantable insulin pump for type I diabetes. *Diabetes Care* 1992; 15: 877–85.
48 Brunetti P, Benedetti MM, Calabrese G, Reboldi GP. Closed loop delivery systems for insulin therapy. *Int J Artificial Organs* 1991; 14:216–26.

49 Brange J, Owens DR, Kang S, Volund A. Monomeric insulins and their experimental and clinical implications. *Diabetes Care* 1990; 13:923–54.
50 Jorgensen LN, Didericksen LH, Drejer K. Carcinogenic effect of the human insulin analogue B10 Asp in female rats. (Abstract) European Association for the Study of Diabetes, 28th Annual Meeting, Prague, Sept, 1992.
51 Salzman R, Manson JE, Griffing GT *et al.* Intranasal aerosolized insulin, mixed meal studies and long-term use in type I diabetes. *N Engl J Med* 1985; 312: 1078–84.
52 Frauman AG, Cooper ME, Parsons BJ *et al.* Long-term use of intranasal insulin in insulin-dependent diabetic patients. *Diabetes Care* 1987; 10:573–8.
53 Saffran M, Kumar GS, Savariar C *et al.* A new approach to the oral administration of insulin and other peptide drugs. *Science* 1986; 233: 1081–4.
54 Gruessner RWG, Dunn DL, Tzardis PJ *et al.* Simultaneous pancreas and kidney transplants versus single kidney transplants and previous kidney transplants in uremic patients and single pancreas transplants in nonuremic diabetic patients: comparison of rejection, morbidity, and long-term outcome. *Transplant Proc* 1990; 22:622–3.
55 Scharp DW, Lacy PE, Santiago JV *et al.* Insulin independence after islet transplantation into type I diabetic patient. *Diabetes* 1990; 39: 515–18.
56 Lanza RP, Sullivan SJ, Chick WL. Islet transplantation with immunoisolation. *Diabetes* 1992; 41: 1503–10.
57 Faustman D, Coe C. Prevention of xenograft rejection by masking donor HLA class I antigens. *Science* 1991; 252: 1700–2.
58 MacLaren NK. How, when, and why to predict IDDM. *Diabetes* 1988; 37: 1591–4.
59 Eisenbarth GS, Verge CF, Allen H, Rewers MJ. The design of trials for prevention of IDDM. *Diabetes* 1993; 42: 941–47.
60 Jenner M, Bradish G, Stiller C *et al.* Cyclosporin A treatment of young children with newly-diagnosed type I diabetes mellitus. *Diabetologia* 1992; 35: 884–8.

# Appendix Sample Patient Rules for Insulin Adjustment

## INSULIN ADJUSTMENT WHEN TESTING BLOOD SUGAR BEFORE MEALS: INCREASE

Many times your insulin dosage needs to be changed. Before making changes you need to make sure you:

(a) have maintained consistency in your diet
(b) have monitored your blood sugar consistently
(c) are not ill
(d) have not had an insulin reaction.

The goals for your blood sugar control are:
Fasting less than ________
All others less than ________

Guidelines:

### Adjust only one insulin dosage at a time

Be sure the blood sugar is higher than acceptable for **2 days** in a row before making the appropriate adjustment.

| If your blood sugar: | Increase your: |
|---|---|
| Before breakfast is over ________ | Evening NPH/Lente by ________ units |
| Before lunch is over ________ | Morning regular by ________ units |
| Before dinner | Noon regular or morning NPH/Lente by ________ units |
| Before bedtime is over ________ | Evening regular by ________ units |

If you adjust your intermediate insulin by 8 units or your short-acting by 4 units without adequate results, please call your doctor for evaluation.

### Insulin adjustment: decrease

When the insulin dosage needs to be decreased, it is necessary to follow basic guidelines. You must determine if the low blood sugar may be due to any of the following:

(a) a skipped meal
(b) eating less at a meal than usual
(c) an increase in exercise
(d) an inaccurate amount of insulin.

Guidelines:

### Adjust only one insulin dosage at a time

If there is no explanation for an insulin reaction or a blood sugar less than ________, decrease the appropriate insulin dose the next day according to the following guidelines.

| For a reaction or low blood sugar: | Decrease: |
|---|---|
| Between 2 am and breakfast | Evening NPH/Lente by ________ units |
| Between breakfast and lunch | Morning regular by ________ units |
| Between lunch and supper | Noon regular or morning NPH/Lente by ________ units |
| Between supper and 2 am | Evening regular by ________ units |

## INSULIN PUMP ADJUSTMENT WHEN TESTING BLOOD SUGAR BEFORE MEALS: INCREASE

Many times your insulin dosage needs to be changed. Before making changes you need to make sure you:

(a) have maintained consistency in your diet
(b) have monitored your blood sugar consistently
(c) are not ill
(d) have not had an insulin reaction.

The goals for your blood sugar control are:
Fasting less than
All others less than

Guidelines:

**Only adjust one insulin dosage at a time**

Do not change both the basal and bolus doses on the same day unless you have been specifically instructed to do so. Be sure the blood sugar is higher than acceptable for **2 days** in a row before making the appropriate adjustment.

| If your blood sugar: | Increase your: |
|---|---|
| Before breakfast is over ________ | Basal rate by ________ units |
| Before breakfast is between ________ and ________, but pre-meals tests are over ________, the bolus doses should be adjusted as follows: | |
| Before lunch is over ________ | Pre-breakfast bolus by ________ units |
| Before dinner is over ________ | Pre-lunch bolus by ________ units |
| Before bedtime is over ________ | Pre-dinner bolus by ________ units |

## INSULIN PUMP ADJUSTMENT: DECREASE

When the insulin dosage needs to be decreased, it is necessary to follow basic guidelines. You must determine if the low blood sugar may be due to any of the following:

(a) a skipped meal
(b) eating less at a meal than usual
(c) an increase in exercise
(d) an inaccurate amount of insulin.

Guidelines:

**Only adjust one insulin dosage at a time**

If there are no explanation for an insulin reaction or a blood sugar less than, decrease the appropriate insulin dose the next day according to the following guidelines.

| For a reaction or low blood sugar: | Decrease: |
|---|---|
| Between 2 am and breakfast | Basal rate by ________ units |
| Between breakfast and lunch | Pre-breakfast bolus by ________ units |
| Between lunch and supper | Pre-lunch bolus by ________ units |
| Between supper and bedtime | Pre-dinner bolus by ________ units |
| Between bedtime and 2 am | Bedtime bolus by ________ units |

# 33 Rationale in the Management of Non-insulin-dependent Diabetes

Harold E. Lebovitz

## GOALS FOR MANAGEMENT OF PATIENTS WITH NIDDM

Goals for the management of patients with NIDDM are frequently described in tables which list good, acceptable and unsatisfactory numerical values for parameters such as fasting and postprandial plasma glucose, glycosylated haemoglobin, serum LDL- and HDL-cholesterol, and fasting plasma triglycerides (1, 2). While this approach provides simplicity, it also shackles the physician with sometimes unobtainable and perhaps unnecessary targets and disregards factors which may be of equal, or greater, importance.

An alternative approach to creating management goals for NIDDM patients would be to define desired clinical endpoints that need to be achieved by the individual patient. Using knowledge which is available about the pathogenetic events leading to the clinical endpoints allow metabolic targets to be set which will achieve the desired clinical outcomes.

Clinical outcomes in the management of NIDDM patients are: (1) elimination of symptoms and promotion of a sense of well-being; (2) prevention of acute metabolic complications; (3) prevention or minimising the development of the unique microvascular and neuropathic complications of diabetes mellitus; (4) reduction of macrovascular disease morbidity and mortality rates to those of the non-diabetic population. For patients who have a probable life expectancy, independent of NIDDM, of less than 10 years, the desired clinical outcomes would be eliminating symptoms, promoting well-being and preventing acute complications. A newly diagnosed NIDDM patient under the age of 60 years presents the challenge of achieving all of the desired clinical outcomes. In contrast, a newly diagnosed NIDDM patient over the age of 65 years may benefit only marginally from measures designed to reduce macrovascular disease morbidity and mortality rates to those of the non-diabetic population.

## INCREASED MORBIDITY AND MORTALITY IN NIDDM

Non-insulin-dependent diabetes mellitus is associated with a marked increase in mortality in all populations (3–10). A ten-year follow-up of 1012 Oklahoma Indians who at baseline had a mean age of 52 years and a duration of diagnosed diabetes of 7 years yielded mortality rates of 4.99% per year in men and 4.17% per year in women (7). The ratio of observed deaths to expected deaths (derived from the non-diabetic population) was 2.92 in men and 4.17 in women. The leading cause of death was cardiovascular diseases. Prospective and retrospective studies with such diverse NIDDM populations as Pima Indian (8), Mexican–American (6), Japanese (10), Scottish (11), Australian (9), English (5) and American (USA) show approximately a 40% mortality in 8 to 10 years of follow up. The mortality rate for these NIDDM populations compared to their non-diabetic populations averages about 2.0 (range 1.4 to 4.0). The average life expectancy at 60 years in the NIDDM population in western Australians is reduced an average of 5 years compared to the non-diabetic population (9). The younger the age of onset of NIDDM in the population the greater is the increase in mortality rate.

The major causes of the increased mortality in NIDDM populations are diseases involving the cardiovascular system. Ischaemic heart disease accounts for most of the increased mortality in US and European NIDDM populations (3–5). In contrast, diabetic nephropathy is the leading cause of the increased mortality in Pima Indians with NIDDM (12). Japanese NIDDM patients have increased mortality resulting equally from ischaemic heart disease or diabetic nephropathy (10). It appears that the frequency of the various chronic complications of NIDDM are significantly influenced by racial and ethnic factors.

The reasons for increased cardiovascular disease morbidity and mortality in NIDDM patients are unclear. The duration of diabetes (13), and the presence of proteinuria (14, 15) and/or retinopathy (6,16,17) are significant risk factors. While some studies implicate the classic risk factors of hypercholesterolaemia, hypertriglyceridaemia, hypertension and obesity, other studies such as those in Mexican–Americans (18) and the Whitehall study (19) do not support the link between these classic risk factors and ischaemic heart disease in NIDDM populations. Unfortunately most of our current concepts about macrovascular disease in NIDDM are extrapolated from studies in non-diabetics (13).

The relationship between glycaemic control and the development and progression of macrovascular disease in NIDDM patients is complex. Individuals with impaired glucose tolerance have a two- to three-fold increase in ischaemic heart disease in spite of minimal or no hyperglycaemia and normal haemoglobin $A_{lc}$ (3, 4, 19). Newly diagnosed NIDDM patients have a surprisingly high prevalence of macrovascular disease (two- to three-fold increased compared to age–sex matched non-diabetic controls) (3,13). Chronic moderate to severe hyperglycaemia is, however, associated with an increased incidence and greater severity of ischaemic heart disease. Glycaemic control, therefore, may not be the major determinant in the accelerated atherosclerosis of NIDDM but does appear to contribute to it.

The increase in ischaemic heart disease in newly diagnosed NIDDM patients and in IGT individuals indicate that the accelerated atherosclerosis of NIDDM starts many years prior to the onset of hyperglycaemia. This has led to the very controversial hypothesis that insulin resistance and hyperinsulinaemia may play a major role in this process (see Chapter 14). The task of reducing cardiovascular morbidity and mortality in NIDDM patients is greatly complicated by our lack of understanding of its pathogenesis and by the onset of the process years before the patient seeks medical attention.

Knowledge about the pathogenesis and the relationship of hyperglycaemia to the microvascular and neuropathic complications of NIDDM has advanced significantly in recent years. Epidemiological studies have shown that retinopathy in NIDDM patients is positively correlated with the duration of diabetes and the magnitude of hyperglycaemia as reflected both in fasting plasma glucose and glycosylated haemoglobin levels (20). Some intervention studies in IDDM patients comparing intensive insulin treatment to ordinary insulin treatment indicate that good glycaemic control decreases the progression of background retinopathy to the more serious proliferative retinopathy (21, 22). Several intervention studies in IDDM patients with microalbuminuria show that intensive insulin administration will prevent the progression of most of these patients to clinical diabetic nephropathy during an 8 year follow-up (21, 23). From the few small well-controlled studies that were available, it appeared that a target mean HbAlc value (average of measurement every 3 or 4 months) of less than 7.0% would significantly slow the rate of progression of microvascular disease. The results of the Diabetes Control and Complication Trial (DCCT) in the US which were recently presented (22) show unequivocally that such glycaemic control reduces proliferative retinopathy 47%, the development of clinical nephropathy 56% and neuropathy 60% during a mean follow-up of 5 years when compared to ordinary glycaemic control (mean haemoglobulin $A_{1c}$ 9.0%). The UK Prospective Study of type 2 diabetes which is to be completed in 1996 or 1997 should provide data on the relationship between glycaemic control and chronic complications in NIDDM patients (24–26). It is becoming possible now to define glycaemic goals in terms of clinical end points on the basis of data rather than speculation.

The prevention of microvascular disease or slowing its progression will have some benefit in slowing the progression of ischaemic heart disease. Microalbuminuria is a known risk factor in NIDDM patients for ischaemic heart disease and peripheral vascular disease. Several studies have linked diabetic retinopathy to increased cardiovascular mortality. Finally, diabetic nephropathy markedly accelerates atherosclerosis.

## INCREASED PHYSICAL ACTIVITY AND DIET: THE FIRST APPROACH TO TREATMENT OF NIDDM

A relationship between physical activity and the development of NIDDM has become firmly established by several epidemiological and prospective studies. A survey of the population of Mauritius showed a strong correlation between reported physical activity of an individual and his or her likelihood to develop NIDDM (27). A large prospective study of approximately 6000 University of Pennsylvania male alumni using a questionnaire showed an inverse correlation between leisure time physical activity and the development of NIDDM in 202 individuals over a 14-year period (28). Leisure-time physical activity was defined as kilocalories expended per week in walking, stair-climbing and sports. For each 500 kcal increment in energy expediture, the age-adjusted risk of NIDDM was reduced by 6%. A similar 8-year prospective study in 87 253 normal US women aged 34 to 59 years showed that women who exercised vigorously at least once a week had an age-adjusted relative rate of NIDDM of 0.67 (29). Both studies showed effects independent of obesity, age or family history of diabetes. The protective effect of exercise appears greatest in those with an increased risk of NIDDM. These studies provide strong support for increased physical activity as primary prevention of NIDDM.

Short-term metabolic studies show that increased physical activity improves glucose metabolism and decreases insulin resistance (30). Unfortunately, it has been difficult to demonstrate a beneficial effect of such programmes in the long-term treatment of patients with NIDDM. In a recently completed clinical study 6956 47- to 49-year-old males from Malmo were screened for NIDDM and IGT (31). Over 5 years, 41 early NIDDM patients and 181 IGT individuals were identified and put into a 5-year treatment protocol of dietary intervention and increased physical activity. The treated group had a reduction of body weight of 2.3 to 3.7% and an increase in maximal oxygen uptake of 10 to 14% while a non-randomised, no intervention group gained 0.5 to 1.7% body weight and decreased maximal oxygen uptake by 5–9%. During the study, 50% of the IGT group normalised their glucose tolerance, and only 10.6% progressed to NIDDM. Of the initial NIDDM group, 50% were in remission after a mean follow-up of 6 years. As might be expected, blood pressure, blood lipid levels and hyperinsulinaemia were reduced. Improvement in glucose tolerance was correlated to both weight reduction and increased fitness.

Thus, it appears that increased physical activity can be both a primary preventative and a secondary treatment. In all of these studies, however, it is difficult to separate the primary effects of physical activity from its effect in increasing caloric expenditure and causing weight loss. Increased physical activity must usually be coupled with some type of dietary intervention if it is to be practically effective in either preventing or treating NIDDM.

Virtually every treatise on the management of NIDDM starts by emphasizing that diet is the cornerstone of all therapeutic programmes. This is based on the observations that: (1) obesity in every population is associated with an increased prevalence of NIDDM; (2) the incidence of NIDDM decreases in populations when food is restricted such as during war or famine; (3) the prevalence of NIDDM increases in populations which change their traditional life-style and eating patterns to those of western civilisations; (4) obesity causes insulin resistance; (5) short-term dietary intervention studies have been shown to decrease hyperglycaemia (32–40).

Clinical practice, however, has shown that only a small percentage of the NIDDM population can achieve appropriate target goals of glycaemic control by dietary management with or without increased physical activity (41–44). This has been attributed to both patient and physican failure in obtaining compliance to an appropriate programme.

The UK Prospective Diabetes Study has published data recently on the result of dietary management of 3044 newly diagnosed NIDDM patients. This study gives insight into some of the major difficulties of dietary management (45). The patients were treated with a diet containing 50% carbohydrate (mostly complex), 30% fat and 20% protein. The caloric intake was adjusted for the degree of obesity (1672 kcal/day for patients with less than 110% ideal body weight to 1098 kcal/day for patients with greater than 150% ideal body weight). Of patients 15% were primary diet failures in the first 3 months and had to be given pharmacological therapy because of continuing symptoms and/or fasting plasma glucoses (FPG) greater than 15 mmol/l. Of the remaining 2597, only 482 (16%) achieved an FPG <6 mmol/l at 3 months. They remained on diet therapy alone. Of the 2115 who had an FPG of >6 mmol/l, 341 were allocated to remain on diet therapy. The results of dietary therapy on glycaemia were analysed at 3 months and 15 months and were correlated with initial body weight and degree of hyperglycaemia and weight change during therapy.

The major factors predicting glycaemic response were the level of FPG at diagnosis and the absolute weight loss during treatment. The degree of initial obesity had little effect. Maintenance of glycaemic control required continued caloric restriction since weight maintenance after achieving adequate glycaemic control was associated with a rising FPG. Of patients presenting with an FPG of 6.0 to 8.0 mmol/l 50% achieved FPG <6 mmol/l while only 10% of those presenting with an FPG of 16 to 22 mmol/l were successful. Average weight loss necessary at 3 months to achieve an FPG <6 mol/l was 10 kg for those presenting with an FPG of 6–8 mmol/l and rose approximately 4 kg for each 2 mmol/l increase in presenting FPG. The average patient presenting with a FPG of 10 to 12 mmol/l had to lose 18 kg to attain an FPG <6 mmol/l at 3 months. Only 8% of patients who failed to attain an FPG <6 mmol/l at 3 months attained it at 15 months. Of those who achieved an FPG of 6 mmol/l at 3 months, only 54% maintained it over the next 12 months.

The insights into dietary management of NIDDM that can be gleaned from the UK Prospective Diabetes Study are: (1) three months of dietary treatment is an adequate trial; (2) reduction of hyperglycaemia occurs most rapidly in the first month or two; (3) response to dietary therapy is mostly determined by the magnitude of fasting hyperglycaemia; (4) substantial absolute weight loss is necessary for achieving near normoglycaemia and is relatively independent of the degree of initial obesity; (5) maintenance of near normoglycaemia requires continued caloric restriction and (6) caloric restriction rather than weight loss is probably the major determinant of the benefit of dietary therapy.

While caloric content seems to be the most important aspect of dietary management, alterations in the composition of the diet do play some modulating role in fasting and postprandial hyperglycaemia. Jenkins and his co-workers have repeatedly emphasised that foods can be classified as having low or high glycaemic indices as determined by the plasma glucose curve after ingestion of comparable amounts. Short-term studies show that a diet with a low glycaemic index results in better glucose regulation and lower serum cholesterol in NIDDM patients than an isocaloric diet with a higher glycaemic index (46–48). O'Dea and her colleagues assessed metabolic control in 10 NIDDM men on four isocaloric diets for two weeks (49). The most significant improvement in metabolic control was obtained with a high fibre, high carbohydrate, low fat diet or a low carbohydrate, high protein, low fat diet. Metabolic control was not affected by a low fibre, high carbohydrate, low fat diet but deteriorated on a high fat, low carbohydrate diet. The value of a high carbohydrate, relatively low fat diet for treating most NIDDM patients is supported by many studies (50).

In a small subset of obese NIDDM patients, diets high in carbohydrate may increase hyperglycaemia and serum triglycerides and decrease serum HDL-cholesterol. In such patients, substitution of carbohydrate by mono-unsaturated fats has been shown to reverse these detrimental effects (51, 52). The use of this high mono-unsaturated fat, low carbohydrate diet for the treatment of ordinary NIDDM patients remains controversial (53). Most experts reserve this diet for the small subset that show detrimental metabolic effects on high carbohydrate diets.

The supplementation of *n*-3 fatty acids to the diet of NIDDM patients is not useful since they increase fasting plasma glucose, haemoglobin $A_{1c}$, serum LDL-cholesterol and plasminogen activator inhibitor -1 (54, 55). Some studies show a decrease in insulin action. Their serum triglyceride lowering effect is not sufficient to warrant the other detrimental metabolic effects.

The use of very low calorie diets supplemented with essential nutrients is advocated by some investigators as an initial form of dietary therapy (56). This intensive calorie deprivation must be done under careful medical supervision since safety has been an issue. Additionally, it must be coupled with behavioural modification. Some studies suggest that short courses of treatment (8 weeks) with slow re-introduction of food have continued benefit on glycaemic control at 1 year in spite of some weight regain (57). Successive courses of very low calorie diets may not be as successful as first courses probably as a result of poorer compliance (58). More long-term studies of the effects of very low calorie diets are needed.

## PHARMACOLOGICAL MANAGEMENT OF HYPERGLYCAEMIA IN NIDDM

As noted in the preceding section, about 85 to 90% of diet-treated NIDDM patients do not achieve long-term near normoglycaemic regulation even under the most favourable clinical research conditions. Population-based studies of NIDDM patients being treated with pharmacological agents for hyperglycaemia have shown that good metabolic control defined as a haemoglobin $A_{1c} \leq 7\%$ or its equivalent is infrequently achieved (usually only 10–20% of the population) (11, 20). Management of glycaemia by diet even when effective frequently does not ameliorate the increased cardiovascular risk factors associated with NIDDM (43, 59). More distressing are the observations that many newly diagnosed NIDDM patients already have significant microvascular and macrovascular disease. These observations taken as a whole indicate that: (1) adequate therapy of NIDDM patients must begin when hyperglycaemia commences not when it becomes symptomatic; (2) treat-

Table 33.1. *Primary modes of action of anti-hyperglycaemic drugs*

| | Sulphonylureas | Metformin | Alpha-glucosidase inhibitors | Insulin |
|---|---|---|---|---|
| Increase insulin binding to its receptor | 0 | 0 | 0 | 0 |
| Increase glucose transport and metabolism by cells | 0 | 1 to 2+ | 0 | 4+ |
| Decrease basal hepatic glucose production | 2+ | 1+ | 1+ | 4+ |
| Increase endogenous insulin secretion | 4+ | 0 | 0 | 0 |
| Potentiate insulin action on glucose uptake and metabolism | 1 to 2+ | 2+ | 0 | 0 |
| Decrease hepatic clearance of insulin | 2+ | 0 | 0 | 0 |
| Decrease carbohydrate digestion and/or absorption | 0 | ? | 4+ | 0 |

0 = no effect. 4+ = marked effect.

ment of hyperglycaemia should be aggressively pursued when possible; (3) associated cardiovascular risk factors must also be considered when implementing an appropriate therapeutic regimen for hyperglycaemia.

## Mechanism of action

The classes of pharmacological agents that are available for the management of hyperglycaemia are sulphonylureas (60), biguanides (61), alpha-glucosidase inhibitors (62) and insulins (63). Each of these classes of agents has a different mode of action and each has its advantages and disadvantages. The management of an individual patient should involve matching the patient's requirements with the agent's profile of action. Since the mode of action differs among the classes, there is also the option of combining agents to achieve better glycaemic control with less adverse effects in specific patients.

Table 33.1 defines what is thought to be the mechanism of action for each class of pharmacological agents. Sulphonylureas exert their major action by stimulating the beta cell to secrete more insulin in both the basal and postprandial state (60, 64). This action occurs through the binding of the sulphonylurea to its receptor on the cell surface of the beta cell with subsequent changes in ion fluxes through the cell which trigger insulin release (65, 66). The ion changes which occur are a decrease in K+ efflux, a depolarisation of the plasma membrane and an influx of extracellular $Ca^{+2}$. The rise in cytosolic $Ca^{+2}$ stimulates insulin granule exocytosis. This sulphonylurea stimulation of insulin secretion occurs even though glucose-stimulated insulin secretion is impaired. Sulphonylureas have extrapancreatic effects such as potentiating insulin action on glucose uptake and metabolism of muscle, adipose tissue and liver cells and decreasing hepatic clearance of insulin (60, 67), which contribute to the anti-hyperglycaemic action of sulphonylureas, but the major action is stimulation of insulin secretion.

Metformin which is the only biguanide commercially available exerts its anti-hyperglycaemic effects through direct action in stimulating glucose uptake and metabolism, potentiating insulin action on peripheral tissues and decreasing basal hepatic glucose production (61). The exact biochemical mechanisms by which these effects occur are still controversial. Metformin does not stimulate insulin secretion and does not cause hypoglycaemia.

The alpha-glucosidase inhibitors are competitive inhibitors that bind to the various alpha-glucosidases in the brush border of intestinal enterocytes and interfere with the digestion of starch, sucrose and malto-trioses. As a result, monosaccharides are generated and absorbed through the length of the small intestine rather

Table 33.2. *Major clinical effects of anti-hyperglycaemic drugs*

| | Sulphonylureas | Metformin | Alpha-glucosidase inhibitors | Insulin |
|---|---|---|---|---|
| Decrease fasting plasma glucose | 2–3 mM | 2–3 mM | 1 mM | No limit |
| Decrease post-prandial plasma glucose | 2–3 mM | 2–3 mM | 2–3 mM | No limit |
| Decrease $HbA_{1c}$ | 1.5–2.0 | 1.5–2.0 | 1.0 | No limit |
| Decrease plasma LDL-chol. | ± | + | 0 | ± |
| Raise plasma HDL-chol. | 0 | 0 | 0 | ± |
| Decrease plasma triglyceride | + | + | + | + |
| Lower blood pressure | 0 | 0 | 0 | 0 |
| Increase body wt | + | | 0 | 2+ |
| Decrease body wt | | + | | |

0 = no effect. 4+ = marked effect.

than in the proximal jejunum. The net result is a decrease in the rate of postprandial plasma glucose rise. The small effect on fasting plasma glucose and basal hepatic glucose production is probably the result of improved insulin action from the decrease in mean 24-hour plasma glucose (62, 68, 69).

Insulin preparations act through decreasing hepatic glucose production and increasing glucose uptake and metabolism by the normal physiological mechanisms (63). The main differences between pharmacological treatment and physiological regulation with insulin are: (1) the portal vein: peripheral vein gradient is 1:1 rather than 3:1; (2) insulin action is slow in onset and very prolonged rather than rapid and brief; (3) peripheral hyperinsulinaemia always occurs and (4) portal vein and peripheral plasma insulin levels can not be rapidly altered.

## Clinical effects

Table 33.2 summarises the salient effects, of monotherapy of NIDDM with these pharmacological agents which have been consistently observed in large, randomised, placebo–controlled studies. Unfortunately, clinical conclusions have frequently been drawn from studies which involve 10 to 50 patients, last for 6 to 26 weeks and may not have been randomised and placebo controlled. Such conclusions are unwarranted and frequently prove to be incorrect. Insulin therapy if designed properly, i.e. several times a day and with preparations of different durations of action, can lower fasting and postprandial glycaemia to any desired level. Insulin treatment therefore can be effective regardless of the magnitude of hyperglycaemia and can lower the $HbA_{1c}$ to whatever level is desired (70–72). It will lower plasma triglycerides and may have some small beneficial effects on plasma LDL- and HDL-cholesterol. A major effect of insulin treatment is significant weight gain (70–73). This is highly undesirable in an already obese NIDDM individual.

Sulphonylurea therapy is initially effective in lowering glycaemia in about three-quarters of NIDDM patients (60, 74). The mean maximal decrease in fasting and postprandial plasma glucoses that can be expected are 2 to 3 mmol/l. This is when compared to a randomised placebo-treated control NIDDM population. The mean maximal decrease in $HbA_{1c}$ is between 1.5 and 2.0%. When combined with dietary therapy, sulphonylurea therapy can decrease mean glycaemia 3 to 5 mmol/l and $HbA_{1c}$ 3 to 3.5% in the untreated NIDDM patient. A mean weight gain of 1.5 to 3.0 kg is ordinarily observed with sulphonylurea treatment. Sulphonylurea treatment alters lipid metabolism only through its

Table 33.3. *Side-effects of anti-hyperglycaemic drugs*

| | Sulphonylureas | Metformin | Alpha-glucosidase inhibitors | Insulin |
|---|---|---|---|---|
| Hypoglycaemia | 1+ to 3+ | 0 | 0 | 3+ |
| Weight gain | 1+ | 0 | 0 | 3+ |
| GI distress | ± | 2+ | 2+ | 0 |
| Nausea | | | | |
| Bloating | | | | |
| Diarrhoea | | | | |
| Lactic acidosis | 0 | 1+ | 0 | 0 |
| Hyperinsulinaemia | 1+ | 0 | 0 | 4+ |
| Hypertension | 0 | 0 | 0 | ? |

0 = no effect. 4+ = marked effect.

improvement in glycaemia. Sulphonylurea therapy is only effective in NIDDM patients who have significant residual insulin secretory function.

Metformin therapy usually decreases fasting and postprandial glycaemia about 2 to 3 mmol/l (61, 75). This results in a 1.5 to 2.0% decrease in $HbA_{1c}$. Metformin can cause some anorexia and chronic therapy results in a mean weight loss of 1.0 to 2.0 kg. The mechanism responsible for the weight loss is unknown. Metformin treatment can result in a decrease in fasting plasma triglycerides and LDL-cholesterol. Plasma insulin levels may decrease with metformin therapy.

Treatment with alpha-glucosidase inhibitors selectively reduces postprandial hyperglycaemia by 2.5 to 3.0 mmol/l (62, 76). The fasting plasma glucose is reduced about 1 mmol/l probably as the result of an increase in insulin sensitivity due to decreased 24 h glycaemia. Associated with alpha-glucosidase treatment is a reduction in postprandial levels of insulin, gastric inhibitory polypeptide (GIP) and other GI hormones. Steatorrhoea, malabsorption and weight loss do not occur during alpha-glucosidase therapy.

## Side-effects

The major side-effects occurring during the treatment of NIDDM with the various pharmacological agents are given in Table 33.3. Insulin treatment of NIDDM subjects frequently requires multiple daily injections and large quantities of insulin. As near-normoglycaemia is achieved, severe and frequent hypoglycaemia becomes more common. In a recent primary care system where insulin treatment was used to obtain ordinary control, the hospitalisation rate for severe hypoglyaemia was 9.1 per 1000 patient years (77). Long-term treatment of NIDDM patients with insulin (6 months to 5 years) consistently show weight gains of approximately 10 kg (70–73). Several studies of insulin treatment of NIDDM patients have found an increase in systolic and diastolic blood pressure (78). In all of these studies it is not possible to separate the blood pressure elevations from the gain in body weight. The major side-effects of insulin treatment are therefore hypoglycaemia, marked weight gain, and a progressive increase in insulin resistance. Hyperinsulinaemia always accompanies insulin treatment and if it is causally related to hypertension and macrovascular disease (see Chapter 14) it can be considered a complication of treatment.

Sulphonylurea therapy is also complicated by hypoglycaemia and weight gain. This is not surprising since such therapy stimulates endogenous insulin secretion. Mild episodes of hypoglycaemia either recognised or asymptomatic occur with relative frequency in patients well controlled on sulphonylurea therapy (79). These episodes are of limited consequence. Occasionally, however, severe and sometimes fatal hypoglycaemia occurs with sulphonylurea therapy (60, 77, 80, 81). This happens in patients who are predisposed to hypoglycaemia (elderly individuals who are poorly nourished, forget to eat or have cardiovascular, kidney or liver disease). Long-acting sulphonylureas such as glibenclamide and chlorpropamide are most often the offending sulphonylureas. The severe form of hypoglycaemia ordinarily occurs with average doses of sulphonylureas. A good general guideline is to prescribe relatively short-acting sulphonylureas such as glipizide, gliclizide or tolbutamide for patients who are at increased risk for hypoglycaemia and to start treatment with the lowest recommended dose. The weight gain which occurs with sulphonylurea therapy is less than that which occurs with insulin treatment and usually amounts to 1 to 3 kg. Chlorpropamide by virtue of its unique structure can cause free water retention and hyponatraemia (60). Alcohol induced flushing occurs primarily with chlorpropamide treatment (60).

Metformin, if used in the proper doses and not administered to contraindicated patients, has relatively mild side-effects consisting of GI distress and diarrhoea (61, 75, 82). These can be minimised by initiating therapy with low doses and increasing the dose over several weeks. Though low serum $B_{12}$ levels have been reported in patients taking metformin, pernicious anaemia is quite rate. The major complication of metformin therapy is the development of lactic acidosis. Biguanide therapy increases lactate production. Normally the lactate is oxidised and/or utilised through metabolic pathways. In the presence of renal disease, metformin clearance is severely reduced and lactic acidosis may ensue. Likewise in cardiovascular failure or pulmonary disease which predispose to cellular hypoxia, metformin should be avoided since it may facilitate the development of lactic acidosis.

The alpha-glucosidase inhibitor acarbose is relatively non-absorbable and its major side-effects are abdominal discomfort, bloating and flatulence (62, 76). These symptoms can be minimized by starting therapy with a low dose and increasing the dose slowly over several weeks. The GI symptoms appear to decrease with chronic therapy.

## Treatment strategies for using pharmacological agents

The initial decisions concerning the pharmacological treatment of hyperglycaemia in a patient with NIDDM is whether the prescribed dietary management and increased physical activity programme have achieved their maximal practical beneficial effects and whether the effects have resulted in the target goals set for that patient. An 80 year-old modestly obese individual (BMI 29 kg/m$^2$) may achieve a fasting plasma glucose of 8 mmol/l and a haemogloblin $A_{1c}$ of 7.5% after 3 months on a dietary and increased physical activity programme and that is all that may be required. The same result in an otherwise healthy 40 year-old NIDDM patient would be considered inadequate treatment. As noted previously, those patients who achieve good glycaemic control on a dietary programme usually show significant improvement in hyperglycaemia within the first six weeks of treatment and near target values by 3 months. Thus, failure to achieve significant improvement in hyperglycaemia by six weeks of dietary therapy is reasonable justification for the addition of pharmacological agents to the treatment program of NIDDM patients to control hyperglycaemia.

The addition of an alpha glucosidase inhibitor, metformin or a sulphonylurea is indicated if the NIDDM patient persists with symptoms and/or has a FPG of 6 to 15 mmol/l after the trial of dietary therapy. If the FPG remains greater than 15 mmol/l, it would be advisable to start insulin therapy. Patients with markedly elevated fasting plasma glucoses on a dietary regimen are significantly insulin deficient and are also experiencing 'glucose toxicity'. The order of ascending antidiabetic potency of the pharmacological agents are: alpha-glucosidase inhibitors, metformin sulphonylureas and insulin (Fig. 33.1).

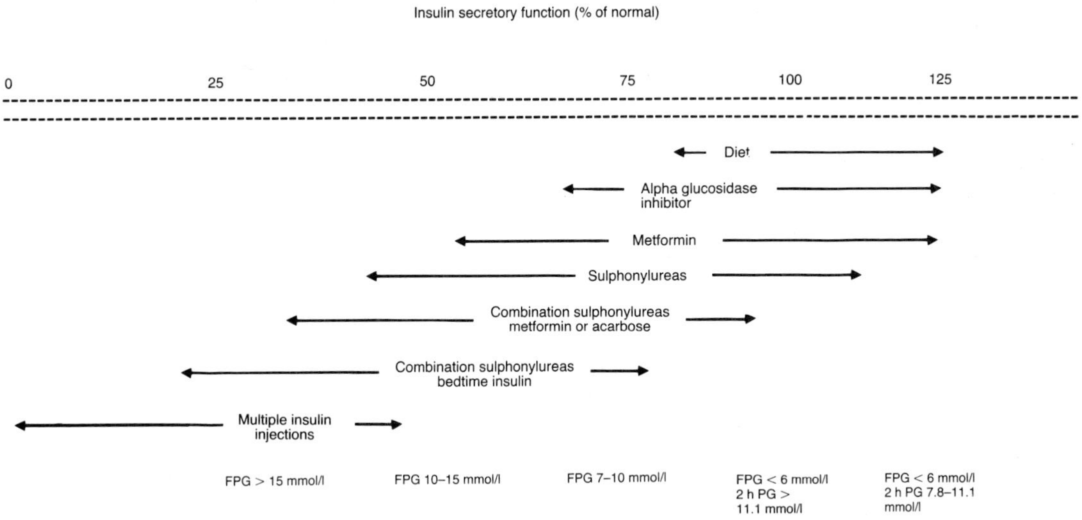


Fig. 33.1. Relationships among insulin secretory capacity, glycaemic regulation and therapeutic regimens.

Monotherapy with a particular oral antidiabetic agent should achieve near normoglycaemia (FPG $<7$ mmol/l and haemogloblin $A_{1c} \leqslant 7.0\%$). If not, therapy should be switched to another class of oral antidiabetic agent. In the event that monotherapy does not achieve appropriate glycaemic control, the various oral antidiabetic agents can be combined. Combinations usually include sulphonylureas plus either metformin or an alpha–glucosidase inhibitor. Combination sulphonylurea-metformin results in a 20 to 30% reduction in fasting plasma glucose from monotherapy with either alone and as many as 40% of patients on such combination therapy achieve good glycaemic control (FPG 7 to 8 mmol/l) (83–88). Addition of the alpha-glucosidase inhibitor, acarbose, to NIDDM patients inadequately controlled on sulphonylureas has been reported to lower haemogloblin $A_{1c}$ by 0.5 to 1.0% (89–90).

Therapy with oral agents alone or in combination are only effective in NIDDM patients who have reasonably well-preserved beta cell insulin secretory function. If insulin secretory function is marginal, then combinations of insulin and oral agents may be effective and, if insulin secretion is markedly impaired, then complete replacement therapy with multiple daily insulin administration is necessary.

Combination insulin–sulphonylurea therapy has been examined by innumerable investigators (91, 92). Most studies have been seriously flawed in their design and in the use of inadequate doses of sulphonylureas. Several recent excellent studies, however, clearly show that the administration of intermediate-acting insulin at bedtime and sulphonylureas during the day can markedly improve glycaemic control (decrease haemoglobulin $A_{1c}$ 1.0 to 1.5%) with minimal weight gain and elevation of plasma free insulin (93–95).

Thus a logical scheme for the management of NIDDM patients can be developed which is based on their residual insulin secretory capacity. Fig. 33.1 is a schematic representation of the relationship between insulin secretory function, glycaemic levels and the potential value of each therapeutic treatment regimen for hyperglycaemia. The doses of the various pharmacological agents to be used in the management of hyperglycaemia in NIDDM patients are given in Table 33.4.

Table 33.4. *Pharmacological agents for treatment of hyperglycaemia*

| Class | Agent | Initial dose | Therapeutic dose range |
|---|---|---|---|
| Alpha-glucosidase inhibitor | Acarbose | 50 mg immediately before each meal | 50–200 mg immediately before each meal |
| Biguanide | Metformin | 850 mg once a day or 500 mg twice a day | 1500 to 2500 mg/day in two or three divided doses |
| Sulphonylurea | Tolbutamide | 500 mg twice a day | 1000 to 3000 mg/day in two or three divided doses |
| | Chlorpropamide | 100 mg/day | 100 to 500 mg once daily |
| | Glipizide | 2.5 to 5.0 mg once daily | 2.5 to 30 mg daily |
| | Glibenclamide | 1.25 to 2.5 mg once daily | 1.25 to 20 mg daily |
| | Gliclizide | 40 to 80 mg once daily | 40–320 mg daily |
| Insulin | Regular<br>Semi-lente<br>Lente<br>NPH<br>Ultra-lente | Type, species, doses, times and combinations to be individually determined | |

## MANAGEMENT OF ASSOCIATED METABOLIC ABNORMALITIES IN NIDDM

While the initial focus of management in NIDDM patients is the amelioration of hyperglycaemia, it is important to recognise that NIDDM is usually associated with other interrelated metabolic disorders such as hypertension and dyslipidaemias. Chronic complications of NIDDM cannot be minimised without concomitant treatment of these associated metabolic disturbances.

The control of blood pressure is necessary to decrease macrovascular disease and prevent the development and progression of microvascular disease (96, 97). Though definitive proof is lacking, most investigators set a target diastolic blood pressure in NIDDM patients between 80 and 85 mm of Hg. Considerable controversy exists about the antihypertensive drugs of choice in diabetic patients. Diuretic therapy as sole management is likely to be associated with hypokalaemia, an elevation in serum LDL-cholesterol and a deterioration of endogenous insulin secretion (98, 99). Beta-adrenergic antagonists can interfere with endogenous insulin secretion, recovery from hypoglycaemia and may increase serum LDL cholesterol (97, 99). Alpha-adrenergic antagonists are neutral as far as effects on glucose and lipid and lipoprotein metabolism (97, 99). Angiotensin converting enzyme inhibitors have conclusively been shown to have specific renal protective effects in diabetic patients in addition to their blood pressure lowering actions (100–103). They do not possess any detrimental effects on carbohydrate and lipid metabolism. Calcium channel antagonists have not been as extensively studied in diabetic patients as angiotensin converting enzyme inhibitors. Current data suggest the angiotension converting enzyme inhibitors alone, or in combination with other antihypertensives, are the agents of choice for the management of hypertension in diabetic patients (100–103).

The management of hypercholesterolaemia, hypertriglyceridaemia and low serum HDL-cholesterol levels in NIDDM patients starts with glycaemic control and dietary management (104, 105). Most recommendations are that NIDDM patients without known cardiovascular disease should be maintained with serum LDL-cholesterol below 3.4 mmol/l and with known cardiovascular disease below 2.6 mmol/l (105).

The recommendations for serum triglyceride levels are not as firm but generally would best be kept below 2.25 mmol/l (105). The use of bile acid binding resins or HMG-CoA reductase inhibitors are recommended for elevated serum LDL-cholesterol levels (106). Fibrates are the treatment of choice for hypertriglyceridaemia (107). Nicotinic acid is generally contra-indicated in NIDDM patients because of its hyperglycaemic action (108).

## CONCLUSION

The rationale approach to the management of NIDDM patients is based on reducing morbidity and mortality to that of the non-diabetic. This requires very early diagnosis of hyperglycaemia and its related metabolic disturbances (hypertension, dylipidaemias) and intensive management based on an understanding of the pathophysiology.

## REFERENCES


1 *Physician's guide to non-insulin-dependent (Type II) Diabetes: diagnosis and treatment.* 2nd edn, Lebovitz HE, ed. American Diabetes Association, Alexandria VA, 1988.

2 Alberti KGMM, Gries FA. Management of non-insulin-dependent diabetes mellitus in Europe: a consensus view. *Diabetic Med* 1988; 5: 275–81.

3 Harris MI. Undiagnosed NIDDM: clinical and public health issues. *Diabetes Care* 1993; 16: 642–52.

4 Eschwege E, Richard JL, Thibult N *et al.* Coronary heart disease mortality in relation with diabetes, blood glucose and plasma insulin levels, the Paris Prospective Study Ten Years Later. *Hormone Metab Res* 1985; 15 (Suppl.): 41–6.

5 Jarrett RJ, Shipley MJ. Type II (non-insulin-dependent) diabetes mellitus and cardiovascular disease-putative association via common antecedents: further evidence from the Whitehall Study. *Diabetologia* 1988; 31: 737–40.

6 Hanis CL, Chu HH, Lawson K *et al.* Mortality of Mexican Americans with NIDDM. Retinopathy and other predictors in Starr County, Texas. *Diabetes Care* 1993; 16: 82–9.

7 Lee ET, Russel D, Jorge N, Kenny S, Yu ML. A follow-up study of diabetic Oklahoma Indians. Mortality and causes of death. *Diabetes Care* 1993; 16: 300–5.

8 Sievers ML, Nelson RG, Knowler WC, Bennett PH. Impact of NIDDM on mortality and causes of death in Pima Indians. *Diabetes Care* 1992; 15: 1541–9.

9 Knuiman MW, Welborn TA, Whittall DE. An analysis of excess mortality rates for persons with non-insulin-dependent diabetes mellitus in Western Australia using the cox proportional hazards regression model. *Am J Epidemiol* 1992; 135: 638–48.

10 Sasaki A, Horiuchi N, Hasegawa K, Uehara M. Mortality and causes of death in Type 2 diabetic patients. A long-term follow up study in Osaka District Japan. *Diabetes Res Clin Pract* 1989; 71: 33–40.

11 Duncan C, Charlmers J, Campbell IW, Jones IG. An audit of non-insulin-dependent diabetics attending a district general hospital diabetic clinic: implications for shared care between hospital and general practice. *Health Bull* 1992; 50: 302–8.

12 Nelson RG, Newman JM, Knowler WC, Sievers ML, Kunzelman CL, Pettitt DJ, Moffett CD, Teutsch SM, Bennett PH: Incidence of end-stage renal disease in Type 2 (non-insulin-dependent) diabetes mellitus in Pima Indians. *Diabetologia* 1988; 31: 730–6.

13 Uusitupa MIJ. Niskanen LK, Siitonen O, Voutilainen E, Pyorala K. 5-year incidence of atherosclerotic vascular disease in relation to general risk factors, insulin level, and abnormalities in lipoprotein composition in non-insulin-dependent diabetic and non-diabetic subjects. *Circulation* 1990, 82: 27–36.

14 Deckert T, Kofoed-Enevoldsen A, Norgaard K, Borch-Johnsen K, Feldt-Rasmussen B, Jensen T. Microalbuminuria: implications for micro-and macrovascular disease. *Diabetes Care* 15: 1992, 1181–91.

15 Mattock MB, Morrish NJ, Viberti G, Keen H, Fitzgerald AP, Jackson G. Prospective study of microalbuminuria as a predictor of mortality. *Diabetes* 1992, 41: 736–41.

16 Davis MD, Hiller R, Magli YLM *et al.* Prognosis for life in patients with diabetes: relation to severity of retinopathy. *Trans Am Opthalmol Soc* 1979; 77: 144–70.

17 Sharma NH, Archer DB, Hadden DR *et al.* Morbidity and mortality in patients with diabetic retinopathy. *Eye* 1980; 100: 83–9.

18 Mitchell BD, Stern MP, Haffner SM *et al.* Risk factors for cardiovascular mortality in Mexican–Americans and Non-Hispanic Whites. *Am J Epidemiol* 1990; 131: 423–33.

19 Fitzgerald AP, Jarrett RJ. Are conventional risk factors for mortality relevant in Type 2 diabetes? *Diabetic Med* 1991; 8: 475–80.

20 Klein R, Klein BE, Moss SE, Davis MD, DeMets DL. Glycosylated hemoglobin predicts the incidence and progression of diabetic retinopathy. *JAMA* 1988; 260: 2864–71.

21 Reichard P, Nilsson B-Y, Rosenqvist U. The effect of long-term intensified insulin treatment on the development of microvascular complications of diabetes mellitus. *N Engl J Med* 1993; 329: 304–9.

22 Diabetic Control and Complications Trial Research Group. The effect of intensive treatment of diabetes on the development and progression of long-term complications in insulin-dependent diabetes mellitus. *N Engl J Med.* 1993; 329: 977–86.

23 Feldt-Rasmussen B, Mathiesen ER, Jensen T, Deckert R. Effect of improved metabolic control on loss of kidney function in Type 1 (insulin-dependent) diabetic patients. *Diabetologia* 1991; 34: 164–70.

24 UK Prospective Diabetes Study. I Effect of diet, sulphonylurea, insulin or biguanide therapy on fasting plasma glucose and body weight over one year. *Diabetologia* 1983; 24: 404–11.

25 UK Prospective Diabetes Study. II Reduction in $HBA_{1c}$ with basal insulin supplement, sulfonylurea or biguanaide therapy in maturity-onset diabetes. *Diabetes* 1985; 34: 793–8.
26 UK Prospective Diabetes Study Group. UK Prospective Diabetes Study VIII Study design, progress and performance. *Diabetologia* 1991; 34: 877–90.
27 Dowse GK, Zimmet PZ, Gareebo H *et al.* Abdominal obsesity and physical inactivity as risk factors for NIDDM and impaired glucose tolerance in Indian, Creole and Chinese Mauritians. *Diabetes Care* 1991; 14: 271–82.
28 Helmrich SP, Ragland DR, Leung RW, Paffenbarger RS Jr. Physical activity and reduced occurrence of non-insulin-dependent diabetes mellitus. *N Engl J Med* 1991; 325: 147–52.
29 Manson JAE, Rimm EB, Stampfer MJ, Colditz GA, Willett WC, Krolewski AS, Rosner B, Hennekens CH, Speizer FE. Physical activity and incidence of non-insulin-dependent diabetes mellitus in women. *Lancet* 1991; 338: 774–8.
30 Horton ES. Exercise and decreased risk of NIDDM. *N Engl J Med* 1991; 325: 196–8.
31 Eriksson K-F, Lindgarde F. Prevention of Type 2 (non-insulin dependent) diabetes mellitus by diet and physical exercise. *Diabetologia* 1991; 34: 891–8.
32 Cowie CC, Harris MI, Silverman RE, Johnson EW, Rust KF. Effect of multiple risk factors on differences between blacks and whites in the prevalence of non-insulin-dependent diabetes mellitus in the United States. *Am J Epidemiol* 1993; 137: 719–32.
33 Bouchardat A. De la glycosurie ou diabete sucre. Paris 1985 Germer-Baillière Vol II.
34 Zimmet PZ. Challenges in diabetes epidemiology – from west to the rest. *Diabetes Care* 1992; 15: 232–52.
35 Carter Center of Emory University. Closing the gap. The problem of diabetes mellitus in the United States. *Diabetes Care* 1985; 8; 391–406.
36 Zimmet P, Donse G, Finch C, Serjeantson S, King H. The epidemiology and natural history of NIDDM – lessons from the South Pacific. *Diabetes Metab Rev* 1990; 6: 91–124.
37 Bogardus C, Lillioja S, Mott DM, Hollenbeck C, Reaven GM. Relationship between degree of obesity and *in vivo* insulin action in man. *Am J Physiol* 1985; 248: E286–91.
38 Yki-Jarvinen H, Koivisto VA. Effects of body composition on insulin sensitivity. *Diabetes* 1983; 32: 965–9.
39 Wilson EA, Hadden DR, Merrett JD, Montgomery DAD, Weaver JA. Dietary management of maturity-onset diabetes. *Br Med J* 1980; 1: 1367–9.
40 Newburgh LH. Control of the hyperglycemia of obese diabetics by weight reduction. *Ann Intern Med* 1942; 17: 935–42.
41 Stalhammar J, Bergman U, Boman K, Dahlen M. Metabolic control in three Swedish areas with high, medium and low sales of antidiabetic drugs. *Diabetes Care* 1991; 14: 12–19.
42 Wolffenbuttel BH, Weber RF, Van Koetsveld PM, Verschoor L. Limitations of diet therapy in patients with non-insulin-dependent diabetes mellitus. *Int J Obesity* 1989; 13: 173–82.
43 Takeda N, Horiya T, Yasuda K *et al.* Comparative effects of diet or glibenclamide on insulin secretion and action in non-obese NIDDM. *Diabetes Res and Clin Pract* 1991; 11: 99–106.
44 Lebovitz HE. Is diet the therapy of choice in adult non-insulin-dependent diabetes mellitus? Negative. *Debates Med* 1991; 4: 172–8, 184–7.
45 UKPDS Group. UK Prospective Diabetes Study? Response of fasting plasma glucose to diet therapy in newly presenting type II diabetic patients. *Metabolism* 1990; 39: 905–12.
46 Wolever TM, Jenkins DJ, Vuksan V, Jenkins AL, Wong GS, Josse RG. Beneficial effect of low-glycemic index diet in overweight NIDDM subjects. *Diabetes* 1992; 15: 562–4.
47 Wolever TW, Jenkins DJ, Vuksan V *et al.* Beneficial effect of a low glycaemic index diet in Type 2 diabetes. *Diabetic Med* 1992; 9: 451–8.
48 Fontvieille AM, Rizkalla SW, Penfornis A, Acosta M, Bornet FR, Slama G: The use of low glycaemic index foods improves metabolic control of diabetic patients over five weeks. *Diabetic Med* 1992; 9: 444–50.
49 O'Dea K, Traianedes K, Ireland P *et al.* The effects of diet differing in fat, carbohydrate, and lipid metabolism in type II diabetes. *J Am Dietetic Assoc* 1989; 89: 1076–86.
50 Howard BV, Abbott WG, Swinburn BA. Evaluation of metabolic effects of substitution of complex carbohydrates for saturated fat in individuals with obesity and NIDDM. *Diabetes Care* 1991; 14: 786–95.
51 Grundy SM. Dietary therapy in diabetes mellitus. Is there a single best diet? *Diabetes Care* 1991; 14: 796–801.
52 Parillo M, Rivellese AA, Ciardullo AV *et al.* A high monounsaturated-fat/low carbohydrate diet improves peripheral insulin sensitivity in non-insulin-dependent diabetic patients. *Metab. Clin Exper* 1992; 41: 1373–8.
53 Franz MJ. How enthusiastically should the use of monounsaturated fats be encouraged. *Diabetes Educator* 1989; 15: 494–7.
54 Vessby B, Boberg M. Dietary supplementation with n-3 fatty acids may impair glucose homeostasis in patients with non-insulin-dependent diabetes mellitus. *J Int Med* 1990; 228: 165–71.
55 Boberg M, Pollare T, Siegbahn A, Vessby B. Supplementation with *n*-3 fatty acids reduces triglycerides but increases PA1–1 in non-insulin-dependent diabetes mellitus. *Eur Clin Invest* 1992; 22: 645–50.
56 Henry RR, Gumbiner B. Benefits and limitations of very low calorie diet theraphy in obese NIDDM. *Diabetes Care* 1991; 14: 802–23.
57 Wing RR, Marcus MD, Salata R, Epstein LH, Miaskiewicz S. Effects of a very low calorie diet (VLCD) in type 2 diabetic subjects. *Arch Int Med* 1991; 151: 1334–40.
58 Smith DE, Wing RR. Diminished weight loss and behavioral compliance during repeated diets in obese patients with type 2 diabetes. *Health Psych* 1991; 10: 378–83.
59 Marsiaj HI, Catalano C, Sum CF, Home PD, Alberti KG. Management of newly diagnosed non-insulin-dependent (type 2) diabetes: a retrospective audit. *Diabetes Res Clin Pract* 1991; 12: 129–36.
60 Lebovitz HE. *Oral antidiabetic agents in Joslin's diabetes mellitus* 13th edn, Kahn R, Weir GC eds. Lea and Febiger Philadelphia, 1993.

61 Bailey CJ. Biguanides and NIDDM. *Diabetes Care* 1992; 15: 755–72.
62 Lebovitz HE. Oral antidiabetic agents. The emergence of alpha-glucosidase inhibitors. *Drugs* 1992; 44 (Suppl 3): 21–28
63 Genuth S. Insulin use in NIDDM. *Diabetes Care* 1990, 13: 1240–64.
64 McIntyre HD, Ma A, Bird DM, Patterson CA, Cameron DP. Chronic sulfonylurea therapy augments basal and meal-stimulated insulin secretion while attenuating insulin responses to sulfonylurea *per se*. *Diabetes Care* 1992; 15: 1534–40.
65 Gaines KL, Hamilton S, Boyd AE III. Characterization of the sulfonylurea receptor on beta cell membranes. *J Biol Chem* 1988; 263: 2589–2592
66 Siconolfi-Baez L, Banerji MA, Lebovitz HE. Characterization and significance of sulfonylurea receptors. *Diabetes Care* 1990; 13 (Suppl 3): 2–8.
67 Pedersen O, Hother-Nielsen O, Bak J, Hjollund E, Beck-Nielsen H. Effects of sulfonylureas on adipocyte and skeletal muscle insulin action in patients with non-insulin-dependent diabetes mellitus. *Am J Med* 1991; 90 (Suppl 6A): 225–85.
68 Holman RR, Steemson J, Turner RC. Post-prandial glyceamic reduction by an alpha-glucosidase inhibitor in type 2 diabetic patients with therapeutically attained basal normoglycemia. *Diabetes Res* 1991; 18: 149–53.
69 Kingman PJ, Menheere PP, Sels JP, Nieuwenhuijzen Kruseman AC. Alpha-glucosidase inhibition by miglitol in NIDDM patients. *Diabetes Care* 1992; 15: 478–83.
70 Henry RR, Gumbiner B, Ditzler T, Wallace P, Lyon R, Glauber HS. Intensive conventional insulin therapy for type II diabetes. Metabolic effects during a 6 month outpatient trial. *Diabetes Care* 1993; 16: 21–31.
71 Lindstrom TH, Arnqvist HJ, Von Schenck HH. Effect of conventional and intensified insulin therapy on free-insulin profiles and glycemic control in NIDDM. *Diabetes Care* 1992; 15: 27–34.
72 Kudlacek S, Schernthaner G. The effect of insulin treatment on $HBA_{1c}$, body weight and lipids in type 2 diabetic patients with secondary failure to sulfonylureas. A five year follow-up study. *Hormone Metab Res* 1992; 24: 478–83.
73 Hickey ME, Hall TR. Insulin therapy and weight change in Native-American NIDDM patients. *Diabetes Care* 1993; 16: 364–8.
74 Lebovitz HE, ed. *Sulfonylurea drugs in therapy for diabetes mellitus and related disorders*. American Diabetes Association, Alexandria, VA, 1994: 116–23.
75 Lebovitz HE, ed. *Metformin in therapy for diabetes mellitus and related disorders*. American Diabetes Association, Alexandria, VA, 1994: 124–7.
76 Lebovitz HE, ed. *Alpha-glucosidase inhibitors in treatment of hyperglycemia in therapy for diabetes mellitus and related disorders*. American Diabetes Association, Alexandria, VA, 1994: 128–30.
77 Sugarman JR. Hypoglycemia associated hospitalizations in a population with a high prevalence of non-insulin-dependent diabetes mellitus. *Diabetes Res Clin Prac* 1991; 14: 139–47.
78 Randeree HA, Omar MA, Motala AA, Seedat MA. Effect of insulin therapy on blood pressure in NIDDM patients with secondary failure. *Diabetes Care* 1992; 15: 1258–63.
79 Jennings AM, Wilson RM, Ward JD. Symptomatic hypoglycemic in NIDDM patients treated with oral hypoglycemic agents. *Diabetes Care* 1989; 12: 203–208.
80 Berger W, Casuff F, Pasquet M, Rump A. Relative incidence of severe hypoglycemia induced by sulfonylureas in the last 25 years in Switzerland. *Schweiz Med Wsch* 1986; 116: 145–51.
81 Ferner RE, Haw N. Sulfonylureas and hypoglycemia. *Br Med J* 1988; 296–50.
82 Dornan TL, Heller SR, Peck GM, Tattersall RB. Double-blind evaluation of efficacy and tolerability of metformin in NIDDM. *Diabetes Care* 1991; 14: 342–4.
83 Clarke BF, Marshall AM, McGill RC, McCuish AC, Duncan LJP. A 3 year evaluation of combined sulphonylurea-metformin treatment in 200 diabetic ketoacidisis resistant sulphonylurea failures. Tolbutamide . . . after 10 years. WJH Butterworth and W Van Westering. *Excerpta Medica NY* 1967: 312–20.
84 Herman LS, Kjellstrom T, Nilsson-Ehle P. Effects of metformin and glibenclamide alone and in combination on serum lipids and lipoprotein in patients with non-insulin-dependent diabetes mellitus. *Diabete Metab* 1991; 17: 174–9.
85 Elkeles RS. The effects of oral hypoglycaemic drugs on serum lipids and lipoproteins in non-insulin-dependent diabetes (NIDDM). *Diabete Metab* 1991; 17: 197–200.
86 Haupt E, Knick B, Koschinsky T, Liebermeister H, Schneider J, Hirche H. Oral antidiabetic combination therapy with sulphonylureas and metformin. *Diabete Metab* 1991; 17: 224–31.
87 Reaven GM, Johnston P, Hollenbeck CB *et al*. Combined metformin-sulfonylurea treatment of patients with non-insulin-dependent diabetes in fair to poor glycemic control. *J Clin Endocrinol Metab* 1992; 74: 1020–26.
88 Trischitta V, Italia S, Mazzarino S *et al*. Comparison of combined therapies in treatment of secondary failure to sulfonylureas. *Diabetes Care* 1992; 15: 539–42.
89 Coniff RF, Krol AE, Shapiro JA, Seaton TB, Lebovitz HE. Long-term efficacy and safety of Acarbose as adjunctive therapy in NIDDM inadequately controlled by maximal sulfonylurea therapy: a multicenter double blind placebo-controlled study. Submitted for publication.
90 Spengler M. Unpublished observations.
91 Lebovitz HE, Pasmantier RM. Combination insulin-sulfonylurea therapy. *Diabetes Care* 1990; 13: 667–75.
92 Pugh JA, Wagner ML, Sawyer J, Ramirez G, Tuley M, Friedberg SJ. Is combination sulfonylurea and insulin therapy useful in NIDDM patients? *Diabetes Care* 1992; 15: 953–8.
93 Yki-Jarvinen J, Kauppila M, Kujansuu E, Lahti J, Marjanen T *et al*. Comparison of insulin regimens in patients with non-insulin-dependent diabetes mellitus. *N Engl J Med* 1992; 327: 1426–33.
94 Seigler DE, Olsson GM, Skyler JS. Morning versus bedtime isophane insulin in type 2 (non-insulin-dependent) diabetes mellitus. *Diabetic Med* 1992; 9: 826–33.
95 Sane T, Helve E, Yki-Jarvinen H, Taskinen MR. One year response to evening insulin therapy in non-insulin-dependent diabetes. *J Int Med* 1992; 23: 253–60.
96 Tjoa HI, Kaplan NM. Nonpharmacologic treatment of hypertension in diabetes mellitus. *Diabetes Care* 1991; 14: 449–60.

97 Stein PP, Black HR. Drug treatment of hypertension in patients with diabetes mellitus. *Diabetes Care* 1991; 14: 425–48.

98 Murphy MB, Lewis PJ, Kohner E, Schumer B, Dollery CT. Glucose intolerance in hypertensive patients treated with diuretics: a fourteen year follow-up. *Lancet* 1982; ii: 1293–5.

99 Ames RP. The effects of antihypertensive drugs on serum lipids and lipoprotein II non-diuretic drugs. *Drugs* 1986; 32: 335–7.

100 Bjorck S, Mulec H, Johnsen SA, Norden G, Aurell M. Renal protective effect of enalapril in diabetic nephropathy. *Br Med J* 1992; 304: 339–43.

101 Kasiske BL, Kalil RSN, Ma JZ, Liao M, Keane WF. Effect of antihypertensive therapy on the kidney in patients with diabetes: a meta-regression analysis. *Ann Intern Med* 1993; 118: 129–38.

102 Lewis EJ, Hunsicker LG, Bain RP, Rhode RD. The effect of angiotensin-converting-enzyme inhibition on diabetic nephropathy. N Engl J Med 1993; 329: 1456–62.

103 Lebovitz HE, Wiegmann TB, Cnaan A, Shahinfar S *et al*. Renal protective effects of enalapril in hypertensive NIDDM: role of baseline albuminuria. *Kidney Int* 1994; 45 (Suppl 45): 5150–5.

104 Garg A, Grundy SM. Management of dyslipidemia in NIDDM. *Diabetes Care* 1990; 13: 153–69.

105 Consensus Statement of the American Diabetes Association. Detection and management of lipid disorders in diabetes. *Diabetes Care* 1993, 16 (Suppl 2): 106–12.

106 Garg A, Grundy SM. Lovastatin for lowering cholesterol levels in non-insulin-dependent diabetes mellitus. *N Engl J Med* 1988, 318: 81–5.

107 Garg A, Grundy SM. Gemfibrozil alone or in combination with lovastatin for the treatment of hypertriglyceridemia in NIDDM. *Diabetes* 1989; 38: 364–72.

108 Garg A, Grundy SM. Nicotinic acid as therapy for dyslipidemia in non-insulin-dependent diabetes mellitus. *JAMA* 1990; 264: 723–6.f

# 34 Psychosocial Aspects of Diabetes Care

Mark Peyrot and Richard R. Rubin

Modern diabetes treatment carries tremendous potential for preventing adverse health consequences, whether they be acute (ketoacidotic, hyperosmolar, and hypoglycaemic coma) or long-term (amputations, blindness, kidney failure, heart disease). However, implementation of effective treatment ultimately depends on the behaviour of diabetic patients and their support networks. It is therefore incumbent upon health care professionals (HCPs) to become aware of the psychosocial factors implicated in diabetes treatment.

There are two approaches to identifying the role of psychosocial factors in diabetes treatment: (a) review basic psychosocial principles and concepts, and then apply them to diabetes care, and (b) identify diabetes care problems and issues which have a psychosocial component, and then review the way in which psychosocial principles and concepts can be applied to those problems. Because this publication is oriented toward care providers, we have chosen the second alternative. We will therefore describe the psychosocial problems involved with diabetes and the interventions which have been found successful.

Before identifying the psychosocial problems which will be the focus of this chapter, we would like to describe some of the assumptions which provide the foundation. It is important to distinguish between problems/issues facing children and those facing adults, not only because the problems are different, but also because the resources for solving them differ. Children are heavily dependent on caretakers for the management of their disease. Although this dependence decreases as the patient matures, it never disappears completely, and adults are at least partially dependent upon spouses, room-mates, co-workers, and others.

The developmental distinction is partially confounded with another important distinction, disease type. Adults can have both insulin dependent diabetes mellitus (IDDM) and non-insulin dependent diabetes mellitus (NIDDM), while children have only the former. We distinguish between these two biological conditions because they can present quite different problems for patients. Elsewhere, one of us has argued that the critical distinction is whether diabetes is treated with insulin or not, since insulin treatment produces its own set of psychosocial problems and issues (1).

One of the primary principles of clinical medicine is differential diagnosis, the concept that treatment must be tailored to a specific disorder, and, therefore, the disorder to be treated must be identified before treatment can proceed. While this may be something of an oversimplification, it is the basis of this chapter. For the purpose of clarity, we will group psychosocial problems into three categories, each containing one or more specific problems. The three categories are: psychiatric, behavioural, and motivational.

*Psychiatric* problems include several diagnosable disorders such as eating disorders, depression, obsessive–compulsive disorder, and a variety of other neurotic and psychotic disorders. In addition, we include behavioural syndromes which reflect underlying psychiatric disorders. These conditions may present either in terms of medical symptoms (e.g. recurrent diabetic ketoacidosis, frequent and severe hyperglycaemia and hypoglycaemia, life-threatening/disabling complications) or psychiatric symptoms (e.g. depression, anxiety, phobia). Interventions for these problems are traditional psychiatric modalities, with some diabetes-specific modifications.

*Behavioural* problems include knowledge-based non-compliance, and the inability to employ state-of-the-art self-management techniques. Also included is sub-optimal distribution of self-care responsibilities between parents and children. Interventions for these problems are educational.

*Motivational* problems include attitudinal problems in managing the day-to-day hassles of living with diabetes. Patients may have problems dealing with the demands of the diabetes regimen, especially if the individual's regimen is demanding and requires great personal sacrifice. One of the special problems involves obese patients who must follow a very strict weight management regimen in order to control their diabetes. Also included in this category are interpersonal difficulties. Interpersonal conflicts may create problems for the patient, or for those in the patient's social network (e.g. parents, spouses, siblings, friends, etc.). Interventions for this category of problems are behavioural weight management programs and coping skills training.

We discuss the psychosocial problems in the order listed above. Thus, we move from the most serious, but least common, problems to those less serious but more common.

## PSYCHIATRIC PROBLEMS AND INTERVENTIONS

The relationship between diabetes and psychiatric disorders has received increased attention in the past decade. A recent comprehensive review (2) describes psychiatric disorders often associated with diabetes, and the interventions used to treat these disorders. Patients with diabetes may suffer disproportionately from certain psychiatric problems, and the course and consequences of psychiatric disorders may be more severe in diabetic patients (3).

Patients with both NIDDM and IDDM may suffer from psychiatric problems, but these problems are expressed most dramatically in patients who have IDDM. In IDDM patients, psychiatric problems may lead to serious lapses in adherence to the treatment regimen resulting in immediate, life-threatening medical crises. Patients suffering from these problems generally present to HCPs as cases of chronically poor metabolic control, often with glycaemic fluctuations so precipitous as to require frequent hospitalisation (4, 5). Since patients whose care is defined by a series of medical crises often suffer from underlying severe psychosocial problems, no effective medical management is possible until the associated psychosocial factors are assessed and treated. Without effective psychosocial intervention by a mental health professional experienced in treating patients with diabetes, care of these patients represents a 'revolving door' of emergency treatment and hospital admissions.

Severe behavioural or emotional problems are the most common aetiological factors in recurrent diabetic ketoacidosis (RDKA) and 'brittle diabetes' (frequent incapacitating episodes of hypoglycaemia or hyperglycaemia). Psychosocial factors, including communication disorders, malingering, and factitious disease, have been identified as the cause of brittle diabetes in 75% of all cases; physiological factors were identified in only 25% of cases (6). Unfortunately, it may often be impossible for HCPs to identify the causes of RDKA and brittle diabetes in their patients during office visits, because establishing a definitive aetiology requires a comprehensive diagnostic approach and close observation of patients, generally in an inpatient setting. Since an accurate diagnosis is critical to the effective treatment of RDKA and brittle diabetes, HCPs may refer these patients to a centre equipped to evaluate such problems. Specific treatment should be applied as appropriate to the aetiology of each patient's glycaemic derangement, but mental health consultation or treatment is almost always indicated. Severe psychosocial disturbance may require intensive, long-term psychological or psychiatric treatment (7, 8), often on a residential basis and including family therapy.

Eating disorders are often the cause of RDKA and brittle diabetes in young women (9–11), so anorexia nervosa and bulimia nervosa should be considered as a possible aetiology in cases of severe metabolic derangement, especially if the patient is a young woman between the ages of 14 and 30. Behaviours associated with eating disorders, including severe restriction of caloric intake, binge-eating, and purging, can dramatically compromise glycaemic control and medical management. One of the special manifestations of eating disorders in young women is manipulation of insulin doses for the purpose of weight control. This behaviour is common among young women with IDDM, and it has devastating effects on glycaemia and overall health (12–14).

Diagnosis of an eating disorder can be difficult because patients suffering with these problems generally resist acknowledging their existence. HCPs should consider the possibility of an eating disorder in patients with poorly controlled IDDM and substantial weight loss over a short period of time. Other signs of eating disorders include unrealistically low goals for ideal weight, and chronic complaints about body shape. Some patients, who may not acknowledge other eating disordered behaviour, will acknowledge skipping insulin shots or reducing dosages.

When HCPs find signs that an eating disorder is present, they should consider referring patients for definitive diagnosis, and for treatment. The diagnosis and treatment of clinical eating disorders requires the skills of a mental health professional who understands diabetes and has experience treating these disorders. Because these disorders are so severe and resistant to treatment, successful resolution requires intensive psychotherapy, often on an in-patient basis, and, in many cases, family therapy.

Other medical events experienced by patients with NIDDM as well as those with IDDM should alert HCPs to the possible coexistence of psychological problems. These events include the diagnosis of the disease itself, and onset of any of the long-term complications of diabetes. The period immediately following diabetes onset and diagnosis can be a time of crisis for patients. Studies of children (15, 16) show that emotional disturbances sufficient to warrant a psychiatric diagnosis are fairly common after diabetes onset. Similar reactions are often seen in adults. HCPs should closely monitor emotional reactions to diagnosis in their patients, so that efforts to reduce distress may be applied at the outset, when such treatment is most useful. Restoring emotional equilibrium has two potential benefits. First, it is a worthy goal in its own right. Secondly, it may improve health status directly, by reducing negative neuroendocrine and physiological effects of stress and, indirectly, by re-establishing emotional states that facilitate learning and positive patterns of self-care (17–19).

The onset of complications can trigger emotional disturbances such as depression, anxiety disorder, or obsessive compulsive disorder, which may, in turn, seriously compromise medical management of the complication (20, 21). HCPs should recognise that most patients need full information and extensive psychosocial support at the outset in order to accommodate well to a diabetes-related complication. Unfortunately, many HCPs offer less than patients need at this time. For example, ophthalmologists may participate in a 'conspiracy of silence' with patients who have been diagnosed with proliferative diabetic retinopathy (PDR) (22, 23). The onset of any complication may be a critical period for psychosocial interventions, as it seems to be for PDR. HCPs can help by fully discussing facts and feelings associated with onset of complications, and by referring patients to mental health professionals when such treatment is indicated. Effective intervention not only enhances patients' emotional well-being, it also contributes to an increased capacity for coping with the added regimen demands which often follow from the diagnosis of complications.

One diabetes-related complication, erectile impotence, often involves psychological causes as well as psychiatric sequelae. Psychological problems, including anxiety and depression, potentiate and are by potentiated by organic pathology in the development and maintenance of this sexual dysfunction (24). The fact that diabetes-related erectile impotence often has a demonstrable organic basis should not lead HCPs to overlook potentially meaningful psychological factors and interventions. HCPs should take a thorough sexual history, with particular attention to psychosocial factors, and refer for sex therapy when indicated. Before referring diabetic patients who are impotent for implant surgery, HCPs should consider one or more of the less physically invasive behavioural interventions. These interventions can improve long-term functioning and adjustment (2).

One important reason for attention to psychiatric problems is the fact that some of these problems, most notably depression, can complicate medical management of diabetes. Feelings of hopelessness and helplessness often associated with depression may contribute to a negative cycle of poor self-care, worsened glycaemia, and deeper depression. In addition, some (25) have suggested that symptoms of depression and hyperglycaemia may exacerbate one another at a neuroendocrine level. There is evidence that the natural course of depression may be more severe in patients with diabetes than in depressed patients who have no other medical problems (26–28).

HCPs should consider the possibility of depression in patients who present with symptoms such as insomnia, fatigue, appetite disturbances, and lack of interest in sex. Unfortunately, some of these symptoms overlap with those of chronic hyperglycaemia, which complicates the task of reaching a diagnosis. Since depressed diabetic patients are often chronically hyperglycaemic, cognitive symptoms of depression, including sadness, anhedonia, and self-blame are particularly useful for accurate diagnosis of the depression. Consultation with a mental health professional may be helpful in this regard.

There are no reliable studies to indicate whether standard methods of pharmacotherapy and psychotherapy are as effective in treating patients with diabetes as they are in the treatment of non-diabetic individuals. Despite the lack of data, psychotherapy is indicated for depressed patients with diabetes, given its generally demonstrated efficacy. HCPs should keep in mind the fact that most conventional antidepressant agents have side-effect profiles that may create problems for some patients with diabetes (3). Tricyclic agents often have side-effects such as sedation, and cardiovascular effects such as conduction delays and arrhythmias, orthostasis, weight gain, and sexual dysfunction. Fluoxetine apparently causes substantially less incidence of these side-effects, but it can cause non-specific gastrointestinal distress (29). HCPs must decide whether these potential difficulties with pharmacotherapy outweigh their benefits for patients with diabetes.

## BEHAVIOURAL PROBLEMS AND INTERVENTIONS

Although psychiatric problems represent the most dramatic challenge faced by diabetes HCPs, the more common challenge is patients who exhibit no severe disorder, yet fail to meet the expectations of HCPs regarding self-care and metabolic control. Many HCPs equate suboptimal glycaemic control with patient non-compliance. However, it is inappropriate to equate glycaemic control with self-care. There are many reasons for poor glycaemic control. We view non-compliance not as a patient trait but as a particular type of behaviour. Research indicates that non-compliance in diabetes is very common (i.e many patients exhibit sub-optimal self-care) and that quality of self-care ranges from very high to quite low (30). Compliance is not a global construct, however, since correlations are low among levels of compliance with different elements of the treatment regimen (31, 32).

We reserve the term 'non-compliance' for a very specific type of sub-optimal self-care. 'Non-compliance' can occur only when a patient has been asked to comply with a specific standard (33). (Unfortunately, most research on patient self-care does not compare patient behaviour to their prescribed regimen, but to some unarticulated ideal.) Patients who do not meet HCPs' standards for exercise should not be regarded as 'non-compliant' unless a specific exercise regimen has been prescribed and communicated to the patient. Therefore, the first thing to do for patients exhibiting suboptimal self-care is to make sure they have explicit instructions regarding their regimen, including specific behaviours and the situations in which they are to be performed. Studies have shown that explicit communication is essential to regimen compliance (34). Moreover, patient understanding should be verified, as research has shown that patients understand and remember less than HCPs believe (35).

Often implementation of self-care behaviour requires more than a prescription; patients must be educated about self-care. Health care settings with multidisciplinary teams may implement the instructional process over an extended series of patient visits, using a process customised to individual patients. Specialised education for children is often available through diabetes camps (36). Another popular approach is the comprehensive education program. Increasingly delivered on an outpatient basis over a short to medium period (days or weeks), these programmes cover all aspects of self-care, including diet, exercise, medication, self-monitoring of blood glucose (SMBG), sick day and hypoglycaemia management, etc. It is becoming apparent that all educational programs are not equally effective. Didactic programmes which emphasise textbook aspects of diabetes are not likely to yield dramatic improvements in self-care and metabolic control (37). However, programmes which emphasise pragmatic information about how to manage diabetes have shown great success (38–40).

Several behavioural techniques have been used to promote learning of self-care skills. These approaches are designed not only to transfer information about how to manage diabetes, but also to prepare patients to perform self-care behaviours and motivate them to do so. *Behavioural rehearsal* is an effective means of insuring that patients actually know how to enact the desired behaviours (41). Moreover, rehearsal establishes familiar behavioural routines with which patients feel more comfortable. *Contingency contracting*, in which patients sign a contract to perform certain behaviours – often in return for some token reward, can be an effective technique for motivating patients to implement their self-care training (42).

Many HCPs believe that tight glycaemic control (euglycaemia) is a worthwhile goal for at least some of their patients. However, for insulin-treated patients, tight control imposes a greater burden than loose control because there is a much smaller margin of error in terms of glycaemic excursions (1). With tight control, patients must restrict elevations in glucose, and must maintain glucose levels relatively close to hypoglycaemia. Many patients are fearful of attempting tight control because of increased risk of hypoglycaemia (43). This fear is clinically appropriate for those with compromised counterregulatory systems or inadequate cognitive skills (44). However, it is possible to teach patients (including adolescents) how to 'micromanage' their diabetes through self-monitoring of blood glucose and situational adjustment of insulin dosage (45–47).

The simplest form of micro-management is the so-called 'sliding scale' technique in which insulin dosage is increased or decreased by a certain amount for each increment above or below a target SMBG reading. A more sophisticated approach is to adjust not only based on current glucose levels but also by projecting future glucose levels and insulin needs based on current glucose levels and an assessment of behaviours in the immediate past and future which can effect glucose levels (48). This dynamic, retrospective–prospective adjustment process requires a more sophisticated ability to assess one's own glucose metabolism. This approach is currently under investigation, based on the blood glucose awareness training (BGAT) program of Cox *et al.*(49).

Micro-management is an approach which 'empowers' patients (50), thereby increasing their motivation to optimise self-care. Patients respond well to self-management training, and find it more easily implemented and maintained than changing life-style behaviours such as diet and exercise (51). Other aspects of empowerment include training patients to take the initiative in dealing with health care professionals, whether taking one's shoes off before an office visit to facilitate foot examinations, asking specific questions of one's HCPs, or negotiating treatment decisions. This patient activation can produce improvement in metabolic control and quality of life (52).

An alternative to patient empowerment is intensive supervision by HCPs. Patients may be asked to record SMBG data in a memory meter and transmit the data electronically to HCPs for periodic review and medicat˙ )n adjustment or there may be more frequent contacts between patient and HCPs. There is some question regarding the efficacy of this approach when used as an alternative to conventional management (53), but it has been effective in the Diabetes Control and Complications Trial (DCCT) when used in conjunction with patient-oriented micro-management (44). HCPs should be cautioned not to equate intensive supervision with attempting to control patient behaviour; control-oriented communication has been associated with worsening of glycaemic control (54). Currently, it is not clear what contribution intensive supervision makes, nor what mechanism might make it effective. While intensive supervision may permit fine tuning of the treatment regimen, we speculate that intensive supervision often serves to cue and motivate better self-care. Simply getting patients to pay attention to their behaviour (e.g. by having to record and report it) can have a desirable impact. In any case, it is probably wise for HCPs to emphasise that they are available to patients for telephone consultations and office appointments. Also, intensive supervision is facilitated if HCPs have lab tests available when they see patients (i.e. obtain a test before the office visit or use quick, in-office tests).

Behavioural issues can differ depending on stage of development. For young patients, parents must bear a major portion of the responsibility for self-care. Very young patients may not even be able to co-operate with the treatment regimen, let alone administer it by themselves. For these patients, parents must be encouraged to follow treatment recommendations even if children cry and resist shots and finger-sticks for SMBG. As young patients develop, they become increasingly capable of handling regimen behaviours (55, 56). And as patients take on more responsibilities, parents must relinquish theirs. However, a major problem results when parents relinquish their responsibilities in anticipation of increased patient responsibility which does not occur. This pattern can result in a 'self-care gap' in which neither patient nor parent takes responsibility for some aspects of the regimen, and metabolic control deteriorates (57).

Several interventions have been suggested to deal with the changing division of self-care responsibilities between parent and child. These interventions are oriented toward two goals: (1) defining age-appropriate division of responsibility, and (2) enhancing effective parent–child communication. One of the most important issues in the division of responsibility is how parents should phase out their efforts. Parents should continue to monitor children's behaviours, even after children have taken responsibility for performing the behaviours. In effect, parents must continue to act as 'tutors' in diabetes management (and must be knowledgeable enough to handle this role). Of course, at some point, parents must relinquish this responsibility as well, unless non-compliance or adverse health consequences indicate otherwise. Communication is required so that parent and child can coordinate the shifting of responsibilities with a clear understanding of who is expected to do what.

An often overlooked factor in diabetes management is the relationship between patients and HCPs. Most research on this relationship has examined physician HCPs, but much of the research is directly applicable to relationships with other HCPs. In addition to explicit communication (noted above), several aspects of the patient–HCP relationship have been found to contribute to better self-care. One important aspect is the establishment of a positive and supportive relationship. HCPs should encourage patients and support their efforts; a punitive or critical orientation is seldom productive. Maintenance of this type of relationship creates a situation in which patients strive to meet the expectations of HCPs (58).

HCPs should form collaborative relationships with patients, including negotiation of goals for treatment. While HCPs may feel that certain measures are imperative, they must depend on patients' willingness to implement these measures. Patients are more likely to follow through on HCPs' recommendations if they have had a role in making the decision. HCPs should play an 'authoritative' role rather than an 'authoritarian' role (59), basing their participation on 'expert' knowledge, but recognising that patient considerations should also be factored into decisions (60). Research shows that patients generally place greater emphasis on short-term considerations such as quality of life, while HCPs place greater emphasis on long-term considerations such as avoiding complications (1). Conversely, HCPs are less likely to take into account the burden imposed by treatment recommendations. Although it is not possible for HCPs to impose their will on patients, it may be possible to identify effective measures that patients are willing to implement. For example, patients may not be willing to endure the burden of restricting caloric intake at every meal, but may be willing to adjust insulin to 'cover' the resulting glucose elevations (51). Moreover, since regimen complexity is an important determinant of compliance (61), it is necessary to determine what level of complexity patients are willing to implement.

There are special issues in HCPs' relationships with young patients (55, 62). For preadolescents HCPs should meet with patients and parents together. Diabetes management responsibilities must be closely coordinated between patients and parents. However, as patients reach the teen years, they must be treated at least partly as independent individuals. Patients must be seen individually, as well as with parents. If conflict increases within the family, HCPs must be careful not to be cast in the role of parent surrogate, nor should they form coalitions with parents against patients.

## MOTIVATIONAL PROBLEMS AND INTERVENTIONS

Even after patients have been educated and treatment regimens have been prescribed and fully communicated, many do not closely follow their regimens. The primary cause of the low levels of regimen adherence in adequately educated patients may be motivational problems. Identifying and addressing motivational issues is crucially important, since current treatment regimens, which are more intensive and directed toward achieving tighter metabolic control, place increased demands on patients and require greater effort on their part. To consistently and continuously expend this effort, patients must be highly motivated and motivational problems may undermine patients' efforts to follow their self-care regimens. Motivational barriers or obstacles fall into two categories: self-defeating beliefs and attitudes about diabetes and its treatment, and interpersonal hassles which undermine motivation. HCPs should learn to identify specific motivational barriers in their patients, as a first step to successfully addressing motivational problems.

Motivation for self-care is influenced by patients' beliefs concerning diabetes and its treatment. Patients will be highly motivated to take good care of their diabetes if they believe that diabetes is:

- a serious disease with potentially serious consequences,
- but which they can control,
- through their own efforts and/or those of HCPs,
- with the benefits of those efforts outweighing their costs (63, 64).

On the other hand, converse beliefs will reduce patients' motivation for self-care. HCPs must balance an emphasis on the seriousness of the disease with an emphasis on the benefits of controlling diabetes. Fear will not motivate compliance without hope, and excessive fear and anxiety can produce denial and avoidance rather than increased motivation (65).

Patients' social environment also may support or undermine motivation for diabetes self-care (66). Social support may help patients mobilise positive coping strategies for dealing with the demands of life with diabetes, or it may buffer the effects of stress on these patients. Patients are more highly motivated when their social networks provide instrumental (practical) and emotional support for their diabetes self-management efforts. Other patients, whose social networks are unsupportive either instrumentally or emotionally, are less motivated to take good care of their diabetes. Thus, it is important for HCPs to determine the involvement of other important people in their patients' lives with diabetes. For children with diabetes, parents are major influencers of patterns of self-care and metabolic control (67, 68). As children age into adolescence, peer relationships increase in importance and may also affect self-care. For adults with diabetes, support provided by spouses, other family members, friends, and co-workers are probably critical in motivating compliance (69, 70).

In order to help patients manage their support networks, HCPs should determine what practical and emotional help patients receive from their social networks, what barriers to self-care other individuals represent, and what changes patients need in the area of social support. HCPs may find it useful to include important members of patients' social networks in education and treatment plans. Some comprehensive education programs operate on this format, as do most support groups. Several efforts to provide education for parents of adolescents with diabetes led to improved self-care and glycaemic control in these young people (45, 71). HCPs may refer patients and their families for such interventions, or they may offer this kind of counselling in their own offices.

Facilitating self-motivation is the key to helping patients effectively manage their diabetes. The diabetes regimen is demanding: it is pervasive, affecting every aspect of patients' lives; it is persistent, requiring attention 24 hours a day, 365 days a year; it is unpleasant, involving finger-sticks, food restrictions, and, in many cases, insulin injections; it involves risks, with tight control increasing the likelihood of hypoglycaemia; and, it does not guarantee good glycaemic control, since some of the factors which affect glycaemia may not be completely under patients' control. Because diabetes can be so demanding, patients often feel overwhelmed, and lapses in care are inevitable. To effectively manage the diabetes regimen, with its dozens of clinically relevant decisions each day, its continuing frustrations, and its predictable lapses, patients must find within themselves the motivation to persevere. The most constructive role for HCPs is that of facilitator, helping patients identify intrapersonal and interpersonal motivational barriers to effective self-care, and providing motivational 'boosters' at those times when patients find their self-motivation inadequate. HCPs may also encourage patients to participate in programs for developing coping skills which will allow them to sustain their motivation without ongoing support from others.

Coping skills training is designed to prepare participants to deal effectively with the hassles of daily life. The goals of diabetes-specific coping skills training are two-fold: (a) to help patients overcome attitudinal and emotional barriers to the application of self-care skills and (b) to help patients deal more effectively with diabetes-related interpersonal experiences. Interventions that attempt to promote effective coping occur in a variety of settings including one-to-one interactions between HCPs and patients, therapy groups, self-help groups, support groups, and diabetes camps for children and adolescents. Coping skills training in group settings has the advantage of permitting peer modeling, group problem-solving, and role-play.

While different approaches have been used in different settings, most formal efforts share common strategies (72, 73). Patients learn that certain thoughts or attitudes trigger constructive problem-solving behaviour in difficult situations, while other thoughts and attitudes trigger unconstructive behaviour. Patients are then taught how to implement a procedure for achieving a positive approach to those diabetes-related events they find most troublesome, and they practise this approach. A final component of coping skills training is relapse prevention, offering protection against the possibility that the inevitable slips in self-care may trigger a full-blown relapse. Positive results of coping skills training include: greater emotional well-being (74, 75), enhanced coping skills (36, 76, 77), better regimen adherence (45), and improved glycaemic control (75, 78).

Since many patients with diabetes can benefit from coping skills training, and since training in a group setting may have special advantages, HCPs should consider referring any patients with motivational problems to a diabetes education programme which offers such training. One such programme positively affected emotional well-being, self-care skills, and glycaemic control at 6-month and 12-month follow-ups (38, 41, 51). When such a referral is not possible, HCPs might consider learning some diabetes-specific problem-solving skills (72, 73) and helping patients apply them. Alternatively, HCPs might consult with a cognitive–behavioural therapist for help in improving patients' general coping skills. Finally, HCPs might help patients find support groups where some coping skills might be addressed.

Some patients, particularly obese individuals with NIDDM, face motivational challenges so severe and pervasive that they require highly structured support to successfully manage their problems. Obesity in patients with NIDDM is a serious problem which contributes to hyperglycaemia, insulin insensitivity, hypertension, and hyperlipidaemia, and is therefore a risk factor for many of the long-term complications of diabetes (79–81). Obesity is also highly resistant to change, and even once weight is lost, relapse is common (82). Without highly structured support, few obese patients are sufficiently motivated to make and maintain the behavioural changes required to lose weight and not regain it.

HCPs should consider referring obese NIDDM patients to specialised treatment programs as an adjunct to regular diabetes care. Providing the degree of structured support these patients require may be impossible in an office-based practice. In the early stages of treatment, this support involves intensive medical supervision on a very low calorie diet. The initial intensive phase of obesity treatment is designed to facilitate rapid weight loss and improved glycaemia, leading to marked gains in physical functioning, self-confidence, and self-esteem. These improvements are a source of self-motivation for many patients, as compared to slow weight loss on traditional (higher calorie) diets.

Initial weight loss provides the foundation for the long-term maintenance phase. Support should be provided on a continuing basis, based on the fact that obesity is a chronic disease, much like diabetes and hypertension, that may require life-long treatment and may never be cured. The long-term maintenance therapy obese diabetic patients may need includes combinations of the following strategies: continued professional guidance through ongoing therapist contact (in person or by mail or telephone) for months or even years; coping skills training to help the patient effectively manage specific situations which pose a high risk for abandoning weight-reducing behaviours; self-help groups to provide the patient with enhanced social support; and, exercise programs to provide the patient with positive physical and psychological effects that may enhance long-term success (83).

HCPs may treat some obese NIDDM patients without referring them to specialised programs. HCPs who make this choice should try to apply the principles and strategies employed in structured programmes (e.g. continuing contact and support, active problem solving, and referral to self-help groups). In addition, the prescribed regimens should be specific, concrete, and not overly ambitious, if patients are to follow them successfully. Patients and HCPs should collaboratively establish small, incremental changes in weight as a goal, and try to protect themselves from demoralisation, since at least occasional disappointment is inevitable. Finally, treating obesity in patients with diabetes requires special care, so patients (especially those receiving insulin and/or oral hypoglycaemic medication) should be counselled against participating in popular commercial weight loss plans without supervision by diabetes HCPs.

## CONCLUDING REMARKS

This chapter has provided an overview of psychosocial issues in diabetes care. This overview has emphasised breadth over depth, a fact which can be illustrated by comparing the coverage of psychosocial issues in this volume with that of biological issues. Consider the depth of coverage of biological issues that would result if only one chapter were devoted to biological topics. Although we commend the editors for their foresight in soliciting a chapter on psychosocial issues, we make this comparison to illustrate that any number of the topics we have discussed could have been the subject of an entire chapter of its own.

In spite of our limited depth of coverage, we were not able to cover all psychosocial topics. For example, we did not discuss psychosocial stress, which can worsen glycaemic control either by disrupting self-care or by metabolic disregulation (65), nor did we describe the ways in which coping resources (84) and stress management (85) can ameliorate the negative effects of stress. We have not exhaustively examined determinants of self-care behaviour, in part because some factors are beyond the influence of HCPs, e.g. personality characteristics. Similarly, we have not made a special effort to review family characteristics that are associated with self-care or glycaemic control, although we have noted such characteristics where they fall within our larger framework. Our inability to examine these and other aspects within the constraints of this chapter is not meant to imply that they are not worth considering.

Perhaps the most important point of this chapter is that psychosocial treatment is a specialty in its own right. HCPs should not expect to be experts on all aspects of diabetes management, and psychosocial problems are no exception. HCPs should refer patients to psychosocial specialists in the same way as they would refer to a medical specialist. Moreover, there are multiple psychosocial specialists: some have behavioural nutrition practices for treating obese

NIDDM patients, some help train patients in micro-management, some specialise in treating adolescents, some treat eating disorders and brittle diabetes, some provide psychiatric treatment for emotional disorders, and still others offer coping skills training. HCPs should develop a referral network of psychosocial specialists and make referrals based on their preliminary assessment of patients' psychosocial needs. Likewise, they should seek psychosocial consultations when appropriate.

In conclusion, we believe that the importance of psychosocial factors will grow in the future. Some might feel that the importance of psychosocial issues in diabetes treatment will decrease over time; however, recent advances in clinical science have made psychosocial issues more important rather than less. Motivation will play an even larger role in future efforts to control glycaemia and enhance quality of life, as continuing advances in technology lead to more complex and demanding regimens. On the prevention front, as genetic risk screening becomes more prevalent, so will the psychosocial consequences of being identified as being at risk for diabetes. Genetic counselling will need to address this potential crisis.

Although HCPs must be knowledgeable in the biomedical aspects of diabetes, the majority of diabetes care is implemented by patients who are not HCPs. Thus, HCPs must develop an understanding of the psychosocial issues which are central to patients. We hope that the issues identified in this chapter will help HCPs in caring for their diabetic patients.

## REFERENCES


1 Peyrot M, McMurry JF, Hedges R. Living with diabetes: the role of personal and professional knowledge in symptom and regimen management. In: Roth JA, Conrad P, eds. *Research in the sociology of health care, Volume 6*, Greenwich, CT: JAI Press, 1987; 107–46.
2 Rubin RR, Peyrot M. Psychosocial problems and interventions in diabetes: a review of the literature. *Diabetes Care* 1992; 16: 1640–57.
3 Lustman PJ, Griffith LS, Gavard JA, Clouse RE. Depression in adults with diabetes. *Diabetes Care* 1992; 15: 1631–9.
4 Cohen AS, Vance VK, Runyan JW, Hurwitz D. Diabetic acidosis: an evaluation of the cause, course, and therapy of 73 cases. *Ann Int Med* 1960; 52: 55–86.
5 Schade DS, Drumm DA, Duckworth WC, Eaton RP. The etiology of incapacitating, brittle diabetes. *Diabetes Care* 1985; 8: 12–20.
6 Schade DS, Burge MR, Hardy KJ. Brittle diabetes: an update. *Clin Diabetes* November/December 1992; 83–6.
7 Boehnert CE, Popkin MK. Psychological issues in treatment of severely noncompliant diabetics. *Psychosomatics* 1986; 27: 11–20.
8 Nathan SW. Psychological aspects of recurrent diabetic ketoacidosis in preadolescent boys. *Am J Psychotherapy* 1985; 39: 193–205.
9 Fairburn CG, Peveler RC, Davies B, Mann JI, Mayou RA. Eating disorders in young adults with insulin dependent diabetes mellitus: a controlled study. *Br Med J* 1991; 303: 17–20.
10 Stancin T, Link DL, Reuter JM. Binge eating and purging in young women with IDDM. *Diabetes Care* 1989; 12: 601–3.
11 Steel JM, Young RJ, Lloyd GG. Abnormal eating attitudes in young insulin-dependent diabetics. *Br J Psychiat* 1989; 155: 515–21.
12 Birk R, Spencer ML. The prevalence of anorexia nervosa, bulimia, and induced glycosuria in IDDM females. *Diabetes Educator* 1989; 15: 336–41.
13 LaGreca A, Schwartz L, Satin W, Rafkin-Mervis L, Enfield G, Goldberg R. Binge eating among women with IDDM: associations with weight dissatisfaction, adherence and metabolic control (Abstract). *Diabetes* 1990; 39 (Suppl 1): 164A.
14 Littlefield C, Rodin G, Craven J, Danemen D. Eating disorders: a source of poor compliance and control in female adolescents with IDDM (Abstract). *Diabetes* 1989; 38 (Suppl 1): 8A.
15 Jacobson AM, Hauser ST, Wertlieb D, Wolfsdorf JI, Orleans J, Vierya M. Psychological adjustment of children with recently diagnosed diabetes mellitus. *Diabetes Care* 1986; 9: 323–9.
16 Kovacs M, Feinberg TL, Paulauskas S, Finkelstein R, Pollock M, Crouse-Novak M. Initial coping responses and psychosocial characteristics of children with insulin-dependent diabetes mellitus. *J Pediatrics* 1985; 106: 827–34.
17 Brown SA. Diabetes and grief. *Diabetes Educator* 1985; 11: 53–7.
18 Hamburg BA, Inoff GE. Coping with predictable crises of diabetes. *Diabetes Care* 1983; 6: 409–16.
19 Holmes DM. The person with diabetes in psychosocial context. *Diabetes Care* 1986; 9: 194–206.
20 Bently FR, Jung S, Garrison RN. Neuropathy and psychosocial adjustment after pancreas transplant in diabetes. *Transpl Proc* 1990; 22: 691–5.
21 D'Elia JA, Piening S, Kaldany A *et al.* Psychosocial crisis in diabetic renal failure. *Diabetes Care* 1981; 4: 99–103.
22 Jacobson AM, Rand LI, Hauser ST. Psychological stress and glycemic control: a comparison of patients with and without proliferative diabetic retinopathy. *Psychosom Med* 1985; 47: 372–81.
23 Oehler-Giarratana J. Reactions to complications. In: Hamburg BA, Lipsett LF, Inoff GE, Drash SL, eds. *Proceedings of the National Conference*, U.S. Department of

Health and Human Services (PHS Publication No. NIH 80–1993), 1979; 193–7.
24 Schiava PC, Hogan B. Sexual problems in diabetes mellitus: psychological aspects. *Diabetes Care* 1979; 2: 9–17.
25 Lustman PJ, Griffith LS, Clouse RE. Depression in adults with diabetes: results of a 5-year follow-up study. *Diabetes Care* 1988; 11: 605–12.
26 Keller MB, Klerman GL, Lavori PW, Coryell W, Endicott J, Taylor J. Longterm outcome of episodes of major depression: clinical and public health significance. *JAMA* 1984; 252: 788–92.
27 Keller MB, Shapiro KW, Lavori PW, Wolfe N. Recovery in major depressive disorder. *Arch Gen Psychiat* 1982; 39: 905–10.
28 Keller MB, Shapiro KW, Lavori PW, Wolfe N. Relapse in major depressive disorder. *Arch Gen Psychiat* 1982; 39: 911–15.
29 Cole JO, Bodkin JA. Antidepressant drug side-effects. *J Clin Psychiat* (Suppl 1) 1990; 51: 21–6.
30 Watkins JD, Roberts DE, Williams TF *et al.* Observations of medication errors made by diabetic patients in the home. *Diabetes* 1967; 16: 882–5.
31 Orme CM, Binik YM. Consistency of adherence across regimen demands. *Hlth Psychol* 1989; 8: 27–43.
32 Glasgow RE, Wilson W, McCaul KD. Regimen adherence: a problematic construct in diabetes research. *Diabetes Care* 1985; 8: 300–1.
33 Anderson RM. Is the problem of noncompliance all in our heads? *Diabetes Educator* 1985; 11: 31–4.
34 Ley P, Spelman M. *Communicating with the Patient.* Staples, London; 1967.
35 Boyd JR, Covington TR, Stanaszek WF, Coussons RT. Drug-defaulting. II. Analysis of noncomplaince patterns. *Am J Hosp Pharmacy* 1974; 31: 485–91.
36 Smith KE, Schreiner B, Jackson C, Travis LB. Teaching assertive communication skills to adolescents with diabetes: evaluation of a camp curriculum. *Diabetes Educator* 1993; 19: 136–41.
37 Watts FN. Behavioral aspects of the management of diabetes mellitus: education, self-care and metabolic control. *Beh Res Therapy* 1980; 18: 171–80.
38 Rubin RR, Peyrot M, Saudek CD. Effect of diabetes education on self-care, metabolic control, and emotional wellbeing. *Diabetes Care* 1989; 12: 673–9.
39 Vinicour F, Cohen SJ, Mazzuca SA *et al.* Diabetes: a randomized trial of the effects of physician and/or patient education on diabetes patient outcomes. *J Chronic Dis* 1987; 40: 2345–56.
40 Wise PH, Dowlatshani DC, Farrant S, Fromson S, Meadows KA. Effect of computer based learning on diabetes and control. *Diabetes Care* 1986; 9: 504–8.
41 Rubin RR, Peyrot M, Saudek CD. The effect of a diabetes education program incorporating coping skills training on emotional well-being and diabetes self-efficacy. *Diabetes Educator* 1993; 19: 210–14.
42 Carney RM, Schecter K, Davis T. Improving adherence to blood glucose testing in insulin-dependent diabetic children. *Beh Therapy* 1983; 24: 247–54.
43 Cox DJ, Irvine AI, Gonder-Frederick L, Nowacek G, Butterfield J. Fear of hypoglycemia: quantification, validation, and utilization. *Diabetes Care* 1987; 10: 617–21.
44 The DCCT Research Group. Diabetes Control and Complications Trial (DCCT): update. *Diabetes Care* 1990; 13: 427–33.
45 Anderson BJ, Wolf FM, Burkhart MT, Cornell RG, Bacon GE. Effects of peer-group intervention on metabolic control of adolescents with IDDM: randomized outpatient study. *Diabetes Care* 1989; 12: 179–83.
46 Ingersoll GM, Orr DP, Herrold AJ, Golden MP. Cognitive maturity and self-management among adolescents with insulin-dependent diabetes mellitus. *J Pediatr* 1986; 108: 620–3.
47 Peyrot M, Rubin RR. Insulin self-adjustment predicts better glycemic control (Abstract). *Diabetes* 1988; 37 (Suppl 1): 53A.
48 Guthrie DW, Guthrie RA. Approach to management. *Diabetes Educator* 1990; 16: 401–6.
49 Cox DJ, Gonder-Frederick LA, Lee JH, Julian DM, Carter WR, Clarke WL. Effects and correlates of blood glucose awareness training among patients with IDDM. *Diabetes Care* 1989; 12: 313–1.
50 Anderson RM, Funnell MM, Barr PA, Dedrick RF, Davis WK. Learning to empower patients: the results for professional education program for diabetes educators. *Diabetes Care* 1991; 14: 584–90.
51 Rubin RR, Peyrot M, Saudek CD. Differential effect of diabetes education on self-regulation and life-style behaviors. *Diabetes Care* 1991; 14, 335–8.
52 Greenfield S, Kaplan SH, Ware JE, Yano EM, Frank HJ. Patients' participation in medical care: effects on blood sugar control and quality of life in diabetes. *J Gen Intern Med* 1988; 3: 448–57.
53 Marrero D, Vandagriff J, Fineberg N, Golden M. Using telecommunication technology to manage children with Type I diabetes (Abstract). *Diabetes* 1990; 40 (Suppl 1): 363A.
54 Street RL, Piziak VK, Carpenter WS *et al.* Provider–patient communication and metabolic control. *Diabetes Care* 1993; 16: 714–21.
55 Anderson BJ, Wolfsdorf JI, Jacobson AM. Psychosocial adjustment in children with type I diabetes. In: Lebokitz HE, ed. *Therapy for Diabetes Mellitus and Related Disorders*, American Diabetes Association, Alexandria, VA, 1991; 51–8.
56 Wysoki T, Meinhold PA, Abrams KC *et al.* Parental and professional estimates of self-care independence of children and adolescents with IDDM. *Diabetes Care* 1992; 15; 43–52.
57 Anderson BJ, Auslander WF, Jung KC, Miller JP, Santiago JV. Assessing family sharing of diabetes responsibilities. *J Pediatr Psychol* 1990; 15: 477–92.
58 Rodin J, Janis IL. The social power of health-care practitioners as agents of change. *J Soc Issues* 1979; 35: 60–81.
59 Baumrind D. Current patterns of parental authority. *Dev Psychol Monogr* 1971; 4: 1–107
60 Stone GC. Patient compliance and the role of the expert. *J Soc Issues* 1979; 35: 34–59
61 Hulka BS, Cassel JC, Kupper LL, Burdette JA. Communication, compliance, and concordance between physicians and patients with prescribed medications. *Am J Pub Hlth* 1976; 84: 646–51.
62 Sperling MA. *Physician's guide to insulin-dependent (type I) diabetes: diagnosis and treatment.* American Diabetes Association, Alexandria, VA, 1988.
63 Bradley C, Lewis KS, Jennings AM, Ward JD. Scales to measure perceived control developed specifically for people with tablet-treated diabetes. *Diabetic Med* 1990; 7: 685–94.
64 Nagasawa M, Smith MC, Barnes JH, Fincham JE. Meta-

analysis of diabetes patients' compliance with prescribed medications. *Diabetes Educator* 1990; 16: 192–200.

65 Peyrot M, McMurry JF. Psychosocial factors in diabetes control: adjustment of insulin-treated adults. *Psychosom Med* 1985; 47: 542–57.

66 Peyrot M, McMurry JF, Hedges R. Marital adjustment to adult diabetes: interpersonal congruence and spouse satisfaction. *J Marriage Family* 1988; 50: 363–76.

67 Anderson BJ, Miller JP, Auslander, WF, Santiago JV. Family characteristics of diabetic adolescents: relationship to metabolic control. *Diabetes Care* 1981; 4: 580–94.

68 Hanson CL, Henggeler SW, Burghen GA. Social competence and parental support as mediators of the link between stress and metabolic control in adolescents with insulin-dependent diabetes mellitus. *J Consult Clin Psychol* 1987; 55: 529–33.

69 Schlenk EA, Hart LA. Relationship between health locus of control, health value, and social support and compliance of persons with diabetes mellitus. *Diabetes Care* 1984; 7: 566–74.

70 Ruggiero L, Spirito A, Bond A, Coustan D, McGarvey S. Impact of social support and stress on compliance in women with gestational diabetes. *Diabetes Care* 1990; 13: 441–3.

71 Satin W, LaGreca AM, Zigo MA, Skyler JS. Diabetes in adolescence: effects of multifamily group intervention and parental simulation of diabetes. *J Ped Psychol* 1989; 15: 477–92.

72 Rubin RR, Walen S, Ellis A. Living with diabetes: a rational-emotive therapy perspective. *J Rational-Emotive Cognitive-Behavioral Therapy* 1991; 8: 21–39.

73 Rubin RR, Biermann J, Toohey B. *Psyching out diabetes*, Lowell House, Los Angeles, 1992.

74 Rabin C, Amir S, Nardi R, Ovadia B. Compliance and control: issues in group training of diabetics. *Hlth Soc Work* 1986; 11: 141–51.

75 Warren-Boulton E, Anderson BJ, Schwartz NL, Drexler AJ. A group approach to the management of diabetes in adolescents and young adults. *Diabetes Care* 1981; 4: 620–3.

76 Gross AM, Heimann L, Shapiro R, Schultz RM. Children with diabetes: social skills training and hemoglobin $A_{1c}$ levels. *Beh Modification* 1983; 7: 151–64.

77 Smith KE, Schreiner BJ, Brouhard BH, Travis LB. Impact of a camp experience on choice of coping strategies by adolescents with insulin-dependent diabetes mellitus. *Diabetes Educator* 1991; 17: 49–53.

78 Cigrang JA, Shuster ML, Hanson CL, Burghen GA, Harris MA, Shinkel AM. Psychosocial intervention for youths with IDDM: a controlled study of the metabolic and psychosocial effects of group therapy (Abstract). *Diabetes* 1991; 41 (Suppl 1): 531A.

79 Olefsky J, Reaven GM, Farquhar JW. Effects of weight reduction on obesity: studies of lipid and carbohydrate metabolism in normal and hypolipoproteinemic subjects. *J Clin Invest* 1974; 53: 64–76.

80 Wing RR, Epstein LH, Nowalk MP, Koeske R, Hagg S. Behavior change, weight loss, and psychological improvements in type II diabetic patients. *J Consult Clin Psychol* 1985; 53: 111–22.

81 Wing RR, Koeske R, Epstein LH, Nowalk MP, Gooding W, Becker D. Long-term effects of modest weight loss in type II diabetic patients. *Arch Int Med* 1987; 147: 1749–53.

82 Wing RR. Behavioral treatment of obesity: its application to type II diabetes. *Diabetes Care* 1993; 16: 193–9.

83 Perri MG, Sears SF, Clark JE. Strategies for improving maintenance of weight loss: toward a continuous care model of obesity management. *Diabetes Care* 1993; 16: 200–9.

84 Peyrot M, McMurry JF. Stress buffering and glycemic control: the role of coping styles. *Diabetes Care* 1992; 15: 842–6.

85 Surwit RS, Feinglos MN. The effects of relaxation on glucose tolerance in noninsulin dependent diabetes mellitus. *Diabetes Care* 1983; 6: 176–9.

# Index

pancreatectomy, islet autotransplantation after 431